1994

Health
United
States
1992

and

Healthy People
2000 Review

U.S. DEPARTMENT OF HEALTH
AND HUMAN SERVICES

Public Health Service
Centers for Disease Control and Prevention
National Center for Health Statistics

Hyattsville, Maryland
August 1993

DHHS Pub. No. (PHS) 93-1232

U.S. Department of Health and Human Services

Donna E. Shalala
Secretary

Public Health Service

Philip R. Lee, M.D.
Assistant Secretary for Health

Centers for Disease Control and Prevention (CDC)

Walter R. Dowdle, Ph.D.
Acting Director

National Center for Health Statistics

Manning Feinleib, M.D., Dr. P.H.
Director

Preface

Health, United States, 1992 is the 17th report on the health status of the Nation submitted by the Secretary of Health and Human Services to the President and Congress of the United States in compliance with Section 308 of the Public Health Service Act. This volume also contains the 1992 *Healthy People 2000 Review*, first in a series of profiles tracking the Year 2000 objectives, submitted by the Secretary of Health and Human Services to the President and the Congress of the United States in compliance with the Health Services and Centers Amendments of 1978. These reports were compiled by the National Center for Health Statistics, Centers for Disease Control and Prevention (CDC). The National Committee on Vital and Health Statistics served in a review capacity.

Health, United States, 1992 presents national trends in public health statistics. The 145 detailed tables in this year's report are organized around four major subject areas—health status and determinants, utilization of health resources, health care resources, and health care expenditures. The detailed tables are designed to show trends in health statistics. A major criterion used in selecting the detailed tables is the availability of comparable national data over a period of several years. Similar tables appear in each volume of *Health, United States* to enhance the use of this publication as a standard reference source. Data are reported for selected years to highlight major trends. Several tables in *Health, United States, 1992* present data according to race and/or Hispanic origin consistent with department-wide emphasis on expanding racial and ethnic detail in the presentation of health data. The large differences in health status according to race and Hispanic origin that are documented in this report may be explained by several factors including socioeconomic status, health practices, psychosocial stress and resources, environmental exposures, and access to health care.

To use *Health, United States, 1992* most effectively, the reader should become familiar with the two appendixes immediately following the detailed tables. Appendix I describes each data source used in this report and provides references for further information about the sources. Appendix II is an alphabetical listing of the terms used in the report. It also contains the standard populations used for age adjustment and *International Classification of Diseases* codes for cause of death and diagnostic and procedure categories.

Healthy People 2000 Review begins a series of annual profiles of the Nation's health as an integral part of the Department's disease prevention and health promotion initiative for the year 2000. *Healthy People 2000 Review* continues the work of its predecessor, *Prevention Profile*, which monitored progress toward the 1990 goals and objectives. This prevention initiative was unveiled in September 1990 by the Secretary of Health and Human Services, with the release of *Healthy People 2000: National Health Promotion and Disease Prevention*

Objectives. In this first year, the report provides tracking data, if available, for objectives and subobjectives in all 22 priority areas. The year 2000 objectives will be tracked annually throughout the decade in this publication.

Acknowledgments

Overall responsibility for planning and coordinating the content of this volume rested with the Office of Analysis and Epidemiology, National Center for Health Statistics, under the general direction of Jacob J. Feldman.

Health, United States was prepared under the direction of Kate Prager and Diane M. Makuc. Detailed tables were prepared by Margaret A. Cooke, Virginia M. Freid, and Rebecca A. Placek, with assistance from Lois A. Fingerhut, Kenneth Schoendorf, and Diane K. Wagener. Systems design and computer programming were provided by Mitchell B. Pierre, Jr., Andrew W. Gordon, Ildy I. Shannon, and Patricia A. Knapp. Statistical assistance was provided by Mavis B. Prather and Michael K. Pisarcik. Production planning and coordination were managed by Rebecca A. Placek with typing assistance from Carole J. Hunt.

The *Healthy People 2000 Review* was prepared by Kathleen M. Turczyn, with assistance from Susan E. Schober, Fred Seitz, Susan Hawk, and Christine M. Plepys under the guidance of Richard J. Klein and Mary Anne Freedman. Cheryl V. Rose, Christine M. Plepys, Mitchell B. Pierre, Jr., Ildy I. Shannon, Patricia A. Knapp, and Jean Williams provided computer programming assistance, and Gail R. Jones and Cheryl V. Rose provided statistical and graphic assistance.

Publications management and editorial review were provided by Thelma W. Sanders and Rolfe W. Larson. Production was managed by Linda L. Bean, assisted by Jacqueline M. Davis, Annette F. Gaidurgis, and Zung Le. Printing was managed by Patricia L. Wilson. Graphics were supervised by Stephen L. Sloan. The designer was Sarah M. Hinkle.

Publication of *Health, United States* and *Healthy People 2000 Review* would not have been possible without the contributions of numerous staff members throughout the National Center for Health Statistics and several other agencies. These people gave generously of their time and knowledge, providing data from their surveys and programs; their cooperation and assistance are gratefully acknowledged.

Contents

Preface_____ iii
Acknowledgments_____ iv

Health, United States, 1992

Highlights_____ 3
Geographic Regions and Divisions of the
  United States_____ 8
List of Detailed Tables_____ 9
Detailed Tables_____ 14
  Health Status and Determinants
    Population_____ 14
    Fertility and Natality_____ 17
    Mortality_____ 33
    Determinants and Measures
      of Health_____ 87
  Utilization of Health Resources
    Ambulatory Care_____ 117
    Inpatient Care_____ 122
  Health Care Resources
    Personnel_____ 140
    Facilities_____ 153
  Health Care Expenditures
    National Health Expenditures_____ 160
    Sources and Types of Payment_____ 166
    Health Care Coverage and
      Major Federal Programs_____ 182

Appendixes

Contents_____ 194
  I. Sources and Limitations of Data_____ 196
  II. Glossary_____ 215

Index to Health, United States, 1992
Detailed Tables_____ 385

Symbols

- - -   Data not available

. . .   Category not applicable

-   Quantity zero

0.0   Quantity more than zero but less than 0.05

*   Figure does not meet standard of reliability or precision

---

Healthy People 2000 Review, 1992

List of Figures_____ 233
List of Tables_____ 234
Introduction_____ 235
  Background and Summary_____ 235
  Organization and Scope of This Review_____ 236
  Data Issues_____ 237
    Revised Baselines_____ 237
    Minority Group Subobjectives_____ 238
    Age Adjustment_____ 238
    Data Source Comparability_____ 239
    Cause-of-Death Terminology and Codes___ 239
    Years of Healthy Life_____ 239
Year 2000 Goals and Age-Related Objectives___ 241
  1. Physical Activity and Fitness_____ 245
  2. Nutrition_____ 252
  3. Tobacco_____ 260
  4. Alcohol and Other Drugs_____ 266
  5. Family Planning_____ 271
  6. Mental Health and Mental Disorders_____ 275
  7. Violent and Abusive Behavior_____ 279
  8. Educational and Community-based
     Programs_____ 283
  9. Unintentional Injuries_____ 287
  10. Occupational Safety and Health_____ 293
  11. Environmental Health_____ 297
  12. Food and Drug Safety_____ 303
  13. Oral Health_____ 306
  14. Maternal and Infant Health_____ 313
  15. Heart Disease and Stroke_____ 319
  16. Cancer_____ 327
  17. Diabetes and Chronic Disabling Conditions__ 333
  18. HIV Infection_____ 341
  19. Sexually Transmitted Diseases_____ 346
  20. Immunization and Infectious Diseases___ 350
  21. Clinical Preventive Services_____ 357
  22. Surveillance and Data Systems_____ 363
Information Tables
  A. Priority area lead agencies_____ 366
  B. Mortality objective cause-of-death
     categories_____ 367
  C. Data sources for Healthy People 2000
     objectives and subobjectives_____ 370
  D. Health Status Indicators_____ 384

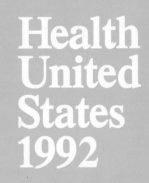

Health
United
States
1992

Highlights
Health, United States, 1992

Health Status and Determinants

■ Between 1980 and 1990 the **elderly population** in the United States grew more rapidly than other age groups. The population aged 85 years and over increased by 35 percent to 3 million and the population aged 75–84 years, by 30 percent to 10 million. During this period the total U.S. population increased by about 10 percent (table 1).

■ In 1990 the **fertility rate** was 70.9 live births per 1,000 women 15–44 years of age, 4 percent higher than in 1980 but 19 percent lower than in 1970. Between 1986 and 1990 the fertility rate increased at an average annual rate of 2 percent. The increase was greatest for women aged 35–44 years (7–8 percent) and for teens aged 15–17 years (5 percent) (tables 3 and 4).

■ The overall percent of live-born **infants weighing less than 2,500 grams** has remained generally stable between 1980 and 1990 at 7 percent. However, the proportion of **infants weighing less than 1,500 grams** (those at greatest risk of death and disability) increased 18 percent for infants of black mothers and 6 percent for infants of white mothers during this period. In 1990 the percent of black infants weighing less than 1,500 grams was 3 times that for white infants (2.92 compared with 0.95 percent) (table 8).

■ Between 1980 and 1990 the percent of mothers who began **prenatal care** in the first trimester of pregnancy remained stable at 76 percent. Large differences among racial and ethnic groups in use of prenatal care continued in 1990. In the United States early prenatal care was received by only 58 percent of Mexican-American and American Indian mothers and 61–64 percent of black, Central and South American, and Puerto Rican-origin mothers compared with 81–87 percent of Chinese, non-Hispanic white, Cuban, and Japanese-origin mothers (table 9).

■ Between 1980 and 1990 the percent of live births to **unmarried mothers** increased steadily from 18 to 28 percent, continuing the upward trend of the 1970's. In 1990 two-thirds of black mothers of live-born infants and more than half of Puerto Rican (56 percent) and American Indian (54 percent) mothers were unmarried compared with 5 and 10 percent of mothers of Chinese and Japanese ancestry and 17 percent of white non-Hispanic mothers (table 10).

■ Between 1989 and 1991 the **poverty** rate for female-headed households with children increased from 43 to 47 percent and the poverty rate for children increased from 19 to 21 percent. In 1991 poverty among black children (46 percent) was almost 3 times that for white children (16 percent) and poverty among Hispanic children (40 percent) was 2.5 times that for white children (table 2).

■ **Infant mortality** for the 1985–87 birth cohort was lowest among infants of Chinese-American mothers (6.0 infant deaths per 1,000 live births) and highest for infants of American Indian and black mothers (13.3 and 18.2 infant deaths per 1,000 live births). High infant mortality for black infants was due to elevated neonatal (12.0) and postneonatal (6.2) mortality that was more than twice the neonatal and postneonatal rates for white infants (5.5 and 3.0). High infant mortality for American Indian infants was mainly due to elevated postneonatal mortality (7.2) that was 2.4 times that for white infants (table 18).

■ In 1990 the **infant mortality** rate was 9.2 deaths per 1,000 live births, a record low. Between 1980 and 1990 infant mortality decreased by 30 percent for infants of white mothers to 7.6 deaths per 1,000 live births and by 19 percent for infants of black mothers to 18.0 deaths per 1,000 live births (table 20).

■ In 1989 **infant mortality** in the United States was more than twice as high and feto-infant mortality was 64 percent higher than in Japan. Postneonatal mortality in the United States was 88 percent higher than in Finland. The feto-infant mortality rate is an alternative measure of pregnancy outcome that substantially reduces the effect of international differences in distinguishing between fetal and infant deaths (table 25).

■ In 1989 **life expectancy** at birth in the United States was shorter than in Japan by 4.4 years for males and 3.9 years for females. Life expectancy at 65 years in the United States was also shorter than in Japan by 1.3 years for men and 1.9 years for women (table 26).

■ Between 1980 and 1990 overall **life expectancy** at birth increased from 73.7 to 75.4 years, a gain of 1.7 years. However, increases in life expectancy over the decade ranged from 0.7 year for black males to 2 years for white males, thereby widening the gap in life expectancy between the black and white populations. In 1990 life expectancy for white males was 8.2 years longer than for black males (72.7 compared with 64.5 years). Life expectancy for white females was 5.8 years longer than for black females (79.4 compared with 73.6 years) (table 27).

■ **Years of potential life lost** (YPLL) per 100,000 population under 65 years of age is a measure of premature mortality. Between 1987 and 1990 the YPLL rate due to HIV infection increased by 78 percent. Increases were greatest for black females (97 percent), followed by white females (84 percent), white males (77 percent), and black males (70 percent) (table 29).

■ In 1988–90 the age-adjusted death rate for heart disease for **Asian persons in the United States** aged 45 years and over (290.1 deaths per 100,000 population) was about 25 percent lower than the rate for **Hispanics** and **American Indians**, close to half the rate for white persons, and 63 percent lower than the rate for black persons. In 1988–90 the age-adjusted death rates for cancer for American Indians, Asians, and Hispanics aged 45 years and over were similar (265.0, 271.9, and 278.3 deaths per 100,000) and were considerably lower than the rates for white persons or black persons (456.4 and 621.1 deaths per 100,000) (table 31).

■ In 1988–90 the motor vehicle crash-related death rate for **American Indian children** 1–14 years of age (10.5 deaths per 100,000 population) was about 1.5 times the rate for black, white, and **Hispanic children**, and more than twice the rate for **Asian children in the**

United States. Similarly the motor vehicle crash-related death rate for American Indian youth aged 15–24 years (56.4 deaths per 100,000) was 1.5 times the rate for white youth, 1.8 times the rate for Hispanic youth, 2.4 times the rate for black youth, and 3.2 times the rate for Asian youth aged 15–24 years (table 31).

■ In 1988–90 the suicide rate for **American Indian youth** 15–24 years of age (26.8 deaths per 100,000) was nearly twice the rate for white youth, about 3 times the rates for black and **Hispanic youth**, and 3.6 times the rate for **Asian youth in the United States**. In 1988–90 the homicide rate for young black persons 15–24 years of age (67.6 deaths per 100,000) was 2.5–3.6 times the rates for Hispanic and American Indian youth and 7.9–9.1 times the rates for white and Asian youth (table 31).

■ In 1988–90 the age-adjusted death rate for residents of **large core metropolitan** counties (569 deaths per 100,000 population) was 19 percent greater than for **large fringe metropolitan** counties (479 deaths per 100,000) and the age-adjusted death rate for residents of **rural** counties (537 deaths per 100,000) was 12 percent greater than for fringe counties. Between 1980–82 and 1988–90 the age-adjusted death rate declined by 10 percent for large fringe metropolitan counties, by 6 percent for rural counties, and by 5 percent for large core metropolitan counties (table 32).

■ **Educational attainment** is inversely associated with mortality. In 1989–90 among men and women 25–44 years of age death rates for those with less than a high school education were about 3 times those for college graduates. Among middle aged men and women 45–64 years of age death rates for those who did not complete high school were almost twice those for college graduates (table 33).

■ Between 1980 and 1990 the age-adjusted death rate for **heart disease**, the leading cause of death for men and women, declined 25 percent, continuing the downward trend of the 1970's. Since 1980 heart disease mortality declined 27 percent for white men, 23 percent for white women, and 16 percent for black men and black women. In 1990 heart disease mortality was almost twice as great for white men as for white women and more than 60 percent greater for black men than for black women (table 35).

■ Between 1980 and 1990 the age-adjusted death rate for **stroke**, the third leading cause of death, declined by 32 percent, continuing the downward trend of the 1970's. Declines in stroke mortality since 1980 ranged from 28 percent for black males to 34 percent for white males. In 1990 the age-adjusted death rate for stroke was twice as great for black men as for white men and almost 80 percent greater for black women as for white women (table 36).

■ Between 1980 and 1990 the age-adjusted death rate for **lung cancer** increased by 41–46 percent for black women and white women, 11 percent for black men, and remained stable for white men. In 1990 lung cancer death rates for black men and white men (91.0 and 59.0 deaths per 100,000 population) were 2–3 times those for black women and white women (27.5 and 26.5 deaths per 100,000) (table 38).

■ In 1990 the age-adjusted death rate for **human immunodeficiency virus (HIV) infection** increased by 13

percent, a smaller increase than in 1989 (30 percent) and in 1988 (22 percent). In 1990 the age-adjusted HIV infection death rate for black men was almost 3 times that for white men (44.2 and 15.0 deaths per 100,000 population) and the HIV death rate for black women was 9 times that for white women (9.9 and 1.1 deaths per 100,000). Provisional data indicate that HIV infection was the ninth leading cause of death in 1991 (tables 40 and 49).

■ Between 1985 and 1990 the age-adjusted **homicide** rate increased 23 percent to 10.2 deaths per 100,000 population after having declined by a similar amount in the first half of the decade. The largest increases since 1985 were for black males and white males 15–24 years of age with homicide rates rising 110 percent and 40 percent. In 1990 the homicide rate for these young black males was 9 times the rate for white males (138.3 compared with 15.4 deaths per 100,000) (table 43).

■ Between 1980 and 1990 **suicide** rates increased 32–33 percent for elderly white men 75 years and over to 60–70 deaths per 100,000 population. In 1990 suicide rates for white men 75 years and over were 9 times those for white women (table 44).

■ Between 1985 and 1990 the age-adjusted death rate for **firearm injuries** increased 14 percent to 14.6 deaths per 100,000 population following a decline of similar magnitude during the previous 5-year period. The firearm death rate for those 15–24 years of age increased more than for any other age group, 50 percent from 1985 to 1990. The 1990 firearm death rate for black males aged 15–24 years was almost 5 times the rate for young white males (138.0 compared with 29.5 per 100,000 population). For these young persons homicide by firearm was the leading cause of firearm death (exceeding firearm deaths from suicide and unintentional injuries). At ages 75–84 years, however, the firearm death rate for white males was more than twice that for black males (49.8 compared with 22.4 deaths per 100,000). Between 1985 and 1990 the increase in the firearm death rate among elderly white males was due to an increase in suicide by firearm (table 45).

■ Between 1980 and 1989 the **death rate for occupational injuries** decreased at an average annual rate of 5 percent with declines occurring in all industries. Between 1983 and 1990 the **lost workday rate for occupational injuries** increased at an average annual rate of almost 5 percent following a period of decline. During the 1980's the same industries had the highest death rates and the highest lost workday rates for occupational injuries: mining; construction; transportation, communication, and public utilities; and agriculture, fishing, and forestry (tables 47 and 75).

■ In 1991 **vaccination levels** for children 1 to 4 years of age were 78 percent for MMR (measles-mumps-rubella), 66 percent for DTP (diphtheria-tetanus-pertussis), and 51 percent for polio. The proportion of children immunized for DTP and polio was 25 percent greater for white children than for those of other races whereas the proportion of children immunized for MMR did not vary by race (table 51).

■ Between 1988 and 1991 the number of reported **tuberculosis** cases increased 17 percent, to 26,000 cases. In 1991 the number of reported **measles** cases decreased

65 percent to 9,000 cases following a sharp increase in measles between 1988 and 1990 (table 52).

■ In 1992 the number of **AIDS cases** per 100,000 population among black non-Hispanic men (115.3) was more than 4 times that for white non-Hispanic men (27.5) and the risk of AIDS among Hispanic men (63.0) was more than twice that for white non-Hispanic men. The risk of AIDS among black non-Hispanic women (27.8) was more than 15 times that for white non-Hispanic women (1.8) and the risk of AIDS among Hispanic women (12.2) was nearly 7 times that for white non-Hispanic women (table 53).

■ In 1991, 44 percent of noninstitutionalized persons 75 years of age and over reported some **limitation of activity due to chronic conditions** with 18 percent limited outside their major activity, 15 percent limited in the amount or kind of their major activity, and 11 percent unable to carry on their major activity. These percents have remained stable over the 5-year period 1986–91 (table 61).

■ In 1991 the health status of black Americans continued to lag behind that of white Americans. The age-adjusted proportion reporting **fair or poor health** was 76 percent greater for black persons than for white persons (15.1 compared with 8.6 percent). The age-adjusted proportion **unable to carry on their major activity** due to chronic conditions was 66 percent greater for black persons than for white persons (6.3 compared with 3.8 percent) (tables 61 and 63).

■ In 1991 the age-adjusted prevalence of **current cigarette smoking** among persons 25 years of age and over ranged from 14 percent for college graduates to 37 percent for persons with less than a high school education. Between 1985 and 1991 the prevalence of current smoking declined by 25 percent for college graduates while declining by 7–9 percent for those with 12 or fewer years of education (table 65).

■ Between 1980 and 1991 the percent of **high school seniors who used cocaine** in the past month dropped from 5 to 1 percent; the percent who used **marijuana** in the past month dropped from 34 to 14 percent; and the percent who used **alcohol** in the past month dropped from 72 to 54 percent. During this period the percent of high school seniors who **smoked cigarettes** in the past month remained stable at 31–32 percent for white seniors while dropping from 25 to 9 percent for black high school seniors (table 67).

■ In 1991 the number of **cocaine-related emergency room episodes** increased by 28 percent following a decline of similar magnitude in 1990. Increases in 1991 occurred among Hispanic, black non-Hispanic, and white non-Hispanic males and females. In 1991 black non-Hispanic persons accounted for more than half of cocaine-related emergency room episodes (table 68).

■ In 1990, 72 percent of men and 51 percent of women were current drinkers of **alcohol**, down 5 percentage points for both groups since 1985. Between 1985 and 1990 the percent of current drinkers who consumed alcohol at heavier levels declined from 17 to 14 percent for men and from 5 to 3 percent for women (table 69).

■ Between 1960–62 and 1988–91 the age-adjusted mean **serum total cholesterol level** for adults ages 20–74 years declined from 220 mg/dL to 205 mg/dL. During the same time period the percent of adults ages 20–74 years with high serum total cholesterol levels (greater than or equal to 240 mg/dL) declined from 32 percent to 20 percent (table 72).

Utilization of Health Resources

■ In 1991, 89 percent of both white and black Americans had a physician contact within the past 2 years. However, the age-adjusted average annual number of **ambulatory physician contacts** was lower for black persons than for white persons (5.2 compared with 5.8 contacts) and **inpatient hospital days of care** per 1,000 population was 35 percent greater for black persons than for white persons (tables 78, 79, and 83).

■ In 1990 among children under 15 years of age, 80 percent of **visits to office-based physicians** were to pediatricians or general and family practitioners. Half of all office visits among elderly persons 65 years of age and over were to internists or general and family practitioners (table 80).

■ Between 1988 and 1991 the age-adjusted **discharge rate from nonfederal short-stay hospitals** declined by 4 percent. The average length of stay remained stable at 6.3 days (table 84).

■ Between 1988 and 1991 the short-stay **hospital discharge rate for HIV infection** increased by 69 percent. In 1991 men 20 to 49 years of age accounted for 67 percent of all HIV discharges, down from 77 percent in 1988; and women 20 to 49 years of age accounted for 20 percent of all HIV discharges, up from 14 percent in 1988 (table 85).

■ After a 38 percent increase in the proportion of deliveries by **cesarean section** between 1980 and 1985, the cesarean section rate has remained stable at about 24 percent through 1991 (table 88).

■ Between 1985 and 1991 the number of **inpatient admissions** to short-stay hospitals decreased by 8 percent to 32.6 million in 1991. During the same time period **outpatient visits** in short-stay hospitals grew by 38 percent to 376 million in 1991 (table 90).

■ In 1991, 52 percent of all surgery performed in short-stay hospitals was on an outpatient basis, 3 times the level of **outpatient surgery** performed in 1980 (table 90).

Health Care Resources

■ Between 1990 and 1991 **employment in the health services industry** increased by 4 percent to 9.8 million workers, while total civilian employment decreased by 0.9 percent. In 1991, 49 percent of all health workers were employed in hospitals, 17 percent in nursing homes, and 12 percent in physicians' offices (table 97).

■ Between 1985 and 1990 the number of active nonfederal **patient care physicians** grew by 8 percent to 19.5 per 10,000 civilian population. In 1990 the patient care physician to population ratio was lowest in Idaho, Mississippi, Wyoming, and South Dakota (12.0 to 13.2 per 10,000 population) and highest in New York, Maryland, and Massachusetts (27.6 to 28.6 per 10,000 population) (table 98).

■ In 1990 the **medical specialties** of general/family practice and internal medicine each accounted for 16 percent of all active nonfederal office-based physicians; and pediatricians, general surgeons, and obstetrician/gynecologists each accounted for 7 percent of the total. Between 1985 and 1990 the numbers of general/family practitioners, obstetrician/gynecologists, and internists each increased by 7–10 percent, while pediatricians increased by 18 percent, and general surgeons decreased by 1 percent (table 100).

■ Between 1986 and 1990 the number of full-time equivalent (FTE) **employees in community hospitals** increased by 13 percent to 3.4 million with nursing personnel comprising 36 percent of the total. Between 1986 and 1990 FTE's for ancillary nursing staff increased by 18 percent, registered nurses increased by 10 percent, and licensed practical nurses decreased by 4 percent (table 102).

■ After a 25 percent decline between 1985 and 1989, the number of **registered nurse (RN) graduates** increased by 17 percent between 1989 and 1991. In 1991, 27 percent of RN graduates received baccalaureate degrees, 65 percent received associate degrees, and 9 percent were graduates of diploma programs (table 104).

■ Between 1980–81 and 1990–91 **dental school enrollment** declined by almost one-third to 16,000 students. During this period minority enrollment increased from 12 to 29 percent of dental students, primarily due to a 2.4-fold increase in the number of Asian dental students. In 1990–91, 16 percent of dental students were Asian, 7 percent were Hispanic, and 6 percent were black (table 105).

■ Between 1980–81 and 1990–91 the proportion of **female medical students** increased from 27 to 37 percent. In 1990–91, the proportion of female medical students varied by race and ethnicity with 56 percent female among black medical students, 38–39 percent among Asian and Hispanic medical students, and 35 percent among white medical students (table 106).

■ Between 1980 and 1991 the total number of short-stay **hospital beds** in the United States declined by 7 percent with beds in State and local government hospitals experiencing the largest decline (20 percent). Between 1980 and 1986 beds in proprietary hospitals grew by 23 percent followed by a 7 percent decline from 1986 to 1991 (table 107).

■ In 1990 there were 3.8 community **hospital beds** per 1,000 civilian population in the United States, a 16 percent decline since 1980. Between 1980 and 1985 **occupancy rates** in community hospitals fell 13 percent and then rose slightly to 67 percent in 1990. Between 1980 and 1990 the number of full-time equivalent **employees** per 100 average daily patients in community hospitals grew by 43 percent to 563 (tables 110–112).

■ Community hospital resources and utilization vary substantially among the States. In 1990 the number of community **hospital beds** per 1,000 population ranged from 2.3 in Alaska to 7.0 in North Dakota. Community hospital **occupancy rates** ranged from 50 percent in Alaska to 86 percent in New York (tables 110 and 111).

Health Care Expenditures

■ In 1991 **national health care expenditures** in the United States totaled $752 billion, an average of $2,868 per person. Health expenditures comprised 13.2 percent of the gross domestic product (GDP) in 1991, up from 12.2 percent in 1990. GDP increased by 2.8 percent in 1991 and national health expenditures by 11.4 percent; total federal expenditures increased by 4.6 percent and federal health expenditures by 14.6 percent; State and local expenditures increased by 8.8 percent and State and local health expenditures by 18.3 percent (table 114).

■ In 1991 health spending in the United States accounted for a larger **share of gross domestic product** (GDP) than in any other major industrialized country and the gap has continued to widen since 1985. The United States devoted 13.2 percent of GDP to health in 1991, up from 12.2 percent in 1990 and 10.5 percent in 1985. Canada, the country with the second highest health share of GDP in 1991, devoted 10 percent of GDP to health (table 115).

■ In 1991 rising prices explained the largest portion (54 percent) of growth in **personal health care expenditures**. Nine percent of the growth was attributed to population increase and 37 percent to changes in the use or kinds of services and supplies (table 117).

■ In 1991 the rate of increase in the medical care component of the **Consumer Price Index** (CPI) was 8.7 percent, more than twice the overall inflation rate of 4.2 percent. In 1992 the medical care component of the CPI increased by 7.4 percent, nearly 2.5 times the overall inflation rate of 3.0 percent. Hospital services increases, 10.2 percent in 1991 and 9.1 percent in 1992, outpaced other items in the medical care component of the CPI (tables 118 and 119).

■ **Expenses in nonfederal short-stay hospitals** increased at an average annual rate of 10.2 percent from 1987 to 1991, following a period of slower growth from 1983 to 1987 (averaging 7 percent annually). In 1991 employee costs accounted for 53.8 percent of total hospital costs. Personnel per 100 patients continued its gradual rise to 427 in 1991 (table 120).

■ In 1991, 22 percent of **personal health expenditures** were paid out-of-pocket; health insurance paid 32 percent; and the federal government paid 31 percent. In 1965 when Medicare and Medicaid were introduced, 53 percent of personal health care expenditures were paid out-of-pocket; private health insurance paid 24 percent; and the federal government paid 8 percent. The State and local governments' share of personal health care expenditures was 12 percent in both 1965 and 1991 (table 123).

■ In 1991 the major **sources of funds** for hospital care were the government (56 percent) and private health insurance (35 percent). Medicare provided a quarter of the total funds for hospital care. In contrast, in 1991 nursing home care was financed primarily by Medicaid (47 percent) and out-of-pocket payments (43 percent).

Physician services were funded by private health insurance (47 percent), Medicare (23 percent), and out-of-pocket payments (18 percent) (table 125).

■ Between 1980 and 1991 funding for **health research and development** has increased at an average annual rate of 11.2 percent in the United States with funding by industry (including drug research) increasing by 15.5 percent per year and funding by the federal government increasing by 7.7 percent per year. Industry's share of health research and development funding grew from 31 percent in 1980 to 47 percent in 1991 while the federal government's share has declined from 59 to 42 percent (table 128).

■ Between 1980 and 1991 the share of **federal funding for health research and development** contributed by the Department of Health and Human Services increased steadily from 78 to 86 percent. The share contributed by the National Institutes of Health rose from 67 percent in 1980 to nearly 75 percent in 1988, and then declined to 72 percent of the total in 1991 (table 129).

■ Expenditures for **human immunodeficiency virus (HIV)**-related activities by the federal government increased 22 percent between 1990 and 1991 to $3.65 billion. Of the total in 1991, 43 percent was for medical care, 35 percent for research, 14 percent for education and prevention, and 8 percent for cash assistance (Disability Insurance and Supplemental Security Income). Between 1990 and 1991 expenditures for medical care grew by 39 percent, cash assistance by 36 percent, research by 10 percent, and education and prevention by 7 percent (table 130).

■ Enrollment in **health maintenance organizations (HMO's)** increased from 34 to 36 million persons between 1991 and 1992. In 1992 about one quarter of the population was enrolled in an HMO in the West compared with 8 percent in the South (table 137).

■ In 1991 the **Medicare** program had nearly 35 million enrollees and expenditures totaling $121.3 billion. Between 1990 and 1991 Medicare expenditures under Hospital Insurance (HI) rose 8 percent to $72.6 billion, with the largest increases occurring for home health agencies (46 percent) and hospices (40 percent). Expenditures under Supplementary Medical Insurance (SMI) rose 11 percent to $48.8 billion with the largest increase occurring for group practice prepayment (25 percent) (table 138).

■ Of the nearly 31 million **Medicare** enrollees age 65 years and over in 1990 almost 11 percent were 85 years and over, up from 7 percent in 1967. Medicare payments rise with age of enrollee; in 1990 average payment per enrollee for those aged 85 years and over ($3,962) was more than double that for those aged 65–66 years ($1,854) (table 139).

■ In 1991 **Medicaid** payments totaled $77 billion for 28.3 million recipients. Children in families receiving Aid to Families with Dependent Children (AFDC) comprised 46 percent of Medicaid recipients but accounted for only 15 percent of expenditures. The aged, blind, and disabled accounted for 26 percent of recipients and 70 percent of expenditures. Average payment per recipient ranged from $892 for children in AFDC families to $7,577 for the aged (table 141).

■ In 1991 more than one quarter of **Medicaid** payments went to nursing facilities, another quarter to general hospitals, and 10 percent to intermediate care facilities for the mentally retarded. Early and periodic screening, rural health clinics, and family planning services combined received 1 percent of Medicaid funds. Payments per recipient ranged from $81 for early and periodic screening for children to $52,750 for intermediate care facility services for the mentally retarded (table 142).

■ Between 1990 and 1991 spending on health care by the **Department of Veterans Affairs** increased by 8 percent to $12.4 billion. In 1991, 57 percent of the total was for inpatient hospital care, 26 percent for outpatient care, and 10 percent for nursing home care. Veterans with service connected disabilities accounted for 39 percent of both inpatients and outpatients. Low income veterans with no service connected disability accounted for 55 percent of inpatients and 42 percent of outpatients (table 143).

■ In 1990 **State mental health agency per capita expenditures** averaged $48 and ranged from $17 in Iowa and $20 in Idaho to $84 in Massachusetts and $118 in New York. States with the greatest average annual percent increases in per capita expenditures during 1981–90 were Arizona, Maine, and Massachusetts (11.4 to 11.7 percent). States with the smallest changes were Montana, New Mexico, and North Dakota (–0.3 to 1.5 percent). The average annual increase in State mental health agency expenditures among all States during 1981–90 was 6.7 percent (table 145).

Geographic Regions and Divisions of the United States

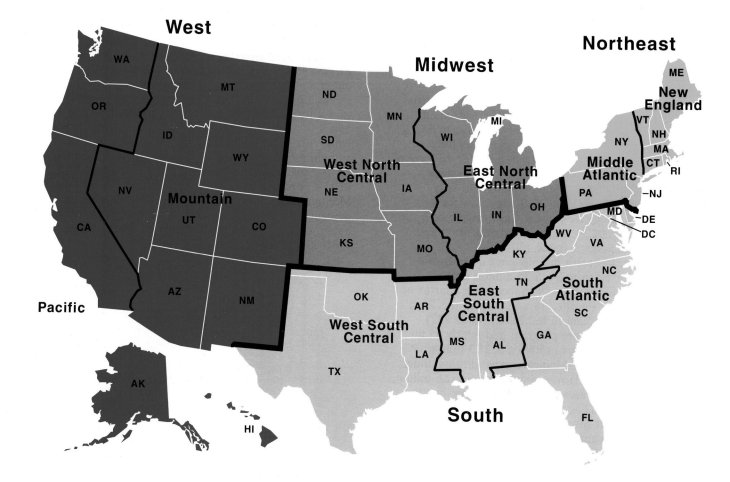

List of Detailed Tables

Population

1. **Resident population**, according to age, sex, detailed race, and Hispanic origin: United States, selected years 1950–90 _____ 14

2. Persons and families below **poverty** level, according to selected characteristics, race, and Hispanic origin: United States, selected years 1973–91 _____ 16

Fertility and Natality

3. Live births, crude **birth rates**, and birth rates by age of mother, according to race: United States, selected years 1950–91 _____ 17

4. **Fertility rates**, according to live-birth order and race: United States, selected years 1950–91 _____ 18

5. **Completed fertility rates** and parity distribution for women 50–54 years of age at the beginning of selected years 1930–91, according to race of child and birth cohort: United States, selected birth cohorts 1876–80 to 1937–41 _____ 19

6. **Lifetime births expected** by currently married women and percent of expected births already born, according to age and race: United States, selected years 1967–90 _____ 20

7. **Live births**, according to detailed race of mother and Hispanic origin of mother: United States, selected years 1970–90 _____ 21

8. **Low-birth-weight** live births, according to detailed race of mother and Hispanic origin of mother: United States, selected years 1970–90 _____ 22

9. **Prenatal care and maternal education** for live births, according to detailed race of mother and Hispanic origin of mother: United States, selected years 1970–90 _____ 23

10. **Maternal age and marital status** for live births, according to detailed race of mother and Hispanic origin of mother: United States, selected years 1970–90 _____ 25

11. **Low-birth-weight** live births, according to race of mother, geographic division, and State: United States, average annual 1978–80, 1983–85, and 1988–90 _____ 26

12. **Very low-birth-weight** live births, according to race of mother, geographic division, and State: United States, average annual 1978–80, 1983–85, and 1988–90 _____ 27

13. Legal **abortion ratios**, according to selected patient characteristics: United States, selected years 1973–90 _____ 28

14. Legal **abortions**, according to selected characteristics: United States, selected years 1973–90 _____ 29

15. Legal abortions, **abortion-related deaths**, and abortion-related death rates, according to period of gestation: United States, 1973–75, 1976–78, 1979–81, 1982–84, and 1985–87 _____ 30

16. Methods of **contraception** for ever-married women 15–44 years of age, according to race and age: United States, 1973, 1982, and 1988 _____ 31

17. Methods of **contraception** for women 15–44 years of age, according to race and marital status: United States, 1982 and 1988 _____ 32

Mortality

18. **Infant, neonatal, and postneonatal mortality rates**, according to detailed race of mother and Hispanic origin of mother: United States, 1960 and 1983–87 birth cohorts _____ 33

19. **Infant mortality rates**, according to birth weight, detailed race of mother, and Hispanic origin of mother: United States, 1960 and 1983–87 birth cohorts _____ 34

20. **Infant mortality rates**, fetal death rates, and perinatal mortality rates, according to race: United States, selected years 1950–91 _____ 35

21. **Infant mortality rates**, according to race, geographic division, and State: United States, average annual 1978–80, 1983–85, and 1988–90 _____ 37

22. **Neonatal mortality rates**, according to race, geographic division, and State: United States, average annual 1978–80, 1983–85, and 1988–90 _____ 38

23. **Postneonatal mortality rates**, according to race, geographic division, and State: United States, average annual 1978–80, 1983–85, and 1988–90 _____ 39

24. **Fetal death rates**, according to race, geographic division, and State: United States, average annual 1978–80, 1983–85, and 1988–90 _____ 40

25. **Infant mortality rates**, feto-infant mortality rates, and postneonatal mortality rates, and average annual percent change: Selected countries, 1984 and 1989 _____ 41

26. **Life expectancy** at birth and at 65 years of age, according to sex: Selected countries, 1984 and 1989 _____ 42

27. **Life expectancy** at birth and at 65 years of age, according to race and sex: United States, selected years 1900–91 _____ 44

28. **Age-adjusted death rates** for selected causes of death, according to sex and race: United States, selected years 1950–90 _____ 45

29. **Years of potential life lost** before age 65 for selected causes of death, according to sex and race: United States, selected years 1970–90 _____ 47

30. **Numbers of deaths and rank** for selected causes of death, according to sex and detailed race: United States, 1985–90 _____ 49

31. **Death rates** for selected causes of death, according to detailed race, Hispanic origin, age, and sex: United States, 1980–82, 1985–87, and 1988–90 _____ 52

32. Age-adjusted death rates, according to race, sex, region, and **urbanization**: United States, average annual 1980–82, 1984–86, and 1988–90 _____ 59

33. Death rates for persons 25–64 years of age, for all races and the white population, according to sex, age, and **educational attainment**: Selected States, 1989–90 _____ 61

34. **Death rates** for all causes, according to sex, race, and age: United States, selected years 1950–90 _____ 62

35. Death rates for **diseases of heart**, according to sex, race, and age: United States, selected years 1950–90 _____ 64

36. Death rates for **cerebrovascular diseases**, according to sex, race, and age: United States, selected years 1950–90 _____ 66

37. Death rates for **malignant neoplasms**, according to sex, race, and age: United States, selected years 1950–90 _____ 68

38. Death rates for **malignant neoplasms of respiratory system**, according to sex, race, and age: United States, selected years 1950–90 _____ 70

39. Death rates for **malignant neoplasm of breast** for females, according to race and age: United States, selected years 1950–90 _____ 71

40. Death rates for human immunodeficiency virus (**HIV**) infection, according to sex, race, and age: United States, 1987–90 _____ 72

41. **Maternal mortality rates** for complications of pregnancy, childbirth, and the puerperium, according to race and age: United States, selected years 1950–90 _____ 73

42. Death rates for **motor vehicle crashes**, according to sex, race, and age: United States, selected years 1950–90 _____ 74

43. Death rates for **homicide** and legal intervention, according to sex, race, and age: United States, selected years 1950–90 _____ 76

44. Death rates for **suicide**, according to sex, race, and age: United States, selected years 1950–90 _____ 78

45. Death rates for **firearm injuries**, according to sex, race, and age: United States, selected years 1970–90 _____ 80

46. Deaths for selected **occupational diseases** for males, according to age: United States, selected years 1970–90 _____ 82

47. **Occupational injury deaths**, according to industry: United States, 1980–89 _____ 83

48. **Provisional death rates** for all causes, according to race, sex, and age: United States, 1989–91 _____ 84

49. **Provisional death rates** for selected causes of death: United States, 1989–91 _____ 85

50. **Provisional death rates** for the three leading causes of death, according to age: United States, 1989–91 _____ 86

Determinants and Measures of Health

51. **Vaccinations** of children 1–4 years of age for selected diseases, according to race and residence in metropolitan statistical area (MSA): United States, 1970, 1976, 1983–85, and 1991 _____ 87

52. Selected **notifiable disease rates**, according to disease: United States, selected years 1950–91 _____ 88

53. Acquired immunodeficiency syndrome (**AIDS**) cases, according to age at diagnosis, sex, detailed race, and Hispanic origin: United States, 1985–92 _____ 89

54. Deaths among acquired immunodeficiency syndrome (**AIDS**) cases, according to age at death, sex, detailed race, and Hispanic origin: United States, 1985–92 _____ 90

55. Acquired immunodeficiency syndrome (**AIDS**) cases, according to race, Hispanic origin, sex, and transmission category for persons 13 years of age and over at diagnosis: United States, 1985–92 _____ 91

56. Deaths among acquired immunodeficiency syndrome (**AIDS**) cases, according to race, Hispanic origin, sex, and transmission category for persons 13 years of age and over at diagnosis: United States, 1985–92 _____ 93

57. Acquired immunodeficiency syndrome (**AIDS**) cases, according to geographic division and State: United States, 1985–92 _____ 95

58. Deaths among acquired immunodeficiency syndrome (**AIDS**) cases, according to geographic division and State: United States, 1985–92 _____ 96

59. Age-adjusted **cancer incidence rates** for selected cancer sites, according to sex and race: Selected geographic areas, selected years 1973–90 _____ 97

60. Five-year relative **cancer survival rates** for selected sites, according to race and sex: Selected geographic areas, 1974–76, 1977–79, 1980–82, and 1983–89 _____ 98

61. **Limitation of activity** caused by chronic conditions, according to selected characteristics: United States, 1986 and 1991 _____ 99

62. **Disability days** associated with acute conditions and incidence of acute conditions, according to age: United States, 1983–91 _____ 100

63. **Self-assessment of health**, according to selected characteristics: United States, 1986 and 1991 _____ 101

64. Current **cigarette smoking** by persons 18 years of age and over, according to sex, race, and age: United States, selected years 1965–91 _____ 102

65. Age-adjusted prevalence of current **cigarette smoking** by persons 25 years of age and over, according to sex, race, and education: United States, selected years 1974–91 _____ 103

66. **Use of selected substances** in the past month by youths 12–17 years of age and young adults 18–25 years of age, according to age, sex, race, and Hispanic origin: United States, selected years 1974–91 _____ 104

67. **Use of selected substances** in the past month by high school seniors, according to sex, race, and average parental education: United States, 1980–91 _____ 106

68. **Cocaine-related emergency room episodes**, according to age, sex, race, and Hispanic origin: Selected metropolitan areas, 1985–89 and United States, 1989–91 _____ 107

69. **Alcohol consumption** by persons 18 years of age and over, according to sex, race, Hispanic origin, and age: United States, 1985 and 1990 _____ 108

70. **Elevated blood pressure** among persons 20–74 years of age, according to race, sex, and age: United States, 1960–62, 1971–74, and 1976–80 _____ 109

71. **Hypertension** among persons 20–74 years of age, according to race, sex, and age: United States, 1960–62, 1971–74, and 1976–80 _____ 110

72. Persons 20 years of age and over with high **serum cholesterol levels** and mean serum cholesterol levels, according to sex, age, race, and Hispanic origin: United States, 1960–62, 1971–74, 1976–80, and 1988–91 _____ 111

73. **Overweight persons** 20–74 years of age, according to race, sex, and age: United States, 1960–62, 1971–74, and 1976–80 _____ 112

74. **Air pollution**, according to source and type of pollutant: United States, selected years 1970–91 _____ 113

75. **Occupational injuries** with lost workdays in the private sector, according to industry: United States, 1980–90 _____ 114

76. Production employees with potential **exposure to elemental lead or to continuous noise**, according to industry and size of facility: United States, 1972–74 and 1981–83 _____ 115

77. **Health and safety services** available in nonagricultural industries, according to size of facility: United States, 1972–74 and 1981–83——————————————— 116

Utilization of Health Resources

Ambulatory Care

78. **Physician contacts**, according to place of contact and selected patient characteristics: United States, 1986 and 1991——————————————————————— 117

79. **Interval since last physician contact**, according to selected patient characteristics: United States, 1964, 1986, and 1991——————————————————— 118

80. **Office visits** to physicians, according to physician specialty and selected patient characteristics: United States, 1985 and 1990————————————— 119

81. **Office visits** to physicians, according to selected patient and visit characteristics and physician specialty: United States, 1985 and 1990————————— 120

82. **Dental visits** and interval since last visit, according to selected patient characteristics: United States, 1964, 1983, and 1989——————————————————— 121

Inpatient Care

83. **Discharges**, days of care, and average length of stay in short-stay hospitals, according to selected characteristics: United States, 1964, 1986, and 1991————— 122

84. **Discharges**, days of care, and average length of stay in nonfederal short-stay hospitals, according to selected characteristics: United States, selected years 1980–91———— 123

85. **Discharges**, days of care, and average length of stay in nonfederal short-stay hospitals for discharges with the diagnosis of human immunodeficiency virus (**HIV**) and for all discharges: United States, 1984–91——————— 124

86. **Rates of discharges** and days of care in nonfederal short-stay hospitals, according to sex, age, and selected first-listed diagnosis: United States, 1980, 1985, 1990, and 1991——————————————————————— 125

87. **Discharges** and average length of stay in nonfederal short-stay hospitals, according to sex, age, and selected first-listed diagnosis: United States, 1980, 1985, 1990, and 1991——————————————————————— 127

88. **Operations** for inpatients discharged from nonfederal short-stay hospitals, according to sex, age, and surgical category: United States, 1980, 1985, 1990, and 1991————— 129

89. Diagnostic and other **nonsurgical procedures** for inpatients discharged from nonfederal short-stay hospitals, according to sex, age, and procedure category: United States, 1980, 1985, 1990, and 1991————————— 131

90. Admissions, average length of stay, outpatient visits, and percent **outpatient surgery** in short-stay hospitals, according to type of ownership and size of hospital: United States, selected years 1960–91————————— 133

91. **Nursing home** and personal care home **residents** 65 years of age and over and rate per 1,000 population, according to age, sex, and race: United States, 1963, 1973–74, 1977, and 1985———————————— 134

92. **Nursing home residents**, according to selected functional status and age: United States, 1977 and 1985__ 135

93. **Additions to mental health organizations** and rate per 100,000 civilian population, according to type of service and organization: United States, selected years 1975–88————————————————————— 136

94. Inpatient and residential treatment **episodes in mental health organizations**, rate per 100,000 civilian population, and inpatient days, according to type of organization: United States, selected years 1975–88————— 137

95. **Additions** to selected inpatient **psychiatric organizations** and rate per 100,000 civilian population, according to sex, age, and race: United States, 1975, 1980, and 1986——————————————————— 138

96. **Additions** to selected inpatient **psychiatric organizations**, according to selected primary diagnoses and age: United States, 1975, 1980, and 1986——————— 139

Health Care Resources

Personnel

97. **Persons employed** in health service sites: United States, selected years 1970–91——————————————— 140

98. Active nonfederal **physicians** per 10,000 civilian population, according to geographic division, State, and primary specialty: United States, 1975, 1985, 1987, and 1990——————————————————————— 141

99. Active **physicians**, according to type of physician, and number per 10,000 population: United States and outlying U.S. areas, selected years 1950–90 and projections for year 2000————————————————— 143

100. **Physicians**, according to activity and place of medical education: United States and outlying U.S. areas, selected years 1970–90——————————————— 144

101. Active **health personnel** and number per 100,000 population, according to occupation and geographic region: United States, 1970, 1980, and 1990——————— 145

102. Full-time equivalent **employment in** selected occupations for **community hospitals**: United States, 1981 and 1986–90————————————————————— 146

103. Full-time equivalent patient care **staff in mental health organizations**, according to type of organization and staff discipline: United States, selected years 1984–88 147

104. First-year enrollment and **graduates of health professions schools** and number of schools, according to profession: United States, selected years 1950–91 and projections for year 2000————————————————— 149

105. First-year and total **enrollment of minorities** in schools for selected health occupations, according to detailed race and Hispanic origin: United States, academic years 1980–81 and 1990–91——————————— 150

106. First-year and total **enrollment of women** in schools for selected health occupations, according to detailed race and Hispanic origin: United States, academic years 1971–72, 1980–81, and 1990–91———————————— 152

Facilities

107. **Short-stay hospitals**, beds, and occupancy rates, according to type of ownership and size of hospital: United States, selected years 1960–91——————————— 153

108. **Long-term hospitals**, beds, and occupancy rates, according to type of hospital and ownership: United States, selected years 1970–91 _____ 154

109. Inpatient and residential treatment **beds in mental health organizations** and rate per 100,000 civilian population, according to type of organization: United States, selected years 1970–88 _____ 155

110. **Community hospital beds** per 1,000 population and average annual percent change, according to geographic division and State: United States, selected years 1940–90_ 156

111. **Occupancy rates** in community hospitals and average annual percent change, according to geographic division and State: United States, selected years 1940–90_ 157

112. Full-time equivalent **employees** per 100 average daily patients in community hospitals and average annual percent change, according to geographic division and State: United States, selected years 1960–90 _____ 158

113. **Nursing homes** with 25 or more beds, beds, and bed rates, according to geographic division and State: United States, 1976, 1982, and 1986 _____ 159

Health Care Expenditures

National Health Expenditures

114. Gross domestic product, **national health expenditures**, and Federal and State and local government expenditures: United States, selected years 1960–91 _____ 160

115. **Total health expenditures** as a percent of gross domestic product and per capita expenditures in dollars: Selected countries and years 1960–91 _____ 161

116. **National health expenditures**, percent distribution, and average annual percent change, according to type of expenditure: United States, selected years 1960–91 _____ 162

117. **Personal health care expenditures** average annual percent change and percent distribution of factors affecting growth: United States, 1960–91 _____ 163

118. **Consumer Price Index** and average annual percent change for all items and selected items: United States, selected years 1950–92 _____ 164

119. **Consumer Price Index** and average annual percent change for all items and medical care components: United States, selected years 1950–92 _____ 165

Sources and Types of Payment

120. **Hospital expenses** and personnel and average annual percent change in nonfederal short-stay hospitals: United States, 1971–91 _____ 166

121. **Hospital expenses** in short-stay hospitals, according to type of ownership and size of hospital: United States, selected years 1970–91 _____ 167

122. **National health expenditures** and average annual percent change, according to source of funds: United States, selected years 1929–91 _____ 168

123. **Personal health care expenditures** and percent distribution, according to source of funds: United States, selected years 1929–91 _____ 169

124. **Expenditures for health services** and supplies and percent distribution, by type of payer: United States, selected calendar years 1965–91 _____ 170

125. **Expenditures on hospital care**, nursing home care, physician services, and all other personal health care expenditures and percent distribution, according to source of funds: United States, selected years 1960–91___ 172

126. **Nursing home average monthly charges** per resident and percent of residents, according to primary source of payments and selected facility characteristics: United States, 1977 and 1985 _____ 173

127. **Nursing home average monthly charges** per resident and percent of residents, according to selected facility and resident characteristics: United States, 1964, 1973–74, 1977, and 1985 _____ 174

128. National **funding for health research** and development and average annual percent change, according to source of funds: United States, selected years 1960–91 _____ 175

129. Federal **funding for health research** and development and percent distribution, according to agency: United States, selected fiscal years 1970–91 _____ 176

130. Federal spending for human immunodeficiency virus (**HIV**)-related activities according to agency and type of activity: United States, fiscal years 1982–91 _____ 177

131. **Public health expenditures** by State and territorial health agencies, according to source of funds and program area: United States, selected fiscal years 1976–89 _____ 178

132. **Personal health care per capita expenditures** and average annual percent change, according to geographic division and State: United States, selected years 1966–82_ 179

133. **Hospital care per capita expenditures** and average annual percent change, according to geographic division and State: United States, selected years 1966–82 _____ 180

134. **Nursing home care per capita expenditures** and average annual percent change, according to geographic division and State: United States, selected years 1966–82_ 181

Health Care Coverage and Major Federal Programs

135. **Health care coverage** for persons under 65 years of age, according to type of coverage and selected characteristics: United States, 1980, 1984, and 1989 _____ 182

136. **Health care coverage** for persons 65 years of age and over, according to type of coverage and selected characteristics: United States, 1980, 1984, and 1989 _____ 183

137. **Health maintenance organizations** and enrollment, according to model type, geographic region, and Federal program: United States, selected years 1976–92 _____ 184

138. **Medicare** enrollees and expenditures and percent distribution, according to type of service: United States and other areas, selected years 1967–91 _____ 185

139. **Medicare** enrollment, persons served, and payments for Medicare enrollees 65 years of age and over, according to selected characteristics: United States and other areas, selected years 1967–90 _____ 186

140. Hospital utilization and benefit payments for aged and disabled **Medicare** enrollees in nonfederal short-stay hospitals, according to geographic division: United States, 1980, 1985, and 1990 _____ 187

141. **Medicaid** recipients and medical vendor payments, according to basis of eligibility: United States, selected fiscal years 1972–91 _____ 188

142. **Medicaid** recipients and medical vendor payments, according to type of service: United States, selected fiscal years 1972–91 _____ 189

143. **Department of Veterans Affairs** health care expenditures and use, and persons treated according to selected characteristics: United States, selected fiscal years 1965–91 _____ 191

144. **Mental health expenditures**, percent distribution, and per capita expenditures, according to type of mental health organization: United States, selected years 1969–88 _____ 192

145. **State mental health agency** per capita expenditures for mental health services, and average annual percent change, according to State: United States, selected fiscal years 1981–90 _____ 193

Table 1 (page 1 of 2). Resident population, according to age, sex, detailed race, and Hispanic origin: United States, selected years 1950–90

[Data are based on decennial census updated by data from multiple sources]

Sex, race, Hispanic origin, and year	Total resident population	Under 1 year	1–4 years	5–14 years	15–24 years	25–34 years	35–44 years	45–54 years	55–64 years	65–74 years	75–84 years	85 years and over
All persons						Number in thousands						
1950	150,697	3,147	13,017	24,319	22,098	23,759	21,450	17,343	13,370	8,340	3,278	577
1960	179,323	4,112	16,209	35,465	24,020	22,818	24,081	20,485	15,572	10,997	4,633	929
1970	203,212	3,485	13,669	40,746	35,441	24,907	23,088	23,220	18,590	12,435	6,119	1,511
1980	226,546	3,534	12,815	34,942	42,487	37,082	25,635	22,800	21,703	15,581	7,729	2,240
1985	237,923	3,679	14,163	33,692	39,992	41,696	31,691	22,459	22,135	16,859	8,890	2,667
1986	240,134	3,700	14,263	33,573	39,557	42,372	33,009	22,659	21,994	17,137	9,128	2,742
1987	242,289	3,703	14,349	33,807	38,890	42,841	34,226	23,096	21,751	17,427	9,376	2,823
1988	244,499	3,757	14,439	34,256	38,151	43,130	35,180	23,949	21,514	17,626	9,612	2,885
1989	246,819	3,858	14,650	34,714	37,391	43,236	36,414	24,633	21,241	17,864	9,850	2,968
1990	248,710	3,946	14,812	35,095	37,013	43,161	37,435	25,057	21,113	18,045	10,012	3,021
White male												
1950	67,129	1,400	5,845	10,860	9,689	10,430	9,529	7,836	6,180	3,736	1,406	218
1960	78,367	1,784	7,065	15,659	10,483	9,940	10,564	9,114	6,850	4,702	1,875	331
1970	86,721	1,501	5,873	17,667	15,232	10,775	9,979	10,090	7,958	4,916	2,243	487
1980	94,976	1,487	5,402	14,773	18,123	15,940	11,010	9,774	9,151	6,096	2,600	621
1985	98,635	1,535	5,897	14,013	16,828	17,698	13,538	9,538	9,290	6,628	2,982	688
1986	99,374	1,538	5,927	13,926	16,605	17,959	14,076	9,610	9,213	6,751	3,065	704
1987	100,072	1,530	5,950	13,998	16,276	18,106	14,572	9,791	9,097	6,877	3,154	721
1988	100,786	1,543	5,968	14,167	15,921	18,170	14,929	10,167	8,990	6,958	3,242	731
1989	101,535	1,569	6,030	14,332	15,565	18,156	15,417	10,455	8,870	7,056	3,335	750
1990	102,143	1,604	6,071	14,467	15,389	18,071	15,819	10,624	8,813	7,127	3,397	760
White female												
1950	67,813	1,341	5,599	10,431	9,821	10,851	9,719	7,868	6,168	4,031	1,669	314
1960	80,465	1,714	6,795	15,068	10,596	10,204	11,000	9,364	7,327	5,428	2,441	527
1970	91,028	1,434	5,615	16,912	15,420	11,004	10,349	10,756	8,853	6,366	3,429	890
1980	99,835	1,412	5,127	14,057	17,653	15,896	11,232	10,285	10,325	7,951	4,457	1,440
1985	103,397	1,457	5,599	13,288	16,236	17,435	13,699	9,909	10,378	8,536	5,104	1,756
1986	104,056	1,460	5,627	13,204	15,965	17,656	14,207	9,963	10,278	8,657	5,232	1,807
1987	104,697	1,453	5,648	13,269	15,604	17,790	14,674	10,128	10,121	8,785	5,363	1,862
1988	105,342	1,465	5,666	13,422	15,214	17,850	15,005	10,495	9,968	8,867	5,484	1,906
1989	106,005	1,492	5,724	13,579	14,817	17,830	15,457	10,780	9,793	8,968	5,604	1,961
1990	106,561	1,524	5,762	13,706	14,599	17,757	15,834	10,946	9,698	9,048	5,687	2,001
Black male												
1950	7,300	- - -	- - -	1,442	1,162	1,105	1,003	772	460	299	- - -	- - -
1960	9,114	281	1,082	2,185	1,305	1,120	1,086	891	617	382	137	29
1970	10,748	245	975	2,784	2,041	1,226	1,084	979	739	461	169	46
1980	12,585	269	967	2,614	2,807	1,967	1,235	1,024	854	567	228	53
1985	13,505	276	1,067	2,599	2,768	2,391	1,543	1,069	887	586	257	62
1986	13,687	280	1,076	2,594	2,769	2,452	1,629	1,082	889	591	262	63
1987	13,869	287	1,086	2,612	2,750	2,507	1,707	1,105	888	596	267	64
1988	14,057	297	1,103	2,640	2,723	2,550	1,789	1,132	885	602	271	65
1989	14,258	315	1,135	2,671	2,687	2,579	1,883	1,157	881	609	275	66
1990	14,420	322	1,164	2,700	2,669	2,592	1,962	1,175	878	614	277	66
Black female												
1950	7,745	- - -	- - -	1,446	1,300	1,260	1,112	796	443	322	- - -	- - -
1960	9,758	283	1,085	2,191	1,404	1,300	1,229	974	663	430	160	38
1970	11,832	243	970	2,773	2,196	1,456	1,309	1,134	868	582	230	71
1980	14,046	266	951	2,578	2,937	2,267	1,488	1,258	1,059	776	360	106
1985	15,063	271	1,045	2,547	2,845	2,711	1,828	1,298	1,121	833	431	133
1986	15,256	275	1,053	2,541	2,830	2,767	1,921	1,313	1,128	844	446	138
1987	15,456	281	1,061	2,557	2,803	2,820	2,007	1,336	1,133	854	460	144
1988	15,667	291	1,079	2,583	2,771	2,863	2,094	1,366	1,133	864	474	149
1989	15,887	309	1,110	2,613	2,726	2,892	2,195	1,395	1,132	876	486	153
1990	16,063	316	1,137	2,641	2,700	2,905	2,279	1,416	1,135	884	495	156
American Indian or Alaskan Native male												
1980	702	17	59	153	161	114	75	53	37	22	9	2
1985	848	20	75	171	181	144	104	66	47	26	11	3
1986	882	20	78	176	185	151	112	70	48	27	12	3
1987	919	21	81	183	188	158	120	74	50	29	12	3
1988	952	21	82	191	189	166	127	78	52	30	13	3
1989	992	23	85	200	190	176	135	83	53	31	13	3
1990	1,024	24	88	206	192	183	140	86	55	32	13	3

See footnotes at end of table.

Table 1 (page 2 of 2). Resident population, according to age, sex, detailed race, and Hispanic origin: United States, selected years 1950–90

[Data are based on decennial census updated by data from multiple sources]

Sex, race, Hispanic origin, and year	Total resident population	Under 1 year	1–4 years	5–14 years	15–24 years	25–34 years	35–44 years	45–54 years	55–64 years	65–74 years	75–84 years	85 years and over
American Indian or Alaskan Native female						Number in thousands						
1980	718	16	57	149	158	118	79	57	41	27	12	4
1985	867	19	73	165	172	149	111	71	52	33	17	5
1986	899	20	76	169	174	155	120	74	54	34	18	5
1987	935	20	79	177	176	162	128	78	56	36	18	5
1988	971	21	80	184	177	170	136	82	58	38	19	6
1989	1,011	23	82	193	178	179	143	88	60	39	20	6
1990	1,041	24	85	200	178	186	148	92	61	41	21	6
Asian or Pacific Islander male												
1980	1,693	31	117	297	306	339	239	152	106	70	29	5
1985	2,741	52	205	463	499	559	409	244	160	99	43	8
1986	2,923	54	216	490	534	593	444	263	169	106	45	9
1987	3,103	57	225	515	566	628	479	283	179	113	48	10
1988	3,292	61	234	544	600	661	517	305	188	120	51	11
1989	3,493	66	246	574	636	696	557	327	198	127	55	11
1990	3,652	68	258	598	665	718	588	347	208	133	57	12
Asian or Pacific Islander female												
1980	1,807	30	115	285	302	401	258	186	122	68	32	9
1985	2,866	50	201	445	463	608	459	265	200	117	46	12
1986	3,055	51	211	472	494	639	500	283	215	127	50	13
1987	3,240	54	219	497	526	670	540	302	228	137	53	14
1988	3,433	58	226	526	557	699	583	325	240	147	57	15
1989	3,641	63	237	553	593	730	629	349	253	157	61	16
1990	3,805	65	247	578	621	749	664	371	264	166	65	17
Hispanic male												
1980	7,280	173	675	1,530	1,646	1,255	761	570	364	201	86	19
1985	9,275	208	783	1,823	2,022	1,852	1,060	674	479	239	111	24
1986	9,691	219	814	1,873	2,099	1,969	1,134	695	497	250	115	26
1987	10,113	229	847	1,937	2,161	2,079	1,214	722	512	265	119	28
1988	10,558	240	886	2,006	2,234	2,179	1,300	755	525	280	123	30
1989	11,017	262	937	2,074	2,304	2,260	1,394	791	538	298	128	31
1990	11,388	279	980	2,128	2,376	2,310	1,471	818	551	312	131	32
Hispanic female												
1980	7,329	166	648	1,482	1,547	1,249	805	615	411	257	116	30
1985	9,094	199	749	1,755	1,814	1,704	1,092	719	540	317	163	42
1986	9,462	210	779	1,800	1,867	1,794	1,160	740	562	332	172	46
1987	9,834	219	811	1,860	1,908	1,877	1,231	769	580	349	181	49
1988	10,229	231	849	1,926	1,949	1,958	1,304	803	599	366	192	52
1989	10,632	252	897	1,989	1,986	2,025	1,382	840	617	386	202	56
1990	10,966	268	939	2,039	2,028	2,073	1,448	868	632	403	209	59

NOTES: The race groups, white and black, include persons of both Hispanic and non-Hispanic origin. Conversely, persons of Hispanic origin may be of any race. Population figures are census counts as of April 1 for 1950, 1960, 1970, 1980, and 1990 and estimates as of July 1 for other years. Data for the 1980's are intercensal population estimates and differ from postcensal population estimates in previous editions of Health, United States. See Appendix I, Department of Commerce.

SOURCES: U.S. Bureau of the Census: 1950 Nonwhite Population by Race. Special Report P-E, No. 3B. Washington. U.S. Government Printing Office, 1951; Population estimates and projections. Current Population Reports. Series P-25, Nos. 499, 1022, 1045, 1046, and 1057. Washington. U.S. Government Printing Office, May 1973, Mar. 1988, Sept. 1989, Jan. 1990, and Mar. 1990; U.S. Bureau of the Census, U.S. Census of Population: 1960, Number of Inhabitants, PC(1)-A1, United States Summary, 1964. U.S. Bureau of the Census, U.S. Census of Population: 1970, Number of Inhabitants, Final Report PC(1)-A1, United States Summary, 1971; U.S. Bureau of the Census, U.S. Census of Population: 1980, General Population Characteristics, PC80-1-B1, United States Summary, May 1983; U.S. Bureau of the Census, U.S. Census of Population: 1990, Population and Housing, CPH-L-74, Aug. 1991; Unpublished data from the U.S. Bureau of the Census.

Table 2. Persons and families below poverty level, according to selected characteristics, race, and Hispanic origin: United States, selected years 1973–91

[Data are based on household interviews of the civilian noninstitutionalized population]

Selected characteristics, race, and Hispanic origin	1973	1980 [1]	1985	1986	1987	1988	1989	1990	1991
All persons	Percent below poverty								
All races	11.1	13.0	14.0	13.6	13.4	13.0	12.8	13.5	14.2
White	8.4	10.2	11.4	11.0	10.4	10.1	10.0	10.7	11.3
Black	31.4	32.5	31.3	31.1	32.4	31.3	30.7	31.9	32.7
Hispanic	21.9	25.7	29.0	27.3	28.0	26.7	26.2	28.1	28.7
Related children under 18 years of age in families									
All races	14.2	17.9	20.1	19.8	19.7	19.0	19.0	19.9	21.1
White	9.7	13.4	15.6	15.3	14.7	14.0	14.1	15.1	16.1
Black	40.6	42.1	43.1	42.7	44.4	42.8	43.2	44.2	45.6
Hispanic	27.8	33.0	39.6	37.1	38.9	37.3	35.5	37.7	39.8
Families with female householder, no husband present, and children under 18 years of age									
All races	43.2	42.9	45.4	46.0	45.5	44.7	42.8	44.5	47.1
White	35.2	35.9	38.7	39.8	38.3	38.2	36.1	37.9	39.6
Black	58.8	56.0	58.9	58.0	58.6	56.2	53.9	56.1	60.5
Hispanic	- - -	57.3	64.0	59.5	60.9	59.2	57.9	58.2	60.1
All persons	Number below poverty in thousands								
All races	22,973	29,272	33,064	32,370	32,221	31,745	31,528	33,585	35,708
White	15,142	19,699	22,860	22,183	21,195	20,715	20,785	22,326	23,747
Black	7,388	8,579	8,926	8,983	9,520	9,356	9,302	9,837	10,242
Hispanic	2,366	3,491	5,236	5,117	5,422	5,357	5,430	6,006	6,339
Related children under 18 years of age in families									
All races	9,453	11,114	12,483	12,257	12,275	11,935	12,001	12,715	13,658
White	5,462	6,817	7,838	7,714	7,398	7,095	7,164	7,696	8,316
Black	3,822	3,906	4,057	4,037	4,234	4,148	4,257	4,412	4,637
Hispanic	1,364	1,718	2,512	2,413	2,606	2,576	2,496	2,750	2,977
Families with female householder, no husband present, and children under 18 years of age									
All races	1,987	2,703	3,131	3,264	3,281	3,294	3,190	3,426	3,767
White	1,053	1,433	1,730	1,812	1,742	1,740	1,671	1,814	1,969
Black	905	1,217	1,336	1,384	1,437	1,452	1,415	1,513	1,676
Hispanic	- - -	288	493	489	527	510	491	536	584

[1] Data for Hispanic families with female householder, no husband present, and children under 18 years are for 1979.

NOTES: The race groups, white and black, include persons of both Hispanic and non-Hispanic origin. Conversely, persons of Hispanic origin may be of any race. Some numbers in this table have been revised and differ from previous editions of Health, United States.

SOURCE: U.S. Bureau of the Census: Poverty in the United States 1991. Current Population Reports. Series P-60, No. 181. Washington. U.S. Government Printing Office, Aug. 1992.

Table 3. Live births, crude birth rates, and birth rates by age of mother, according to race: United States, selected years 1950–91

[Data are based on the National Vital Statistics System]

Race and year	Live births	Crude birth rate [1]	10–14 years	15–17 years	18–19 years	20–24 years	25–29 years	30–34 years	35–39 years	40–44 years	45–49 years
All races						Live births per 1,000 women					
1950	3,632,000	24.1	1.0	40.7	132.7	196.6	166.1	103.7	52.9	15.1	1.2
1960	4,257,850	23.7	0.8	43.9	166.7	258.1	197.4	112.7	56.2	15.5	0.9
1970	3,731,386	18.4	1.2	38.8	114.7	167.8	145.1	73.3	31.7	8.1	0.5
1975	3,144,198	14.6	1.3	36.1	85.0	113.0	108.2	52.3	19.5	4.6	0.3
1980	3,612,258	15.9	1.1	32.5	82.1	115.1	112.9	61.9	19.8	3.9	0.2
1985	3,760,561	15.8	1.2	31.0	79.6	108.3	111.0	69.1	24.0	4.0	0.2
1986	3,756,547	15.6	1.3	30.5	79.6	107.4	109.8	70.1	24.4	4.1	0.2
1987	3,809,394	15.7	1.3	31.7	78.5	107.9	111.6	72.1	26.3	4.4	0.2
1988	3,909,510	16.0	1.3	33.6	79.9	110.2	114.4	74.8	28.1	4.8	0.2
1989	4,040,958	16.4	1.4	36.4	84.2	113.8	117.6	77.4	29.9	5.2	0.2
1990	4,158,212	16.7	1.4	37.5	88.6	116.5	120.2	80.8	31.7	5.5	0.2
Provisional data:											
1989 [2]	4,021,000	16.2	- - -	- - -	- - -	- - -	- - -	- - -	- - -	- - -	- - -
1990 [2]	4,179,000	16.7	- - -	- - -	- - -	- - -	- - -	- - -	- - -	- - -	- - -
1991	4,111,000	16.2	- - -	- - -	- - -	- - -	- - -	- - -	- - -	- - -	- - -
Race of child [3]: White											
1950	3,108,000	23.0	0.4	31.3	120.5	190.4	165.1	102.6	51.4	14.5	1.0
1960	3,600,744	22.7	0.4	35.5	154.6	252.8	194.9	109.6	54.0	14.7	0.8
1970	3,091,264	17.4	0.5	29.2	101.5	163.4	145.9	71.9	30.0	7.5	0.4
1975	2,551,996	13.6	0.6	28.0	74.0	108.2	108.1	51.3	18.2	4.2	0.2
1980	2,898,732	14.9	0.6	25.2	72.1	109.5	112.4	60.4	18.5	3.4	0.2
1985	2,991,373	14.8	0.6	24.0	69.2	102.4	110.7	68.9	22.9	3.6	0.2
1986	2,970,439	14.6	0.6	23.3	68.7	101.0	109.9	69.8	23.5	3.7	0.2
1987	2,992,488	14.6	0.6	24.0	67.3	100.4	110.7	71.9	25.5	4.1	0.2
1988	3,046,162	14.8	0.6	25.3	67.8	101.6	113.0	74.3	27.2	4.4	0.2
1989	3,131,991	15.1	0.7	27.4	70.9	104.6	115.9	76.9	29.2	4.8	0.2
1990	3,225,343	15.5	0.7	28.6	75.6	107.2	118.8	80.4	30.9	5.1	0.2
Race of mother [4]: White											
1989	3,192,355	15.4	0.7	28.1	72.9	106.9	117.8	78.1	29.7	4.9	0.2
1990	3,290,273	15.8	0.7	29.5	78.0	109.8	120.7	81.7	31.5	5.2	0.2
Race of child [3]: Black											
1960	602,264	31.9	4.3	- - -	- - -	295.4	218.6	137.1	73.9	21.9	1.1
1970	572,362	25.3	5.2	101.4	204.9	202.7	136.3	79.6	41.9	12.5	1.0
1975	511,581	20.7	5.1	85.6	152.4	142.8	102.2	53.1	25.6	7.5	0.5
1980	589,616	22.1	4.3	73.6	138.8	146.3	109.1	62.9	24.5	5.8	0.3
1985	608,193	21.3	4.6	70.7	136.4	140.7	105.9	61.4	25.5	4.9	0.3
1986	621,221	21.5	4.7	71.1	140.0	143.5	106.8	63.0	25.4	5.0	0.3
1987	641,567	21.9	4.8	74.2	141.4	149.2	110.2	64.4	26.2	5.2	0.2
1988	671,976	22.6	4.9	78.1	149.4	157.1	114.4	67.1	27.3	5.5	0.3
1989	709,395	23.5	5.2	84.4	159.4	165.2	120.9	70.6	28.6	5.8	0.3
1990	724,576	23.8	4.9	85.4	161.6	170.0	122.3	73.3	30.2	5.9	0.3
Race of mother [4]: Black											
1989	673,124	22.3	5.1	81.9	151.9	156.8	114.4	66.3	26.7	5.4	0.3
1990	684,336	22.4	4.9	82.3	152.9	160.2	115.5	68.7	28.1	5.5	0.3

[1] Live births per 1,000 population.
[2] Includes births of nonresidents of the United States.
[3] Live births are tabulated by race of child.
[4] Live births are tabulated by race of mother.

NOTES: Data are based on births adjusted for underregistration for 1950 and on registered births for all other years. Beginning in 1970, births to nonresidents of the United States are excluded. Final data for the 1980's have been revised based on intercensal population estimates and differ from previous editions of Health, United States. Provisional data for 1989–91 were calculated using 1980's-based postcensal population estimates. Differences between provisional and final data are due to differences in both the numerator and denominator. See Appendix I, National Center for Health Statistics and Department of Commerce.

SOURCES: Centers for Disease Control and Prevention, National Center for Health Statistics: Vital Statistics of the United States, 1990, Vol. I, Natality. Public Health Service. Washington. U.S. Government Printing Office, 1992; and Births, marriages, divorces, and deaths for 1991. Monthly Vital Statistics Report. Vol. 40, No. 12. DHHS Pub. No. (PHS) 92-1120. April 15, 1992. Public Health Service. Hyattsville, Md.

Table 4. Fertility rates, according to live-birth order and race: United States, selected years 1950–91

[Data are based on the National Vital Statistics System]

Race and year	Total	Live-birth order				
		1	2	3	4	5 or higher
All races		Live births per 1,000 women 15–44 years of age				
1950	106.2	33.3	32.1	18.4	9.2	13.2
1960	118.0	31.1	29.2	22.8	14.6	20.3
1970	87.9	34.2	24.2	13.6	7.2	8.7
1975	66.0	28.1	20.9	9.4	3.9	3.7
1980	68.4	29.5	21.8	10.3	3.9	2.9
1985	66.3	27.6	22.0	10.4	3.8	2.5
1986	65.4	27.2	21.6	10.3	3.8	2.5
1987	65.8	27.2	21.6	10.5	3.9	2.5
1988	67.3	27.6	22.0	10.9	4.1	2.7
1989	69.2	28.4	22.4	11.3	4.3	2.8
1990	70.9	29.0	22.8	11.7	4.5	3.0
Provisional data:						
1989 [1]	68.8	- - -	- - -	- - -	- - -	- - -
1990 [1]	71.1	- - -	- - -	- - -	- - -	- - -
1991	69.6	- - -	- - -	- - -	- - -	- - -
Race of child [2]: White						
1950	102.3	33.3	32.3	17.9	8.4	10.4
1960	113.2	30.8	29.2	22.7	14.1	16.4
1970	84.1	32.9	23.7	13.3	6.8	7.4
1975	62.5	26.7	20.3	8.8	3.5	3.1
1980	64.7	28.4	21.0	9.5	3.4	2.4
1985	63.2	26.6	21.5	9.7	3.3	2.0
1986	62.1	26.1	21.0	9.7	3.3	1.9
1987	62.3	26.0	21.0	9.8	3.4	1.9
1988	63.4	26.3	21.2	10.2	3.6	2.1
1989	65.1	27.1	21.5	10.5	3.8	2.2
1990	66.9	27.8	22.0	10.8	3.9	2.3
Race of mother [3]: White						
1989	66.4	27.6	21.9	10.7	3.8	2.2
1990	68.3	28.4	22.4	11.1	4.0	2.4
Race of child [2]: Black						
1960	153.5	33.6	29.3	24.0	18.6	48.0
1970	115.4	43.3	27.1	16.1	10.0	18.9
1975	87.9	36.9	24.2	12.6	6.3	8.0
1980	88.1	35.2	25.7	14.5	6.7	6.0
1985	82.4	32.5	24.5	14.0	6.3	5.1
1986	82.6	32.6	24.6	14.1	6.4	4.9
1987	84.1	33.0	25.0	14.5	6.5	5.0
1988	87.0	33.7	25.9	15.1	6.9	5.2
1989	90.8	34.9	26.8	16.0	7.4	5.7
1990	91.9	34.6	27.1	16.4	7.7	6.0
Race of mother [3]: Black						
1989	86.2	32.9	25.4	15.3	7.1	5.5
1990	86.8	32.4	25.6	15.6	7.4	5.8

[1]Includes births of nonresidents of the United States.
[2]Live births are tabulated by race of child.
[3]Live births are tabulated by race of mother.

NOTES: Data are based on births adjusted for underregistration for 1950 and on registered births for all other years. Beginning in 1970, births to nonresidents of the United States are excluded. Figures for live-birth order not stated are distributed. Final data for the 1980's have been revised based on intercensal population estimates and differ from previous editions of Health, United States. Provisional data for 1989–91 were calculated using 1980's-based postcensal population estimates. Differences between provisional and final data are due to differences in both the numerator and denominator. See Appendix I, National Center for Health Statistics and Department of Commerce.

SOURCES: Centers for Disease Control and Prevention, National Center for Health Statistics: Vital Statistics of the United States, 1990, Vol. I, Natality. Public Health Service. Washington. U.S. Government Printing Office, 1992; and Births, marriages, divorces, and deaths for 1991. Monthly Vital Statistics Report. Vol. 40, No. 12. DHHS Pub. No. (PHS) 92-1120. April 15, 1992. Public Health Service. Hyattsville, Md.

Table 5. Completed fertility rates and parity distribution for women 50–54 years of age at the beginning of selected years 1930–91, according to race of child and birth cohort: United States, selected birth cohorts 1876–80 to 1937–41

[Data are based on the National Vital Statistics System]

Race of child and birth cohort of mother	Age 50–54 as of January 1,–	Completed fertility rate [1]	Parity (number of children born alive)								
			Total	0	1	2	3	4	5	6	7 or more
			Distribution of women [2]								
All races											
1876–80	1930	3,531.9	1,000.0	216.8	123.2	132.0	114.0	93.0	72.0	64.5	184.5
1886–90	1940	3,136.8	1,000.0	210.4	148.5	153.2	129.7	99.5	68.0	55.4	135.3
1896–1900	1950	2,675.9	1,000.0	194.6	200.7	195.2	136.6	87.8	53.5	41.5	90.1
1906–10	1960	2,285.8	1,000.0	215.6	225.1	218.7	131.4	77.5	44.6	29.2	57.9
1916–20	1970	2,574.0	1,000.0	149.0	179.0	251.7	174.6	102.8	55.8	32.0	55.1
1921–25	1975	2,857.0	1,000.0	108.5	152.1	248.7	197.0	123.5	68.0	39.5	62.7
1926–30	1980	3,079.2	1,000.0	105.5	113.7	226.5	209.6	143.5	81.9	47.6	71.7
1927–31	1981	3,118.0	1,000.0	104.1	107.3	222.4	212.0	147.6	84.6	49.2	72.8
1928–32	1982	3,152.7	1,000.0	101.1	102.2	219.7	214.7	151.3	87.0	50.8	73.2
1929–33	1983	3,182.8	1,000.0	96.3	98.9	218.0	217.7	154.9	89.2	52.0	73.0
1930–34	1984	3,199.6	1,000.0	91.5	96.8	217.8	220.9	157.9	90.7	52.6	71.8
1931–35	1985	3,201.4	1,000.0	87.2	96.3	218.8	224.0	160.0	91.4	52.5	69.8
1932–36	1986	3,182.4	1,000.0	84.8	97.0	221.0	226.9	160.8	91.3	51.7	66.5
1933–37	1987	3,146.4	1,000.0	84.0	98.7	224.4	229.5	160.6	90.2	50.2	62.4
1934–38	1988	3,092.6	1,000.0	85.0	100.8	229.7	232.0	159.2	87.7	48.1	57.5
1935–39	1989	3,026.3	1,000.0	86.9	103.8	236.6	234.2	156.6	84.2	45.6	52.1
1936–40	1990	2,949.7	1,000.0	89.6	107.1	245.7	236.1	152.6	79.9	42.4	46.6
1937–41	1991	2,863.8	1,000.0	93.1	111.3	256.5	237.1	147.1	75.1	38.8	41.0
White											
1876–80	1930	3,444.4	1,000.0	218.2	121.9	136.1	116.9	94.8	74.0	64.2	173.9
1886–90	1940	3,092.9	1,000.0	209.1	144.3	160.3	132.4	100.2	70.3	54.8	128.6
1896–1900	1950	2,631.5	1,000.0	193.1	192.1	205.9	141.4	89.0	55.2	41.1	82.2
1906–10	1960	2,248.9	1,000.0	207.9	218.0	233.2	138.8	79.6	44.7	28.0	49.8
1916–20	1970	2,526.7	1,000.0	134.6	175.9	268.7	185.1	106.5	55.3	30.3	43.6
1921–25	1975	2,793.7	1,000.0	94.2	150.6	264.6	208.8	127.9	67.9	36.9	49.1
1926–30	1980	2,986.0	1,000.0	94.1	114.1	240.2	222.3	148.8	81.2	44.5	54.8
1927–31	1981	3,022.6	1,000.0	92.5	108.2	236.8	223.9	153.1	83.9	46.0	55.6
1928–32	1982	3,057.9	1,000.0	89.5	103.2	232.9	227.6	157.2	86.5	47.2	55.9
1929–33	1983	3,087.2	1,000.0	85.0	99.8	231.2	230.5	161.1	88.6	48.2	55.6
1930–34	1984	3,102.5	1,000.0	81.2	97.6	230.5	233.6	164.1	90.0	48.5	54.5
1931–35	1985	3,101.2	1,000.0	78.5	96.8	231.1	236.4	166.0	90.5	48.2	52.5
1932–36	1986	3,080.0	1,000.0	77.9	97.0	232.9	239.2	166.3	89.9	47.3	49.5
1933–37	1987	3,042.3	1,000.0	78.6	98.5	236.2	241.6	165.5	88.1	45.5	46.0
1934–38	1988	2,990.0	1,000.0	80.7	100.6	241.2	243.9	163.3	85.2	43.1	42.0
1935–39	1989	2,926.9	1,000.0	83.2	103.6	248.4	245.7	159.8	81.3	40.3	37.7
1936–40	1990	2,854.7	1,000.0	86.3	107.1	257.6	247.1	154.9	76.5	37.2	33.3
1937–41	1991	2,773.8	1,000.0	90.2	111.5	268.6	247.4	148.5	71.1	33.6	29.1
All other											
1876–80	1930	4,254.7	1,000.0	207.7	134.0	99.5	87.4	79.9	54.7	64.8	272.0
1886–90	1940	3,451.4	1,000.0	231.9	175.9	105.9	96.6	93.3	52.4	58.0	186.0
1896–1900	1950	2,967.7	1,000.0	227.4	255.0	114.1	97.5	74.3	38.8	42.6	150.3
1906–10	1960	2,529.1	1,000.0	287.5	266.6	114.5	73.2	60.1	43.5	35.6	119.0
1916–20	1970	2,924.2	1,000.0	266.2	202.0	120.9	91.2	72.5	57.8	44.9	144.5
1921–25	1975	3,316.0	1,000.0	217.7	163.5	131.7	108.2	89.0	68.7	56.4	164.8
1926–30	1980	3,718.9	1,000.0	187.4	110.8	130.2	121.0	106.4	85.7	69.3	189.2
1927–31	1981	3,756.0	1,000.0	185.7	102.5	129.1	123.0	109.1	88.1	71.5	191.0
1928–32	1982	3,779.4	1,000.0	181.6	96.7	129.4	126.5	111.4	90.2	73.5	190.7
1929–33	1983	3,805.1	1,000.0	172.4	93.2	132.3	130.1	114.4	93.1	75.1	189.4
1930–34	1984	3,822.2	1,000.0	160.3	92.2	136.0	135.3	117.5	95.5	76.9	186.3
1931–35	1985	3,836.2	1,000.0	145.1	93.4	140.8	140.4	121.8	98.2	78.4	181.9
1932–36	1986	3,830.3	1,000.0	131.0	96.4	145.5	145.5	125.9	100.5	79.9	175.3
1933–37	1987	3,805.9	1,000.0	119.4	99.8	150.3	150.2	129.9	102.4	80.6	167.4
1934–38	1988	3,745.8	1,000.0	113.8	102.8	154.9	155.3	132.7	102.7	80.6	157.2
1935–39	1989	3,661.6	1,000.0	111.5	105.4	160.6	160.4	135.3	102.4	79.2	145.2
1936–40	1990	3,556.1	1,000.0	111.8	107.6	168.2	165.6	137.2	101.3	76.9	131.4
1937–41	1991	3,438.0	1,000.0	112.7	110.6	177.6	170.6	139.0	99.5	73.3	116.7

[1] Number of children born alive to each 1,000 women who have completed their reproductive histories (women 50–54 years of age).
[2] Proportional distribution of each 1,000 women in the cohort by the number of children born alive to them.

NOTES: Example of use of table—For every 1,000 women 50–54 years of age in 1980, an average of 3,079.2 children were born alive (about 3 children per woman). About 10 percent of the women in this cohort reached 50–54 years of age having had no children, about 11 percent had 1 child, and about 12 percent had 6 children or more.

SOURCES: Centers for Disease Control and Prevention, National Center for Health Statistics: Fertility Tables for Birth Cohorts by Color, United States, 1917–73 by R. Heuser. DHEW Pub. No. (HRA) 76-1152. Health Resources Administration. Washington. U.S. Government Printing Office, Apr. 1976; Data computed from Vital Statistics of the United States, 1990, Vol. I, Natality. Public Health Service. Washington. U.S. Government Printing Office, 1992.

Table 6. Lifetime births expected by currently married women and percent of expected births already born, according to age and race: United States, selected years 1967–90

[Data are based on reporting of birth expectations by currently married women of the civilian noninstitutionalized population]

Race and year	All ages 18–34 years	18–19 years	20–21 years	22–24 years	25–29 years	30–34 years
All races	Expected births per currently married woman					
1967.	3.1	2.7	2.9	2.9	3.0	3.3
1971.	2.6	2.3	2.4	2.4	2.6	3.0
1975.	2.3	2.2	2.2	2.2	2.3	2.6
1980.	2.2	2.1	2.2	2.1	2.2	2.2
1985.	2.2	2.1	2.2	2.2	2.2	2.2
1986.	2.3	2.2	2.2	2.3	2.3	2.2
1987.	2.2	2.1	2.2	2.2	2.2	2.2
1988.	2.2	2.1	2.2	2.2	2.3	2.2
1990.	2.3	2.1	2.2	2.3	2.3	2.3
White						
1967.	3.0	2.7	3.0	2.8	3.0	3.2
1971.	2.6	2.3	2.4	2.4	2.6	2.9
1975.	2.3	2.2	2.1	2.1	2.2	2.6
1980.	2.2	2.1	2.2	2.1	2.1	2.2
1985.	2.2	2.0	2.2	2.2	2.2	2.1
1986.	2.2	2.1	2.2	2.3	2.2	2.2
1987.	2.2	2.0	2.2	2.2	2.2	2.2
1988.	2.2	2.1	2.2	2.2	2.2	2.2
1990.	2.3	2.1	2.2	2.3	2.3	2.3
Black						
1967.	3.5	*	2.5	3.0	3.4	4.3
1971.	3.1	*	2.4	2.8	3.1	3.7
1975.	2.8	*	2.6	2.5	2.6	3.2
1980.	2.4	*	2.2	2.1	2.4	2.5
1985.	2.4	*	*	2.3	2.3	2.5
1986.	2.4	*	*	2.4	2.3	2.6
1987.	2.3	*	*	2.2	2.3	2.3
1988.	2.3	*	*	2.2	2.3	2.3
1990.	2.5	2.1	2.4	2.6	2.4	2.6
All races	Percent of expected births already born					
1967.	70.2	26.9	33.2	47.8	76.1	92.7
1971.	69.4	25.3	32.5	46.7	74.4	93.7
1975.	68.8	27.5	30.7	43.9	70.9	93.0
1980.	67.0	29.5	32.9	44.9	64.7	89.7
1985.	64.2	27.0	30.9	41.8	60.2	84.4
1986.	64.7	29.0	30.4	41.8	59.5	84.8
1987.	66.5	27.8	36.4	43.0	62.0	83.8
1988.	65.3	25.0	33.4	40.9	58.9	83.6
1990.	64.5	29.9	33.1	44.2	57.5	81.1
White						
1967.	68.9	24.2	30.1	46.2	75.1	92.9
1971.	68.9	23.7	31.4	45.3	74.1	93.8
1975.	68.2	24.9	29.4	42.3	70.5	93.2
1980.	66.3	28.6	31.8	43.5	64.0	90.0
1985.	63.3	25.7	30.6	40.4	59.4	84.1
1986.	63.8	28.6	28.7	40.5	58.6	84.8
1987.	65.6	27.0	36.0	42.0	60.9	83.6
1988.	64.4	24.0	32.6	38.9	58.2	83.2
1990.	63.6	26.8	30.0	43.1	56.2	80.8
Black						
1967.	82.8	*	65.7	67.9	87.9	92.3
1971.	74.8	*	43.0	57.5	81.0	93.4
1975.	76.4	*	43.3	61.0	78.2	91.8
1980.	74.7	*	46.1	58.9	73.8	90.9
1985.	77.1	*	*	62.3	72.8	91.4
1986.	75.7	*	*	59.7	70.2	90.0
1987.	77.8	*	*	55.4	76.6	89.7
1988.	75.5	*	*	61.4	70.1	89.9
1990.	74.1	49.0	54.8	56.6	71.9	85.0

*Estimates based on 50 or fewer subjects are not shown.

NOTE: Data for 1989 are not available.

SOURCE: U.S. Bureau of the Census: Population characteristics. Current Population Reports. Series P-20, Nos. 301, 375, 406, 421, 427, 436, and 454. Washington. U.S. Government Printing Office, Nov. 1976, Oct. 1982, June 1986, Dec. 1987, May 1988, May 1989, and Oct. 1991.

Table 7. Live births, according to detailed race of mother and Hispanic origin of mother: United States, selected years 1970–90

[Data are based on the National Vital Statistics System]

Race of mother and Hispanic origin of mother	1970	1975	1980	1985	1986	1987	1988	1989	1990
				Total number of live births					
All races	3,731,386	3,144,198	3,612,258	3,760,561	3,756,547	3,809,394	3,909,510	4,040,958	4,158,212
White	3,109,956	2,576,818	2,936,351	3,037,913	3,019,175	3,043,828	3,102,083	3,192,355	3,290,273
Black	561,992	496,829	568,080	581,824	592,910	611,173	638,562	673,124	684,336
American Indian or Alaskan Native	22,264	22,690	29,389	34,037	34,169	35,322	37,088	39,478	39,051
Asian or Pacific Islander	- - -	- - -	74,355	104,606	107,797	116,560	129,035	133,075	141,635
Chinese	7,044	7,778	11,671	16,405	16,701	17,818	21,322	20,982	22,737
Japanese	7,744	6,725	7,482	8,035	7,938	8,054	8,658	8,689	8,674
Filipino	8,066	10,359	13,968	20,058	21,237	22,134	23,207	24,585	25,770
Other Asian or Pacific Islander [1]	- - -	- - -	41,234	60,108	61,921	68,554	75,848	78,819	84,454
Hispanic origin (selected States) [2,3]	- - -	- - -	307,163	372,814	389,048	406,153	449,604	532,249	595,073
Mexican American	- - -	- - -	215,439	242,976	246,174	251,189	271,170	327,233	385,640
Puerto Rican	- - -	- - -	33,671	35,147	36,588	38,139	46,232	56,229	58,807
Cuban	- - -	- - -	7,163	10,024	9,924	9,987	10,189	10,842	11,311
Central and South American	- - -	- - -	21,268	40,985	45,026	50,350	57,610	72,443	83,008
Other and unknown Hispanic	- - -	- - -	29,622	43,682	51,336	56,488	64,403	65,502	56,307
Non-Hispanic white (selected States) [2]	- - -	- - -	1,245,221	1,394,729	1,388,251	1,399,129	1,664,239	2,526,367	2,626,500
Non-Hispanic black (selected States) [2]	- - -	- - -	299,646	336,029	342,179	355,644	434,843	611,269	661,701

[1]Includes Hawaiians and part Hawaiians.

[2]Trend data for Hispanics and non-Hispanics are affected by expansion of the reporting area for an Hispanic-origin item on the birth certificate and by immigration. These two factors affect numbers of events, composition of the Hispanic population, and maternal and infant health characteristics. The number of States in the reporting area increased from 22 in 1980, to 23 plus the District of Columbia (D.C.) in 1983, 30 plus D.C. in 1988, 47 plus D.C. in 1989, and 48 plus D.C. in 1990 (see Appendix I, National Vital Statistics System).

[3]Includes mothers of all races.

NOTES: The race groups, white and black, include persons of both Hispanic and non-Hispanic origin. Conversely, persons of Hispanic origin may be of any race.

SOURCE: Centers for Disease Control and Prevention, National Center for Health Statistics: Data computed by the Division of Analysis from data compiled by the Division of Vital Statistics.

Table 8. Low-birth-weight live births, according to detailed race of mother and Hispanic origin of mother: United States, selected years 1970–90

[Data are based on the National Vital Statistics System]

Birth weight, race of mother, and Hispanic origin of mother	1970	1975	1980	1981	1982	1983	1984	1985	1986	1987	1988	1989	1990
Low birth weight (less than 2,500 grams)						Percent of live births							
All mothers	7.93	7.38	6.84	6.81	6.75	6.82	6.72	6.75	6.81	6.90	6.93	7.05	6.97
White	6.85	6.27	5.72	5.69	5.64	5.69	5.61	5.65	5.66	5.70	5.67	5.72	5.70
Black	13.90	13.19	12.69	12.72	12.61	12.82	12.58	12.65	12.77	12.98	13.26	13.51	13.25
American Indian or Alaskan Native	7.97	6.41	6.44	6.27	6.06	6.17	6.15	5.86	5.94	6.15	6.00	6.26	6.11
Asian or Pacific Islander	- - -	- - -	6.68	6.74	6.74	6.57	6.57	6.16	6.47	6.41	6.31	6.51	6.45
Chinese	6.67	5.29	5.21	5.55	5.26	5.07	5.05	4.98	4.85	5.02	4.63	4.89	4.69
Japanese	9.03	7.47	6.60	6.22	6.09	6.05	5.91	6.21	6.03	6.49	6.69	6.67	6.16
Filipino	10.02	8.08	7.40	7.50	7.15	7.28	7.78	6.95	7.42	7.30	7.15	7.35	7.30
Other Asian or Pacific Islander [1]	- - -	- - -	6.87	6.89	7.03	6.77	6.65	6.22	6.64	6.47	6.48	6.66	6.69
Hispanic origin (selected States) [2,3]	- - -	- - -	6.12	6.12	6.23	6.29	6.15	6.16	6.13	6.24	6.17	6.18	6.06
Mexican American	- - -	- - -	5.62	5.61	5.72	5.77	5.68	5.77	5.62	5.74	5.60	5.60	5.55
Puerto Rican	- - -	- - -	8.95	9.01	9.11	8.90	8.88	8.69	9.22	9.30	9.42	9.50	8.99
Cuban	- - -	- - -	5.62	5.83	5.76	5.65	5.86	6.02	5.46	5.89	5.94	5.77	5.67
Central and South American	- - -	- - -	5.76	5.73	5.61	6.20	5.81	5.68	5.69	5.74	5.58	5.81	5.84
Other and unknown Hispanic	- - -	- - -	6.96	7.00	7.30	7.23	6.89	6.83	6.87	6.91	6.85	6.74	6.87
Non-Hispanic white (selected States) [2]	- - -	- - -	5.67	5.63	5.62	5.64	5.53	5.60	5.58	5.63	5.62	5.62	5.61
Non-Hispanic black (selected States) [2]	- - -	- - -	12.71	12.79	12.60	12.83	12.54	12.61	12.85	13.10	13.28	13.61	13.32
Very low birth weight (less than 1,500 grams)													
All mothers	1.17	1.16	1.15	1.16	1.18	1.19	1.19	1.21	1.21	1.24	1.24	1.28	1.27
White	0.95	0.92	0.90	0.91	0.92	0.93	0.93	0.94	0.93	0.94	0.93	0.95	0.95
Black	2.40	2.40	2.48	2.52	2.56	2.60	2.60	2.71	2.73	2.79	2.86	2.95	2.92
American Indian or Alaskan Native	0.98	0.95	0.92	0.89	1.06	1.07	1.02	1.01	0.99	1.13	1.00	1.00	1.01
Asian or Pacific Islander	- - -	- - -	0.92	0.93	0.91	0.88	0.93	0.85	0.86	0.83	0.84	0.90	0.87
Chinese	0.80	0.52	0.66	0.68	0.70	0.77	0.70	0.57	0.63	0.65	0.57	0.61	0.51
Japanese	1.48	0.89	0.94	0.75	0.94	0.63	0.81	0.84	0.86	0.80	0.92	0.86	0.73
Filipino	1.08	0.93	0.99	1.03	0.89	0.98	0.97	0.86	0.87	0.94	0.91	1.12	1.05
Other Asian or Pacific Islander [1]	- - -	- - -	0.97	0.99	0.95	0.90	0.98	0.92	0.92	0.84	0.89	0.91	0.92
Hispanic origin (selected States) [2,3]	- - -	- - -	0.98	0.98	0.99	1.03	1.01	1.01	1.02	1.06	1.01	1.05	1.03
Mexican American	- - -	- - -	0.92	0.92	0.93	0.96	0.93	0.97	0.94	0.96	0.89	0.94	0.92
Puerto Rican	- - -	- - -	1.29	1.43	1.54	1.46	1.49	1.30	1.47	1.63	1.61	1.71	1.62
Cuban	- - -	- - -	1.02	1.17	0.90	0.97	1.04	1.18	1.09	0.97	1.17	1.13	1.20
Central and South American	- - -	- - -	0.99	0.93	0.83	0.99	1.04	1.01	1.04	1.02	0.97	1.05	1.05
Other and unknown Hispanic	- - -	- - -	1.01	0.93	1.03	1.08	1.05	0.96	1.08	1.15	1.11	1.04	1.09
Non-Hispanic white (selected States) [2]	- - -	- - -	0.86	0.87	0.89	0.90	0.88	0.90	0.89	0.91	0.89	0.93	0.93
Non-Hispanic black (selected States) [2]	- - -	- - -	2.46	2.50	2.53	2.57	2.56	2.66	2.68	2.73	2.82	2.97	2.93

[1] Includes Hawaiians and part Hawaiians.

[2] Trend data for Hispanics and non-Hispanics are affected by expansion of the reporting area for an Hispanic-origin item on the birth certificate and by immigration. These two factors affect numbers of events, composition of the Hispanic population, and maternal and infant health characteristics. The number of States in the reporting area increased from 22 in 1980, to 23 plus the District of Columbia (D.C.) in 1983, 30 plus D.C. in 1988, 47 plus D.C. in 1989, and 48 plus D.C. in 1990 (see Appendix I, National Vital Statistics System).

[3] Includes mothers of all races.

NOTES: The race groups, white and black, include persons of both Hispanic and non-Hispanic origin. Conversely, persons of Hispanic origin may be of any race.

SOURCE: Centers for Disease Control and Prevention, National Center for Health Statistics: Data computed by the Division of Analysis from data compiled by the Division of Vital Statistics.

Table 9 (page 1 of 2). Prenatal care and maternal education for live births, according to detailed race of mother and Hispanic origin of mother: United States, selected years 1970–90

[Data are based on the National Vital Statistics System]

Prenatal care, education, race of mother, and Hispanic origin of mother	1970	1975	1980	1981	1982	1983	1984	1985	1986	1987	1988	1989	1990
Prenatal care began during 1st trimester						Percent of live births							
All mothers	68.0	72.4	76.3	76.3	76.1	76.2	76.5	76.2	75.9	76.0	75.9	75.5	75.8
White	72.3	75.8	79.2	79.3	79.2	79.3	79.6	79.3	79.1	79.3	79.3	78.9	79.2
Black	44.2	55.5	62.4	62.1	61.1	61.2	61.9	61.5	61.2	60.8	60.7	60.0	60.6
American Indian or Alaskan Native	38.2	45.4	55.8	56.6	57.7	56.6	57.4	57.5	58.2	57.6	58.1	57.9	57.9
Asian or Pacific Islander	- - -	- - -	73.7	73.2	73.3	73.9	74.7	74.1	74.9	75.0	75.5	74.8	75.1
Chinese	71.8	76.7	82.6	82.6	81.9	80.4	81.5	82.0	82.2	81.5	82.3	81.5	81.3
Japanese	78.1	82.7	86.1	85.2	85.6	86.6	87.0	84.7	85.7	86.6	86.3	86.2	87.0
Filipino	60.6	70.6	77.3	77.5	76.8	77.4	77.8	76.5	78.2	77.9	78.4	77.6	77.1
Other Asian or Pacific Islander [1]	- - -	- - -	67.6	67.4	68.9	69.9	70.2	69.7	70.3	71.0	71.5	70.8	71.4
Hispanic origin (selected States) [2,3]	- - -	- - -	60.2	60.6	61.0	61.0	61.5	61.2	60.3	61.0	61.3	59.5	60.2
Mexican American	- - -	- - -	59.6	60.1	60.7	60.2	60.4	60.0	58.9	60.0	58.3	56.7	57.8
Puerto Rican	- - -	- - -	55.1	54.2	54.5	55.1	57.4	58.3	57.2	57.4	63.2	62.7	63.5
Cuban	- - -	- - -	82.7	80.1	79.3	81.2	82.2	82.5	81.8	83.1	83.4	83.2	84.8
Central and South American	- - -	- - -	58.8	58.3	58.5	59.3	61.1	60.6	58.8	59.1	62.8	60.8	61.5
Other and unknown Hispanic	- - -	- - -	66.4	66.9	66.0	66.6	66.7	65.8	66.6	65.5	67.3	66.0	66.4
Non-Hispanic white (selected States) [2]	- - -	- - -	81.2	81.3	81.1	81.3	81.6	81.4	81.5	81.7	81.8	82.7	83.3
Non-Hispanic black (selected States) [2]	- - -	- - -	60.7	60.7	59.7	59.9	60.6	60.1	60.1	60.0	60.4	59.9	60.7
Prenatal care began during 3d trimester or no prenatal care													
All mothers	7.9	6.0	5.1	5.2	5.5	5.6	5.6	5.7	6.0	6.1	6.1	6.4	6.1
White	6.3	5.0	4.3	4.3	4.5	4.6	4.7	4.8	5.0	5.0	5.0	5.2	4.9
Black	16.6	10.5	8.9	9.2	9.7	9.8	9.7	10.2	10.7	11.2	11.0	11.9	11.3
American Indian or Alaskan Native	28.9	22.4	15.2	14.7	14.0	14.4	13.8	12.9	12.9	13.1	13.2	13.4	12.9
Asian or Pacific Islander	- - -	- - -	6.5	6.6	6.6	6.5	6.4	6.5	6.2	6.3	5.9	6.1	5.8
Chinese	6.5	4.4	3.7	3.8	3.5	4.6	4.2	4.4	4.2	4.2	3.4	3.6	3.4
Japanese	4.1	2.7	2.1	2.5	2.5	2.4	2.6	3.1	3.1	2.8	3.3	2.7	2.9
Filipino	7.2	4.1	4.0	3.6	3.8	4.1	4.3	4.8	4.5	4.9	4.8	4.7	4.5
Other Asian or Pacific Islander [1]	- - -	- - -	9.0	9.0	8.5	8.2	8.1	8.1	7.8	7.8	7.3	7.6	7.2
Hispanic origin (selected States) [2,3]	- - -	- - -	12.0	11.6	12.1	12.5	12.6	12.4	13.0	12.7	12.1	13.0	12.0
Mexican American	- - -	- - -	11.8	11.6	12.0	12.7	13.0	12.9	13.4	13.0	13.9	14.6	13.2
Puerto Rican	- - -	- - -	16.2	15.8	17.2	17.4	16.3	15.5	17.4	17.1	10.2	11.3	10.6
Cuban	- - -	- - -	3.9	4.2	4.9	4.0	4.0	3.7	4.2	3.9	3.6	4.0	2.8
Central and South American	- - -	- - -	13.1	12.4	13.4	13.3	12.6	12.5	13.8	13.5	9.9	11.9	10.9
Other and unknown Hispanic	- - -	- - -	9.2	8.3	9.3	9.0	9.1	9.4	9.0	9.3	8.8	9.3	8.5
Non-Hispanic white (selected States) [2]	- - -	- - -	3.5	3.6	3.8	3.9	3.9	4.0	4.1	4.1	4.1	3.7	3.4
Non-Hispanic black (selected States) [2]	- - -	- - -	9.7	9.9	10.6	10.7	10.6	10.9	11.4	11.8	11.0	12.0	11.2
Education of mother less than 12 years													
All mothers	30.8	28.6	23.7	22.9	22.3	21.7	20.9	20.6	20.4	20.2	20.4	23.2	23.8
White	27.1	25.1	20.8	19.9	19.3	18.7	18.1	17.8	17.7	17.4	17.6	21.6	22.4
Black	51.2	45.3	36.4	35.7	35.1	34.5	33.4	32.6	31.9	31.6	31.4	30.4	30.2
American Indian or Alaskan Native	60.5	52.7	44.2	43.0	41.8	41.3	40.0	39.0	39.2	38.5	37.9	37.2	36.4
Asian or Pacific Islander	- - -	- - -	21.0	23.0	23.3	21.7	20.2	19.4	17.9	17.9	17.9	19.5	20.0
Chinese	23.0	16.5	15.2	16.1	17.3	18.2	18.2	15.5	12.3	13.5	14.2	14.9	15.8
Japanese	11.8	9.1	5.0	4.7	4.3	4.0	3.5	4.8	4.0	3.1	3.5	3.3	3.5
Filipino	26.4	22.3	16.4	16.0	15.6	15.0	13.4	13.9	12.6	12.3	11.8	10.2	10.3
Other Asian or Pacific Islander [1]	- - -	- - -	26.4	29.3	29.3	26.6	24.8	23.5	22.2	21.7	21.7	26.1	26.2
Hispanic origin (selected States) [2,3]	- - -	- - -	51.1	49.5	48.0	46.5	44.9	44.5	43.4	42.8	42.5	52.8	53.9
Mexican American	- - -	- - -	62.8	61.9	60.5	59.4	58.7	59.0	58.9	58.4	56.9	61.3	61.4
Puerto Rican	- - -	- - -	55.3	53.9	52.9	50.0	48.2	46.6	44.8	44.3	45.2	43.7	42.7
Cuban	- - -	- - -	24.1	26.9	27.0	24.6	22.4	21.1	19.7	18.7	18.1	17.9	17.8
Central and South American	- - -	- - -	41.2	39.3	39.2	39.5	37.1	37.0	35.9	34.1	31.8	43.6	44.2
Other and unknown Hispanic	- - -	- - -	40.1	39.5	38.7	38.9	36.0	36.5	33.7	34.3	34.1	34.5	33.3
Non-Hispanic white (selected States) [2]	- - -	- - -	18.3	17.4	17.3	16.7	15.9	15.8	15.7	15.3	16.7	15.3	15.2
Non-Hispanic black (selected States) [2]	- - -	- - -	37.4	36.6	36.4	35.4	34.2	33.5	32.6	32.2	31.8	29.9	30.0

See footnotes at end of table.

[Data are based on the National Vital Statistics System]

Prenatal care, education, race of mother, and Hispanic origin of mother	1970	1975	1980	1981	1982	1983	1984	1985	1986	1987	1988	1989	1990
Education of mother 16 years or more						Percent of live births							
All mothers.	8.6	11.4	14.0	14.8	15.3	15.8	16.4	16.7	17.1	17.6	17.7	17.4	17.5
White.	9.6	12.7	15.5	16.4	16.9	17.6	18.3	18.6	19.2	19.8	20.1	19.2	19.3
Black.	2.8	4.3	6.2	6.5	6.7	6.7	6.9	7.0	7.1	7.1	7.1	7.2	7.2
American Indian or Alaskan Native.	2.7	2.2	3.5	3.7	3.6	3.4	3.6	3.7	3.8	3.7	3.7	4.3	4.4
Asian or Pacific Islander	- - -	- - -	30.8	29.4	29.3	30.0	30.4	30.3	31.4	32.0	31.7	31.2	31.0
Chinese	34.0	37.8	41.5	40.8	38.2	38.0	36.4	35.2	36.8	36.8	36.4	40.5	40.3
Japanese.	20.7	30.6	36.8	35.2	38.4	38.8	39.8	38.1	41.3	41.8	42.3	43.6	44.1
Filipino.	28.1	36.6	37.1	36.8	36.6	35.8	35.8	35.2	35.4	36.9	35.5	36.0	34.5
Other Asian or Pacific Islander [1]	- - -	- - -	25.5	24.2	24.2	25.6	26.4	27.1	28.0	28.8	28.6	25.3	25.7
Hispanic origin (selected States) [2,3]	- - -	- - -	4.2	4.6	5.0	5.2	5.7	6.0	6.5	6.6	7.0	5.1	5.1
Mexican American.	- - -	- - -	2.2	2.4	2.8	2.8	2.9	3.0	3.3	3.2	3.7	3.2	3.3
Puerto Rican.	- - -	- - -	3.0	3.4	3.7	3.9	4.3	4.6	4.9	5.4	5.3	6.3	6.5
Cuban	- - -	- - -	11.6	10.7	11.2	12.4	13.7	15.0	15.4	17.3	18.2	19.2	20.4
Central and South American.	- - -	- - -	6.1	6.8	7.1	6.6	7.6	8.1	8.4	8.8	10.1	8.2	8.6
Other and unknown Hispanic	- - -	- - -	5.5	6.0	6.0	6.4	7.0	7.2	8.7	7.6	8.0	7.7	8.5
Non-Hispanic white (selected States) [2]	- - -	- - -	16.4	17.2	17.6	18.3	18.9	19.3	19.8	20.4	20.4	22.0	22.6
Non-Hispanic black (selected States) [2]	- - -	- - -	5.7	6.1	6.3	6.3	6.5	6.7	6.9	6.8	6.9	7.2	7.3

[1]Includes Hawaiians and part Hawaiians.

[2]Trend data for Hispanics and non-Hispanics are affected by expansion of the reporting area for an Hispanic-origin item on the birth certificate and by immigration. These two factors affect numbers of events, composition of the Hispanic population, and maternal and infant health characteristics. The number of States in the reporting area increased from 22 in 1980, to 23 plus the District of Columbia (D.C.) in 1983, 30 plus D.C. in 1988, 47 plus D.C. in 1989, and 48 plus D.C. in 1990 (see Appendix I, National Vital Statistics System).

[3]Includes mothers of all races.

NOTES: Excludes births that occurred in States not reporting education and/or prenatal care (see Appendix I). The race groups, white and black, include persons of both Hispanic and non-Hispanic origin. Conversely, persons of Hispanic origin may be of any race.

SOURCE: Centers for Disease Control and Prevention, National Center for Health Statistics: Data computed by the Division of Analysis from data compiled by the Division of Vital Statistics.

Table 10. Maternal age and marital status for live births, according to detailed race of mother and Hispanic origin of mother: United States, selected years 1970–90

[Data are based on the National Vital Statistics System]

Age, marital status, race of mother, and Hispanic origin of mother	1970	1975	1980	1981	1982	1983	1984	1985	1986	1987	1988	1989	1990
Age of mother less than 18 years						Percent of live births							
All mothers	6.3	7.6	5.8	5.4	5.2	5.0	4.8	4.7	4.8	4.8	4.8	4.8	4.7
White	4.8	6.0	4.5	4.3	4.1	3.9	3.7	3.7	3.7	3.7	3.7	3.6	3.6
Black	14.8	16.3	12.5	11.7	11.4	11.2	10.8	10.6	10.6	10.7	10.6	10.5	10.1
American Indian or Alaskan Native	7.5	11.2	9.4	9.1	8.5	8.7	7.9	7.6	8.0	7.9	7.8	7.5	7.2
Asian or Pacific Islander	- - -	- - -	1.5	1.6	1.7	1.6	1.6	1.6	1.7	1.8	1.8	2.0	2.1
Chinese	1.1	0.4	0.3	0.2	0.3	0.3	0.2	0.3	0.2	0.2	0.3	0.3	0.4
Japanese	2.0	1.7	1.0	1.0	1.3	0.7	0.8	0.9	0.9	0.9	0.8	0.9	0.8
Filipino	3.7	2.4	1.6	1.6	1.6	1.8	2.0	1.6	1.7	1.8	1.7	1.9	2.0
Other Asian or Pacific Islander [1]	- - -	- - -	1.8	2.0	2.0	1.9	2.0	2.1	2.2	2.3	2.4	2.6	2.7
Hispanic origin (selected States) [2,3]	- - -	- - -	7.4	7.3	7.2	7.0	6.7	6.4	6.5	6.6	6.6	6.7	6.6
Mexican American	- - -	- - -	7.7	7.7	7.5	7.5	7.2	6.9	6.9	7.0	7.0	6.9	6.9
Puerto Rican	- - -	- - -	10.0	9.8	9.9	9.3	8.5	8.5	8.4	8.7	9.2	9.4	9.1
Cuban	- - -	- - -	3.8	3.6	3.2	2.6	2.5	2.2	2.3	2.1	2.2	2.7	2.7
Central and South American	- - -	- - -	2.4	2.4	2.6	2.6	2.4	2.4	2.4	2.7	2.7	3.0	3.2
Other and unknown Hispanic	- - -	- - -	6.5	6.5	6.9	7.1	7.0	7.0	7.3	7.7	7.6	8.0	8.0
Non-Hispanic white (selected States) [2]	- - -	- - -	4.0	3.8	3.6	3.4	3.2	3.2	3.2	3.2	3.2	3.0	3.0
Non-Hispanic black (selected States) [2]	- - -	- - -	12.7	11.9	11.6	11.2	10.9	10.7	10.6	10.7	10.8	10.5	10.2
Age of mother 18–19 years													
All mothers	11.3	11.3	9.8	9.4	9.0	8.7	8.3	8.0	7.8	7.6	7.7	8.1	8.1
White	10.4	10.3	9.0	8.6	8.2	7.9	7.4	7.1	7.0	6.8	6.9	7.2	7.3
Black	16.6	16.9	14.5	14.1	13.7	13.6	13.3	12.9	12.6	12.2	12.3	12.9	13.0
American Indian or Alaskan Native	12.8	15.2	14.6	13.9	13.8	13.3	13.1	12.4	12.1	11.8	11.4	12.1	12.3
Asian or Pacific Islander	- - -	- - -	3.9	4.1	4.1	3.7	3.4	3.4	3.4	3.3	3.4	3.7	3.7
Chinese	3.9	1.7	1.0	1.0	0.8	0.6	0.5	0.6	0.5	0.6	0.5	0.7	0.8
Japanese	4.1	3.3	2.3	2.6	2.5	2.3	2.3	1.9	1.9	1.6	1.8	1.8	2.0
Filipino	7.1	5.0	4.0	3.9	4.3	3.8	3.5	3.7	3.4	3.4	3.8	4.0	4.1
Other Asian or Pacific Islander [1]	- - -	- - -	4.9	5.2	4.9	4.5	4.3	4.2	4.3	4.1	4.3	4.6	4.5
Hispanic origin (selected States) [2,3]	- - -	- - -	11.6	11.2	11.1	10.6	10.3	10.1	9.9	9.7	9.8	10.0	10.2
Mexican American	- - -	- - -	12.0	11.7	11.5	10.9	10.8	10.6	10.5	10.3	10.3	10.5	10.7
Puerto Rican	- - -	- - -	13.3	13.3	13.1	13.2	12.8	12.4	12.5	11.8	12.2	12.6	12.6
Cuban	- - -	- - -	9.2	9.2	8.2	6.8	5.7	4.9	4.5	4.1	3.9	4.3	5.0
Central and South American	- - -	- - -	6.0	5.8	6.4	6.0	5.7	5.8	5.7	5.3	5.4	5.6	5.9
Other and unknown Hispanic	- - -	- - -	10.8	10.4	11.3	11.2	10.9	10.5	10.0	10.5	10.8	11.2	11.1
Non-Hispanic white (selected States) [2]	- - -	- - -	8.5	8.1	7.8	7.4	6.8	6.6	6.4	6.2	6.6	6.5	6.6
Non-Hispanic black (selected States) [2]	- - -	- - -	14.7	14.1	13.9	13.5	13.4	12.9	12.6	12.2	12.4	13.0	13.0
Unmarried mothers													
All mothers	10.7	14.3	18.4	18.9	19.4	20.3	21.0	22.0	23.4	24.5	25.7	27.1	28.0
White	5.5	7.1	11.2	11.8	12.3	12.9	13.6	14.7	15.9	16.9	18.0	19.2	20.4
Black	37.5	49.5	56.1	56.9	57.7	59.2	60.3	61.2	62.4	63.4	64.7	65.7	66.5
American Indian or Alaskan Native	22.4	32.7	39.2	41.2	42.6	45.3	46.1	46.8	48.8	51.1	51.7	52.7	53.6
Asian or Pacific Islander	- - -	- - -	7.3	7.0	7.9	8.6	9.2	9.5	10.0	11.0	11.5	12.4	13.2
Chinese	3.0	1.6	2.7	2.4	2.5	3.3	3.4	3.0	3.5	4.5	3.9	4.2	5.0
Japanese	4.6	4.6	5.2	6.2	7.1	7.2	6.9	7.9	7.9	7.9	8.8	9.4	9.6
Filipino	9.1	6.9	8.6	9.1	9.9	10.3	10.8	11.4	12.0	12.7	13.6	14.8	15.9
Other Asian or Pacific Islander [1]	- - -	- - -	8.5	7.7	8.7	9.5	10.4	10.9	11.4	12.4	13.2	14.2	14.9
Hispanic origin (selected States) [2,3]	- - -	- - -	23.6	24.5	25.6	27.5	28.3	29.5	31.6	32.6	34.0	35.5	36.7
Mexican American	- - -	- - -	20.3	20.7	21.9	23.7	24.2	25.7	27.9	28.9	30.6	31.7	33.3
Puerto Rican	- - -	- - -	46.3	48.0	49.0	49.5	50.8	51.1	52.6	53.0	53.3	55.2	55.9
Cuban	- - -	- - -	10.0	14.3	15.9	16.1	16.2	16.1	15.8	16.1	16.3	17.5	18.2
Central and South American	- - -	- - -	27.1	29.0	30.2	33.0	34.0	34.9	38.0	37.1	36.4	38.9	41.2
Other and unknown Hispanic	- - -	- - -	22.4	25.0	26.3	28.2	30.0	31.1	31.9	34.2	35.5	37.0	37.2
Non-Hispanic white (selected States) [2]	- - -	- - -	9.6	10.0	10.5	11.0	11.5	12.4	13.5	14.3	15.2	16.1	16.9
Non-Hispanic black (selected States) [2]	- - -	- - -	57.3	58.0	59.0	60.5	61.5	62.1	63.3	64.2	64.8	66.0	66.7

[1]Includes Hawaiians and part Hawaiians.

[2]Trend data for Hispanics and non-Hispanics are affected by expansion of the reporting area for an Hispanic-origin item on the birth certificate and by immigration. These two factors affect numbers of events, composition of the Hispanic population, and maternal and infant health characteristics. The number of States in the reporting area increased from 22 in 1980, to 23 plus the District of Columbia (DC) in 1983, 30 plus DC in 1988, 47 plus DC in 1989, and 48 plus DC in 1990 (see Appendix I, National Vital Statistics System).

[3]Includes mothers of all races.

NOTES: Data for 1970 and 1975 exclude births that occurred in States not reporting marital status (see Appendix I). The race groups, white and black, include persons of both Hispanic and non-Hispanic origin. Conversely, persons of Hispanic origin may be of any race.

SOURCE: Centers for Disease Control and Prevention, National Center for Health Statistics: Data computed by the Division of Analysis from data compiled by the Division of Vital Statistics.

Table 11. Low-birth-weight live births, according to race of mother, geographic division, and State: United States, average annual 1978–80, 1983–85, and 1988–90

[Data are based on the National Vital Statistics System]

Geographic division and State	All races			White			Black		
	1978–80	1983–85	1988–90	1978–80	1983–85	1988–90	1978–80	1983–85	1988–90
	Percent of live births weighing less than 2,500 grams								
United States	6.95	6.76	6.98	5.82	5.65	5.69	12.79	12.68	13.34
New England	6.28	5.95	5.95	5.87	5.50	5.37	12.31	12.27	12.06
Maine	5.67	5.39	4.96	5.67	5.35	4.95	*	*	*
New Hampshire	5.63	5.01	4.96	5.62	4.99	4.93	*	*	*
Vermont	6.10	5.98	5.25	6.08	5.98	5.22	*	*	*
Massachusetts.	6.20	5.85	5.92	5.82	5.45	5.34	11.65	11.38	11.06
Rhode Island	6.43	6.26	6.16	6.00	5.83	5.70	*12.56	*11.62	*10.45
Connecticut	6.88	6.56	6.75	6.06	5.65	5.71	13.06	13.35	13.80
Middle Atlantic	7.24	6.92	7.37	5.98	5.68	5.79	13.16	12.61	13.99
New York	7.55	7.07	7.68	6.23	5.76	5.99	12.86	12.04	13.78
New Jersey	7.33	7.00	7.11	5.80	5.64	5.52	13.41	12.75	13.53
Pennsylvania	6.72	6.64	7.04	5.75	5.58	5.65	13.65	13.99	14.96
East North Central.	6.81	6.64	7.08	5.63	5.43	5.60	13.43	13.46	14.15
Ohio	6.82	6.59	7.00	5.83	5.64	5.83	13.21	12.62	13.48
Indiana	6.41	6.35	6.58	5.71	5.70	5.84	12.36	12.01	12.63
Illinois	7.35	7.16	7.58	5.58	5.37	5.56	13.86	13.93	14.45
Michigan	7.02	6.93	7.49	5.78	5.52	5.67	13.42	14.19	14.84
Wisconsin	5.46	5.28	5.69	4.97	4.69	4.81	12.96	12.88	13.89
West North Central	5.78	5.65	5.85	5.26	5.11	5.20	13.00	12.74	13.00
Minnesota	5.18	4.94	4.98	5.00	4.73	4.57	*12.73	*12.02	13.45
Iowa	5.08	5.01	5.42	4.90	4.86	5.21	*12.97	*11.66	*12.16
Missouri	6.75	6.70	6.96	5.65	5.56	5.72	13.11	13.09	13.16
North Dakota	5.14	4.80	5.09	4.95	4.66	4.98	*	*	*
South Dakota	5.12	5.23	5.03	4.95	4.92	4.92	*	*	*
Nebraska.	5.67	5.37	5.53	5.30	5.00	5.08	*13.39	*12.09	*12.91
Kansas	6.16	6.09	6.17	5.63	5.53	5.57	12.52	12.57	12.61
South Atlantic	8.03	7.78	7.99	6.12	5.93	5.92	12.61	12.51	13.05
Delaware.	7.53	7.30	7.49	5.57	5.71	5.75	14.01	12.63	13.21
Maryland	7.89	7.60	7.97	5.94	5.50	5.68	12.58	12.57	13.07
District of Columbia	12.85	12.95	15.13	*6.42	5.90	6.33	14.15	14.72	17.67
Virginia	7.40	7.12	7.13	5.90	5.63	5.49	12.11	12.01	12.26
West Virginia	6.77	6.83	6.70	6.53	6.61	6.47	*12.85	*12.40	*12.70
North Carolina	8.05	7.86	8.04	6.21	6.01	6.01	12.33	12.51	12.80
South Carolina.	8.78	8.67	8.96	6.05	6.09	6.32	12.86	12.80	13.15
Georgia	8.62	8.25	8.46	6.28	6.05	6.02	12.74	12.42	12.85
Florida.	7.71	7.47	7.59	6.12	5.97	5.96	12.34	12.20	12.82
East South Central	7.89	7.87	8.07	6.22	6.24	6.33	12.31	12.30	12.61
Kentucky.	6.95	6.95	6.89	6.38	6.42	6.35	12.66	12.38	12.00
Tennessee.	8.01	7.94	8.10	6.51	6.46	6.47	13.21	13.16	13.39
Alabama	8.07	7.97	8.24	5.87	5.90	6.11	12.09	11.95	12.29
Mississippi.	8.69	8.77	9.23	5.84	5.96	6.37	11.82	12.02	12.43
West South Central	7.37	7.17	7.32	6.10	5.96	6.02	12.74	12.79	13.05
Arkansas.	7.52	7.78	8.23	5.91	6.23	6.63	12.31	12.70	13.39
Louisiana.	8.68	8.61	9.04	6.13	5.78	6.01	12.75	13.24	13.42
Oklahoma	6.78	6.48	6.53	6.19	5.94	5.99	12.63	12.14	11.80
Texas	7.07	6.84	6.93	6.10	5.97	5.96	12.87	12.53	12.86
Mountain	6.69	6.58	6.70	6.50	6.40	6.46	13.53	13.02	13.95
Montana	5.71	5.70	5.90	5.68	5.60	5.85	*	*	*
Idaho	5.39	5.40	5.45	5.36	5.34	5.39	*	*	*
Wyoming.	7.48	7.06	7.23	7.42	7.05	7.17	*	*	*
Colorado.	8.22	7.77	7.87	7.89	7.46	7.45	15.24	13.99	14.60
New Mexico.	8.18	7.41	7.19	8.13	7.54	7.26	*14.14	*12.62	*12.08
Arizona	6.10	6.14	6.31	5.89	5.92	6.09	*12.11	12.98	13.01
Utah	5.41	5.61	5.69	5.38	5.52	5.64	*	*	*
Nevada	7.05	6.85	7.32	6.43	6.27	6.49	*12.75	*11.59	15.02
Pacific	5.89	5.82	5.87	5.27	5.18	5.16	11.89	12.15	13.10
Washington	5.26	5.20	5.38	5.02	4.89	5.01	11.38	11.34	12.19
Oregon	5.07	5.10	5.15	4.90	4.94	4.94	*11.85	*11.82	*11.91
California.	6.04	5.96	5.97	5.36	5.26	5.20	11.98	12.26	13.25
Alaska.	5.48	4.80	4.91	4.98	4.41	4.37	*7.39	*7.84	*9.91
Hawaii.	7.05	6.92	7.03	5.82	5.74	5.68	*9.93	*10.94	*10.83

*Data for States with fewer than 5,000 live births for the 3-year period are considered unreliable. Data for States with fewer than 1,000 live births are considered highly unreliable and are not shown.

SOURCE: Centers for Disease Control and Prevention, National Center for Health Statistics: Data computed by the Division of Analysis from data compiled by the Division of Vital Statistics.

Table 12. Very low-birth-weight live births, according to race of mother, geographic division, and State: United States, average annual 1978–80, 1983–85, and 1988–90

[Data are based on the National Vital Statistics System]

Geographic division and State	All races			White			Black		
	1978–80	1983–85	1988–90	1978–80	1983–85	1988–90	1978–80	1983–85	1988–90
	Percent of live births weighing less than 1,500 grams								
United States	1.15	1.20	1.27	0.91	0.93	0.95	2.45	2.64	2.91
New England	1.10	1.05	1.10	0.99	0.94	0.95	2.73	2.78	2.83
Maine	1.32	0.97	0.82	1.32	0.96	0.82	*	*	*
New Hampshire	0.93	0.85	0.89	0.93	0.85	0.89	*	*	*
Vermont	0.99	0.91	0.73	0.98	0.92	0.72	*	*	*
Massachusetts	1.01	1.01	1.09	0.90	0.91	0.96	2.47	2.36	2.51
Rhode Island	1.23	1.08	1.12	1.09	0.98	1.02	*3.09	*2.51	*2.33
Connecticut	1.21	1.26	1.34	0.99	1.00	1.05	2.91	3.28	3.38
Middle Atlantic	1.21	1.25	1.41	0.94	0.95	1.00	2.52	2.64	3.18
New York	1.28	1.27	1.44	0.98	0.95	1.00	2.48	2.51	3.09
New Jersey	1.24	1.26	1.38	0.92	0.95	1.00	2.54	2.58	3.06
Pennsylvania	1.11	1.22	1.36	0.90	0.95	0.99	2.57	3.04	3.51
East North Central	1.18	1.22	1.32	0.92	0.93	0.96	2.66	2.84	3.09
Ohio	1.16	1.20	1.27	0.94	0.97	0.99	2.57	2.68	2.88
Indiana	1.06	1.09	1.18	0.89	0.92	0.99	2.54	2.51	2.70
Illinois	1.33	1.33	1.43	0.94	0.94	0.96	2.80	2.87	3.05
Michigan	1.21	1.30	1.47	0.94	0.96	0.96	2.63	3.08	3.50
Wisconsin	0.95	0.97	1.03	0.86	0.84	0.82	2.37	2.74	2.91
West North Central	0.95	0.97	1.01	0.85	0.85	0.86	2.51	2.60	2.69
Minnesota	0.89	0.88	0.87	0.86	0.84	0.80	*2.59	*2.47	2.78
Iowa	0.88	0.83	0.89	0.84	0.80	0.84	*2.90	*2.13	*2.63
Missouri	1.10	1.17	1.21	0.87	0.90	0.92	2.46	2.73	2.71
North Dakota	0.91	0.79	0.84	0.87	0.74	0.85	*	*	*
South Dakota	0.71	0.93	0.86	0.70	0.89	0.82	*	*	*
Nebraska	0.90	0.89	0.95	0.82	0.80	0.85	*2.61	*2.60	*2.53
Kansas	0.97	1.02	1.07	0.85	0.92	0.93	2.47	2.33	2.69
South Atlantic	1.42	1.49	1.57	0.98	1.01	1.02	2.49	2.71	2.94
Delaware	1.36	1.48	1.59	0.84	1.08	1.07	3.08	2.85	3.31
Maryland	1.52	1.57	1.71	1.03	1.01	1.04	2.71	2.94	3.21
District of Columbia	2.74	3.25	3.80	*0.79	1.33	1.38	3.13	3.74	4.47
Virginia	1.29	1.32	1.38	0.97	0.93	0.94	2.30	2.58	2.78
West Virginia	1.06	1.12	1.16	1.02	1.06	1.10	*2.12	*2.82	*2.77
North Carolina	1.47	1.48	1.62	1.00	1.01	1.07	2.56	2.68	2.93
South Carolina	1.52	1.68	1.72	0.91	1.08	1.10	2.44	2.65	2.70
Georgia	1.51	1.62	1.64	0.98	1.04	1.01	2.44	2.70	2.79
Florida	1.30	1.36	1.42	0.96	1.00	1.00	2.33	2.49	2.81
East South Central	1.25	1.38	1.48	0.91	1.01	1.04	2.15	2.37	2.62
Kentucky	1.04	1.21	1.18	0.91	1.06	1.03	2.26	2.71	2.60
Tennessee	1.28	1.40	1.50	0.98	1.04	1.07	2.32	2.64	2.87
Alabama	1.32	1.40	1.59	0.87	0.95	1.07	2.14	2.26	2.59
Mississippi	1.38	1.54	1.64	0.81	0.95	0.94	2.00	2.20	2.43
West South Central	1.15	1.20	1.25	0.87	0.93	0.94	2.32	2.49	2.65
Arkansas	1.15	1.38	1.32	0.81	1.05	0.95	2.19	2.44	2.55
Louisiana	1.41	1.53	1.68	0.90	0.91	0.96	2.24	2.56	2.73
Oklahoma	1.01	1.06	1.04	0.90	0.92	0.94	2.17	2.44	2.12
Texas	1.09	1.12	1.17	0.86	0.92	0.93	2.44	2.45	2.67
Mountain	0.90	0.94	0.98	0.86	0.89	0.92	2.57	2.56	2.64
Montana	0.83	0.77	0.87	0.82	0.71	0.86	*	*	*
Idaho	0.72	0.80	0.87	0.72	0.78	0.87	*	*	*
Wyoming	0.91	1.01	0.91	0.88	0.99	0.93	*	*	*
Colorado	1.04	1.00	1.01	0.96	0.93	0.93	2.81	2.60	2.43
New Mexico	1.02	1.01	0.97	1.00	1.00	0.96	*3.17	*2.68	*2.11
Arizona	0.91	1.03	1.04	0.87	0.97	0.99	*2.12	2.73	3.01
Utah	0.73	0.77	0.80	0.74	0.75	0.79	*	*	*
Nevada	1.07	0.96	1.17	0.92	0.85	0.98	*2.59	*2.22	2.88
Pacific	0.97	1.01	1.00	0.85	0.88	0.85	2.29	2.61	2.79
Washington	0.82	0.91	0.87	0.77	0.85	0.79	1.81	2.35	2.71
Oregon	0.80	0.86	0.82	0.77	0.85	0.80	*1.69	*2.01	*1.81
California	1.02	1.05	1.03	0.88	0.90	0.87	2.35	2.65	2.81
Alaska	0.84	0.81	0.97	0.77	0.74	0.78	*1.38	*2.06	*2.90
Hawaii	0.91	1.02	1.01	0.73	0.92	0.93	*1.39	*2.13	*2.73

*Data for States with fewer than 5,000 live births for the 3-year period are considered unreliable. Data for States with fewer than 1,000 live births are considered highly unreliable and are not shown.

SOURCE: Centers for Disease Control and Prevention, National Center for Health Statistics: Data computed by the Division of Analysis from data compiled by the Division of Vital Statistics.

Table 13. Legal abortion ratios, according to selected patient characteristics: United States, selected years 1973–90

[Data are based on reporting by State health departments and by facilities]

Characteristic	1973	1975	1980	1981	1982	1983	1984	1985	1986	1987	1988	1989	1990[1]
	Abortions per 100 live births												
Total	19.6	27.2	35.9	35.8	35.4	34.9	36.4	35.4	35.4	35.6	35.2	34.6	34.4
Age													
Under 15 years	74.3	101.5	122.7	126.4	120.0	133.6	145.8	141.2	130.5	131.3	90.5	83.5	81.5
15–19 years.	31.7	46.4	66.4	66.8	66.5	67.3	71.4	71.7	70.2	72.6	61.2	54.8	50.7
20–24 years.	17.9	25.0	37.5	37.9	38.0	38.1	41.2	40.4	41.0	42.0	36.9	36.1	37.5
25–29 years.	12.3	16.6	23.0	23.2	23.5	23.0	23.9	23.2	24.0	23.9	21.1	20.9	21.6
30–34 years.	16.5	22.1	23.3	23.7	23.0	22.0	22.3	21.4	21.5	21.4	18.6	18.4	18.9
35–39 years.	26.7	37.5	40.3	40.3	37.1	35.4	35.2	33.4	33.4	31.7	27.7	26.8	27.1
40 years and over	40.2	59.9	78.3	77.6	75.0	69.1	66.7	63.8	59.8	56.2	51.3	49.4	50.1
Race													
White	17.5	22.7	31.3	31.2	30.4	29.5	30.8	29.6	30.0	30.0	25.7	24.8	25.3
All other.	28.9	46.5	54.7	54.4	55.6	56.0	58.2	57.6	55.8	55.7	45.5	46.1	47.5
Marital status													
Married	6.2	8.3	10.2	9.8	9.7	9.3	9.6	8.7	9.3	9.8	8.1	7.8	8.1
Unmarried	109.8	141.1	149.9	147.5	142.2	135.2	137.1	129.5	120.6	114.9	97.1	88.4	90.2
Number of previous live births [2]													
0.	23.0	30.2	48.6	48.6	48.2	46.9	49.3	47.7	47.1	46.3	37.4	37.2	35.9
1.	12.1	17.3	21.9	21.9	22.0	22.1	23.0	22.8	23.8	24.7	21.0	21.2	22.5
2.	19.6	29.7	32.8	32.6	32.4	32.5	34.0	33.0	33.5	34.5	29.3	28.6	31.2
3.	25.8	39.8	33.5	33.5	32.2	31.9	32.8	32.1	32.4	33.2	27.7	27.8	29.8
4 or more	26.4	40.8	27.3	26.6	25.4	24.8	24.9	23.7	24.2	24.2	20.2	19.9	26.3

[1]Preliminary data.

[2]For 1973–75, data indicate number of living children.

NOTE: Ratios exclude cases for which selected characteristic was unknown and are based on abortions reported to the Centers for Disease Control and Prevention.

SOURCES: Centers for Disease Control and Prevention: Abortion Surveillance, 1973–75. Public Health Service, DHHS, Atlanta, Ga., May 1977–Nov. 1980; Abortion Surveillance, 1980. Public Health Service, DHHS, Atlanta, Ga., May 1983; CDC Surveillance Summaries. Abortion Surveillance, United States: 1984–85, Vol. 38, No. SS-2, Sept. 1989; 1986 and 1987, Vol. 39, No. SS-2, June 1990; 1988, Vol. 40, No. SS-2, July 1991; 1989, Vol. 41, No. SS-5, Sept. 1992. Public Health Service, DHHS, Atlanta, Ga.; and Abortion Surveillance: Preliminary Analysis, United States, 1990, Vol. 41, No. 50. Public Health Service, DHHS, Atlanta, Ga., Dec. 1992.

Table 14. Legal abortions, according to selected characteristics: United States, selected years 1973–90

[Data are based on reporting by State health departments and by facilities]

Characteristic	1973	1975	1980	1981	1982	1983	1984	1985	1986	1987	1988	1989	1990[1]
	Number of legal abortions reported in thousands												
Centers for Disease Control and Prevention	616	855	1,298	1,301	1,304	1,269	1,334	1,329	1,328	1,354	1,371	1,397	1,430
Alan Guttmacher Institute [2]	745	1,034	1,554	1,577	1,574	1,575	1,577	1,589	1,574	1,559	1,591	- - -	- - -
	Percent distribution												
Total	100.0	100.0	100.0	100.0	100.0	100.0	100.0	100.0	100.0	100.0	100.0	100.0	100.0
Period of gestation													
Under 9 weeks.	36.1	44.6	51.7	51.2	50.6	49.7	50.5	50.3	51.0	50.4	48.7	49.8	51.6
9–10 weeks	29.4	28.4	26.2	26.8	26.7	26.8	26.4	26.6	25.8	26.0	26.4	25.8	25.3
11–12 weeks	17.9	14.9	12.2	12.1	12.4	12.8	12.6	12.5	12.2	12.4	12.7	12.6	11.7
13–15 weeks	6.9	5.0	5.2	5.2	5.3	5.8	5.8	5.9	6.1	6.2	6.6	6.6	6.4
16–20 weeks	8.0	6.1	3.9	3.7	3.9	3.9	3.9	3.9	4.1	4.2	4.5	4.2	4.0
21 weeks and over.	1.7	1.0	0.9	1.0	1.1	1.0	0.8	0.8	0.8	0.8	1.1	1.0	1.0
Type of procedure													
Curettage	88.4	90.9	95.5	96.1	96.4	96.8	96.8	97.5	97.0	97.2	98.6	98.8	98.8
Intrauterine instillation.	10.4	6.2	3.1	2.8	2.5	2.1	1.9	1.7	1.4	1.3	1.1	0.9	0.8
Hysterotomy or hysterectomy	0.7	0.4	0.1	0.1	0.0	0.0	0.0	0.0	0.0	0.0	0.0	0.0	0.0
Other	0.6	2.4	1.3	1.0	1.0	1.1	1.3	0.8	1.6	1.5	0.3	0.3	0.4
Location of facility													
In State of residence	74.8	89.2	92.6	92.5	92.9	93.3	92.0	92.4	92.3	91.7	91.4	91.0	91.8
Out of State of residence	25.2	10.8	7.4	7.5	7.1	6.7	8.0	7.6	7.7	8.3	8.6	9.0	8.2
Previous induced abortions													
0.	- - -	81.9	67.6	65.3	63.7	62.4	60.5	60.1	59.3	58.5	57.8	58.1	57.2
1.	- - -	14.9	23.5	24.3	24.9	25.0	25.7	25.7	26.3	26.5	26.9	26.5	26.8
2.	- - -	2.5	6.6	7.5	8.2	9.0	9.4	9.8	9.6	10.3	10.4	9.9	10.1
3 or more	- - -	0.7	2.3	2.9	3.2	3.7	4.3	4.4	4.8	4.7	4.9	5.5	5.9

[1]Preliminary data.

[2]No survey was conducted in 1986 and 1989; data for 1986 are projected.

NOTE: For a discussion of the differences in reported legal abortions between the Centers for Disease Control and Prevention and the Alan Guttmacher Institute, see Appendix I. Percent distributions exclude cases for which selected characteristic was unknown and are based on abortions reported to the Centers for Disease Control and Prevention.

SOURCES: Centers for Disease Control and Prevention: Abortion Surveillance, 1980. Public Health Service, DHHS, Atlanta, Ga., May 1983; CDC Surveillance Summaries. Abortion Surveillance, United States: 1984–1985, Vol. 38, No. SS-2, Sept. 1989; 1986 and 1987, Vol. 39, No. SS-2, June 1990; 1988, Vol. 40, No. SS-2, July 1991; 1989, Vol. 41, No. SS-5, Sept. 1992. Public Health Service, DHHS, Atlanta, Ga.; and Abortion Surveillance: Preliminary Analysis, United States, 1990, Vol. 41, No. 50. Public Health Service. DHHS, Atlanta, Ga., Dec. 1992; Sullivan, E., Tietze, C., and Dryfoos, J.: Legal abortions in the United States, 1975–1976. Fam. Plann. Perspect. 9(3):116–129, May–June 1977; Henshaw, S. K., Forrest, J. D., and Blaine, E.: Abortion services in the United States, 1981 and 1982. Fam. Plann. Perspect. 16(3), May–June 1984; Henshaw, S. K., Forrest, J. D., and Van Vort, J.: Abortion services in the United States, 1984 and 1985. Fam. Plann. Perspect. 19(2), Mar.–Apr. 1987; and Henshaw, S. K. and Van Vort, J.: Abortion services in the United States, 1987 and 1988. Fam. Plann. Perspect. 22(3), May–June 1990.

Table 15. Legal abortions, abortion-related deaths, and abortion-related death rates, according to period of gestation: United States, 1973–75, 1976–78, 1979–81, 1982–84, and 1985–87

[Data are based primarily on reporting by State health departments and by facilities]

Period of gestation and year	Number of legal abortions reported	Abortion-related deaths	
		Number	Rate per 100,000 abortions
Total			
1973–75.	2,234,160	80	3.6
1976–78.	3,225,473	37	1.1
1979–81.	3,850,287	[1]39	1.0
1982–84.	3,906,488	[2]34	0.9
1985–87.	4,010,353	[3]26	0.6
Under 9 weeks			
1973–75.	928,731	7	*0.8
1976–78.	1,620,841	6	*0.4
1979–81.	1,989,506	11	*0.6
1982–84.	1,947,672	4	*0.2
1985–87.	1,987,428	3	*
9–10 weeks			
1973–75.	642,922	14	2.2
1976–78.	882,051	7	*0.8
1979–81.	1,025,656	7	*0.7
1982–84.	1,049,486	6	*0.6
1985–87.	1,067,104	1	*
11–12 weeks			
1973–75.	355,304	12	3.4
1976–78.	425,744	2	*
1979–81.	471,921	6	*1.3
1982–84.	497,367	4	*0.8
1985–87.	507,712	3	*
13 weeks and over			
1973–75.	307,203	47	15.3
1976–78.	296,837	22	7.4
1979–81.	363,204	13	3.6
1982–84.	411,963	16	3.9
1985–87.	448,109	13	2.9

[1]1979–81 data includes 2 deaths with weeks of gestation unknown.
[2]1982–84 data includes 4 deaths with weeks of gestation unknown.
[3]1985–87 data includes 6 deaths with weeks of gestation unknown.

*Estimates with relative standard errors greater than 30 percent are considered unreliable. Estimates with relative standard errors greater than 50 percent are considered highly unreliable and are not shown.

SOURCE: Centers for Disease Control and Prevention: Surveillance Summaries, Abortion Surveillance, United States, 1990. Vol. 41, No. SS-4. Public Health Service, DHHS, Atlanta, Ga., Oct. 1992.

Table 16. Methods of contraception for ever-married women 15–44 years of age, according to race and age: United States, 1973, 1982, and 1988

[Data are based on household interviews of samples of women in the childbearing ages]

Method of contraception and age	All races 1973	All races 1982[1]	All races 1988	White 1973	White 1982[1]	White 1988	Black 1973	Black 1982[1]	Black 1988
	Number of ever-married women in thousands								
15–44 years	30,247	34,935	36,842	26,795	30,419	31,465	3,109	3,440	3,614
15–24 years	6,593	5,550	3,971	5,855	4,975	3,495	692	427	343
25–34 years	12,731	15,996	16,889	11,356	31,819	14,371	1,226	1,628	1,666
35–44 years	10,922	13,439	15,982	9,584	11,626	13,599	1,191	1,358	1,606
All methods	Percent of ever-married women using contraception								
15–44 years	66.4	66.9	70.8	67.8	68.0	71.8	55.8	60.4	63.9
15–24 years	66.9	65.4	69.6	67.1	66.8	68.8	65.2	53.3	69.0
25–34 years	70.4	70.0	70.6	71.6	70.7	71.3	59.2	67.7	66.1
35–44 years	61.5	63.9	71.4	63.6	65.3	73.1	46.8	54.0	60.5
Female sterilization	Percent of ever-married contracepting women								
15–44 years	13.6	28.9	34.7	12.5	27.2	32.9	25.4	42.8	54.5
15–24 years	4.3	*6.1	8.4	4.1	*5.7	8.2	6.8	*13.0	*11.0
25–34 years	12.1	24.5	27.6	11.4	22.7	26.2	20.3	37.7	46.9
35–44 years	21.7	44.0	48.5	19.2	42.4	45.9	47.2	59.5	73.6
Male sterilization[2]									
15–44 years	10.4	13.6	15.0	11.2	14.7	16.8	*1.2	*2.2	1.3
15–24 years	2.1	*4.1	*2.8	2.3	*4.4	*3.2	*0.1	*0.5	*–
25–34 years	10.3	11.5	11.8	11.0	12.6	13.1	*2.0	*1.7	*1.6
35–44 years	15.8	20.2	21.3	17.2	21.8	23.9	*1.1	*3.6	*1.4
Birth control pill									
15–44 years	36.6	20.7	21.2	36.1	20.6	21.1	41.8	23.1	22.7
15–24 years	65.3	56.2	61.4	64.4	56.0	59.8	72.4	56.8	74.9
25–34 years	36.2	22.8	28.6	35.8	22.1	28.7	41.6	28.8	29.3
35–44 years	18.3	3.2	3.8	18.2	*3.2	4.0	17.2	*4.3	*2.4
Intrauterine device									
15–44 years	10.2	7.6	2.2	9.8	7.5	2.1	13.8	10.0	3.4
15–24 years	10.8	*3.5	*0.4	10.7	*3.3	*0.5	12.6	*8.2	*–
25–34 years	13.2	9.6	2.1	12.7	9.4	1.8	18.8	14.1	3.8
35–44 years	5.6	6.8	2.8	5.4	7.0	2.7	8.4	*4.5	3.9
Diaphragm									
15–44 years	3.4	6.5	6.0	3.6	6.8	6.2	1.8	4.2	2.3
15–24 years	*1.5	*7.0	3.1	*1.6	*7.2	*3.5	*0.3	*4.5	*1.3
25–34 years	3.1	8.5	6.7	3.2	9.1	7.1	*2.2	3.1	*1.6
35–44 years	5.0	*3.8	5.9	5.3	*3.7	6.0	*2.5	*5.7	3.4
Condom									
15–44 years	12.6	12.1	12.9	13.4	12.6	13.1	4.1	5.0	7.7
15–24 years	7.7	12.7	16.3	8.3	12.9	17.7	*1.8	*6.3	*7.6
25–34 years	12.4	12.4	13.9	13.1	13.0	14.0	3.8	5.0	9.6
35–44 years	16.1	11.4	11.0	17.2	12.0	11.0	6.4	*4.5	5.7

[1]Estimates have been revised and differ from those previously published.
[2]Refers only to currently married couples in 1973.

*Relative standard error greater than 30 percent.

SOURCE: Centers for Disease Control and Prevention, National Center for Health Statistics, Division of Vital Statistics: Data from the National Survey of Family Growth.

Table 17. Methods of contraception for women 15–44 years of age, according to race and marital status: United States, 1982 and 1988

[Data are based on household interviews of samples of women in the childbearing ages]

Marital status and method of contraception	All races		White		Black	
	1982 [1]	1988	1982 [1]	1988	1982 [1]	1988
Marital status	Number of women in thousands					
All marital statuses...............	54,099	57,900	45,367	47,077	6,985	7,679
Currently married	28,231	29,147	25,195	25,426	2,130	2,197
Widowed, separated, or divorced	6,704	7,695	5,224	6,038	1,310	1,417
Never married......................	19,164	21,058	14,948	15,612	3,545	4,065
All methods	Percent of women using contraception					
All marital statuses...............	55.7	60.3	56.7	61.8	52.0	56.7
Currently married	69.7	74.3	70.4	75.3	63.3	67.0
Widowed, separated, or divorced	55.5	57.6	56.3	57.4	55.7	59.0
Never married......................	35.3	41.9	33.6	41.5	43.8	50.4
Female sterilization	Percent of contracepting women					
All marital statuses...............	23.2	27.5	22.1	26.1	30.0	38.1
Currently married	26.9	31.4	25.8	30.2	37.0	48.3
Widowed, separated, or divorced	39.2	50.7	35.2	47.9	53.5	65.4
Never married......................	3.7	6.4	*1.0	2.4	12.8	19.6
Male sterilization						
All marital statuses...............	10.9	11.7	12.2	13.6	1.4	0.9
Currently married	15.5	17.3	16.4	19.1	3.4	2.0
Widowed, separated, or divorced	3.4	3.6	4.3	4.3	*–	*0.1
Never married......................	1.8	1.8	2.3	2.3	*0.4	*0.3
Birth control pill						
All marital statuses...............	28.0	30.7	26.7	29.8	38.0	38.0
Currently married	19.3	20.4	19.0	20.0	24.5	26.0
Widowed, separated, or divorced	28.4	25.3	30.4	27.4	20.4	16.8
Never married......................	53.0	59.0	51.6	60.2	58.1	55.3
Intrauterine device						
All marital statuses...............	7.1	2.0	6.9	1.8	9.1	3.1
Currently married	6.9	2.0	6.8	1.8	9.3	2.3
Widowed, separated, or divorced	11.5	3.6	11.8	3.3	11.4	5.4
Never married......................	5.4	1.3	4.3	*0.9	7.9	2.7
Diaphragm						
All marital statuses...............	8.1	5.7	8.8	6.2	3.5	1.9
Currently married	6.5	6.2	6.7	6.4	5.1	2.4
Widowed, separated, or divorced	6.7	5.3	7.8	5.6	*2.5	*2.1
Never married......................	13.4	4.9	16.8	6.1	2.6	1.5
Condom						
All marital statuses...............	12.0	14.6	12.7	14.9	6.2	10.3
Currently married	14.1	14.3	14.5	14.3	6.8	9.8
Widowed, separated, or divorced	*1.5	5.9	*1.5	6.3	*1.6	4.1
Never married......................	11.6	19.6	12.8	21.4	7.9	13.2

[1] Estimates have been revised and differ from those previously published.

*Relative standard error greater than 30 percent.

SOURCE: Centers for Disease Control and Prevention, National Center for Health Statistics, Division of Vital Statistics: Data from the National Survey of Family Growth.

Table 18. Infant, neonatal, and postneonatal mortality rates, according to detailed race of mother and Hispanic origin of mother: United States, 1960 and 1983–87 birth cohorts

[Data are based on the National Linked Files of Live Births and Infant Deaths]

Race of mother and Hispanic origin of mother	Birth cohort						
	1960[1]	1983	1984	1985	1986	1987	1985–87
	Infant deaths per 1,000 live births						
All mothers	25.1	10.9	10.4	10.4	10.1	9.8	10.1
White	22.2	9.3	8.9	8.9	8.5	8.2	8.5
Black	42.1	19.2	18.2	18.6	18.2	17.8	18.2
American Indian or Alaskan Native	- - -	15.2	13.4	13.1	13.9	13.0	13.3
Asian or Pacific Islander	- - -	8.3	8.9	7.8	7.8	7.3	7.6
Chinese	- - -	9.5	7.2	5.8	5.9	6.2	6.0
Japanese	- - -	*	*	*6.0	*7.2	*6.6	6.6
Filipino	- - -	8.4	8.5	7.7	7.2	6.6	7.2
Other Asian or Pacific Islander[2]	- - -	8.3	9.7	8.6	8.6	7.9	8.3
Hispanic origin[3,4]	- - -	9.5	9.3	8.8	8.4	8.2	8.5
Mexican American	- - -	9.1	8.9	8.5	7.9	8.0	8.1
Puerto Rican	- - -	12.9	12.9	11.1	11.7	9.9	10.9
Cuban	- - -	*7.5	*8.1	8.5	*7.5	7.1	7.7
Central and South American	- - -	8.5	8.3	8.0	7.8	7.8	7.8
Other and unknown Hispanic	- - -	10.6	9.6	9.5	9.2	8.7	9.1
Non-Hispanic white[4]	- - -	9.2	8.7	8.7	8.4	8.1	8.4
Non-Hispanic black[4]	- - -	19.1	18.1	18.3	18.0	17.4	17.9
	Neonatal deaths per 1,000 live births						
All mothers	18.4	7.1	6.8	6.8	6.5	6.2	6.6
White	16.9	6.1	5.8	5.8	5.5	5.2	5.5
Black	27.3	12.5	11.9	12.3	11.9	11.8	12.0
American Indian or Alaskan Native	- - -	7.5	6.4	6.1	6.1	6.2	6.1
Asian or Pacific Islander	- - -	5.2	5.7	4.8	4.8	4.5	4.7
Chinese	- - -	5.5	4.4	3.3	3.1	3.7	3.4
Japanese	- - -	*	*	*3.1	*4.7	*4.0	3.9
Filipino	- - -	5.6	5.3	5.1	4.9	4.1	4.7
Other Asian or Pacific Islander[2]	- - -	5.2	6.5	5.4	5.3	4.9	5.2
Hispanic origin[3,4]	- - -	6.2	6.2	5.7	5.5	5.3	5.5
Mexican American	- - -	5.9	5.8	5.4	5.1	5.1	5.2
Puerto Rican	- - -	8.7	8.6	7.6	7.6	6.7	7.3
Cuban	- - -	*5.0	*6.4	6.2	*5.1	5.3	5.5
Central and South American	- - -	5.8	5.9	5.6	5.2	5.0	5.2
Other and unknown Hispanic	- - -	6.4	6.5	5.6	6.0	5.6	5.7
Non-Hispanic white[4]	- - -	6.0	5.7	5.7	5.4	5.0	5.4
Non-Hispanic black[4]	- - -	12.1	11.5	11.9	11.5	11.3	11.6
	Postneonatal deaths per 1,000 live births						
All mothers	6.7	3.8	3.6	3.6	3.6	3.5	3.6
White	5.3	3.2	3.1	3.1	3.0	3.0	3.0
Black	14.8	6.7	6.3	6.3	6.3	6.1	6.2
American Indian or Alaskan Native	- - -	7.7	7.0	7.0	7.8	6.8	7.2
Asian or Pacific Islander	- - -	3.1	3.1	2.9	3.0	2.8	2.9
Chinese	- - -	*	*	*2.5	*2.8	*2.5	2.6
Japanese	- - -	*	*	*	*2.5	*	2.7
Filipino	- - -	*2.8	*3.2	*2.7	2.3	2.5	2.5
Other Asian or Pacific Islander[2]	- - -	3.1	3.2	3.1	3.3	3.0	3.2
Hispanic origin[3,4]	- - -	3.3	3.1	3.2	2.9	2.9	3.0
Mexican American	- - -	3.2	3.2	3.2	2.8	2.9	2.9
Puerto Rican	- - -	4.2	4.3	3.5	4.2	3.2	3.6
Cuban	- - -	*	*1.7	*	*2.4	*	2.2
Central and South American	- - -	2.6	2.4	2.4	2.6	2.8	2.6
Other and unknown Hispanic	- - -	4.2	3.1	3.9	3.2	3.2	3.4
Non-Hispanic white[4]	- - -	3.2	3.0	3.0	3.0	3.0	3.0
Non-Hispanic black[4]	- - -	7.0	6.6	6.4	6.5	6.2	6.3

[1]Data are shown by race of child in 1960.
[2]Includes Hawaiians and part Hawaiians.
[3]Includes mothers of all races.
[4]Data shown only for States with an Hispanic-origin item on their birth certificates. In 1983–87, 23 States and the District of Columbia included this item.

*Infant and neonatal mortality rates for groups with fewer than 10,000 births are considered unreliable. Postneonatal mortality rates for groups with fewer than 20,000 births are considered unreliable. Infant and neonatal mortality rates for groups with fewer than 7,500 births are considered highly unreliable and are not shown. Postneonatal mortality rates for groups with fewer than 15,000 births are considered highly unreliable and are not shown.

SOURCE: Centers for Disease Control and Prevention, National Center for Health Statistics: Data computed by the Division of Analysis from data compiled by the Division of Vital Statistics for the National Linked Files of Live Births and Infant Deaths.

Table 19. Infant mortality rates, according to birth weight, detailed race of mother, and Hispanic origin of mother: United States, 1960 and 1983–87 birth cohorts

[Data are based on the National Linked Files of Live Births and Infant Deaths]

Birth weight, race of mother, and Hispanic origin of mother	Birth cohort						
	1960[1]	1983	1984	1985	1986	1987	1985–87
Birth weight less than 1,500 grams	Infant deaths per 1,000 live births						
All mothers	752.6	393.6	383.5	381.0	364.8	351.4	365.2
White	769.4	402.4	389.5	385.1	369.8	354.8	369.6
Black	706.4	378.7	372.5	370.5	353.6	346.5	356.2
American Indian or Alaskan Native	- - -	376.1	356.7	388.9	422.6	334.2	379.3
Asian or Pacific Islander	- - -	352.9	363.4	384.4	347.2	299.3	341.9
Chinese	- - -	*	*	*369.6	*	*	320.3
Japanese	- - -	*	*	*238.8	*	*	*294.4
Filipino	- - -	*321.0	*287.3	*350.9	*285.7	214.6	279.6
Other Asian or Pacific Islander [2]	- - -	342.4	408.7	414.9	370.4	334.5	371.8
Hispanic origin [3,4]	- - -	382.2	381.7	359.8	347.1	328.7	344.2
Mexican American	- - -	387.1	395.8	360.2	352.3	343.2	351.6
Puerto Rican	- - -	389.9	364.7	351.6	347.6	286.4	324.9
Cuban	- - -	*	*	*	*	*	373.5
Central and South American	- - -	331.2	342.1	347.7	313.2	338.4	332.4
Other and unknown Hispanic	- - -	380.6	368.1	372.3	356.5	296.4	335.8
Non-Hispanic white [4]	- - -	398.8	387.4	384.0	369.4	355.5	369.5
Non-Hispanic black [4]	- - -	372.0	370.6	360.3	345.7	340.4	348.4
Birth weight 1,500–2,499 grams							
All mothers	91.9	30.0	28.9	27.8	27.2	25.5	26.8
White	93.9	31.3	30.8	28.9	28.1	26.2	27.8
Black	85.1	26.6	24.4	25.1	24.2	23.6	24.3
American Indian or Alaskan Native	- - -	*44.7	*45.8	*42.7	*51.6	*35.1	43.0
Asian or Pacific Islander	- - -	25.3	23.8	22.5	25.5	24.5	24.2
Chinese	- - -	*	*	*	*	*	28.8
Japanese	- - -	*	*	*	*	*	*
Filipino	- - -	*	*	*	*	*	18.0
Other Asian or Pacific Islander [2]	- - -	25.8	25.5	22.5	27.6	26.6	25.7
Hispanic origin [3,4]	- - -	26.8	29.1	27.3	25.9	24.6	25.9
Mexican American	- - -	28.0	29.9	27.8	27.9	26.4	27.3
Puerto Rican	- - -	24.5	28.0	26.5	22.9	19.1	22.7
Cuban	- - -	*	*	*	*	*	*
Central and South American	- - -	*24.0	*25.4	*22.4	24.1	21.7	22.7
Other and unknown Hispanic	- - -	28.9	29.3	30.5	22.5	26.1	26.2
Non-Hispanic white [4]	- - -	31.7	30.2	28.8	28.6	26.1	27.8
Non-Hispanic black [4]	- - -	26.7	23.4	26.1	24.5	22.6	24.3
Birth weight 2,500 grams or more							
All mothers	11.2	4.5	4.3	4.2	4.1	4.0	4.1
White	9.7	4.1	3.9	3.9	3.7	3.6	3.7
Black	20.2	6.9	6.3	6.2	6.2	5.9	6.1
American Indian or Alaskan Native	- - -	9.1	7.6	7.3	7.5	7.6	7.5
Asian or Pacific Islander	- - -	3.8	4.1	3.2	3.4	3.5	3.4
Chinese	- - -	*	*	*2.6	*2.5	*3.1	2.7
Japanese	- - -	*	*	*	*	*	2.9
Filipino	- - -	*	*4.5	*3.4	*3.6	3.8	3.6
Other Asian or Pacific Islander [2]	- - -	3.7	4.2	3.5	3.6	3.5	3.5
Hispanic origin [3,4]	- - -	4.2	3.9	3.8	3.5	3.4	3.6
Mexican American	- - -	4.1	3.9	3.7	3.3	3.5	3.5
Puerto Rican	- - -	5.5	5.2	4.5	4.8	3.6	4.3
Cuban	- - -	*	*	*	*	*	2.7
Central and South American	- - -	3.5	3.3	3.3	3.2	3.3	3.3
Other and unknown Hispanic	- - -	4.6	4.0	4.2	3.9	3.7	3.9
Non-Hispanic white [4]	- - -	4.1	3.8	3.8	3.7	3.6	3.7
Non-Hispanic black [4]	- - -	7.1	6.5	6.2	6.4	5.9	6.2

[1] Data are shown by race of child in 1960.
[2] Includes Hawaiians and part Hawaiians.
[3] Includes mothers of all races.
[4] Data shown only for States with an Hispanic-origin item on their birth certificates. In 1983–87, 23 States and the District of Columbia included this item.

*Birth weight specific infant mortality rates are considered unreliable for groups with fewer than 200 births with birth weight less than 1,500 grams, fewer than 2,000 births with birth weight 1,500–2,499 grams, and fewer than 20,000 births with birth weight 2,500 grams or more. Birth weight specific infant mortality rates are considered highly unreliable and are not shown for groups with fewer than 150 births with birth weight less than 1,500 grams, fewer than 1,500 births with birth weight 1,500–2,499 grams, and fewer than 15,000 births with birth weight 2,500 grams or more.

SOURCE: Centers for Disease Control and Prevention, National Center for Health Statistics: Data computed by the Division of Analysis from data compiled by the Division of Vital Statistics for the National Linked Files of Live Births and Infant Deaths.

Table 20 (page 1 of 2). Infant mortality rates, fetal death rates, and perinatal mortality rates, according to race: United States, selected years 1950–91

[Data are based on the National Vital Statistics System]

| Race and year | Infant mortality rate [1] | | | | Fetal death rate [2] | Late fetal death rate [3] | Perinatal mortality rate [4] |
| | Total | Neonatal | | Postneonatal | | | |
		Under 28 days	Under 7 days				
All races	Deaths per 1,000 live births						
1950 [5]	29.2	20.5	17.8	8.7	18.4	14.9	32.5
1960 [5]	26.0	18.7	16.7	7.3	15.8	12.1	28.6
1970	20.0	15.1	13.6	4.9	14.0	9.5	23.0
1975	16.1	11.6	10.0	4.5	10.6	7.8	17.7
1980	12.6	8.5	7.1	4.1	9.1	6.2	13.2
1981	11.9	8.0	6.7	3.9	8.9	5.9	12.6
1982	11.5	7.7	6.4	3.8	8.8	5.9	12.3
1983	11.2	7.3	6.1	3.9	8.4	5.4	11.5
1984	10.8	7.0	5.9	3.8	8.1	5.2	11.0
1985	10.6	7.0	5.8	3.7	7.8	4.9	10.7
1986	10.4	6.7	5.6	3.6	7.7	4.7	10.3
1987	10.1	6.5	5.4	3.6	7.6	4.6	10.0
1988	10.0	6.3	5.2	3.6	7.5	4.5	9.7
1989	9.8	6.2	5.1	3.6	7.5	4.5	9.6
1990	9.2	5.8	4.8	3.4	7.5	4.3	9.1
Provisional data:							
1988 [5]	9.9	6.4	- - -	3.5	- - -	- - -	- - -
1989 [5]	9.7	6.3	- - -	3.5	- - -	- - -	- - -
1990 [5]	9.1	5.7	- - -	3.3	- - -	- - -	- - -
1991	8.9	5.5	- - -	3.4	- - -	- - -	- - -
Race of child [6]: White							
1950 [5]	26.8	19.4	17.1	7.4	16.6	13.3	30.1
1960 [5]	22.9	17.2	15.6	5.7	13.9	10.8	26.2
1970	17.8	13.8	12.5	4.0	12.3	8.6	21.0
1975	14.2	10.4	9.0	3.8	9.4	7.1	16.0
1980	11.0	7.5	6.2	3.5	8.1	5.7	11.9
1981	10.5	7.1	5.9	3.4	8.0	5.4	11.3
1982	10.1	6.8	5.6	3.3	7.9	5.4	11.0
1983	9.7	6.4	5.4	3.3	7.4	5.0	10.3
1984	9.4	6.2	5.1	3.3	7.3	4.8	9.9
1985	9.3	6.1	5.0	3.2	7.0	4.5	9.6
1986	8.9	5.8	4.8	3.1	6.7	4.3	9.1
1987	8.6	5.5	4.5	3.1	6.6	4.2	8.7
1988	8.5	5.4	4.4	3.1	6.4	4.0	8.4
1989	8.2	5.2	4.3	3.0	6.4	4.0	8.3
1990	7.7	4.9	4.0	2.8	6.4	3.8	7.8
Race of child [6]: Black							
1950 [5]	43.9	27.8	23.0	16.1	32.1	- - -	- - -
1960 [5]	44.3	27.8	23.7	16.5	- - -	- - -	- - -
1970	32.6	22.8	20.3	9.9	23.2	- - -	34.5
1975	26.2	18.3	15.7	7.9	16.8	11.4	26.9
1980	21.4	14.1	11.9	7.3	14.4	8.9	20.7
1981	20.0	13.4	11.4	6.6	13.8	8.2	19.4
1982	19.6	13.1	11.1	6.6	13.8	8.1	19.1
1983	19.2	12.4	10.6	6.8	13.5	7.7	18.2
1984	18.4	11.8	10.2	6.5	12.7	7.3	17.4
1985	18.2	12.1	10.3	6.1	12.6	7.1	17.4
1986	18.0	11.7	10.1	6.3	12.5	7.0	17.0
1987	17.9	11.7	10.0	6.1	12.8	7.0	16.9
1988	17.6	11.5	9.8	6.2	12.7	6.8	16.5
1989	17.7	11.3	9.6	6.4	12.8	6.7	16.2
1990	17.0	10.9	9.2	6.1	12.9	6.6	15.7

See footnotes at end of table.

Table 20 (page 2 of 2). Infant mortality rates, fetal death rates, and perinatal mortality rates, according to race: United States, selected years 1950–91

[Data are based on the National Vital Statistics System]

| Race and year | Infant mortality rate [1] | | | | Fetal death rate [2] | Late fetal death rate [3] | Perinatal mortality rate [4] |
| | Total | Neonatal | | Postneonatal | | | |
		Under 28 days	Under 7 days				
Race of mother [7]: White	Deaths per 1,000 live births						
1980.	10.9	7.4	6.1	3.5	8.1	5.7	11.8
1981.	10.3	7.0	5.8	3.4	8.0	5.4	11.2
1982.	9.9	6.7	5.6	3.2	7.8	5.4	10.9
1983.	9.6	6.3	5.3	3.3	7.4	5.0	10.2
1984.	9.3	6.1	5.1	3.2	7.3	4.8	9.8
1985.	9.2	6.0	5.0	3.2	6.9	4.5	9.5
1986.	8.8	5.7	4.7	3.1	6.7	4.3	9.0
1987.	8.5	5.4	4.5	3.1	6.6	4.2	8.6
1988.	8.4	5.3	4.3	3.1	6.4	4.0	8.3
1989.	8.1	5.1	4.2	2.9	6.4	4.0	8.2
1990.	7.6	4.8	3.9	2.8	6.4	3.8	7.7
Race of mother [7]: Black							
1980.	22.2	14.6	12.3	7.6	14.7	9.1	21.3
1981.	20.8	14.0	11.8	6.8	14.0	8.3	20.0
1982.	20.5	13.6	11.6	6.9	14.0	8.3	19.7
1983.	20.0	12.9	11.1	7.0	13.7	7.8	18.7
1984.	19.2	12.3	10.6	6.8	12.9	7.3	17.9
1985.	19.0	12.6	10.8	6.4	12.8	7.2	17.9
1986.	18.9	12.3	10.6	6.6	12.7	7.1	17.6
1987.	18.8	12.3	10.5	6.4	13.1	7.1	17.5
1988.	18.5	12.1	10.3	6.5	13.0	6.9	17.1
1989.	18.6	11.9	10.1	6.7	13.1	6.8	16.8
1990.	18.0	11.6	9.7	6.4	13.3	6.7	16.4

[1] Infant mortality rate is deaths under 1 year of age per 1,000 live births. Neonatal deaths occur within 28 days and early neonatal deaths within 7 days of birth; postneonatal deaths occur 28–365 days after birth.
[2] Number of fetal deaths of 20 weeks or more gestation per 1,000 live births plus fetal deaths.
[3] Number of fetal deaths of 28 weeks or more gestation per 1,000 live births plus late fetal deaths.
[4] Number of late fetal deaths plus infant deaths within 7 days of birth per 1,000 live births plus late fetal deaths.
[5] Includes births and deaths of nonresidents of the United States.
[6] Infant deaths and fetal deaths are tabulated by race of decedent; live births are tabulated by race of child (see Appendix II).
[7] Infant deaths are tabulated by race of decedent; fetal deaths and live births are tabulated by race of mother (see Appendix II).

SOURCES: Centers for Disease Control and Prevention, National Center for Health Statistics: Vital Statistics of the United States, Vol. II, Mortality, Part A, for data years 1950–90. Public Health Service. Washington. U.S. Government Printing Office. Annual summary of births, marriages, divorces, and deaths, United States, 1989, 1990, and 1991. Monthly Vital Statistics Report. Vols. 38, 39, and 40, No. 13. DHHS Pub. Nos. (PHS) 90-1120, 91-1120, and 92-1120, Aug. 1990, 1991, and 1992; Public Health Service. Hyattsville, Md.; Data computed by the Division of Analysis from data compiled by the Division of Vital Statistics.

Table 21. Infant mortality rates, according to race, geographic division, and State: United States, average annual 1978–80, 1983–85, and 1988–90

[Data are based on the National Vital Statistics System]

Geographic division and State	All races			White [1]			Black [1]		
	1978–80	1983–85	1988–90	1978–80	1983–85	1988–90	1978–80	1983–85	1988–90
	Infant deaths per 1,000 live births								
United States	13.1	10.9	9.7	11.3	9.4	8.0	22.9	19.4	18.4
New England	11.0	9.4	7.8	10.4	8.7	7.2	21.9	20.3	16.3
Maine	9.8	8.7	7.2	9.8	8.7	7.1	*	*	*
New Hampshire	10.3	9.4	7.8	10.3	9.3	7.8	*	*	*
Vermont	10.9	8.6	6.7	10.9	8.6	6.7	*	*	*
Massachusetts	10.8	9.0	7.5	10.3	8.4	6.9	19.8	19.3	15.1
Rhode Island	12.9	9.9	8.8	11.8	9.4	8.5	*32.3	*17.7	*15.0
Connecticut	11.6	10.1	8.5	10.2	8.8	7.1	22.7	21.4	18.4
Middle Atlantic	13.3	11.0	10.0	11.4	9.4	7.9	22.5	19.0	19.4
New York	13.4	11.1	10.3	11.4	9.5	8.2	21.6	17.5	18.7
New Jersey	12.8	11.0	9.4	10.3	9.1	7.1	23.2	19.7	19.1
Pennsylvania	13.4	10.9	9.9	12.0	9.3	7.8	23.9	22.3	21.6
East North Central	13.4	11.2	10.4	11.4	9.4	8.3	24.9	21.7	20.7
Ohio	13.0	10.6	9.8	11.5	9.4	8.3	22.7	19.0	18.4
Indiana	12.7	11.1	10.3	11.4	10.2	9.2	23.9	19.7	19.4
Illinois	15.2	12.1	11.2	12.1	9.4	8.4	27.3	22.9	21.8
Michigan	13.3	11.6	10.9	11.2	9.3	8.2	24.5	23.7	22.2
Wisconsin	10.7	9.6	8.6	10.2	8.8	7.6	18.5	18.6	17.7
West North Central	12.0	9.7	8.6	11.0	9.0	7.6	25.3	18.7	18.6
Minnesota	10.9	9.2	7.4	10.4	9.0	6.6	*30.0	*21.1	23.4
Iowa	11.7	9.1	8.3	11.3	8.9	7.9	*28.2	*19.4	*22.4
Missouri	13.6	10.5	9.8	11.7	9.0	8.4	25.1	18.7	17.5
North Dakota	12.5	8.5	8.9	11.9	8.1	8.4	*	*	*
South Dakota	11.8	10.2	9.9	10.1	8.5	8.3	*	*	*
Nebraska	12.0	9.7	8.4	11.2	9.2	7.4	*27.9	*18.3	*20.8
Kansas	11.3	9.9	8.4	10.4	9.3	7.5	22.6	18.1	17.5
South Atlantic	15.0	12.3	11.1	11.9	9.6	8.3	22.9	19.7	18.3
Delaware	14.7	11.9	11.2	10.8	9.1	8.5	27.6	21.2	20.4
Maryland	14.4	11.8	10.4	11.5	9.1	7.5	22.1	18.7	17.2
District of Columbia	24.8	20.4	22.2	*11.6	9.4	14.8	27.7	23.4	25.7
Virginia	14.0	11.8	10.2	11.9	9.5	7.6	21.4	20.1	18.9
West Virginia	13.6	10.9	9.4	13.2	10.6	9.1	*24.2	*19.9	*18.6
North Carolina	15.4	12.4	11.4	12.0	9.8	8.7	23.3	19.0	18.1
South Carolina	17.1	14.6	12.2	12.1	10.6	8.9	24.6	21.2	17.6
Georgia	15.0	13.0	12.4	11.3	9.7	9.0	21.6	19.3	18.6
Florida	14.5	11.4	10.0	11.9	9.1	7.9	22.5	18.9	17.0
East South Central	14.6	12.6	10.9	11.7	10.1	8.5	22.4	19.3	17.0
Kentucky	12.4	11.4	9.4	11.5	10.7	8.7	21.3	19.8	16.8
Tennessee	14.0	12.0	10.6	12.1	9.8	8.1	20.6	20.0	18.5
Alabama	15.2	12.9	11.7	11.7	10.1	8.9	21.7	18.3	16.9
Mississippi	17.7	14.4	12.0	11.5	9.9	8.6	24.6	19.5	15.7
West South Central	13.7	10.9	9.2	11.8	9.6	7.9	21.7	17.1	15.5
Arkansas	14.1	11.1	10.0	11.9	9.7	8.3	20.8	15.7	15.9
Louisiana	15.7	12.5	11.2	11.7	9.1	8.2	22.2	18.2	15.7
Oklahoma	13.1	10.9	8.9	12.0	10.4	8.5	21.6	17.2	13.9
Texas	13.1	10.4	8.7	11.8	9.6	7.7	21.4	16.5	15.5
Mountain	11.7	9.8	8.9	11.1	9.4	8.4	23.8	18.9	18.9
Montana	11.6	9.4	9.7	10.7	8.9	8.8	*	*	*
Idaho	10.8	10.3	9.1	10.8	10.3	8.8	*	*	*
Wyoming	11.9	11.0	9.0	11.7	10.9	9.0	*	*	*
Colorado	10.6	9.9	9.0	10.3	9.5	8.7	20.6	19.1	16.6
New Mexico	13.2	10.1	9.2	12.3	9.8	8.8	*26.3	*15.5	*19.7
Arizona	13.0	9.6	9.3	12.0	8.9	8.6	*26.0	20.8	21.7
Utah	10.8	9.2	7.8	10.7	9.1	7.5	*	*	*
Nevada	11.9	9.9	8.3	10.8	9.6	7.5	*23.0	*16.5	17.9
Pacific	11.5	9.7	8.4	10.8	9.0	7.7	20.9	18.8	18.3
Washington	11.9	10.1	8.7	11.5	9.8	8.1	21.5	22.3	21.0
Oregon	11.9	9.8	8.6	11.7	9.6	8.3	*19.1	*19.2	*21.0
California	11.3	9.6	8.3	10.6	8.9	7.6	21.0	18.5	18.2
Alaska	14.2	11.5	10.4	11.5	9.4	8.0	*21.6	*24.5	*16.7
Hawaii	10.5	9.4	7.4	8.0	6.5	4.7	*17.6	*21.8	*13.4

[1]Deaths are tabulated by race of decedent; live births are tabulated by race of mother.

*Data for States with fewer than 5,000 live births for the 3-year period are considered unreliable. Data for States with fewer than 1,000 live births are considered highly unreliable and are not shown.

SOURCE: Centers for Disease Control and Prevention, National Center for Health Statistics: Data computed by the Division of Analysis from data compiled by the Division of Vital Statistics.

Table 22. Neonatal mortality rates, according to race, geographic division, and State: United States, average annual 1978–80, 1983–85, and 1988–90

[Data are based on the National Vital Statistics System]

Geographic division and State	All races			White [1]			Black [1]		
	1978–80	1983–85	1988–90	1978–80	1983–85	1988–90	1978–80	1983–85	1988–90
	Neonatal deaths per 1,000 live births								
United States	8.9	7.1	6.1	7.8	6.1	5.1	15.1	12.6	11.8
New England	8.1	6.7	5.4	7.6	6.2	4.9	16.2	14.7	11.3
Maine	5.9	5.8	4.9	6.0	5.8	4.9	*	*	*
New Hampshire	7.7	6.4	4.7	7.7	6.4	4.7	*	*	*
Vermont	7.1	5.7	4.2	7.0	5.7	4.3	*	*	*
Massachusetts	8.0	6.4	5.2	7.6	5.9	4.7	14.2	13.0	10.6
Rhode Island	9.7	7.3	6.6	9.2	7.0	6.4	*18.6	*12.8	*10.1
Connecticut	8.9	7.7	6.0	7.7	6.6	5.1	18.0	16.5	12.7
Middle Atlantic	9.6	7.5	6.8	8.4	6.6	5.5	15.3	12.2	12.7
New York	9.5	7.6	7.0	8.3	6.7	5.7	14.7	11.1	12.4
New Jersey	9.0	7.5	6.3	7.6	6.5	5.0	15.1	12.2	11.9
Pennsylvania	9.9	7.6	6.7	9.0	6.5	5.4	16.7	15.1	14.3
East North Central	9.1	7.5	6.7	7.9	6.3	5.4	16.3	14.2	13.2
Ohio	8.9	7.1	6.2	8.0	6.3	5.3	15.2	12.3	11.4
Indiana	8.6	7.4	6.4	7.8	6.8	5.7	15.5	12.9	12.4
Illinois	10.4	8.1	7.3	8.6	6.5	5.6	17.5	14.3	13.4
Michigan	9.0	7.9	7.3	7.5	6.3	5.2	16.8	16.9	15.6
Wisconsin	7.2	6.1	5.1	6.9	5.6	4.7	11.0	11.8	9.1
West North Central	8.2	6.1	5.2	7.6	5.7	4.7	17.0	11.8	10.8
Minnesota	7.2	5.7	4.4	7.0	5.6	4.1	*17.8	*13.4	13.5
Iowa	8.0	5.8	5.2	7.8	5.7	4.9	*19.3	*11.8	*15.6
Missouri	9.5	6.7	6.0	8.2	5.7	5.2	17.0	12.0	10.0
North Dakota	8.7	5.3	5.3	8.6	5.2	5.2	*	*	*
South Dakota	6.9	5.6	5.1	6.5	5.2	4.8	*	*	*
Nebraska	8.2	6.3	4.9	7.7	6.0	4.3	*18.3	*11.8	*12.4
Kansas	7.8	6.2	4.9	7.2	5.9	4.4	15.5	10.6	10.0
South Atlantic	10.3	8.3	7.4	8.3	6.4	5.4	15.3	13.2	12.4
Delaware	11.0	8.4	8.1	7.7	6.5	6.1	22.1	14.5	14.7
Maryland	10.5	8.2	6.9	8.4	6.2	4.8	16.1	13.3	11.8
District of Columbia	18.7	15.4	16.2	*9.3	7.6	9.8	20.7	17.6	18.9
Virginia	10.1	8.3	7.0	8.5	6.6	5.0	15.5	14.4	13.4
West Virginia	9.1	7.2	6.2	8.8	6.9	6.0	*17.1	*13.9	*11.1
North Carolina	10.6	8.2	7.6	8.5	6.5	5.6	15.5	12.4	12.4
South Carolina	11.5	9.9	8.1	8.6	7.1	5.9	16.0	14.3	11.6
Georgia	9.9	8.8	8.2	7.9	6.6	5.8	13.6	13.0	12.5
Florida	9.7	7.3	6.5	8.2	6.0	5.2	14.0	11.7	11.0
East South Central	9.7	8.2	6.8	8.0	6.7	5.3	14.4	12.3	10.8
Kentucky	8.2	7.6	5.4	7.6	7.1	4.9	14.1	13.0	10.3
Tennessee	9.6	8.0	6.6	8.2	6.3	5.0	14.3	14.0	12.0
Alabama	10.1	8.4	7.8	8.1	6.9	6.1	13.7	11.4	11.0
Mississippi	11.4	8.9	7.5	8.0	6.5	5.5	15.2	11.7	9.7
West South Central	9.1	6.9	5.6	8.0	6.1	4.8	14.0	10.8	9.5
Arkansas	8.7	6.7	5.9	7.6	6.0	4.9	11.9	9.2	9.3
Louisiana	10.7	8.2	7.0	8.3	6.1	5.2	14.7	11.8	9.8
Oklahoma	8.3	6.9	5.0	7.8	6.6	4.9	13.0	10.9	7.4
Texas	8.8	6.5	5.4	8.0	6.1	4.7	14.2	10.3	9.6
Mountain	7.5	5.7	5.1	7.3	5.5	4.8	14.8	11.4	11.4
Montana	7.4	4.6	4.9	7.1	4.4	4.7	*	*	*
Idaho	6.7	5.7	4.8	6.7	5.7	4.7	*	*	*
Wyoming	7.5	6.2	4.5	7.5	6.1	4.4	*	*	*
Colorado	6.6	5.7	5.3	6.4	5.4	5.0	13.1	11.9	11.4
New Mexico	8.4	5.9	5.6	8.3	5.9	5.5	*14.8	*8.4	*10.2
Arizona	8.8	5.8	5.6	8.5	5.6	5.4	*17.4	12.7	13.7
Utah	7.0	5.5	4.0	7.0	5.4	3.9	*	*	*
Nevada	7.2	5.5	4.1	6.6	5.3	3.8	*13.7	*9.0	8.9
Pacific	7.4	6.0	5.0	6.9	5.6	4.6	13.6	11.9	10.8
Washington	7.3	5.7	4.6	7.2	5.5	4.4	12.0	13.0	11.4
Oregon	7.1	5.2	4.6	7.0	5.1	4.5	*12.1	*10.1	*10.3
California	7.4	6.1	5.1	6.9	5.7	4.7	13.8	11.8	10.8
Alaska	8.5	5.8	4.8	7.4	4.9	3.9	*15.7	*15.0	*8.3
Hawaii	7.2	6.2	4.5	5.6	4.6	2.9	*10.2	*13.0	*8.4

[1] Deaths are tabulated by race of decedent; live births are tabulated by race of mother.

*Data for States with fewer than 5,000 live births for the 3-year period are considered unreliable. Data for States with fewer than 1,000 live births are considered highly unreliable and are not shown.

SOURCE: Centers for Disease Control and Prevention, National Center for Health Statistics: Data computed by the Division of Analysis from data compiled by the Division of Vital Statistics.

Table 23. Postneonatal mortality rates, according to race, geographic division, and State: United States, average annual 1978–80, 1983–85, and 1988–90

[Data are based on the National Vital Statistics System]

Geographic division and State	All races 1978–80	All races 1983–85	All races 1988–90	White [1] 1978–80	White [1] 1983–85	White [1] 1988–90	Black [1] 1978–80	Black [1] 1983–85	Black [1] 1988–90
			Postneonatal deaths per 1,000 live births						
United States	4.2	3.8	3.5	3.5	3.2	2.9	7.7	6.8	6.5
New England	3.0	2.7	2.4	2.8	2.5	2.2	5.7	5.6	5.0
Maine	3.9	2.9	2.2	3.9	2.9	2.2	*	*	*
New Hampshire	2.5	3.0	3.1	2.5	3.0	3.1	*	*	*
Vermont	3.8	3.0	2.5	3.8	2.9	2.5	*	*	*
Massachusetts	2.8	2.7	2.3	2.7	2.4	2.1	5.6	6.3	4.5
Rhode Island	3.1	2.6	2.2	2.5	2.4	2.1	*	*	*4.9
Connecticut	2.7	2.5	2.5	2.5	2.2	2.0	4.7	4.9	5.7
Middle Atlantic	3.7	3.5	3.2	3.0	2.8	2.4	7.2	6.8	6.7
New York	3.9	3.6	3.3	3.1	2.8	2.5	6.9	6.4	6.3
New Jersey	3.8	3.5	3.1	2.7	2.6	2.1	8.1	7.5	7.2
Pennsylvania	3.5	3.3	3.2	3.0	2.8	2.5	7.2	7.2	7.3
East North Central	4.3	3.7	3.8	3.5	3.1	3.0	8.6	7.5	7.6
Ohio	4.1	3.6	3.6	3.6	3.1	3.0	7.6	6.7	7.1
Indiana	4.1	3.8	3.9	3.6	3.4	3.6	8.4	6.8	7.0
Illinois	4.8	4.0	4.0	3.4	2.8	2.8	9.9	8.6	8.4
Michigan	4.3	3.7	3.7	3.7	3.1	2.9	7.7	6.8	6.6
Wisconsin	3.6	3.5	3.5	3.3	3.2	2.9	7.5	6.8	8.5
West North Central	3.9	3.6	3.5	3.4	3.3	3.0	8.4	6.9	7.8
Minnesota	3.7	3.5	3.0	3.4	3.3	2.6	*12.2	*7.7	*9.9
Iowa	3.6	3.3	3.1	3.5	3.2	3.0	*8.9	*7.6	*6.8
Missouri	4.2	3.8	3.8	3.5	3.3	3.1	8.1	6.7	7.5
North Dakota	3.7	3.2	3.6	3.4	2.9	3.1	*	*	*
South Dakota	4.9	4.7	4.8	3.6	3.4	3.5	*	*	*
Nebraska	3.9	3.4	3.5	3.5	3.1	3.1	*9.6	*6.6	*8.4
Kansas	3.6	3.7	3.5	3.3	3.4	3.1	*7.1	*7.5	*7.5
South Atlantic	4.7	4.1	3.7	3.5	3.1	2.9	7.6	6.5	5.9
Delaware	3.7	3.5	3.1	3.2	2.6	2.4	*5.5	*6.7	*5.7
Maryland	3.9	3.7	3.5	3.1	3.0	2.7	5.9	5.4	5.3
District of Columbia	6.2	5.0	6.1	*2.2	*1.8	*5.0	7.0	5.8	6.8
Virginia	3.9	3.5	3.2	3.4	2.9	2.5	5.9	5.7	5.5
West Virginia	4.4	3.7	3.3	4.4	3.6	3.1	*7.0	*6.0	*7.5
North Carolina	4.8	4.2	3.8	3.5	3.3	3.1	7.8	6.6	5.7
South Carolina	5.6	4.8	4.2	3.5	3.5	3.0	8.6	6.9	6.0
Georgia	5.1	4.2	4.3	3.4	3.1	3.2	8.0	6.3	6.2
Florida	4.9	4.1	3.5	3.7	3.1	2.7	8.4	7.2	6.1
East South Central	4.9	4.4	4.1	3.8	3.4	3.3	8.0	7.0	6.1
Kentucky	4.2	3.9	4.0	3.9	3.6	3.8	7.2	6.7	6.5
Tennessee	4.4	4.0	4.0	3.9	3.5	3.2	6.3	6.0	6.5
Alabama	5.1	4.4	3.9	3.6	3.2	2.8	8.0	6.9	5.9
Mississippi	6.3	5.5	4.5	3.5	3.5	3.1	9.4	7.8	6.0
West South Central	4.5	4.0	3.6	3.8	3.5	3.1	7.6	6.3	6.0
Arkansas	5.4	4.4	4.1	4.3	3.7	3.4	8.9	6.5	6.6
Louisiana	5.0	4.2	4.2	3.4	2.9	3.0	7.5	6.4	5.9
Oklahoma	4.8	4.0	3.9	4.1	3.8	3.6	8.6	6.3	6.4
Texas	4.2	3.9	3.4	3.8	3.6	3.0	7.3	6.2	5.8
Mountain	4.2	4.1	3.8	3.8	3.9	3.6	9.0	7.5	7.5
Montana	4.2	4.8	4.8	3.6	4.5	4.1	*	*	*
Idaho	4.1	4.6	4.2	4.1	4.6	4.1	*	*	*
Wyoming	4.4	4.8	4.5	4.2	4.9	4.6	*	*	*
Colorado	4.0	4.1	3.7	3.8	4.1	3.7	*7.6	*7.2	*5.3
New Mexico	4.8	4.2	3.6	4.0	3.9	3.3	*	*	*
Arizona	4.3	3.8	3.6	3.5	3.3	3.2	*8.7	*8.1	*8.0
Utah	3.8	3.7	3.8	3.7	3.7	3.6	*	*	*
Nevada	4.6	4.4	4.2	4.2	4.3	3.7	*9.3	*7.5	*9.1
Pacific	4.1	3.7	3.4	3.9	3.5	3.1	7.3	6.9	7.5
Washington	4.6	4.5	4.1	4.3	4.2	3.7	*9.6	*9.3	*9.6
Oregon	4.8	4.6	4.0	4.8	4.5	3.7	*	*	*10.7
California	3.9	3.5	3.3	3.7	3.2	3.0	7.2	6.7	7.4
Alaska	5.7	5.7	5.6	4.1	4.4	4.1	*	*	*
Hawaii	3.3	3.2	2.9	2.4	1.9	1.8	*	*	*

[1]Deaths are tabulated by race of decedent; live births are tabulated by race of mother.

*Data for States with fewer than 10,000 live births for the 3-year period are considered unreliable. Data for States with fewer than 2,500 live births are considered highly unreliable and are not shown.

SOURCE: Centers for Disease Control and Prevention, National Center for Health Statistics: Data computed by the Division of Analysis from data compiled by the Division of Vital Statistics.

Table 24. Fetal death rates, according to race, geographic division, and State: United States, average annual 1978–80, 1983–85, and 1988–90

[Data are based on the National Vital Statistics System]

Geographic division and State	All races			White [1]			Black [1]		
	1978–80	1983–85	1988–90	1978–80	1983–85	1988–90	1978–80	1983–85	1988–90
	Fetal deaths [2] per 1,000 live births plus fetal deaths								
United States	9.4	8.1	7.5	8.2	7.2	6.4	15.2	13.2	13.1
New England	7.1	6.8	6.3	6.9	6.5	5.8	10.5	12.1	12.3
Maine	8.1	6.7	5.9	7.9	6.7	5.7	*	*	*
New Hampshire	6.1	6.0	6.2	6.1	6.1	6.2	*	*	*
Vermont	6.7	6.8	5.5	6.7	6.7	5.3	*	*	*
Massachusetts	6.0	6.8	6.0	6.0	6.3	5.5	6.2	13.6	11.7
Rhode Island	10.6	7.6	6.9	10.1	7.7	6.7	*19.2	*8.2	*11.5
Connecticut	8.1	6.9	7.0	7.4	6.3	6.2	13.5	11.6	12.6
Middle Atlantic	10.8	9.4	9.1	9.5	8.4	7.6	16.9	14.2	15.7
New York	11.4	9.9	9.9	10.2	8.9	8.1	16.0	14.3	16.6
New Jersey	9.2	8.0	7.9	7.7	6.9	6.3	15.1	13.0	14.4
Pennsylvania	11.0	9.4	8.8	9.6	8.6	7.8	21.1	15.4	14.6
East North Central	8.6	7.3	6.7	7.7	6.6	5.9	13.5	11.3	10.9
Ohio	8.9	7.6	6.9	8.2	7.0	6.4	13.3	12.0	10.2
Indiana	8.8	7.5	7.3	8.2	7.0	6.8	13.9	11.6	11.4
Illinois	9.4	8.1	7.5	8.0	7.0	6.2	14.8	12.5	12.4
Michigan	7.8	6.1	5.4	7.0	5.7	4.6	12.1	8.0	8.6
Wisconsin	6.9	6.6	6.2	6.8	6.1	5.5	8.6	13.4	12.9
West North Central	8.3	7.0	6.4	7.8	6.6	5.9	14.2	11.5	11.5
Minnesota	7.1	6.8	6.3	7.0	6.6	5.9	*11.8	*13.2	13.4
Iowa	7.5	6.7	6.6	7.3	6.7	6.4	*13.0	*9.8	*12.8
Missouri	9.4	7.3	6.6	8.5	6.7	5.7	14.8	11.1	11.1
North Dakota	9.0	6.3	6.8	8.8	6.1	6.7	*	*	*
South Dakota	8.6	7.1	6.3	7.7	6.5	5.8	*	*	*
Nebraska	8.7	7.4	6.5	8.4	7.1	6.1	*14.8	*11.1	*12.2
Kansas	8.4	7.1	5.8	8.0	6.6	5.4	13.1	12.9	10.9
South Atlantic	11.5	10.0	9.1	9.4	8.2	6.9	16.5	14.9	14.6
Delaware	8.0	7.4	6.8	6.9	6.7	5.9	11.5	10.1	9.8
Maryland	8.9	8.6	7.5	7.0	7.0	5.5	13.9	12.7	12.2
District of Columbia	14.2	13.6	13.0	*11.6	8.8	7.0	14.8	14.9	15.3
Virginia	13.9	10.8	9.3	11.9	8.9	7.5	20.7	17.3	15.2
West Virginia	9.9	8.8	7.9	9.5	8.6	7.6	*19.2	*13.3	*15.2
North Carolina	10.7	9.0	8.5	8.5	7.5	6.6	15.8	12.6	13.3
South Carolina	12.6	11.5	10.3	9.4	8.6	7.3	17.3	16.3	15.1
Georgia	14.1	12.2	11.4	11.7	9.8	8.1	18.3	16.9	17.4
Florida	9.8	9.2	8.3	8.3	7.6	6.5	14.2	14.3	13.9
East South Central	11.0	9.5	8.4	8.8	7.8	6.7	16.5	14.1	13.0
Kentucky	9.6	8.3	8.1	9.0	7.7	7.6	14.9	14.5	12.7
Tennessee	9.8	7.5	6.0	8.5	7.0	5.1	14.3	9.4	9.0
Alabama	11.2	10.4	10.3	8.9	8.2	7.8	15.4	14.6	14.9
Mississippi	14.2	12.6	10.3	9.2	8.9	6.6	19.6	16.8	14.4
West South Central	9.0	7.9	7.0	8.0	7.1	6.1	13.5	11.6	10.8
Arkansas	10.3	7.5	7.7	8.5	6.5	6.3	15.4	10.8	11.9
Louisiana	10.4	9.0	8.2	7.7	6.8	6.5	14.9	12.7	10.8
Oklahoma	9.3	8.1	7.5	8.4	7.6	6.8	16.5	10.0	11.9
Texas	8.3	7.7	6.5	7.9	7.2	5.9	11.3	11.1	10.4
Mountain	8.1	7.4	6.3	7.9	7.2	6.0	14.1	12.7	12.3
Montana	7.9	7.2	7.3	7.6	7.0	6.8	*	*	*
Idaho	7.3	7.3	6.7	7.4	7.2	6.6	*	*	*
Wyoming	7.4	6.9	7.2	7.4	6.7	7.1	*	*	*
Colorado	9.9	9.1	7.1	9.5	8.9	6.8	18.9	14.6	11.8
New Mexico	8.2	6.7	4.9	7.9	6.8	4.6	*11.9	*7.7	*8.8
Arizona	7.5	6.7	5.9	7.2	6.4	5.6	*12.1	10.2	11.6
Utah	7.4	6.8	5.4	7.4	6.7	5.4	*	*	*
Nevada	7.9	7.1	8.1	7.3	6.6	7.3	*10.4	*15.5	15.9
Pacific	8.1	6.8	6.5	7.6	6.4	6.0	13.8	11.1	12.2
Washington	7.5	6.4	5.4	7.4	6.2	5.3	13.7	10.3	10.1
Oregon	7.4	6.4	5.8	7.3	6.5	5.7	*10.7	*7.4	*8.0
California	8.1	6.8	6.6	7.6	6.5	6.2	13.9	11.2	12.4
Alaska	8.8	6.0	5.2	7.9	5.9	4.2	*13.6	*12.5	*12.1
Hawaii	11.2	9.0	7.5	12.7	8.3	7.9	*17.3	*10.3	*12.3

[1]Fetal deaths and live births are tabulated by race of mother.
[2]Deaths of fetuses of 20 weeks or more gestation.

*Data for States with fewer than 5,000 live births for the 3-year period are considered unreliable. Data for States with fewer than 1,000 live births are considered highly unreliable and are not shown.

SOURCE: Centers for Disease Control and Prevention, National Center for Health Statistics: Data computed by the Division of Analysis from data compiled by the Division of Vital Statistics.

Table 25. Infant mortality rates, feto-infant mortality rates, and postneonatal mortality rates, and average annual percent change: Selected countries, 1984 and 1989

[Data are based on reporting by countries]

Country [4]	Infant mortality rate [1]			Feto-infant mortality rate [2]			Postneonatal mortality rate [3]		
	1984	1989 [5]	Average annual percent change	1984 [6]	1989 [7]	Average annual percent change	1984 [8]	1989 [9]	Average annual percent change
Japan	5.99	4.59	−5.2	11.77	8.62	−6.0	2.28	2.01	−2.5
Sweden	6.40	5.77	−2.1	10.42	9.39	−2.1	2.29	2.03	−2.4
Finland	6.62	6.03	−1.8	10.58	10.46	−0.2	2.15	1.91	−2.3
Singapore	8.76	6.61	−5.5	14.52	10.92	−5.5	2.62	2.01	−5.2
Netherlands	8.36	6.78	−4.1	14.22	12.53	−2.5	3.24	2.20	−7.5
Northern Ireland	10.51	6.90	−8.1	16.33	11.94	−6.1	3.79	2.91	−5.1
Canada	8.11	7.13	−2.5	12.51	11.23	−2.1	2.96	2.47	−3.6
Switzerland	7.13	7.34	0.6	11.79	11.38	−0.7	2.94	2.91	−0.2
Hong Kong	9.17	7.43	−4.1	13.38	11.92	−2.3	2.93	2.64	−1.7
Federal Republic of Germany	9.64	7.44	−5.0	13.98	10.88	−4.9	4.15	3.45	−3.6
France	8.29	7.54	−1.9	15.84	13.66	−2.9	3.63	3.70	0.4
Ireland	9.63	7.55	−4.8	17.94	13.85	−5.0	3.67	3.21	−2.6
German Democratic Republic	10.05	7.56	−5.5	15.38	12.73	−3.7	3.34	2.89	−2.9
Norway	8.33	7.72	−1.5	13.46	12.58	−1.3	3.96	3.96	0.0
Denmark	7.66	7.95	0.7	12.05	13.01	1.5	2.97	3.31	2.2
Australia	9.25	7.99	−2.9	14.27	13.89	−0.5	3.77	3.29	−2.7
Spain	10.02	8.07	−5.3	16.13	13.30	−4.7	3.20	2.95	−2.7
Austria	11.41	8.31	−6.1	15.92	12.18	−5.2	4.52	3.45	−5.3
England and Wales	9.48	8.45	−2.3	15.11	13.09	−2.8	3.91	3.69	−1.2
Belgium	9.84	8.64	−2.6	16.47	15.58	−1.8	4.04	4.05	0.0
Scotland	10.32	8.73	−3.3	16.05	13.68	−3.1	3.93	4.00	0.4
Italy	11.44	8.80	−5.1	18.41	14.66	−4.5	2.38	2.08	−3.3
Greece	14.34	9.78	−7.4	23.12	17.76	−5.1	3.52	3.15	−2.2
United States	10.79	9.81	−1.9	15.92	14.13	−2.4	3.79	3.59	−1.1
Israel	12.80	9.94	−4.9	18.28	14.81	−4.1	4.96	3.44	−7.1
New Zealand	11.70	10.19	−2.7	16.80	14.72	−2.6	7.13	5.78	−4.1
Cuba	15.01	11.08	−5.9	26.33	22.67	−2.9	5.08	3.91	−5.1
Czechoslovakia	15.32	11.31	−5.9	20.26	15.52	−5.2	4.86	3.47	−6.5
Portugal	16.73	12.18	−6.2	26.31	20.00	−5.3	5.41	4.12	−5.3
Costa Rica	20.25	13.90	−7.2	30.44	23.20	−6.6	8.49	5.32	−11.0
Puerto Rico	15.61	14.27	−1.8	25.97	23.35	−2.1	3.13	3.09	−0.3
Bulgaria	16.09	14.37	−2.2	22.80	20.21	−2.4	7.18	7.05	−0.4
Hungary	20.41	15.74	−5.1	26.61	20.93	−4.7	4.57	4.05	−2.4
Poland	19.23	15.96	−3.7	25.09	21.37	−3.2	5.91	4.44	−5.6
Chile	19.55	17.06	−2.7	25.48	23.36	−1.7	10.31	7.96	−5.0
Kuwait	18.55	17.33	−2.2	27.98	25.14	−5.2	6.96	5.22	−9.1
Yugoslavia	27.67	22.21	−4.3	33.64	27.23	−4.1	12.03	8.92	−5.8
U.S.S.R.	25.92	22.97	−2.4	34.73	34.38	−0.5	14.85	12.87	−6.9
Romania	23.41	26.90	2.8	31.66	34.87	2.0	14.64	19.95	6.4

[1]Number of deaths of infants under 1 year per 1,000 live births.
[2]Number of late fetal deaths plus infant deaths under 1 year per 1,000 live births plus late fetal deaths.
[3]Number of postneonatal deaths per 1,000 live births.
[4]Refers to countries, territories, cities, or geographic areas.
[5]Data for Spain are for 1988 and data for Kuwait are for 1987.
[6]Data for Costa Rica are for 1982 and data for U.S.S.R. are for 1986.
[7]Data for Spain and U.S.S.R. are for 1988. Data for Belgium are for 1987 and data for Kuwait are for 1986.
[8]Data for Hong Kong are for 1983. Data for the U.S.S.R. are for 1987.
[9]Data for Costa Rica and Italy are for 1988. Data for Kuwait and Spain are for 1987.

NOTES: Rankings are from lowest to highest infant mortality rates based on the latest data available for countries or geographic areas with at least 1 million population and with "complete" counts of live births and infant deaths as indicated in the United Nations Demographic Yearbook, 1990. Some of the international variation in infant mortality rates (IMR) is due to variation among countries in distinctions between fetal and infant deaths. The feto-infant mortality rate (FIMR) attempts to reduce international variation due to clinical distinctions between fetal and infant deaths. The United States ranks 24th on the IMR and 21st on the FIMR and 22nd on the postneonatal mortality rate.

SOURCES: World Health Organization: World Health Statistics Annuals. Vols. 1985–1991. Geneva. United Nations: Demographic Yearbook 1985–1990. New York. Centers for Disease Control and Prevention, National Center for Health Statistics: Vital Statistics of the United States, 1984, Vol. II, Mortality, Part A. DHHS Pub. No. (PHS) 88-1101. Public Health Service. Washington. U.S. Government Printing Office, 1989; Vital Statistics of the United States, 1989, Vol. II, Mortality, Part A. DHHS Pub. No. (PHS) 92-1101. Public Health Service. Washington. U.S. Government Printing Office, 1992.

[Data are based on reporting by countries]

Country [1]	At birth		At 65 years	
	1984 [2]	1989 [3]	1984 [2]	1989 [3]
Male	Life expectancy in years			
Japan	74.8	76.2	15.7	16.5
Hong Kong	75.1	74.3	17.2	15.1
Greece	73.8	74.3	15.6	15.6
Sweden	73.9	74.2	14.9	15.0
Switzerland	73.8	74.1	15.5	15.5
Israel	73.2	73.9	15.0	15.2
Netherlands	73.0	73.7	14.1	14.3
Canada	73.0	73.7	15.0	15.3
Spain	73.2	73.6	15.2	15.6
Italy	71.3	73.3	13.7	14.7
Norway	73.0	73.3	14.5	14.7
Australia	72.6	73.3	14.5	14.7
France	71.7	73.1	14.9	15.8
England and Wales	71.9	72.9	13.5	14.0
Federal Republic of Germany	71.3	72.6	13.6	14.3
Kuwait	70.4	72.5	12.9	14.5
Denmark	71.8	72.2	14.0	14.0
Cuba	72.2	72.2	15.3	15.3
Austria	70.1	72.1	13.6	14.5
Costa Rica	74.5	72.1	17.3	14.0
United States	71.2	71.8	14.6	15.2
Ireland	70.8	71.7	12.8	13.0
Northern Ireland	70.3	71.4	12.7	12.9
New Zealand	71.2	71.4	13.9	14.0
Singapore	70.2	71.4	12.9	13.3
Belgium	70.8	71.4	13.3	13.6
Portugal	69.3	71.1	13.6	14.5
Finland	70.5	70.9	13.4	13.9
Scotland	69.9	70.6	12.5	12.7
German Democratic Republic	69.6	70.1	12.5	12.8
Chile	67.4	70.0	12.9	13.7
Puerto Rico	71.6	69.1	16.3	14.9
Yugoslavia	67.1	69.0	12.5	13.4
Bulgaria	68.5	68.3	12.8	12.8
Czechoslovakia	67.1	67.7	11.7	11.9
Poland	66.8	66.7	12.5	12.5
Romania	67.1	66.4	12.8	12.8
Hungary	65.1	65.5	11.8	12.1
U.S.S.R.	62.9	64.2	12.0	12.4
Female				
Japan	80.7	82.5	19.3	20.7
France	80.1	81.5	19.4	20.5
Switzerland	80.8	81.3	19.8	20.0
Netherlands	79.9	81.1	19.0	19.1
Canada	80.1	80.6	19.6	19.8
Spain	79.8	80.3	18.7	19.1
Sweden	80.1	80.1	18.9	18.8
Hong Kong	81.4	80.1	21.0	18.8
Norway	79.8	80.0	18.8	18.9
Italy	77.9	79.9	17.2	18.7
Australia	79.3	79.6	18.7	18.7
Greece	78.6	79.4	17.7	17.9
Federal Republic of Germany	78.1	79.2	17.6	18.2
Finland	79.0	79.0	17.7	17.8
Austria	77.3	78.9	17.0	18.0
United States	78.2	78.6	18.6	18.8
England and Wales	77.9	78.4	17.6	17.8
Portugal	76.2	78.2	16.7	17.9
Belgium	77.8	78.2	17.5	17.8
Denmark	77.8	77.9	18.0	18.0

See footnotes at end of table.

Table 26 (page 2 of 2). Life expectancy at birth and at 65 years of age, according to sex: Selected countries, 1984 and 1989

[Data are based on reporting by countries]

Country [1]	At birth		At 65 years	
	1984 [2]	1989 [3]	1984 [2]	1989 [3]
Female—Con.	Life expectancy in years			
Israel	76.7	77.6	16.5	16.9
New Zealand	77.8	77.3	18.0	17.7
Northern Ireland	76.5	77.3	16.5	16.8
Ireland	76.3	77.2	16.1	16.5
Puerto Rico	78.3	77.2	18.8	17.5
Costa Rica	78.4	76.9	19.0	16.8
Singapore	75.6	76.7	15.9	16.4
German Democratic Republic	75.4	76.4	15.4	15.9
Scotland	75.9	76.2	16.6	16.3
Kuwait	74.5	75.8	14.9	16.2
Chile	74.8	75.7	16.3	16.7
Poland	75.0	75.5	15.9	16.2
Czechoslovakia	74.6	75.4	15.0	15.4
Cuba	75.3	75.3	16.7	16.6
Yugoslavia	73.0	74.8	14.9	15.9
Bulgaria	74.5	74.8	15.1	15.1
U.S.S.R.	72.7	73.9	15.6	16.0
Hungary	73.3	73.9	15.1	15.6
Romania	72.7	72.3	14.7	14.7

[1]Refers to countries, territories, cities, or geographic areas.
[2]Data for Costa Rica, Cuba, Italy, and Yugoslavia are for 1983. Data for Kuwait, Singapore, and Northern Ireland are for 1985.
[3]Data for Costa Rica, Cuba, Israel, Italy, Romania, and Sweden are for 1988. Data for Belgium are for 1986. Data for Denmark and U.S.S.R. are for 1990.

NOTES: Rankings are from highest to lowest life expectancy based on the latest available data for countries or geographic areas with at least 1 million population. This table is based on official mortality data from the country concerned, as submitted to the United Nations Demographic Yearbook or the World Health Statistics Annual.

SOURCES: World Health Organization: World Health Statistics Annuals. Vols. 1984–1990. Geneva. United Nations: Demographic Yearbook 1984 and 1990. New York. Centers for Disease Control and Prevention, National Center for Health Statistics: Vital Statistics of the United States, 1984, Vol. II, Mortality, Part A. DHHS Pub. No. (PHS) 88-1101. Public Health Service. Washington. U.S. Government Printing Office, 1989; Vital Statistics of the United States, 1989, Vol. II, Mortality, Part A. DHHS Pub. No. (PHS) 92-1101. Public Health Service. Washington. U.S. Government Printing Office, 1992.

Table 27. Life expectancy at birth and at 65 years of age, according to race and sex: United States, selected years 1900–91

[Data are based on the National Vital Statistics System]

Specified age and year	All races			White			Black		
	Both sexes	Male	Female	Both sexes	Male	Female	Both sexes	Male	Female
At birth	Remaining life expectancy in years								
1900 [1,2]	47.3	46.3	48.3	47.6	46.6	48.7	[3]33.0	[3]32.5	[3]33.5
1950 [2]	68.2	65.6	71.1	69.1	66.5	72.2	60.7	58.9	62.7
1960 [2]	69.7	66.6	73.1	70.6	67.4	74.1	63.2	60.7	65.9
1970	70.9	67.1	74.8	71.7	68.0	75.6	64.1	60.0	68.3
1975	72.6	68.8	76.6	73.4	69.5	77.3	66.8	62.4	71.3
1980	73.7	70.0	77.4	74.4	70.7	78.1	68.1	63.8	72.5
1981	74.1	70.4	77.8	74.8	71.1	78.4	68.9	64.5	73.2
1982	74.5	70.8	78.1	75.1	71.5	78.7	69.4	65.1	73.6
1983	74.6	71.0	78.1	75.2	71.6	78.7	69.4	65.2	73.5
1984	74.7	71.1	78.2	75.3	71.8	78.7	69.5	65.3	73.6
1985	74.7	71.1	78.2	75.3	71.8	78.7	69.3	65.0	73.4
1986	74.7	71.2	78.2	75.4	71.9	78.8	69.1	64.8	73.4
1987	74.9	71.4	78.3	75.6	72.1	78.9	69.1	64.7	73.4
1988	74.9	71.4	78.3	75.6	72.2	78.9	68.9	64.4	73.2
1989	75.1	71.7	78.5	75.9	72.5	79.2	68.8	64.3	73.3
1990	75.4	71.8	78.8	76.1	72.7	79.4	69.1	64.5	73.6
Provisional data:									
1989 [2]	75.2	71.8	78.5	75.9	72.6	79.1	69.7	65.2	74.0
1990 [2]	75.4	72.0	78.8	76.0	72.6	79.3	70.3	66.0	74.5
1991	75.7	72.2	79.1	76.4	73.0	79.7	70.0	65.6	74.3
At 65 years									
1900–1902 [1,2]	11.9	11.5	12.2	- - -	11.5	12.2	- - -	10.4	11.4
1950 [2]	13.9	12.8	15.0	- - -	12.8	15.1	13.9	12.9	14.9
1960 [2]	14.3	12.8	15.8	14.4	12.9	15.9	13.9	12.7	15.1
1970	15.2	13.1	17.0	15.2	13.1	17.1	14.2	12.5	15.7
1975	16.1	13.8	18.1	16.1	13.8	18.2	15.0	13.1	16.7
1980	16.4	14.1	18.3	16.5	14.2	18.4	15.1	13.0	16.8
1981	16.6	14.3	18.6	16.7	14.4	18.7	15.5	13.4	17.2
1982	16.8	14.5	18.7	16.9	14.5	18.8	15.7	13.5	17.5
1983	16.7	14.4	18.6	16.8	14.5	18.7	15.4	13.2	17.2
1984	16.8	14.5	18.6	16.8	14.6	18.7	15.4	13.2	17.2
1985	16.7	14.5	18.5	16.8	14.5	18.7	15.2	13.0	16.9
1986	16.8	14.6	18.6	16.9	14.7	18.7	15.2	13.0	17.0
1987	16.9	14.7	18.7	17.0	14.8	18.8	15.2	13.0	17.0
1988	16.9	14.7	18.6	17.0	14.8	18.7	15.1	12.9	16.9
1989	17.1	15.0	18.8	17.2	15.1	18.9	15.2	13.0	16.9
1990	17.2	15.1	18.9	17.3	15.2	19.1	15.4	13.2	17.2
Provisional data:									
1989 [2]	17.2	15.2	18.8	17.3	15.2	18.9	15.8	13.8	17.4
1990 [2]	17.3	15.3	19.0	17.3	15.3	19.0	16.1	14.2	17.6
1991	17.5	15.5	19.2	17.6	15.5	19.3	16.1	14.2	17.5

[1]Death registration area only. The death registration area increased from 10 States and the District of Columbia in 1900 to the coterminous United States in 1933.
[2]Includes deaths of nonresidents of the United States.
[3]Figure is for the all other population.

NOTES: Final data for the 1980's have been revised based on intercensal population estimates and differ from previous editions of Health, United States. Provisional data for 1989–91 were calculated using 1980's-based postcensal population estimates. See Appendix I, National Center for Health Statistics and Department of Commerce.

SOURCES: U.S. Bureau of the Census: U.S. Life Tables 1890, 1901, 1910, and 1901–1910, by J. W. Glover. Washington. U.S. Government Printing Office, 1921; Centers for Disease Control and Prevention, National Center for Health Statistics: Vital Statistics Rates in the United States, 1940–1960, by R. D. Grove and A. M. Hetzel. DHEW Pub. No. (PHS) 1677. Public Health Service. Washington. U.S. Government Printing Office, 1968; Annual summary of births, marriages, divorces, and deaths, United States, 1989, 1990, and 1991. Monthly Vital Statistics Report. Vols. 38, 39, and 40, No. 13. DHHS Pub. Nos. (PHS) 90–1120, 91–1120, and 92–1120. 1990, 1991, and 1992; Public Health Service. Hyattsville, Md.; Unpublished data from the Division of Vital Statistics; Data computed by the Office of Research and Methodology from data compiled by the Division of Vital Statistics.

Table 28 (page 1 of 2). Age-adjusted death rates for selected causes of death, according to sex and race: United States, selected years 1950–90

[Data are based on the National Vital Statistics System]

Sex, race, and cause of death	1950[1]	1960[1]	1970	1980	1985	1986	1987	1988	1989	1990
All races				Deaths per 100,000 resident population						
All causes	840.5	760.9	714.3	585.8	548.9	544.8	539.2	539.9	528.0	520.2
Natural causes	766.6	695.2	636.9	519.7	493.0	487.4	483.0	483.2	472.4	465.1
Diseases of heart	307.2	286.2	253.6	202.0	181.4	176.0	170.8	167.7	157.5	152.0
Ischemic heart disease	- - -	- - -	- - -	149.8	126.1	119.5	114.7	111.1	106.2	102.6
Cerebrovascular diseases	88.6	79.7	66.3	40.8	32.5	31.1	30.4	29.9	28.3	27.7
Malignant neoplasms	125.3	125.8	129.8	132.8	134.4	134.1	134.0	134.0	134.5	135.0
Respiratory system	12.8	19.2	28.4	36.4	39.1	39.3	40.0	40.3	40.8	41.4
Colorectal	19.0	17.7	16.8	15.5	14.9	14.5	14.4	14.0	13.7	13.6
Prostate [2]	13.4	13.1	13.3	14.4	14.7	15.2	15.1	15.5	15.9	16.7
Breast [3]	22.2	22.3	23.1	22.7	23.3	23.2	23.0	23.3	23.1	23.1
Chronic obstructive pulmonary diseases	4.4	8.2	13.2	15.9	18.8	18.9	18.9	19.6	19.6	19.7
Pneumonia and influenza	26.2	28.0	22.1	12.9	13.5	13.6	13.2	14.3	13.8	14.0
Chronic liver disease and cirrhosis	8.5	10.5	14.7	12.2	9.7	9.3	9.2	9.1	9.0	8.6
Diabetes mellitus	14.3	13.6	14.1	10.1	9.7	9.7	9.8	10.2	11.6	11.7
Nephritis, nephrotic syndrome, and nephrosis	- - -	- - -	- - -	4.5	4.9	4.9	4.8	4.8	4.5	4.3
Septicemia	- - -	- - -	- - -	2.6	4.1	4.3	4.5	4.6	4.2	4.1
Atherosclerosis	- - -	- - -	- - -	5.7	4.0	3.7	3.6	3.5	3.0	2.7
Human immunodeficiency virus infection	- - -	- - -	- - -	- - -	- - -	- - -	5.5	6.7	8.7	9.8
External causes	73.9	65.7	77.4	66.1	55.9	57.4	56.2	56.7	55.6	55.1
Unintentional injuries	57.5	49.9	53.7	42.3	34.8	35.2	34.7	35.0	33.9	32.5
Motor vehicle crashes	23.3	22.5	27.4	22.9	18.8	19.4	19.4	19.7	18.9	18.5
Suicide	11.0	10.6	11.8	11.4	11.5	11.9	11.7	11.5	11.3	11.5
Homicide and legal intervention	5.4	5.2	9.1	10.8	8.3	9.0	8.6	9.0	9.4	10.2
Drug-induced causes	- - -	- - -	- - -	3.0	3.5	4.0	3.8	4.2	4.1	3.6
Alcohol-induced causes	- - -	- - -	- - -	8.4	7.0	6.7	6.8	7.1	7.3	7.2
White male										
All causes	963.1	917.7	893.4	745.3	693.3	684.9	674.2	671.3	652.2	644.3
Natural causes	860.1	825.8	788.6	651.2	613.4	603.1	594.9	592.2	575.3	567.6
Diseases of heart	381.1	375.4	347.6	277.5	246.2	236.7	228.1	223.0	208.7	202.0
Ischemic heart disease	- - -	- - -	- - -	218.0	182.1	171.3	163.3	157.6	150.2	145.3
Cerebrovascular diseases	87.0	80.3	68.8	41.9	33.0	31.2	30.6	30.3	28.4	27.7
Malignant neoplasms	130.9	141.6	154.3	160.5	160.4	160.2	160.1	159.6	159.4	160.3
Respiratory system	21.6	34.6	49.9	58.0	58.7	58.6	59.2	58.8	58.3	59.0
Colorectal	19.8	18.9	18.9	18.3	17.8	17.3	17.3	16.8	16.5	16.5
Prostate	13.1	12.4	12.3	13.2	13.4	13.9	13.8	14.2	14.7	15.3
Chronic obstructive pulmonary diseases	6.0	13.8	24.0	26.7	28.7	28.3	27.7	28.2	27.2	27.4
Pneumonia and influenza	27.1	31.0	26.0	16.2	17.5	17.6	16.9	18.2	17.1	17.5
Chronic liver disease and cirrhosis	11.6	14.4	18.8	15.7	12.7	12.3	12.2	12.3	12.1	11.5
Diabetes mellitus	11.3	11.6	12.7	9.5	9.2	9.1	9.6	9.7	11.1	11.3
Nephritis, nephrotic syndrome, and nephrosis	- - -	- - -	- - -	4.9	5.4	5.5	5.4	5.3	4.8	4.6
Septicemia	- - -	- - -	- - -	2.8	4.3	4.6	4.6	4.6	4.2	4.2
Atherosclerosis	- - -	- - -	- - -	6.5	4.6	4.3	4.2	4.0	3.5	3.2
Human immunodeficiency virus infection	- - -	- - -	- - -	- - -	- - -	- - -	8.4	10.0	13.2	15.0
External causes	103.0	91.9	104.8	94.1	80.0	81.8	79.2	79.1	76.9	76.7
Unintentional injuries	80.9	70.5	76.2	62.3	50.5	51.2	49.8	50.0	47.8	46.4
Motor vehicle crashes	35.9	34.0	40.1	34.8	27.6	28.7	28.3	28.4	26.7	26.3
Suicide	18.1	17.5	18.2	18.9	19.9	20.6	20.2	19.9	19.7	20.1
Homicide and legal intervention	3.9	3.9	7.3	10.9	8.1	8.4	7.8	7.8	8.1	8.9
Drug-induced causes	- - -	- - -	- - -	3.2	4.0	4.7	4.3	4.9	4.8	4.2
Alcohol-induced causes	- - -	- - -	- - -	10.8	9.2	9.0	9.2	9.5	9.9	9.9
Black male										
All causes	1,373.1	1,246.1	1,318.6	1,112.8	1,053.4	1,061.9	1,063.6	1,083.0	1,082.8	1,061.3
Natural causes	1,209.2	1,093.4	1,095.4	942.6	920.7	922.0	925.0	938.1	936.0	915.2
Diseases of heart	415.5	381.2	375.9	327.3	310.8	306.1	301.0	301.7	289.7	275.9
Ischemic heart disease	- - -	- - -	- - -	196.0	170.4	160.3	158.4	155.1	152.2	147.1
Cerebrovascular diseases	146.2	141.2	122.5	77.5	62.7	61.1	59.7	60.8	57.3	56.1
Malignant neoplasms	126.1	158.5	198.0	229.9	239.9	239.0	240.0	240.4	246.2	248.1
Respiratory system	16.9	36.6	60.8	82.0	87.7	87.9	88.9	88.7	90.8	91.0
Colorectal	13.8	15.0	17.3	19.2	20.2	20.2	20.8	20.1	20.7	21.6
Prostate	16.9	22.2	25.4	29.1	31.2	31.4	31.7	32.0	33.1	35.3
Chronic obstructive pulmonary diseases	- - -	- - -	- - -	20.9	24.8	25.6	25.2	27.4	26.5	26.5
Pneumonia and influenza	63.8	70.2	53.8	28.0	27.5	28.1	27.5	29.2	29.3	28.7
Chronic liver disease and cirrhosis	8.8	14.8	33.1	30.6	23.8	21.3	22.6	21.3	21.2	20.0
Diabetes mellitus	11.5	16.2	21.2	17.7	18.2	18.6	19.2	20.8	24.1	23.6
Nephritis, nephrotic syndrome, and nephrosis	- - -	- - -	- - -	14.2	14.5	14.7	14.0	14.0	14.7	12.9
Septicemia	- - -	- - -	- - -	8.0	12.2	12.8	13.0	12.8	11.8	11.6
Atherosclerosis	- - -	- - -	- - -	7.5	5.2	5.2	4.6	4.8	3.5	3.6
Human immunodeficiency virus infection	- - -	- - -	- - -	- - -	- - -	- - -	25.4	31.6	40.3	44.2

See footnotes at end of table.

[Data are based on the National Vital Statistics System]

Sex, race, and cause of death	1950 [1]	1960 [1]	1970	1980	1985	1986	1987	1988	1989	1990
Black male – Con.			Deaths per 100,000 resident population							
External causes	163.9	152.7	223.2	170.2	132.6	139.8	138.6	144.9	146.8	146.0
Unintentional injuries	105.7	100.0	119.5	82.0	67.6	68.0	68.0	70.4	68.8	62.4
Motor vehicle crashes	39.8	38.2	50.1	32.9	28.0	29.5	28.9	30.1	29.8	28.9
Suicide	7.0	7.8	9.9	11.1	11.5	11.6	12.1	11.9	12.6	12.4
Homicide and legal intervention	51.1	44.9	82.1	71.9	50.2	56.3	54.2	58.6	61.9	68.7
Drug-induced causes	- - -	- - -	- - -	5.8	8.9	10.5	11.3	12.9	11.4	8.4
Alcohol-induced causes	- - -	- - -	- - -	32.4	27.7	25.5	26.7	27.3	27.7	26.6
White female										
All causes	645.0	555.0	501.7	411.1	391.0	388.1	384.8	385.3	376.0	369.9
Natural causes	607.7	522.7	463.8	380.0	363.9	360.6	357.3	358.0	349.3	344.2
Diseases of heart	223.6	197.1	167.8	134.6	121.7	118.9	116.2	114.1	106.6	103.1
Ischemic heart disease	- - -	- - -	- - -	97.4	82.9	79.5	76.8	74.7	71.0	68.6
Cerebrovascular diseases	79.7	68.7	56.2	35.2	27.9	27.0	26.3	25.5	24.2	23.8
Malignant neoplasms	119.4	109.5	107.6	107.7	110.5	110.3	110.0	110.4	111.1	111.2
Respiratory system	4.6	5.1	10.1	18.2	22.7	23.1	23.9	24.9	25.9	26.5
Colorectal	19.0	17.0	15.3	13.3	12.3	12.0	11.8	11.5	11.1	10.9
Breast	22.5	22.4	23.4	22.8	23.4	23.1	22.9	23.1	23.1	22.9
Chronic obstructive pulmonary diseases	2.8	3.3	5.3	9.2	12.9	13.3	13.7	14.5	15.2	15.2
Pneumonia and influenza	18.9	19.0	15.0	9.4	9.9	9.9	9.7	10.7	10.4	10.6
Chronic liver disease and cirrhosis	5.8	6.6	8.7	7.0	5.6	5.4	5.1	5.1	5.0	4.8
Diabetes mellitus	16.4	13.7	12.8	8.7	8.1	8.1	8.1	8.4	9.6	9.5
Nephritis, nephrotic syndrome, and nephrosis	- - -	- - -	- - -	2.9	3.4	3.3	3.3	3.3	3.0	3.0
Septicemia	- - -	- - -	- - -	1.8	3.0	3.2	3.4	3.5	3.1	3.1
Atherosclerosis	- - -	- - -	- - -	5.0	3.5	3.2	3.2	3.0	2.6	2.4
Human immunodeficiency virus infection	- - -	- - -	- - -	- - -	- - -	- - -	0.6	0.7	0.9	1.1
External causes	37.3	32.3	37.9	31.1	27.1	27.5	27.4	27.3	26.7	25.7
Unintentional injuries	30.6	25.5	27.2	21.4	18.4	18.5	18.6	18.9	18.6	17.6
Motor vehicle crashes	10.6	11.1	14.4	12.3	10.8	11.0	11.4	11.6	11.6	11.0
Suicide	5.3	5.3	7.2	5.7	5.3	5.5	5.3	5.1	4.8	4.8
Homicide and legal intervention	1.4	1.5	2.2	3.2	2.9	2.9	2.9	2.9	2.8	2.8
Drug-induced causes	- - -	- - -	- - -	2.6	2.5	2.7	2.5	2.7	2.6	2.5
Alcohol-induced causes	- - -	- - -	- - -	3.5	2.8	2.7	2.6	2.7	2.8	2.8
Black female										
All causes	1,106.7	916.9	814.4	631.1	594.8	594.1	592.4	601.0	594.3	581.6
Natural causes	1,054.8	867.3	757.9	588.4	559.8	557.6	555.4	562.2	556.3	545.1
Diseases of heart	349.5	292.6	251.7	201.1	188.3	186.6	182.6	183.3	175.6	168.1
Ischemic heart disease	- - -	- - -	- - -	116.1	101.6	97.8	94.5	94.1	92.3	88.8
Cerebrovascular diseases	155.6	139.5	107.9	61.7	50.6	47.9	47.1	47.1	45.5	42.7
Malignant neoplasms	131.9	127.8	123.5	129.7	131.8	133.7	133.9	133.5	133.5	137.2
Respiratory system	4.1	5.5	10.9	19.5	22.8	23.7	24.7	25.2	26.0	27.5
Colorectal	15.0	15.4	16.1	15.3	16.2	15.3	15.7	15.1	15.1	15.5
Breast	19.3	21.3	21.5	23.3	25.5	26.2	26.9	27.5	26.5	27.5
Chronic obstructive pulmonary diseases	- - -	- - -	- - -	6.3	8.8	9.0	9.6	10.2	11.1	10.7
Pneumonia and influenza	50.4	43.9	29.2	12.7	12.5	13.2	12.3	13.6	14.0	13.7
Chronic liver disease and cirrhosis	5.7	8.9	17.8	14.4	10.2	9.4	9.2	9.5	8.7	8.7
Diabetes mellitus	22.7	27.3	30.9	22.1	21.3	21.6	21.6	22.5	24.6	25.4
Nephritis, nephrotic syndrome, and nephrosis	- - -	- - -	- - -	10.3	10.6	10.0	9.9	10.5	9.7	9.4
Septicemia	- - -	- - -	- - -	5.4	8.1	8.2	9.2	9.1	8.5	8.0
Atherosclerosis	- - -	- - -	- - -	5.6	3.8	3.5	3.4	3.3	2.9	2.7
Human immunodeficiency virus infection	- - -	- - -	- - -	- - -	- - -	- - -	4.7	6.2	8.1	9.9
External causes	51.9	49.6	56.5	42.7	35.0	36.6	37.0	38.7	38.0	36.6
Unintentional injuries	38.5	35.9	35.3	25.1	20.9	21.2	21.2	22.4	21.9	20.4
Motor vehicle crashes	10.3	10.0	13.8	8.4	8.2	8.5	8.8	9.4	9.3	9.3
Suicide	1.7	1.9	2.9	2.4	2.1	2.4	2.1	2.5	2.4	2.4
Homicide and legal intervention	11.7	11.8	15.0	13.7	10.9	11.9	12.5	12.8	12.7	13.0
Drug-induced causes	- - -	- - -	- - -	2.7	3.3	3.7	4.1	4.4	4.1	3.4
Alcohol-induced causes	- - -	- - -	- - -	10.6	8.0	7.1	7.3	7.9	7.8	7.7

[1]Includes deaths of nonresidents of the United States.
[2]Male only.
[3]Female only.

NOTES: For data years shown, the code numbers for cause of death are based on the then current International Classification of Diseases, which are described in Appendix II, tables IV and V. Categories for the coding and classification of human immunodeficiency virus infection were introduced in the United States beginning with mortality data for 1987. Data for the 1980's have been revised based on intercensal population estimates and differ from previous editions of Health, United States. See Appendix I, Department of Commerce.

SOURCES: Centers for Disease Control and Prevention, National Center for Health Statistics: Vital Statistics Rates in the United States, 1940–1960, by R. D. Grove and A. M. Hetzel. DHEW Pub. No. (PHS) 1677. Public Health Service. Washington. U.S. Government Printing Office, 1968; Vital Statistics of the United States, Vol. II, Mortality, Part A, for data years 1960–90. Public Health Service. Washington. U.S. Government Printing Office; Data computed by the Division of Analysis from data compiled by the Division of Vital Statistics and from table 1.

Table 29 (page 1 of 2). Years of potential life lost before age 65 for selected causes of death, according to sex and race: United States, selected years 1970–90

[Data are based on the National Vital Statistics System]

Sex, race, and cause of death	1970	1980	1982	1983	1984	1985	1986	1987	1988	1989	1990
All races											

Sex, race, and cause of death	1970	1980	1982	1983	1984	1985	1986	1987	1988	1989	1990
All races	Years lost per 100,000 population under 65 years of age										
All causes	8,595.9	6,416.0	5,900.1	5,706.1	5,647.4	5,660.2	5,728.1	5,677.6	5,726.6	5,708.9	5,623.0
Diseases of heart	1,108.9	841.3	792.7	784.9	765.7	752.6	737.5	714.7	692.5	653.0	632.2
Ischemic heart disease	- - -	544.3	508.0	485.3	464.4	448.4	422.3	403.2	380.9	364.3	350.0
Cerebrovascular diseases	241.1	140.8	128.0	124.7	124.6	119.6	116.6	116.6	116.1	110.1	110.7
Malignant neoplasms	1,013.0	907.5	887.7	877.0	878.1	875.3	867.8	854.4	851.8	847.6	848.6
Respiratory system	190.7	211.9	210.5	209.0	208.5	207.6	204.3	205.4	204.7	202.1	203.0
Colorectal	78.9	68.7	66.5	65.8	65.8	65.1	63.1	64.7	62.5	59.4	60.6
Prostate [1]	8.2	8.5	8.3	8.7	8.4	8.4	8.5	8.2	8.5	8.7	8.7
Breast [2]	115.6	105.5	105.3	103.7	108.0	107.1	107.9	107.7	109.0	109.0	109.4
Chronic obstructive pulmonary diseases	73.2	57.2	57.8	60.0	58.8	61.1	60.9	62.0	62.2	62.7	61.0
Pneumonia and influenza	392.1	97.5	79.4	79.5	78.9	81.1	83.1	80.9	84.7	85.3	81.2
Chronic liver disease and cirrhosis	187.8	145.3	122.4	118.1	116.0	113.7	109.7	110.6	110.5	108.0	103.1
Diabetes mellitus	80.6	56.2	53.9	56.4	53.9	54.8	57.4	57.8	62.3	67.3	67.0
Human immunodeficiency virus infection	- - -	- - -	- - -	- - -	- - -	- - -	- - -	170.9	207.3	271.1	303.4
Unintentional injuries	1,599.1	1,373.1	1,172.0	1,115.2	1,101.6	1,087.9	1,117.1	1,084.1	1,083.0	1,034.2	984.7
Motor vehicle crashes	889.4	840.8	694.4	659.9	674.1	660.8	689.8	677.9	676.8	636.1	615.5
Suicide	250.2	309.0	312.8	306.2	313.6	313.5	322.1	315.5	312.8	308.7	312.0
Homicide and legal intervention	271.8	373.6	336.5	299.2	293.2	291.7	322.3	308.5	326.5	340.2	374.3
White male											
All causes	9,757.4	7,611.5	6,988.9	6,729.5	6,670.3	6,697.6	6,770.4	6,632.2	6,646.2	6,559.9	6,503.1
Diseases of heart	1,607.4	1,179.1	1,118.6	1,091.2	1,061.1	1,034.8	1,004.2	967.2	928.9	874.6	847.7
Ischemic heart disease	- - -	869.7	809.4	770.1	734.5	707.8	664.8	629.3	590.7	564.6	545.5
Cerebrovascular diseases	215.0	122.6	111.6	110.0	108.3	104.5	100.2	101.2	100.8	93.7	93.9
Malignant neoplasms	1,036.9	935.1	903.1	888.9	884.7	887.5	881.0	861.5	854.4	842.9	843.1
Respiratory system	287.8	286.0	278.8	271.7	270.8	266.8	261.9	262.6	259.0	251.7	251.6
Colorectal	81.2	73.5	71.8	72.2	72.0	71.2	69.0	70.9	68.8	65.6	66.1
Prostate	14.4	15.2	15.4	16.0	15.5	15.0	15.8	15.2	15.5	16.1	16.2
Chronic obstructive pulmonary diseases	88.8	64.2	63.6	64.4	63.8	63.2	64.0	63.3	63.0	61.7	60.3
Pneumonia and influenza	353.2	88.7	74.1	74.0	75.5	77.6	81.6	77.0	81.4	80.0	76.3
Chronic liver disease and cirrhosis	209.8	166.9	150.4	143.0	141.7	136.8	134.2	136.9	140.6	139.8	132.5
Diabetes mellitus	75.3	52.5	52.6	52.9	52.7	53.9	55.8	58.8	62.0	67.7	65.7
Human immunodeficiency virus infection	- - -	- - -	- - -	- - -	- - -	- - -	- - -	254.3	302.2	401.7	451.2
Unintentional injuries	2,261.3	2,071.0	1,771.5	1,666.9	1,639.4	1,606.9	1,647.6	1,576.3	1,563.9	1,468.9	1,420.1
Motor vehicle crashes	1,296.5	1,301.7	1,071.3	1,005.6	1,019.3	985.2	1,032.7	999.2	989.2	907.4	886.8
Suicide	369.6	509.0	518.6	510.4	526.4	529.4	548.0	533.1	529.9	520.7	532.3
Homicide and legal intervention	201.9	365.4	320.4	286.1	278.6	275.0	292.6	265.4	267.8	279.9	313.3
Black male											
All causes	20,283.5	14,381.9	12,973.6	12,442.4	12,308.9	12,675.5	13,287.7	13,564.8	14,059.5	14,412.5	14,365.8
Diseases of heart	2,022.2	1,661.4	1,510.8	1,552.9	1,538.7	1,561.7	1,556.2	1,514.6	1,514.2	1,458.8	1,387.8
Ischemic heart disease	- - -	800.9	740.0	704.3	697.3	684.9	642.8	621.1	602.7	598.2	552.5
Cerebrovascular diseases	595.6	349.3	309.3	293.6	302.6	295.8	295.1	288.2	300.7	283.2	279.9
Malignant neoplasms	1,216.0	1,175.8	1,160.9	1,141.2	1,167.9	1,141.3	1,121.7	1,093.8	1,109.2	1,125.0	1,131.9
Respiratory system	376.7	400.4	388.2	384.2	390.9	386.0	375.3	366.0	360.6	368.6	378.2
Colorectal	80.8	76.7	79.8	75.9	81.9	79.4	76.8	83.9	82.5	80.7	83.8
Prostate	35.2	34.1	30.0	31.3	30.5	33.1	29.4	28.4	31.1	30.2	30.5
Chronic obstructive pulmonary diseases	146.8	110.8	111.4	114.7	107.8	114.6	116.9	122.4	122.5	120.3	121.9
Pneumonia and influenza	1,308.9	315.2	254.2	257.6	244.2	254.9	249.3	261.3	274.1	275.1	261.4
Chronic liver disease and cirrhosis	463.5	391.9	298.5	288.7	289.5	305.8	282.0	296.8	276.0	269.4	242.4
Diabetes mellitus	144.0	102.2	94.3	106.0	106.4	106.1	108.2	108.6	126.4	139.6	133.7
Human immunodeficiency virus infection	- - -	- - -	- - -	- - -	- - -	- - -	- - -	719.7	892.7	1,124.3	1,224.5
Unintentional injuries	3,500.6	2,308.9	1,948.8	1,865.3	1,874.9	1,891.1	1,979.9	1,985.0	2,003.8	1,945.8	1,807.4
Motor vehicle crashes	1,466.1	1,022.4	857.7	832.5	872.7	893.7	967.7	943.2	964.3	938.7	919.9
Suicide	237.5	323.8	318.3	305.4	324.1	336.9	340.2	356.1	369.2	394.0	376.3
Homicide and legal intervention	2,234.6	2,274.9	2,030.1	1,760.2	1,664.0	1,689.1	1,956.0	1,924.0	2,148.2	2,287.7	2,580.7

See footnotes at end of table.

Table 29 (page 2 of 2). Years of potential life lost before age 65 for selected causes of death, according to sex and race: United States, selected years 1970–90

[Data are based on the National Vital Statistics System]

Sex, race, and cause of death	1970	1980	1982	1983	1984	1985	1986	1987	1988	1989	1990
White female				Years lost per 100,000 population under 65 years of age							
All causes.	5,527.4	3,983.2	3,729.5	3,631.1	3,594.0	3,542.3	3,519.0	3,484.4	3,475.0	3,433.9	3,330.7
Diseases of heart	497.4	401.2	384.0	385.9	377.2	369.4	363.8	357.2	344.1	317.3	309.6
Ischemic heart disease.	- - -	227.9	216.6	211.0	202.4	195.4	185.5	181.5	171.9	160.8	155.9
Cerebrovascular diseases	180.1	111.6	100.7	97.5	98.5	93.0	90.5	89.8	87.2	82.8	84.5
Malignant neoplasms	974.6	858.3	852.3	843.1	847.7	846.4	834.4	827.1	828.8	831.9	829.1
Respiratory system	89.8	132.6	139.1	142.2	141.8	144.9	142.8	145.8	149.4	148.7	150.2
Colorectal.	77.0	64.0	60.1	59.7	59.3	57.9	56.9	56.4	54.1	51.8	52.2
Breast.	233.4	211.7	211.5	207.8	214.8	215.1	213.4	212.7	215.4	217.2	217.5
Chronic obstructive pulmonary diseases.	46.5	43.0	44.7	48.2	47.3	51.8	50.7	52.4	51.6	55.2	52.7
Pneumonia and influenza.	247.2	64.0	49.2	52.6	50.3	52.1	51.8	49.4	51.6	52.0	50.5
Chronic liver disease and cirrhosis	114.7	79.1	64.6	63.7	60.9	58.9	56.9	54.5	54.2	51.3	51.3
Diabetes mellitus.	65.1	45.4	44.2	47.1	42.4	43.2	46.4	44.6	47.7	52.1	52.0
Human immunodeficiency virus infection	- - -	- - -	- - -	- - -	- - -	- - -	- - -	19.0	23.9	31.2	35.0
Unintentional injuries.	755.6	647.8	552.3	538.8	542.9	532.4	542.5	543.1	541.4	534.9	494.2
Motor vehicle crashes	466.5	437.3	364.9	355.1	371.2	364.2	372.8	383.1	383.9	377.4	351.6
Suicide.	157.2	145.4	148.4	142.6	143.0	137.7	140.6	137.7	132.5	127.3	126.3
Homicide and legal intervention	69.7	109.3	107.7	93.1	100.1	98.1	102.7	100.3	99.7	97.6	97.5
Black female											
All causes.	12,188.8	7,927.2	7,194.7	7,057.6	6,958.2	6,961.4	7,108.0	7,211.7	7,455.1	7,542.7	7,382.2
Diseases of heart	1,292.7	937.2	858.2	871.4	853.1	856.7	868.6	832.0	845.7	811.5	782.4
Ischemic heart disease.	- - -	382.7	364.9	349.8	333.2	325.1	310.0	296.2	296.9	287.7	272.3
Cerebrovascular diseases	564.7	289.0	271.7	262.4	250.9	248.8	240.9	243.2	241.5	234.9	235.8
Malignant neoplasms	1,044.8	968.4	946.3	944.2	954.1	936.8	975.7	971.6	960.7	939.9	972.7
Respiratory system	89.3	132.8	132.9	138.8	133.2	137.6	139.5	145.5	137.9	144.8	149.0
Colorectal.	81.4	70.3	75.5	67.9	67.0	74.7	69.3	71.7	72.4	65.7	72.9
Breast.	209.3	210.9	221.5	222.3	247.0	236.4	260.2	263.8	271.5	257.3	264.1
Chronic obstructive pulmonary diseases.	93.3	62.5	71.9	72.1	71.1	74.5	72.3	78.3	86.0	80.4	80.6
Pneumonia and influenza.	888.7	187.4	148.9	133.9	142.6	141.1	154.2	145.9	154.0	163.3	145.6
Chronic liver disease and cirrhosis	295.6	210.9	162.2	159.8	149.0	146.7	139.3	139.9	131.1	118.9	122.7
Diabetes mellitus.	179.7	109.3	99.7	107.6	99.6	100.8	105.4	103.0	113.5	113.8	125.8
Human immunodeficiency virus infection	- - -	- - -	- - -	- - -	- - -	- - -	- - -	170.7	218.0	280.9	336.7
Unintentional injuries.	1,169.9	718.5	651.4	650.9	600.4	616.8	649.3	634.9	692.3	662.3	614.4
Motor vehicle crashes	478.4	296.8	276.1	262.3	269.4	283.1	293.3	304.5	328.2	315.2	305.6
Suicide.	81.9	70.3	65.7	68.0	66.0	59.1	66.1	66.9	74.2	75.0	69.8
Homicide and legal intervention	460.3	492.0	431.0	414.6	421.3	399.8	447.7	467.4	495.8	481.4	509.8

[1]Male only.
[2]Female only.

NOTES: For data years shown, the code numbers for cause of death are based on the International Classification of Diseases, Ninth Revision, described in Appendix II, table V. International Classification of Diseases codes for human immunodeficiency virus infection not available for use with the National Vital Statistics System until 1987. Years of potential life lost before age 65 provides a measure of the impact of mortality on the population under 65 years of age. See Appendix II for method of calculation. Data for the 1980's have been revised based on intercensal population estimates and differ from previous editions of Health, United States. See Appendix I, Department of Commerce.

SOURCES: Centers for Disease Control and Prevention, National Center for Health Statistics: Vital Statistics of the United States, Vol. II, Mortality, Part A, for data years 1970–90. Public Health Service. Washington. U.S. Government Printing Office; Data computed by the Division of Analysis from data compiled by the Division of Vital Statistics and from table 1.

Table 30 (page 1 of 3). Numbers of deaths and rank for selected causes of death, according to sex and detailed race: United States, 1985–90

[Data are based on the National Vital Statistics System]

Sex, race, and cause of death	1985	1986	1987	1988	1989	1990	1985	1986	1987	1988	1989	1990
All races	Number						Rank					
All causes	2,086,440	2,105,361	2,123,323	2,167,999	2,150,466	2,148,463	...	...	...	...	...	...
Diseases of heart	771,169	765,490	760,353	765,156	733,867	720,058	1	1	1	1	1	1
Cerebrovascular diseases	153,050	149,643	149,835	150,517	145,551	144,088	3	3	3	3	3	3
Malignant neoplasms	461,563	469,376	476,927	485,048	496,152	505,322	2	2	2	2	2	2
Chronic obstructive pulmonary diseases	74,662	76,559	78,380	82,853	84,344	86,679	5	5	5	5	5	5
Pneumonia and influenza	67,615	69,812	69,225	77,662	76,550	79,513	6	6	6	6	6	6
Chronic liver disease and cirrhosis	26,767	26,159	26,201	26,409	26,694	25,815	9	9	9	9	9	9
Diabetes mellitus	36,969	37,184	38,532	40,368	46,833	47,664	7	7	7	7	7	7
Nephritis, nephrotic syndrome, and nephrosis	21,349	21,767	22,052	22,392	21,118	20,764	11	11	11	10	12	12
Septicemia	17,182	18,795	19,916	20,925	19,333	19,169	14	13	13	13	14	13
Atherosclerosis	23,926	22,706	22,474	22,086	19,357	18,047	10	10	10	11	13	14
Human immunodeficiency virus infection	- - -	- - -	13,468	16,602	22,082	25,188	- - -	- - -	15	15	11	10
Unintentional injuries	93,457	95,277	95,020	97,100	95,028	91,983	4	4	4	4	4	4
Suicide	29,453	30,904	30,796	30,407	30,232	30,906	8	8	8	8	8	8
Homicide and legal intervention	19,893	21,731	21,103	22,032	22,909	24,932	12	12	12	12	10	11
White male												
All causes	950,455	952,554	953,382	965,419	950,852	950,812	...	...	...	...	...	...
Diseases of heart	355,374	347,967	342,063	341,519	325,397	319,362	1	1	1	1	1	1
Cerebrovascular diseases	51,965	50,365	50,237	50,692	48,563	48,024	4	4	4	4	4	4
Malignant neoplasms	215,079	218,381	221,757	224,514	228,301	232,608	2	2	2	2	2	2
Chronic obstructive pulmonary diseases	43,074	43,341	43,290	44,827	44,046	45,234	5	5	5	5	5	5
Pneumonia and influenza	29,028	29,891	29,284	32,262	30,892	32,101	6	6	6	6	6	6
Chronic liver disease and cirrhosis	14,321	14,099	14,175	14,381	14,414	13,889	8	8	8	8	9	10
Diabetes mellitus	12,758	12,788	13,553	14,008	16,282	16,817	9	9	9	9	8	8
Nephritis, nephrotic syndrome, and nephrosis	8,482	8,754	8,800	8,786	8,093	8,021	10	10	10	11	12	12
Septicemia	6,321	6,962	7,096	7,270	6,728	6,786	14	13	14	14	13	13
Atherosclerosis	8,251	7,767	7,686	7,529	6,652	6,232	11	12	13	13	14	14
Human immunodeficiency virus infection	- - -	- - -	8,700	10,479	14,114	16,106	- - -	- - -	11	10	10	9
Unintentional injuries	53,856	54,864	53,936	54,435	52,691	51,348	3	3	3	3	3	3
Suicide	21,256	22,270	22,188	21,980	21,858	22,448	7	7	7	7	7	7
Homicide and legal intervention	8,122	8,567	7,979	7,994	8,337	9,147	12	11	12	12	11	11
Black male												
All causes	133,610	137,214	139,551	144,228	146,393	145,359	...	...	...	...	...	...
Diseases of heart	38,982	39,076	38,934	39,584	38,321	37,038	1	1	1	1	1	1
Cerebrovascular diseases	8,000	7,938	7,852	8,098	7,739	7,653	4	4	4	5	5	5
Malignant neoplasms	29,028	29,363	29,928	30,321	31,452	31,995	2	2	2	2	2	2
Chronic obstructive pulmonary diseases	3,154	3,302	3,319	3,644	3,593	3,628	8	8	8	9	9	9
Pneumonia and influenza	3,664	3,836	3,795	4,047	4,168	4,161	6	6	6	7	7	7
Chronic liver disease and cirrhosis	2,616	2,404	2,574	2,476	2,517	2,393	9	9	10	11	11	11
Diabetes mellitus	2,230	2,295	2,388	2,640	3,072	3,049	10	10	11	10	10	10
Nephritis, nephrotic syndrome, and nephrosis	1,935	1,963	1,905	1,908	2,047	1,806	11	11	12	12	12	12
Septicemia	1,595	1,697	1,760	1,729	1,643	1,624	12	12	13	13	14	14
Atherosclerosis	758	756	680	739	547	563	16	15	17	17	17	17
Human immunodeficiency virus infection	- - -	- - -	3,301	4,202	5,475	6,097	- - -	- - -	9	6	6	6
Unintentional injuries	8,752	9,035	9,159	9,608	9,503	8,756	3	3	3	3	3	4
Suicide	1,481	1,537	1,635	1,648	1,771	1,737	13	13	14	14	13	13
Homicide and legal intervention	6,616	7,634	7,518	8,314	8,888	9,981	5	5	5	4	4	3
American Indian male												
All causes	4,181	4,365	4,432	4,617	5,066	4,877	...	...	...	...	...	...
Diseases of heart	1,001	999	1,062	1,048	1,184	1,106	1	1	1	1	1	1
Cerebrovascular diseases	157	140	180	171	193	164	7	7	5	7	6	8
Malignant neoplasms	533	522	496	594	706	629	3	3	3	3	3	3
Chronic obstructive pulmonary diseases	89	107	102	112	143	141	10	9	10	10	10	10
Pneumonia and influenza	151	138	153	147	165	170	8	8	8	8	8	7
Chronic liver disease and cirrhosis	173	176	168	193	214	184	4	6	6	4	4	5
Diabetes mellitus	102	97	111	124	155	152	9	10	9	9	9	9
Nephritis, nephrotic syndrome, and nephrosis	36	43	53	50	43	58	13	14	12	13	13	13
Septicemia	30	44	33	35	36	50	14	13	14	14	14	14
Atherosclerosis	12	22	17	19	17	17	16	15	15	16	17	16
Human immunodeficiency virus infection	- - -	- - -	17	26	28	33	- - -	- - -	15	15	15	15
Unintentional injuries	804	871	884	900	885	883	2	2	2	2	2	2
Suicide	172	181	186	192	197	214	5	5	4	5	5	4
Homicide and legal intervention	161	194	158	178	177	177	6	4	7	6	7	6

See footnotes at end of table.

[Data are based on the National Vital Statistics System]

Sex, race, and cause of death	1985	1986	1987	1988	1989	1990	1985	1986	1987	1988	1989	1990
Asian or Pacific Islander male			Number						Rank			
All causes	9,441	9,795	10,496	11,155	11,688	12,211	...	...	...	...	...	...
Diseases of heart	2,837	2,853	3,137	3,225	3,240	3,238	1	1	1	1	1	1
Cerebrovascular diseases	658	718	788	791	821	853	4	4	4	4	3	4
Malignant neoplasms	2,262	2,281	2,454	2,639	2,821	3,021	2	2	2	2	2	2
Chronic obstructive pulmonary diseases	276	308	327	353	391	412	6	6	6	6	6	6
Pneumonia and influenza	315	334	329	376	473	462	5	5	5	5	5	5
Chronic liver disease and cirrhosis	133	115	133	145	161	160	11	12	11	11	12	10
Diabetes mellitus	172	186	183	200	217	244	8	9	9	9	9	9
Nephritis, nephrotic syndrome, and nephrosis	98	101	113	134	134	119	13	13	12	13	13	14
Septicemia	71	82	79	97	81	79	14	14	14	15	15	15
Atherosclerosis	40	42	44	40	38	47	16	16	17	19	20	18
Human immunodeficiency virus infection	- - -	- - -	69	99	132	149	- - -	- - -	15	14	14	12
Unintentional injuries	734	791	827	864	809	935	3	3	3	3	4	3
Suicide	230	237	257	255	270	318	7	7	7	7	8	7
Homicide and legal intervention	164	195	190	221	279	289	9	8	8	8	7	8
White female												
All causes	868,599	878,529	889,685	911,487	902,989	902,442	...	...	...	...	...	...
Diseases of heart	332,778	333,396	333,669	337,007	323,469	318,002	1	1	1	1	1	1
Cerebrovascular diseases	81,067	79,641	79,810	79,383	76,953	76,502	3	3	3	3	3	3
Malignant neoplasms	190,648	193,971	196,716	200,626	205,855	208,977	2	2	2	2	2	2
Chronic obstructive pulmonary diseases	26,364	27,781	29,378	31,846	33,835	34,945	5	5	5	5	5	5
Pneumonia and influenza	31,480	32,432	32,527	37,308	36,961	38,705	4	4	4	4	4	4
Chronic liver disease and cirrhosis	7,871	7,817	7,591	7,543	7,797	7,589	10	11	11	11	11	11
Diabetes mellitus	17,547	17,496	17,842	18,684	21,771	21,879	7	7	7	7	7	7
Nephritis, nephrotic syndrome, and nephrosis	8,564	8,692	8,964	9,129	8,514	8,550	9	9	9	10	10	10
Septicemia	7,419	8,194	8,840	9,673	8,829	8,670	11	10	10	9	9	9
Atherosclerosis	13,770	13,091	13,040	12,732	11,139	10,315	8	8	8	8	8	8
Human immunodeficiency virus infection	- - -	- - -	628	788	981	1,149	- - -	- - -	24	24	23	23
Unintentional injuries	25,155	25,451	25,874	26,656	26,448	25,586	6	6	6	6	6	6
Suicide	5,831	6,167	6,029	5,810	5,566	5,638	12	12	12	12	12	12
Homicide and legal intervention	3,041	3,123	3,149	3,072	2,971	3,006	17	17	16	18	18	18
Black female												
All causes	110,597	113,112	115,263	119,791	121,249	120,139	...	...	...	...	...	...
Diseases of heart	37,702	38,650	38,813	39,882	39,110	38,073	1	1	1	1	1	1
Cerebrovascular diseases	10,341	10,014	10,055	10,381	10,240	9,754	3	3	3	3	3	3
Malignant neoplasms	21,878	22,616	23,099	23,647	24,112	25,082	2	2	2	2	2	2
Chronic obstructive pulmonary diseases	1,505	1,554	1,733	1,832	2,078	2,027	11	11	11	11	9	10
Pneumonia and influenza	2,674	2,864	2,770	3,144	3,417	3,402	7	6	6	6	6	6
Chronic liver disease and cirrhosis	1,439	1,341	1,342	1,427	1,334	1,360	12	12	12	12	12	13
Diabetes mellitus	3,874	4,004	4,109	4,332	4,883	5,065	4	4	4	4	4	4
Nephritis, nephrotic syndrome, and nephrosis	2,109	2,057	2,070	2,249	2,119	2,049	8	8	8	8	8	9
Septicemia	1,662	1,720	1,988	2,011	1,912	1,841	10	10	9	10	11	11
Atherosclerosis	1,022	964	942	955	889	817	13	15	15	15	16	16
Human immunodeficiency virus infection	- - -	- - -	739	995	1,320	1,633	- - -	- - -	16	14	13	12
Unintentional injuries	3,455	3,550	3,618	3,879	3,901	3,663	5	5	5	5	5	5
Suicide	314	355	328	374	382	374	19	19	19	20	19	20
Homicide and legal intervention	1,666	1,861	1,969	2,089	2,074	2,163	9	9	10	9	10	8
American Indian female												
All causes	2,973	2,936	3,170	3,300	3,548	3,439	...	...	...	...	...	...
Diseases of heart	732	683	755	777	860	807	1	1	1	1	1	1
Cerebrovascular diseases	189	175	185	200	181	201	4	4	4	4	5	4
Malignant neoplasms	456	466	549	557	612	646	2	2	2	2	2	2
Chronic obstructive pulmonary diseases	51	46	71	66	85	91	10	12	8	8	8	8
Pneumonia and influenza	99	85	110	131	142	147	7	7	7	7	7	7
Chronic liver disease and cirrhosis	147	124	134	162	172	154	6	6	6	6	6	6
Diabetes mellitus	150	137	158	187	211	198	5	5	5	5	4	5
Nephritis, nephrotic syndrome, and nephrosis	56	74	63	53	59	54	8	8	9	10	11	10
Septicemia	39	33	37	50	35	38	12	14	14	12	13	13
Atherosclerosis	26	26	20	26	29	17	15	15	15	15	15	15
Human immunodeficiency virus infection	- - -	- - -	3	. . .	8	3	- - -	- - -	26	. . .	23	29
Unintentional injuries	306	339	305	306	318	299	3	3	3	3	3	3
Suicide	38	37	39	36	35	38	14	13	13	14	13	13
Homicide and legal intervention	39	55	51	50	72	51	12	11	11	12	10	11

See footnotes at end of table.

Table 30 (page 3 of 3). Numbers of deaths and rank for selected causes of death, according to sex and detailed race: United States, 1985–90

[Data are based on the National Vital Statistics System]

Sex, race, and cause of death	1985	1986	1987	1988	1989	1990	1985	1986	1987	1988	1989	1990
Asian or Pacific Islander female	Number						Rank					
All causes.	6,446	6,719	7,193	7,808	8,354	8,916	. . .	. . .	. . .	. . .	. . .	. . .
Diseases of heart	1,729	1,834	1,875	2,065	2,186	2,360	1	1	2	2	2	1
Cerebrovascular diseases	669	641	719	789	846	924	3	3	3	3	3	3
Malignant neoplasms.	1,649	1,752	1,902	2,115	2,236	2,302	2	2	1	1	1	2
Chronic obstructive pulmonary diseases	146	120	159	168	167	199	6	8	7	7	7	7
Pneumonia and influenza.	201	226	253	242	328	355	5	5	5	5	5	5
Chronic liver disease and cirrhosis	66	78	82	78	79	85	13	13	12	13	13	13
Diabetes mellitus.	132	175	184	188	231	256	7	6	6	6	6	6
Nephritis, nephrotic syndrome, and nephrosis . . .	68	81	83	80	105	103	12	12	11	12	11	12
Septicemia.	44	62	80	59	68	77	15	14	13	14	14	14
Atherosclerosis.	46	37	43	46	46	39	14	15	15	15	15	16
Human immunodeficiency virus infection.	- - -	- - -	10	8	14	16	- - -	- - -	24	27	24	22
Unintentional injuries	380	366	407	433	442	487	4	4	4	4	4	4
Suicide.	123	118	126	109	143	131	9	9	9	10	8	10
Homicide and legal intervention	79	97	79	109	102	107	11	11	14	10	12	11

NOTES: For data years shown, the code numbers for cause of death are based on the International Classification of Diseases, Ninth Revision, described in Appendix II, table V. Categories for the coding and classification of human immunodeficiency virus infection were introduced in the United States beginning with mortality data for 1987. The number of HIV infection deaths based on the National Vital Statistics System differs from the number of deaths among AIDS cases reported to the CDC AIDS Surveillance System. See Appendix I.

SOURCES: Centers for Disease Control and Prevention, National Center for Health Statistics: Vital Statistics of the United States, Vol. II, Mortality, Part A, for data years 1985–90. Public Health Service. Washington. U.S. Government Printing Office; Data computed by the Division of Analysis from data compiled by the Division of Vital Statistics.

Table 31 (page 1 of 7). Death rates for selected causes of death, according to detailed race, Hispanic origin, age, and sex: United States, 1980–82, 1985–87, and 1988–90

[Data are based on the National Vital Statistics System]

Cause of death, race, and age	Both sexes			Male			Female		
	1980–82	1985–87	1988–90	1980–82	1985–87	1988–90	1980–82	1985–87	1988–90
All causes									
All races			Deaths per 100,000 resident population						
All ages, age adjusted [1]	568.6	544.2	528.6	753.7	715.3	690.7	420.9	407.5	397.4
All ages, crude	863.3	876.7	873.0	955.3	944.1	928.9	776.4	812.7	819.9
1–14 years	38.1	33.9	32.3	44.5	39.8	37.3	31.4	27.7	27.1
15–24 years	107.7	97.8	99.1	159.9	143.4	145.7	54.5	50.9	50.5
25–44 years	166.4	166.4	176.5	228.5	232.1	249.6	105.7	101.7	104.3
45–64 years	940.2	884.9	826.1	1,243.5	1,149.5	1,064.1	664.8	642.4	606.4
65–74 years	2,929.6	2,828.1	2,701.6	4,005.3	3,785.9	3,572.7	2,106.0	2,087.2	2,022.9
75–84 years	6,482.6	6,308.9	6,102.4	8,567.3	8,364.9	8,002.9	5,254.7	5,097.5	4,969.6
85 years and over	15,404.8	15,618.5	15,502.3	18,262.5	18,386.5	18,195.4	14,189.5	14,520.4	14,456.3
White									
All ages, age adjusted [1]	544.6	519.5	501.1	724.5	684.1	655.0	401.4	388.0	376.6
All ages, crude	881.4	900.2	896.6	966.0	958.3	941.0	800.9	844.7	854.0
1–14 years	35.6	31.2	29.4	41.7	36.8	34.0	29.2	25.3	24.4
15–24 years	104.9	93.9	91.0	155.7	137.2	132.1	52.7	49.0	47.8
25–44 years	146.0	145.5	152.3	199.6	202.6	215.6	92.5	88.1	88.4
45–64 years	886.8	833.7	772.5	1,174.9	1,083.7	993.8	621.6	601.2	564.6
65–74 years	2,864.1	2,755.6	2,624.5	3,939.3	3,698.7	3,476.4	2,038.5	2,020.3	1,954.4
75–84 years	6,464.5	6,267.2	6,053.9	8,594.6	8,341.9	7,959.3	5,222.1	5,051.3	4,919.8
85 years and over	15,658.7	15,814.9	15,659.4	18,609.3	18,696.9	18,444.1	14,423.8	14,692.4	14,596.0
Black									
All ages, age adjusted [1]	808.5	795.6	800.0	1,070.2	1,059.8	1,073.3	604.9	593.8	591.1
All ages, crude	845.3	863.0	881.0	995.5	999.5	1,018.6	710.8	740.5	757.4
1–14 years	53.0	49.2	49.0	61.7	57.3	56.5	44.2	40.9	41.3
15–24 years	127.6	125.7	152.0	191.7	188.9	236.4	66.1	64.1	68.7
25–44 years	334.1	337.4	371.0	485.3	491.5	543.1	204.5	203.4	219.9
45–64 years	1,523.1	1,446.6	1,406.9	2,045.6	1,931.0	1,888.2	1,099.7	1,055.4	1,019.0
65–74 years	3,811.2	3,854.5	3,794.2	5,034.8	5,149.8	5,063.1	2,928.2	2,947.2	2,911.5
75–84 years	7,080.8	7,193.0	7,077.8	8,862.7	9,275.5	9,228.6	5,968.2	5,968.6	5,860.1
85 years and over	12,917.1	13,956.3	14,376.8	15,240.0	16,200.3	16,674.2	11,771.5	12,934.2	13,384.6
Asian or Pacific Islander [2]									
All ages, age adjusted [1]	298.0	300.2	295.4	391.6	389.3	377.9	214.8	223.1	225.0
All ages, crude	276.9	279.4	280.6	345.6	339.2	334.1	211.6	222.2	229.3
1–14 years	25.5	24.6	24.2	28.3	28.0	26.3	22.6	21.1	22.0
15–24 years	52.0	51.3	50.3	71.4	71.4	70.9	31.6	29.5	28.2
25–44 years	75.7	73.8	74.9	92.9	95.8	98.8	60.2	53.7	52.9
45–64 years	410.5	404.2	392.8	537.3	511.6	487.8	302.5	310.9	309.8
65–74 years	1,516.0	1,504.9	1,472.1	2,087.4	2,036.5	1,983.9	969.9	1,063.5	1,058.4
75–84 years	3,832.7	4,051.2	3,998.3	5,176.0	5,439.1	5,127.6	2,617.7	2,784.3	2,994.7
85 years and over	9,617.6	10,902.5	11,002.3	12,305.2	12,277.8	12,577.4	7,975.6	9,944.1	9,881.9
American Indian or Alaskan Native [3]									
All ages, age adjusted [1]	521.5	459.1	457.6	676.4	590.8	589.9	383.8	344.5	343.3
All ages, crude	453.8	412.1	414.1	553.4	490.1	489.7	356.5	335.7	339.9
1–14 years	48.0	45.2	41.1	57.0	56.3	47.9	38.6	33.7	33.9
15–24 years	186.7	149.9	149.4	276.8	222.2	219.9	94.2	73.3	74.1
25–44 years	289.6	226.5	214.3	400.1	317.6	304.2	184.1	139.6	127.6
45–64 years	846.7	733.5	724.0	1,091.7	911.3	904.4	621.1	569.2	557.5
65–74 years	2,148.9	2,033.4	2,104.6	2,761.2	2,579.8	2,647.6	1,653.7	1,597.7	1,671.5
75–84 years	4,114.0	4,020.8	4,052.9	5,128.3	5,224.7	5,226.5	3,370.9	3,225.9	3,289.3
85 years and over	9,225.3	8,714.0	9,093.6	11,048.4	9,945.4	11,192.6	8,079.3	7,964.7	7,912.7
Hispanic [4]									
All ages, age adjusted [1]	- - -	392.2	405.1	- - -	519.7	536.6	- - -	281.5	289.2
All ages, crude	- - -	313.0	344.4	- - -	373.5	405.7	- - -	250.8	280.4
1–14 years	- - -	27.0	29.7	- - -	31.1	34.1	- - -	22.7	25.2
15–24 years	- - -	95.6	100.5	- - -	148.1	152.5	- - -	36.5	39.7
25–44 years	- - -	161.3	176.8	- - -	242.7	266.2	- - -	75.3	80.4
45–64 years	- - -	565.4	584.7	- - -	744.0	779.8	- - -	402.5	405.7
65–74 years	- - -	1,870.1	1,891.2	- - -	2,467.9	2,437.2	- - -	1,418.8	1,466.4
75–84 years	- - -	4,304.9	4,297.7	- - -	5,507.9	5,537.9	- - -	3,497.3	3,503.7
85 years and over	- - -	10,488.5	11,021.0	- - -	11,886.2	12,534.5	- - -	9,681.6	10,167.6

See footnotes at end of table.

[Data are based on the National Vital Statistics System]

Cause of death, race, and age	Both sexes			Male			Female		
	1980–82	1985–87	1988–90	1980–82	1985–87	1988–90	1980–82	1985–87	1988–90
Diseases of heart									
All races	Deaths per 100,000 resident population								
Age 45 years and over, age adjusted [1] . . .	702.2	631.0	569.6	973.2	862.3	772.3	491.8	451.4	411.6
Age 45 years and over, crude	1,045.7	1,013.2	943.0	1,226.6	1,145.1	1,044.2	898.4	906.3	860.7
45–54 years	175.7	146.9	125.9	274.8	225.3	191.5	82.9	72.7	63.4
55–64 years	481.7	428.7	386.0	725.8	634.1	565.0	267.2	247.0	226.5
65–74 years	1,181.7	1,055.1	939.2	1,676.8	1,480.2	1,314.0	802.6	726.3	647.2
75–84 years	2,880.6	2,615.3	2,391.0	3,707.9	3,381.0	3,078.4	2,393.3	2,164.2	1,981.4
85 years and over	7,494.7	7,276.5	6,927.5	8,460.8	8,031.7	7,603.8	7,083.8	6,976.9	6,664.8
White									
Age 45 years and over, age adjusted [1] . . .	691.5	616.8	553.6	969.2	851.8	758.4	475.3	433.2	392.9
Age 45 years and over, crude	1,056.1	1,022.7	950.7	1,237.0	1,152.2	1,048.4	908.0	917.0	870.4
45–54 years	164.2	135.3	113.9	263.1	212.7	177.8	69.8	60.7	52.0
55–64 years	462.8	408.2	363.9	709.8	614.7	542.4	243.6	223.0	202.3
65–74 years	1,166.7	1,032.0	913.8	1,677.9	1,465.5	1,294.8	774.3	694.0	614.1
75–84 years	2,896.8	2,612.9	2,381.9	3,761.3	3,404.6	3,091.0	2,392.6	2,148.9	1,959.9
85 years and over	7,663.1	7,411.1	7,036.7	8,688.6	8,229.7	7,763.7	7,233.9	7,092.3	6,759.1
Black									
Age 45 years and over, age adjusted [1] . . .	856.0	825.2	779.3	1,094.2	1,058.3	1,002.6	677.5	655.1	618.2
Age 45 years and over, crude	1,063.2	1,074.3	1,031.5	1,256.7	1,243.1	1,179.5	915.9	948.4	922.1
45–54 years	296.3	264.4	247.0	417.8	373.3	349.1	197.0	174.6	162.4
55–64 years	720.3	679.5	643.5	971.2	914.2	871.8	518.9	494.6	466.0
65–74 years	1,430.4	1,410.5	1,316.2	1,813.9	1,811.4	1,697.7	1,153.6	1,129.6	1,050.9
75–84 years	2,895.4	2,842.0	2,689.2	3,406.4	3,408.8	3,240.9	2,576.4	2,508.8	2,376.9
85 years and over	5,814.5	6,070.8	6,042.2	6,405.2	6,519.1	6,452.6	5,523.2	5,866.6	5,865.0
Asian or Pacific Islander [2]									
Age 45 years and over, age adjusted [1] . . .	319.5	309.3	290.1	460.5	426.7	387.8	195.7	209.5	208.7
Age 45 years and over, crude	362.1	352.6	333.1	508.6	466.7	424.8	234.9	254.1	254.4
45–54 years	64.1	53.5	46.0	105.2	83.3	71.8	29.1	25.8	21.8
55–64 years	186.1	178.2	165.6	283.7	277.3	247.2	103.0	100.0	101.4
65–74 years	537.3	492.9	462.0	789.0	701.5	641.5	296.7	319.7	316.9
75–84 years	1,471.3	1,485.8	1,397.2	2,019.6	1,995.7	1,778.4	975.4	1,020.4	1,058.5
85 years and over	4,046.2	4,428.7	4,360.9	5,211.4	4,755.1	4,779.2	3,334.2	4,201.3	4,063.4
American Indian or Alaskan Native [3]									
Age 45 years and over, age adjusted [1] . . .	421.3	402.7	393.5	561.9	548.5	529.3	302.9	282.4	282.7
Age 45 years and over, crude	480.6	466.0	453.6	600.2	579.9	557.1	376.0	367.3	364.2
45–54 years	133.2	128.7	118.8	199.0	197.2	179.0	72.1	64.2	62.1
55–64 years	327.2	308.9	307.0	456.7	432.0	437.2	209.4	198.2	190.5
65–74 years	738.5	689.8	665.7	984.7	959.4	878.7	539.3	474.9	495.9
75–84 years	1,483.3	1,448.6	1,432.7	1,834.8	1,887.3	1,814.7	1,225.8	1,158.9	1,184.2
85 years and over	3,227.5	3,221.3	3,333.1	3,705.7	3,318.8	3,961.7	2,926.9	3,162.0	2,979.4
Hispanic [4]									
Age 45 years and over, age adjusted [1] . . .	- - -	394.4	383.2	- - -	518.6	505.0	- - -	296.1	286.5
Age 45 years and over, crude	- - -	448.2	461.9	- - -	530.2	538.1	- - -	378.0	396.6
45–54 years	- - -	80.2	80.0	- - -	119.5	120.5	- - -	43.4	41.6
55–64 years	- - -	267.1	257.1	- - -	378.2	367.3	- - -	169.5	160.5
65–74 years	- - -	681.3	649.7	- - -	924.9	874.8	- - -	497.4	474.6
75–84 years	- - -	1,662.1	1,602.6	- - -	2,067.0	2,026.7	- - -	1,390.3	1,331.1
85 years and over	- - -	4,514.0	4,660.1	- - -	4,782.9	4,877.4	- - -	4,358.8	4,537.6

See footnotes at end of table.

Table 31 (page 3 of 7). Death rates for selected causes of death, according to detailed race, Hispanic origin, age, and sex: United States, 1980–82, 1985–87, and 1988–90

[Data are based on the National Vital Statistics System]

Cause of death, race, and age	Both sexes			Male			Female		
	1980–82	1985–87	1988–90	1980–82	1985–87	1988–90	1980–82	1985–87	1988–90
Cerebrovascular diseases									
All races			Deaths per 100,000 resident population						
Age 45 years and over, age adjusted [1]	136.3	111.6	101.6	150.0	121.7	111.3	125.8	103.5	94.0
Age 45 years and over, crude	226.2	199.4	186.6	204.2	174.7	162.7	244.1	219.5	206.1
45–54 years	24.6	20.7	18.8	26.4	22.3	20.6	22.9	19.1	17.2
55–64 years	62.4	53.7	49.9	71.2	61.6	57.3	54.7	46.8	43.3
65–74 years	206.0	166.0	149.4	242.8	191.1	172.7	177.8	146.5	131.3
75–84 years	725.5	576.0	519.5	794.9	634.3	572.3	684.6	541.6	488.0
85 years and over	2,127.7	1,802.1	1,677.1	2,043.9	1,679.8	1,581.6	2,163.3	1,850.7	1,714.3
White									
Age 45 years and over, age adjusted [1]	128.2	104.4	94.5	141.0	113.6	103.2	118.5	97.1	87.6
Age 45 years and over, crude	222.4	196.7	183.9	196.9	168.7	156.9	243.2	219.6	206.1
45–54 years	19.6	16.2	14.5	20.8	17.1	15.5	18.5	15.2	13.6
55–64 years	53.5	45.8	42.0	61.0	52.5	48.3	46.8	39.8	36.4
65–74 years	190.3	152.9	136.9	225.5	176.6	158.8	163.3	134.5	119.7
75–84 years	714.1	564.6	507.5	783.3	622.2	560.0	673.7	530.8	476.3
85 years and over	2,164.9	1,830.3	1,697.2	2,081.7	1,711.2	1,602.7	2,199.8	1,876.6	1,733.3
Black									
Age 45 years and over, age adjusted [1]	222.6	185.8	174.0	251.7	210.7	200.1	200.9	167.4	154.7
Age 45 years and over, crude	285.9	249.2	237.1	296.6	252.4	239.9	277.8	246.9	235.0
45–54 years	68.7	58.2	55.1	80.2	69.4	67.7	59.3	49.0	44.7
55–64 years	154.5	132.0	123.9	181.8	156.9	150.6	132.6	112.4	103.1
65–74 years	380.0	311.0	288.8	442.6	362.4	339.0	334.8	275.0	253.9
75–84 years	900.7	736.4	681.3	972.0	801.3	746.9	856.1	698.3	644.1
85 years and over	1,758.8	1,546.0	1,503.8	1,731.2	1,434.4	1,420.2	1,772.4	1,596.8	1,539.9
Asian or Pacific Islander [2]									
Age 45 years and over, age adjusted [1]	94.2	91.0	88.3	107.5	104.4	96.5	81.9	79.5	81.4
Age 45 years and over, crude	108.4	103.8	101.6	120.3	115.6	107.3	98.1	93.6	96.8
45–54 years	19.3	17.6	18.8	20.1	15.7	17.6	18.7	19.3	20.0
55–64 years	46.4	47.4	46.3	55.9	56.5	51.0	38.3	40.3	42.6
65–74 years	148.6	143.3	131.9	177.4	170.4	152.9	121.0	120.8	115.0
75–84 years	471.8	455.0	432.0	555.1	561.9	490.7	396.5	357.3	379.9
85 years and over	1,355.8	1,290.8	1,351.2	1,307.0	1,251.3	1,326.1	1,385.6	1,318.4	1,369.1
American Indian or Alaskan Native [3]									
Age 45 years and over, age adjusted [1]	88.3	75.4	69.9	104.1	84.2	79.5	75.5	67.7	62.9
Age 45 years and over, crude	108.4	91.0	85.2	116.2	91.6	86.5	101.5	90.6	84.1
45–54 years	19.4	17.8	14.3	20.4	21.9	14.5	18.4	13.9	14.1
55–64 years	52.5	44.7	44.1	67.3	53.7	44.8	39.0	36.5	43.5
65–74 years	136.2	139.4	112.5	164.8	161.3	140.1	113.1	121.9	90.6
75–84 years	422.1	310.1	326.9	516.7	322.2	383.9	352.8	302.1	289.8
85 years and over	1,137.9	826.0	832.4	1,088.3	786.0	886.0	1,169.0	850.3	802.2
Hispanic [4]									
Age 45 years and over, age adjusted [1]	- - -	80.8	75.6	- - -	91.5	83.8	- - -	72.3	69.1
Age 45 years and over, crude	- - -	93.3	92.3	- - -	94.9	90.5	- - -	91.9	93.9
45–54 years	- - -	18.8	18.5	- - -	21.9	20.3	- - -	15.9	16.8
55–64 years	- - -	47.4	44.5	- - -	57.3	51.5	- - -	38.7	38.3
65–74 years	- - -	127.5	116.9	- - -	148.6	134.1	- - -	111.5	103.4
75–84 years	- - -	376.8	349.3	- - -	417.3	392.0	- - -	349.6	322.0
85 years and over	- - -	1,020.8	971.6	- - -	1,013.5	916.7	- - -	1,025.0	1,002.6

See footnotes at end of table.

Table 31 (page 4 of 7). Death rates for selected causes of death, according to detailed race, Hispanic origin, age, and sex: United States, 1980–82, 1985–87, and 1988–90

[Data are based on the National Vital Statistics System]

Cause of death, race, and age	Both sexes 1980–82	1985–87	1988–90	Male 1980–82	1985–87	1988–90	Female 1980–82	1985–87	1988–90
Malignant neoplasms									
All races			Deaths per 100,000 resident population						
Age 45 years and over, age adjusted [1]	455.3	465.0	467.3	577.6	584.5	585.6	367.4	379.5	382.4
Age 45 years and over, crude	568.0	603.8	614.9	688.1	724.1	732.3	470.2	506.1	519.4
45–54 years	178.0	167.5	159.6	186.6	172.3	164.3	169.9	162.9	155.1
55–64 years	437.2	452.1	452.2	520.4	534.8	534.9	364.2	379.0	378.5
65–74 years	818.1	852.5	864.5	1,090.0	1,110.4	1,113.5	610.0	653.0	670.5
75–84 years	1,231.4	1,279.3	1,322.6	1,781.9	1,847.0	1,882.7	907.2	944.7	988.7
85 years and over	1,584.2	1,630.4	1,705.5	2,381.3	2,477.7	2,637.5	1,245.3	1,294.2	1,343.5
White									
Age 45 years and over, age adjusted [1]	445.1	454.4	456.4	559.5	565.1	565.1	363.7	375.9	378.9
Age 45 years and over, crude	563.5	600.7	612.4	674.1	710.9	719.2	473.0	510.7	524.7
45–54 years	169.3	159.0	151.2	173.4	159.8	151.5	165.4	158.2	151.0
55–64 years	423.3	439.0	439.2	496.5	511.7	511.6	358.3	373.8	373.6
65–74 years	807.7	840.4	850.6	1,066.1	1,081.3	1,082.2	609.2	652.6	668.3
75–84 years	1,226.0	1,270.0	1,312.2	1,770.1	1,823.1	1,853.5	908.6	945.8	990.0
85 years and over	1,592.4	1,625.2	1,696.3	2,390.7	2,467.5	2,618.8	1,258.2	1,297.1	1,344.0
Black									
Age 45 years and over, age adjusted [1]	589.0	610.9	621.1	812.6	847.0	866.8	426.5	445.8	452.4
Age 45 years and over, crude	667.8	711.6	730.5	902.8	957.5	981.9	488.8	528.0	544.7
45–54 years	269.7	258.4	250.7	329.5	307.3	305.0	220.9	218.1	205.7
55–64 years	616.7	631.3	631.6	820.5	837.4	839.6	453.1	469.0	469.8
65–74 years	987.5	1,063.2	1,105.5	1,441.5	1,557.0	1,599.4	659.9	717.2	762.0
75–84 years	1,366.0	1,465.6	1,534.8	2,050.8	2,272.9	2,418.1	938.3	990.9	1,034.7
85 years and over	1,544.7	1,762.1	1,890.5	2,403.8	2,758.4	3,050.3	1,121.1	1,308.3	1,389.6
Asian or Pacific Islander [2]									
Age 45 years and over, age adjusted [1]	256.4	266.6	271.9	326.6	338.5	340.3	194.3	206.2	216.0
Age 45 years and over, crude	270.7	281.9	287.4	347.3	354.7	353.8	204.1	219.1	230.4
45–54 years	104.6	93.0	93.8	107.3	96.0	92.9	102.4	90.3	94.7
55–64 years	226.2	237.9	239.3	289.1	289.7	290.9	172.7	197.0	198.7
65–74 years	429.7	460.3	476.9	573.4	616.9	642.3	292.3	330.2	343.2
75–84 years	797.7	878.7	891.3	1,085.6	1,217.1	1,180.5	537.3	569.9	634.2
85 years and over	1,180.0	1,272.7	1,340.2	1,681.3	1,715.1	1,763.2	873.7	964.4	1,039.3
American Indian or Alaskan Native [3]									
Age 45 years and over, age adjusted [1]	234.1	240.2	265.0	280.7	281.0	311.5	197.0	210.6	230.6
Age 45 years and over, crude	252.3	261.3	285.5	292.9	293.1	320.2	216.8	233.7	255.5
45–54 years	90.1	89.0	91.8	90.8	85.7	86.0	89.4	92.0	97.1
55–64 years	213.9	216.6	243.5	243.1	228.7	276.5	187.3	205.6	213.9
65–74 years	433.7	446.6	505.2	553.4	539.7	604.9	336.9	372.3	425.7
75–84 years	652.5	691.1	745.6	854.1	972.4	995.6	504.7	505.3	582.9
85 years and over	845.4	933.3	1,048.7	1,102.1	1,266.4	1,517.5	684.1	730.7	785.0
Hispanic [4]									
Age 45 years and over, age adjusted [1]	- - -	258.0	278.3	- - -	318.1	345.4	- - -	214.6	229.4
Age 45 years and over, crude	- - -	273.0	304.8	- - -	317.1	356.5	- - -	235.3	260.4
45–54 years	- - -	84.8	92.3	- - -	81.4	90.8	- - -	88.1	93.7
55–64 years	- - -	227.2	247.0	- - -	255.4	291.5	- - -	202.4	207.9
65–74 years	- - -	472.2	505.5	- - -	624.3	644.2	- - -	357.4	397.7
75–84 years	- - -	831.5	887.0	- - -	1,143.0	1,243.6	- - -	622.5	658.7
85 years and over	- - -	1,191.6	1,326.2	- - -	1,695.2	1,902.6	- - -	900.8	1,001.2

See footnotes at end of table.

Table 31 (page 5 of 7). Death rates for selected causes of death, according to detailed race, Hispanic origin, age, and sex: United States, 1980–82, 1985–87, and 1988–90

[Data are based on the National Vital Statistics System]

Cause of death, race, and age	Both sexes 1980–82	Both sexes 1985–87	Both sexes 1988–90	Male 1980–82	Male 1985–87	Male 1988–90	Female 1980–82	Female 1985–87	Female 1988–90
Motor vehicle crashes									
All races				Deaths per 100,000 resident population					
All ages, age adjusted [1]	21.3	19.2	19.0	31.9	27.9	27.1	11.1	10.7	11.1
All ages, crude	21.8	19.7	19.4	32.8	28.7	27.5	11.5	11.3	11.6
1–14 years	7.6	7.0	6.5	9.3	8.6	7.7	5.9	5.3	5.3
15–24 years	40.9	37.1	35.5	62.2	54.6	51.4	19.3	19.0	19.0
25–44 years	24.0	20.9	20.8	37.6	31.9	31.0	10.7	10.1	10.7
45–64 years	17.0	15.4	15.9	25.0	21.9	22.2	9.7	9.5	10.0
65 years and over	21.8	22.2	23.5	32.6	31.5	32.8	14.5	16.0	17.2
White									
All ages, age adjusted [1]	21.9	19.6	19.2	32.4	28.2	27.2	11.5	11.1	11.4
All ages, crude	22.5	20.1	19.6	33.5	28.9	27.6	12.0	11.7	12.0
1–14 years	7.5	6.9	6.4	9.2	8.4	7.5	5.8	5.3	5.2
15–24 years	44.7	40.1	38.1	67.4	58.6	54.6	21.2	21.0	20.8
25–44 years	24.2	20.8	20.6	37.6	31.4	30.4	10.9	10.1	10.7
45–64 years	16.5	14.9	15.3	23.8	20.7	21.0	9.8	9.5	10.0
65 years and over	21.7	22.3	23.5	31.8	31.0	32.2	14.9	16.4	17.6
Black									
All ages, age adjusted [1]	18.1	17.9	18.7	30.2	28.8	29.5	7.8	8.5	9.3
All ages, crude	17.7	17.8	18.6	28.6	28.1	28.7	7.9	8.6	9.4
1–14 years	8.2	7.6	7.4	10.0	9.8	9.2	6.3	5.4	5.6
15–24 years	19.6	21.7	23.4	31.8	34.4	36.8	7.8	9.3	10.3
25–44 years	23.1	22.7	23.2	39.9	37.6	37.4	8.6	9.8	10.8
45–64 years	21.0	19.8	20.6	36.4	32.8	34.0	8.5	9.4	9.9
65 years and over	21.9	20.8	22.8	40.1	36.3	39.3	9.6	10.8	12.3
Asian or Pacific Islander [2]									
All ages, age adjusted [1]	11.0	11.8	11.7	14.3	15.6	14.7	7.9	8.1	8.7
All ages, crude	10.9	11.6	11.5	14.2	15.4	14.6	7.8	7.9	8.6
1–14 years	5.5	5.2	4.9	6.2	6.2	5.2	4.8	4.3	4.6
15–24 years	14.1	17.6	17.8	20.3	25.7	24.1	7.6	8.8	11.1
25–44 years	11.1	10.8	10.4	14.2	15.2	14.0	8.3	6.9	7.2
45–64 years	10.6	11.5	11.9	12.8	13.7	14.2	8.8	9.6	9.9
65 years and over	24.3	26.5	25.9	33.8	32.5	30.6	15.6	21.4	22.1
American Indian or Alaskan Native [3]									
All ages, age adjusted [1]	47.7	37.8	34.5	68.5	55.0	50.4	28.0	21.2	19.3
All ages, crude	46.6	37.5	33.8	65.8	54.2	49.0	27.9	21.1	18.9
1–14 years	11.9	11.9	10.5	13.0	14.9	11.2	10.8	8.8	9.8
15–24 years	76.3	58.4	56.4	107.7	86.0	80.4	44.0	29.2	30.8
25–44 years	60.7	50.7	44.6	86.4	74.3	67.9	36.1	28.2	22.1
45–64 years	48.9	34.9	31.5	74.0	51.3	45.3	25.8	19.8	18.8
65 years and over	46.2	31.3	31.6	77.2	47.5	55.9	22.3	19.3	13.8
Hispanic [4]									
All ages, age adjusted [1]	- - -	16.8	19.7	- - -	25.9	29.6	- - -	7.5	9.3
All ages, crude	- - -	16.8	19.5	- - -	26.0	29.6	- - -	7.4	9.0
1–14 years	- - -	5.8	6.4	- - -	6.9	7.7	- - -	4.5	5.0
15–24 years	- - -	28.4	32.0	- - -	44.9	48.8	- - -	9.8	12.5
25–44 years	- - -	19.3	23.0	- - -	30.6	36.0	- - -	7.3	9.0
45–64 years	- - -	16.1	19.1	- - -	25.1	28.5	- - -	8.0	10.4
65 years and over	- - -	20.3	25.0	- - -	30.9	39.2	- - -	12.6	14.9

See footnotes at end of table.

Table 31 (page 6 of 7). Death rates for selected causes of death, according to detailed race, Hispanic origin, age, and sex: United States, 1980–82, 1985–87, and 1988–90

[Data are based on the National Vital Statistics System]

Cause of death, race, and age	Both sexes			Male			Female		
	1980–82	1985–87	1988–90	1980–82	1985–87	1988–90	1980–82	1985–87	1988–90
Suicide									
All races			Deaths per 100,000 resident population						
15–24 years	12.2	12.8	13.0	19.9	21.0	21.6	4.4	4.3	4.1
25–44 years	15.8	15.3	15.1	24.1	24.1	24.1	7.7	6.6	6.2
45–64 years	16.3	16.5	15.3	24.2	25.5	23.8	9.2	8.3	7.4
65 years and over	17.7	21.3	20.6	35.0	42.9	41.9	6.1	6.8	6.3
White									
15–24 years	13.1	13.8	13.8	21.2	22.6	22.8	4.7	4.6	4.4
25–44 years	16.6	16.2	15.9	25.0	25.2	25.2	8.3	7.1	6.6
45–64 years	17.5	17.8	16.5	25.7	27.3	25.6	10.0	9.0	8.0
65 years and over	18.8	22.6	22.0	37.3	45.5	44.7	6.5	7.2	6.7
Black									
15–24 years	6.9	7.3	8.9	11.6	12.5	15.4	2.3	2.3	2.6
25–44 years	11.0	10.7	11.3	19.0	19.2	19.9	4.2	3.4	3.8
45–64 years	6.8	7.1	7.1	12.0	12.3	12.0	2.7	2.9	3.0
65 years and over	5.9	8.3	7.1	12.0	17.4	15.6	1.8	2.5	1.8
Asian or Pacific Islander [2]									
15–24 years	7.6	8.5	7.5	10.5	12.1	11.3	4.7	4.5	3.5
25–44 years	8.1	6.5	6.8	10.5	8.9	9.8	6.0	4.3	4.2
45–64 years	8.8	8.0	6.8	10.1	10.4	9.4	7.7	5.9	4.5
65 years and over	13.7	15.9	13.0	18.5	22.5	17.0	9.4	10.4	9.8
American Indian or Alaskan Native [3]									
15–24 years	25.0	22.8	26.8	41.2	37.9	44.9	8.2	6.9	7.5
25–44 years	19.8	18.8	16.9	32.7	32.2	28.7	7.4	6.0	5.4
45–64 years	8.9	8.8	6.7	15.8	13.5	11.8	*2.6	*4.4	*2.0
65 years and over	*5.0	*6.1	7.4	*10.6	*11.1	*12.6	*0.7	*2.3	*3.6
Hispanic [4]									
15–24 years	- - -	8.7	9.4	- - -	14.1	15.0	- - -	2.5	2.9
25–44 years	- - -	8.6	9.8	- - -	14.7	16.0	- - -	2.2	3.2
45–64 years	- - -	7.5	9.1	- - -	12.7	15.8	- - -	2.8	2.9
65 years and over	- - -	9.2	11.8	- - -	18.9	25.2	- - -	2.2	2.2
Homicide and legal intervention									
All races									
15–24 years	14.7	13.2	17.2	22.9	20.5	27.9	6.2	5.7	6.0
25–44 years	16.7	13.6	14.3	27.5	21.4	22.6	6.1	5.9	6.0
45–64 years	8.9	6.9	6.4	14.9	11.0	10.2	3.5	3.1	2.8
White									
15–24 years	9.5	7.7	8.6	14.3	11.4	13.0	4.5	3.9	3.9
25–44 years	10.2	8.4	8.3	16.4	12.8	12.6	4.1	4.1	3.9
45–64 years	6.0	4.8	4.6	9.7	7.4	7.1	2.6	2.4	2.2
Black									
15–24 years	47.2	46.0	67.6	78.7	76.7	117.9	16.9	16.1	17.9
25–44 years	67.5	52.7	57.9	122.3	91.7	100.6	20.6	18.7	20.5
45–64 years	36.1	24.9	22.4	67.4	45.4	40.8	10.8	8.4	7.5
Asian or Pacific Islander [2]									
15–24 years	6.7	6.1	7.4	9.5	8.8	12.3	3.7	3.2	2.3
25–44 years	6.9	5.8	6.8	10.2	8.5	9.8	3.9	3.4	4.1
45–64 years	6.1	5.0	4.8	9.8	7.3	7.3	3.0	3.0	2.6
American Indian or Alaskan Native [3]									
15–24 years	20.7	19.4	19.0	31.6	29.1	27.7	9.5	9.2	9.8
25–44 years	22.2	19.4	18.1	32.7	31.4	29.0	12.1	7.9	7.6
45–64 years	15.8	11.0	8.4	24.2	17.7	12.5	8.1	*4.7	4.5
Hispanic [4]									
15–24 years	- - -	25.2	27.5	- - -	42.5	45.7	- - -	5.6	6.2
25–44 years	- - -	26.1	24.4	- - -	44.1	41.5	- - -	7.2	6.0
45–64 years	- - -	11.1	11.2	- - -	19.8	20.0	- - -	3.1	3.1

See footnotes at end of table.

[Data are based on the National Vital Statistics System]

Cause of death, race, and age	Both sexes			Male			Female		
	1980–82	1985–87	1988–90	1980–82	1985–87	1988–90	1980–82	1985–87	1988–90
Human immunodeficiency virus infection									
All races			Deaths per 100,000 resident population						
25–44 years	- - -	- - -	19.8	- - -	- - -	35.6	- - -	- - -	4.2
45–64 years	- - -	- - -	9.3	- - -	- - -	18.0	- - -	- - -	1.2
White									
25–44 years	- - -	- - -	15.9	- - -	- - -	29.6	- - -	- - -	1.9
45–64 years	- - -	- - -	7.9	- - -	- - -	15.6	- - -	- - -	0.7
Black									
25–44 years	- - -	- - -	52.8	- - -	- - -	90.4	- - -	- - -	19.8
45–64 years	- - -	- - -	23.1	- - -	- - -	44.6	- - -	- - -	5.7
Asian or Pacific Islander									
25–44 years	- - -	- - -	3.8	- - -	- - -	7.3	- - -	- - -	0.6
45–64 years	- - -	- - -	2.9	- - -	- - -	5.6	- - -	- - -	*0.6
American Indian or Alaskan Native									
25–44 years	- - -	- - -	4.0	- - -	- - -	7.2	- - -	- - -	*0.8
45–64 years	- - -	- - -	*1.8	- - -	- - -	*3.2	- - -	- - -	*0.5
Hispanic [4]									
25–44 years	- - -	- - -	28.7	- - -	- - -	48.9	- - -	- - -	6.9
45–64 years	- - -	- - -	16.3	- - -	- - -	31.3	- - -	- - -	2.5

[1]Age adjusted by the direct method based on 11 age groups for all ages and 5 age groups for 45 years and over. See Appendix II.

[2]Interpretation of trends should take into account that the Asian population in the United States more than doubled between 1980 and 1990, primarily due to immigration.

[3]Interpretation of trends should take into account that population estimates for American Indians increased by 45 percent between 1980 and 1990, partly due to better enumeration techniques in the 1990 decennial census and to the increased tendency for people to identify themselves as American Indian in 1990.

[4]Data shown only for States with an Hispanic-origin item on their death certificates. See Appendix I.

*Based on fewer than 20 deaths.

NOTES: The race groups, white, black, Asian or Pacific Islander, and American Indian or Alaskan Native, include persons of both Hispanic and non-Hispanic origin. Conversely, persons of Hispanic origin may be of any race. Consistency of race identification between the death certificate (source of data for numerator of death rates) and data from the Census Bureau (denominator) is high for individual white, black, and Hispanic persons; however, persons identified as American Indian or Asian in data from the Census Bureau are sometimes misreported as white on the death certificate, causing death rates to be underestimated by 22–30 percent for American Indians and by about 12 percent for Asians. (Sorlie, P.D., Rogot, E., and Johnson, N.J.: Validity of demographic characteristics on the death certificate, Epidemiology 3(2):181–184, 1992.)

SOURCE: Centers for Disease Control and Prevention, National Center for Health Statistics: Data computed by the Division of Analysis from data compiled by the Division of Vital Statistics and from intercensal national population estimates from table 1 and intercensal State population estimates for Hispanics provided by the Census Bureau.

Table 32 (page 1 of 2). Age-adjusted death rates, according to race, sex, region, and urbanization: United States, average annual 1980–82, 1984–86, and 1988–90

[Data are based on the National Vital Statistics System]

Sex, region, and urbanization [1]	All races			White			Black		
	1980–82	1984–86	1988–90	1980–82	1984–86	1988–90	1980–82	1984–86	1988–90
Both sexes									
All regions			Deaths per 100,000 resident population						
Large core metropolitan	599.5	577.7	568.7	561.1	539.7	522.8	827.0	809.6	838.5
Large fringe metropolitan	530.1	508.4	479.1	523.0	501.8	471.0	723.6	697.4	681.1
Medium/small metropolitan	563.2	539.3	517.2	541.5	517.8	493.5	812.9	790.4	785.1
Urban nonmetropolitan	570.7	549.1	532.5	551.3	529.9	512.1	806.8	792.6	792.5
Rural	571.9	549.8	537.0	550.6	529.3	513.5	768.1	751.8	765.1
Northeast									
Large core metropolitan	620.4	608.1	608.8	578.1	564.6	554.2	810.3	803.4	836.4
Large fringe metropolitan	538.6	515.1	483.2	531.8	508.5	475.5	713.1	690.7	664.2
Medium/small metropolitan	550.0	527.0	499.4	542.1	517.7	488.2	761.6	764.3	751.7
Urban nonmetropolitan	552.4	538.1	506.4	551.8	537.6	505.8	715.6	733.7	667.0
Rural	548.1	538.6	503.4	548.5	540.0	503.1	*	*	*
South									
Large core metropolitan	609.1	583.3	582.3	546.2	521.7	507.3	861.4	832.3	870.7
Large fringe metropolitan	534.1	512.5	488.1	520.5	500.1	472.5	714.8	682.6	681.3
Medium/small metropolitan	590.5	563.2	543.8	549.8	524.0	502.0	828.6	803.7	798.9
Urban nonmetropolitan	612.8	591.7	579.1	577.6	556.5	542.1	812.4	800.6	802.8
Rural	608.0	592.0	583.0	578.3	562.4	550.9	768.6	754.6	765.7
Midwest									
Large core metropolitan	626.7	600.9	588.4	572.8	544.9	520.2	845.2	824.4	843.8
Large fringe metropolitan	538.7	518.3	484.3	529.6	509.3	474.0	767.4	752.3	726.4
Medium/small metropolitan	544.2	522.8	497.1	531.7	510.3	482.4	777.8	753.6	750.4
Urban nonmetropolitan	527.8	504.8	488.6	525.0	502.3	485.4	754.0	715.6	714.9
Rural	534.1	507.2	493.1	522.9	497.9	481.0	742.6	689.8	792.5
West									
Large core metropolitan	548.8	528.5	513.9	543.6	524.6	509.4	763.9	756.1	779.4
Large fringe metropolitan	488.7	470.4	449.3	493.1	475.1	453.8	688.7	658.7	651.4
Medium/small metropolitan	525.4	505.3	488.7	528.2	507.5	490.7	731.0	707.7	717.9
Urban nonmetropolitan	544.1	516.2	498.9	536.6	509.5	491.9	760.5	*448.0	639.7
Rural	541.4	497.5	478.5	536.7	496.3	473.3	*	*448.0	*929.3
Male									
All regions									
Large core metropolitan	794.6	762.3	750.2	746.3	712.6	688.5	1,104.4	1,091.3	1,146.2
Large fringe metropolitan	691.2	657.9	613.3	683.2	650.1	603.0	928.0	901.4	885.2
Medium/small metropolitan	748.4	710.9	674.4	722.7	685.2	644.6	1,071.0	1,037.9	1,039.0
Urban nonmetropolitan	763.6	727.8	699.0	740.4	704.9	673.5	1,074.0	1,046.3	1,056.8
Rural	764.5	729.5	708.2	738.5	704.3	678.3	1,017.1	995.3	1,019.4
Northeast									
Large core metropolitan	828.1	811.5	816.9	772.8	752.9	740.0	1,099.9	1,103.3	1,173.0
Large fringe metropolitan	701.6	666.2	619.4	693.4	657.9	609.6	930.8	904.9	873.6
Medium/small metropolitan	731.7	696.0	652.2	721.9	684.3	638.0	1,003.1	1,007.5	989.6
Urban nonmetropolitan	730.7	704.9	659.1	730.6	704.9	658.8	857.7	885.9	835.4
Rural	715.7	706.8	656.1	715.8	709.5	656.6	*	*	*
South									
Large core metropolitan	812.5	773.7	778.0	732.0	692.9	677.1	1,152.7	1,121.6	1,196.7
Large fringe metropolitan	701.7	667.9	631.4	686.5	653.3	611.4	912.8	882.4	887.7
Medium/small metropolitan	790.4	746.5	714.1	740.9	698.6	659.8	1,101.0	1,063.0	1,068.8
Urban nonmetropolitan	831.5	795.7	771.7	789.8	753.8	724.5	1,091.8	1,068.4	1,085.4
Rural	822.1	793.0	778.3	787.7	757.7	738.2	1,019.4	1,002.1	1,025.5

See footnotes at end of table.

[Data are based on the National Vital Statistics System]

Sex, region, and urbanization [1]	All races			White			Black		
	1980–82	1984–86	1988–90	1980–82	1984–86	1988–90	1980–82	1984–86	1988–90
Male—Con.									
Midwest			Deaths per 100,000 resident population						
Large core metropolitan	837.6	798.3	777.3	770.4	725.7	686.3	1,124.3	1,107.1	1,145.3
Large fringe metropolitan	705.2	673.4	619.7	694.7	663.0	606.9	984.7	960.9	938.0
Medium/small metropolitan	723.6	690.8	648.0	709.5	676.1	630.2	995.7	975.8	971.5
Urban nonmetropolitan	704.4	667.9	640.9	701.6	665.6	637.7	924.5	871.4	879.2
Rural	708.9	671.1	646.7	695.3	659.4	631.2	930.0	882.6	998.6
West									
Large core metropolitan	716.4	685.7	663.5	711.7	681.3	658.3	994.6	992.1	1,016.4
Large fringe metropolitan	629.2	600.5	565.8	636.4	607.2	571.9	824.6	831.5	803.3
Medium/small metropolitan	683.1	652.8	624.1	689.1	658.1	629.2	923.1	864.5	873.0
Urban nonmetropolitan	705.8	662.2	630.2	697.5	654.1	622.5	932.8	820.3	718.7
Rural	704.2	637.7	605.7	699.0	637.2	599.4	*	*	*767.6
Female									
All regions									
Large core metropolitan	448.0	433.2	422.3	418.2	404.3	388.7	616.3	598.3	606.8
Large fringe metropolitan	403.7	391.2	372.4	397.5	385.6	366.2	559.1	536.6	521.1
Medium/small metropolitan	417.0	404.3	392.0	399.0	386.3	373.2	611.9	601.1	591.5
Urban nonmetropolitan	410.8	402.5	395.3	394.5	386.1	378.9	596.3	596.6	590.4
Rural	401.3	393.1	387.7	383.6	376.2	369.2	558.1	551.2	558.6
Northeast									
Large core metropolitan	465.0	454.1	446.6	432.0	421.3	408.0	604.6	591.6	595.9
Large fringe metropolitan	413.3	399.1	376.6	407.6	393.9	370.7	548.4	528.5	506.2
Medium/small metropolitan	411.6	398.7	381.8	405.5	391.7	373.4	569.7	571.9	562.3
Urban nonmetropolitan	410.8	405.2	384.2	410.1	404.5	383.7	582.6	592.8	515.1
Rural	405.7	394.3	372.2	406.4	394.7	371.4	*	*	*
South									
Large core metropolitan	447.4	431.7	423.5	398.0	384.5	368.2	638.5	614.1	624.4
Large fringe metropolitan	399.3	387.6	371.8	387.1	376.9	359.7	552.5	523.8	520.2
Medium/small metropolitan	432.1	418.5	407.7	397.9	385.4	374.8	620.8	609.8	597.7
Urban nonmetropolitan	433.5	426.6	422.9	402.4	395.2	392.5	596.3	598.2	592.4
Rural	422.6	421.0	416.7	396.2	395.7	390.1	558.0	552.1	557.2
Midwest									
Large core metropolitan	466.8	451.7	443.2	425.9	410.7	394.4	628.5	609.8	617.7
Large fringe metropolitan	407.8	398.1	378.8	400.3	390.6	370.8	588.3	585.3	557.0
Medium/small metropolitan	406.7	394.6	380.8	395.8	384.1	368.8	602.3	579.0	578.6
Urban nonmetropolitan	383.3	373.2	365.3	380.6	370.7	362.4	603.1	577.6	569.8
Rural	377.4	363.0	358.2	368.8	356.1	349.6	596.6	507.3	629.2
West									
Large core metropolitan	414.2	399.4	386.2	409.5	396.0	381.8	575.0	563.7	581.5
Large fringe metropolitan	378.1	365.9	353.7	380.6	369.4	357.0	565.6	506.5	513.5
Medium/small metropolitan	391.0	379.9	372.7	392.9	380.8	373.0	541.1	555.4	568.6
Urban nonmetropolitan	397.0	384.6	379.1	391.5	380.0	373.9	576.3	551.9	568.3
Rural	383.1	362.0	355.6	379.2	360.6	352.3	*	*	*

[1]Urbanization categories for county of residence of decedent are based on classification of counties by the Department of Agriculture. See Appendix II.

*Data for groups with population under 4,000 in the middle year of a 3-year period are considered unreliable. Data for groups with population under 2,000 are considered highly unreliable and are not shown.

SOURCE: Centers for Disease Control and Prevention, National Center for Health Statistics: Data computed by the Division of Analysis using the Compressed Mortality File. See Appendix I, National Vital Statistics System.

Table 33. Death rates for persons 25–64 years of age, for all races and the white population, according to sex, age, and educational attainment: Selected States, 1989–90

[Data are based on the National Vital Statistics System]

Age, race, and educational attainment	Both sexes			Male			Female		
	1989	1990	1989–90	1989	1990	1989–90	1989	1990	1989–90
All races									
25–64 years [1]			Deaths per 100,000 resident population						
0–8 years	474.6	471.0	472.5	617.8	613.7	615.3	314.1	312.2	312.9
9–11 years	502.4	519.5	512.8	728.6	747.1	739.8	308.1	325.0	318.3
12 years	417.9	434.3	427.7	583.3	614.5	602.1	288.9	294.7	292.5
13–15 years	395.3	383.3	388.0	513.3	493.8	501.5	283.4	278.9	280.7
16 years or more	273.5	264.1	267.8	324.3	315.3	318.9	200.1	190.7	194.4
25–44 years of age									
0–8 years	250.5	250.2	250.3	339.9	343.3	341.9	147.0	143.6	145.0
9–11 years	300.9	304.5	303.1	435.1	437.5	436.5	162.7	168.8	166.4
12 years	181.0	189.2	185.9	269.4	285.8	279.2	102.2	103.6	103.0
13–15 years	158.2	156.0	156.9	220.3	217.5	218.6	97.0	95.8	96.3
16 years or more	94.3	94.4	94.4	124.8	126.1	125.6	57.9	57.0	57.4
45–64 years of age									
0–8 years	954.4	942.0	946.9	1,213.9	1,192.7	1,201.1	668.4	667.5	667.8
9–11 years	873.3	912.9	897.2	1,246.7	1,293.2	1,274.7	579.9	615.7	601.5
12 years	809.1	840.3	827.9	1,080.2	1,136.2	1,113.9	606.2	620.3	614.7
13–15 years	761.7	736.4	746.5	959.8	918.0	934.7	574.8	566.3	569.7
16 years or more	536.1	515.0	523.4	630.1	608.5	617.1	394.8	375.8	383.3
White									
25–64 years [1]									
0–8 years	454.7	464.6	460.6	588.0	598.6	594.4	299.6	309.7	305.7
9–11 years	462.8	471.7	468.2	665.7	672.1	669.6	282.4	294.9	289.9
12 years	384.5	394.0	390.2	539.5	562.2	553.2	265.0	265.3	265.2
13–15 years	374.6	358.0	364.6	488.1	463.1	473.0	265.0	257.1	260.2
16 years or more	264.0	254.8	258.4	313.6	304.7	308.2	190.0	181.1	184.6
25–44 years of age									
0–8 years	235.8	244.0	240.7	321.0	332.8	328.1	132.6	137.3	135.4
9–11 years	260.7	258.2	259.2	376.9	370.4	373.0	136.7	139.6	138.4
12 years	161.1	165.1	163.5	239.9	250.4	246.2	90.2	89.0	89.5
13–15 years	146.4	142.1	143.8	206.9	200.5	203.1	86.0	84.3	85.0
16 years or more	90.9	90.9	90.9	120.7	121.9	121.4	54.6	53.5	53.9
45–64 years of age									
0–8 years	925.5	936.6	932.2	1,170.8	1,174.3	1,172.9	648.5	669.7	661.3
9–11 years	843.3	870.6	859.8	1,195.8	1,219.9	1,210.3	556.4	587.6	575.3
12 years	760.1	779.2	771.7	1,016.9	1,059.8	1,042.8	568.9	571.9	570.7
13–15 years	730.4	696.3	709.8	921.7	870.7	890.9	546.5	529.7	536.4
16 years or more	524.4	503.4	511.7	617.4	595.4	604.1	380.3	362.2	369.3

[1] Age adjusted.

NOTES: Based on data from 21 States in 1989 and 29 States in 1990 whose data on educational attainment from the death certificate were at least 90 percent complete. See Appendix I. Data for the black population are not shown because the rates are unstable due to small numbers of deaths in the subgroups. These data will be shown in future editions of Health, United States as the number of States in the reporting area increases.

SOURCE: Centers for Disease Control and Prevention, National Center for Health Statistics: Rates computed by the Division of Analysis from vital statistics data compiled by and population data developed by the Division of Vital Statistics.

Table 34 (page 1 of 2). Death rates for all causes, according to sex, race, and age: United States, selected years 1950–90

[Data are based on the National Vital Statistics System]

Sex, race, and age	1950[1]	1960[1]	1970	1980	1985	1986	1987	1988	1989	1990
All races			Deaths per 100,000 resident population							
All ages, age adjusted	840.5	760.9	714.3	585.8	548.9	544.8	539.2	539.9	528.0	520.2
All ages, crude	963.8	954.7	945.3	878.3	876.9	876.7	876.4	886.7	871.3	863.8
Under 1 year	3,299.2	2,696.4	2,142.4	1,288.3	1,088.1	1,051.1	1,037.2	1,035.7	1,027.9	971.9
1–4 years	139.4	109.1	84.5	63.9	51.8	52.4	52.1	51.5	49.8	46.8
5–14 years	60.1	46.6	41.3	30.6	26.5	26.2	25.9	26.1	25.7	24.0
15–24 years	128.1	106.3	127.7	115.4	94.9	100.9	97.8	100.0	97.6	99.2
25–34 years	178.7	146.4	157.4	135.5	124.4	133.4	134.7	137.1	140.0	139.2
35–44 years	358.7	299.4	314.5	227.9	207.7	213.3	214.6	220.2	222.2	223.2
45–54 years	853.9	756.0	730.0	584.0	519.3	508.2	501.9	490.5	480.1	473.4
55–64 years	1,911.7	1,735.1	1,658.8	1,346.3	1,294.2	1,268.7	1,256.6	1,253.8	1,224.3	1,196.9
65–74 years	4,067.7	3,822.1	3,582.7	2,994.9	2,862.8	2,833.3	2,789.4	2,771.7	2,693.8	2,648.6
75–84 years	9,331.1	8,745.2	8,004.4	6,692.6	6,398.7	6,300.9	6,232.2	6,262.1	6,083.3	6,007.2
85 years and over	20,196.9	19,857.5	16,344.9	15,980.3	15,712.4	15,589.8	15,559.6	15,934.5	15,409.6	15,327.4
White male										
All ages, age adjusted	963.1	917.7	893.4	745.3	693.3	684.9	674.2	671.3	652.2	644.3
All ages, crude	1,089.5	1,098.5	1,086.7	983.3	963.6	958.6	952.7	957.9	936.5	930.9
Under 1 year	3,400.5	2,694.1	2,113.2	1,230.3	1,056.5	993.8	964.9	964.2	940.7	896.1
1–4 years	135.5	104.9	83.6	66.1	52.8	52.6	52.4	51.5	48.3	45.9
5–14 years	67.2	52.7	48.0	35.0	30.1	30.1	30.2	29.2	28.4	26.4
15–24 years	152.4	143.7	170.8	167.0	134.2	143.1	134.2	135.8	128.6	131.3
25–34 years	185.3	163.2	176.6	171.3	158.8	171.0	170.3	172.6	177.0	176.1
35–44 years	380.9	332.6	343.5	257.4	243.1	250.1	251.6	259.5	263.4	268.2
45–54 years	984.5	932.2	882.9	698.9	611.7	595.4	586.4	568.6	556.0	548.7
55–64 years	2,304.4	2,225.2	2,202.6	1,728.5	1,625.8	1,586.3	1,567.0	1,546.7	1,504.1	1,467.2
65–74 years	4,864.9	4,848.4	4,810.1	4,035.7	3,770.7	3,702.1	3,626.3	3,588.1	3,455.1	3,397.7
75–84 years	10,526.3	10,299.6	10,098.8	8,829.8	8,486.1	8,333.5	8,212.2	8,196.7	7,913.4	7,844.9
85 years and over	22,116.3	21,750.0	18,551.7	19,097.3	18,980.1	18,628.8	18,486.0	19,020.8	18,241.7	18,268.3
Black male										
All ages, age adjusted	1,373.1	1,246.1	1,318.6	1,112.8	1,053.4	1,061.9	1,063.6	1,083.0	1,082.8	1,061.3
All ages, crude	1,260.3	1,181.7	1,186.6	1,034.1	989.3	1,002.6	1,006.2	1,026.1	1,026.7	1,008.0
Under 1 year	- - -	5,306.8	4,298.9	2,586.7	2,219.9	2,251.8	2,226.8	2,189.6	2,172.1	2,112.4
1–4 years	- - -	208.5	150.5	110.5	90.1	92.2	92.0	92.1	90.0	85.8
5–14 years	95.1	75.1	67.1	47.4	42.3	43.1	43.9	43.7	43.5	41.2
15–24 years	289.7	212.0	320.6	209.1	173.6	189.8	203.2	222.4	234.5	252.2
25–34 years	503.5	402.5	559.5	407.3	351.9	391.3	396.3	417.4	425.6	430.8
35–44 years	878.1	762.0	956.6	689.8	630.2	661.0	683.4	706.7	718.1	699.6
45–54 years	1,905.0	1,624.8	1,777.5	1,479.9	1,292.9	1,278.2	1,277.3	1,296.9	1,311.5	1,261.0
55–64 years	3,773.2	3,316.4	3,256.9	2,873.0	2,779.8	2,723.1	2,667.3	2,712.7	2,699.9	2,618.4
65–74 years	5,310.3	5,798.7	5,803.2	5,131.1	5,172.4	5,130.3	5,143.0	5,147.7	5,129.7	4,946.1
75–84 years	- - -	8,605.1	9,454.9	9,231.6	9,262.3	9,290.8	9,275.3	9,454.6	9,163.3	9,129.5
85 years and over	- - -	14,844.8	12,222.3	16,098.8	15,774.2	16,471.4	16,415.6	16,643.1	16,751.5	16,954.9
White female										
All ages, age adjusted	645.0	555.0	501.7	411.1	391.0	388.1	384.8	385.3	376.0	369.9
All ages, crude	803.3	800.9	812.6	806.1	840.1	844.3	849.8	865.3	851.8	846.9
Under 1 year	2,566.8	2,007.7	1,614.6	962.5	799.3	772.6	760.3	754.1	739.5	690.0
1–4 years	112.2	85.2	66.1	49.3	40.0	41.0	40.9	40.7	38.8	36.1
5–14 years	45.1	34.7	29.9	22.9	19.5	18.7	18.0	18.7	19.0	17.9
15–24 years	71.5	54.9	61.6	55.5	48.1	50.1	48.7	48.8	48.4	45.9
25–34 years	112.8	85.0	84.1	65.4	59.4	61.0	63.4	62.7	63.1	61.5
35–44 years	235.8	191.1	193.3	138.2	121.9	122.1	120.2	120.1	118.5	117.4
45–54 years	546.4	458.8	462.9	372.7	341.7	332.8	328.5	320.4	310.8	309.3
55–64 years	1,293.8	1,078.9	1,014.9	876.2	869.1	859.3	855.3	858.7	837.5	822.7
65–74 years	3,242.8	2,779.3	2,470.7	2,066.6	2,027.1	2,031.8	2,002.5	1,995.9	1,948.5	1,923.5
75–84 years	8,481.5	7,696.6	6,698.7	5,401.7	5,111.6	5,044.2	5,000.5	5,040.4	4,910.6	4,839.1
85 years and over	19,679.5	19,477.7	15,980.2	14,979.6	14,745.4	14,647.4	14,681.4	15,019.1	14,526.1	14,400.6

See footnotes at end of table.

Table 34 (page 2 of 2). Death rates for all causes, according to sex, race, and age: United States, selected years 1950–90

[Data are based on the National Vital Statistics System]

Sex, race, and age	1950[1]	1960[1]	1970	1980	1985	1986	1987	1988	1989	1990
Black female				Deaths per 100,000 resident population						
All ages, age adjusted	1,106.7	916.9	814.4	631.1	594.8	594.1	592.4	601.0	594.3	581.6
All ages, crude	1,002.0	905.0	829.2	733.3	734.2	741.5	745.7	764.6	763.2	747.9
Under 1 year.	- - -	4,162.2	3,368.8	2,123.7	1,821.4	1,781.5	1,804.3	1,834.0	1,839.8	1,735.5
1–4 years	- - -	173.3	129.4	84.4	71.1	76.8	74.1	71.2	72.9	67.6
5–14 years	72.8	53.8	43.8	30.5	28.6	27.5	25.6	30.6	29.0	27.5
15–24 years	213.1	107.5	111.9	70.5	59.6	64.5	68.1	69.3	68.0	68.7
25–34 years	393.3	273.2	231.0	150.0	137.6	148.1	151.8	157.8	161.0	159.5
35–44 years	758.1	568.5	533.0	323.9	276.5	288.0	293.4	304.8	298.6	298.6
45–54 years	1,576.4	1,177.0	1,043.9	768.2	667.6	671.6	665.2	655.3	640.6	639.4
55–64 years	3,089.4	2,510.9	1,986.2	1,561.0	1,532.5	1,505.0	1,484.6	1,513.3	1,478.3	1,452.6
65–74 years	4,000.2	4,064.2	3,860.9	3,057.4	2,967.8	2,940.3	2,931.7	2,948.1	2,936.0	2,865.7
75–84 years	- - -	6,730.0	6,691.5	6,212.1	6,078.0	5,928.3	5,905.2	5,991.4	5,930.2	5,688.3
85 years and over	- - -	13,052.6	10,706.6	12,367.2	12,703.0	13,144.9	12,997.2	13,461.1	13,509.2	13,309.5

[1]Includes deaths of nonresidents of the United States.

NOTES: Data for the 1980's have been revised based on intercensal population estimates and differ from previous editions of Health, United States. See Appendix I, Department of Commerce.

SOURCES: Centers for Disease Control and Prevention, National Center for Health Statistics: Vital Statistics of the United States, Vol. II, Mortality, Part A, for data years 1950–90. Public Health Service. Washington. U.S. Government Printing Office; Data computed by the Division of Analysis from data compiled by the Division of Vital Statistics and from table 1.

Table 35 (page 1 of 2). Death rates for diseases of heart, according to sex, race, and age: United States, selected years 1950–90

[Data are based on the National Vital Statistics System]

Sex, race, and age	1950[1]	1960[1]	1970	1980	1985	1986	1987	1988	1989	1990
All races				Deaths per 100,000 resident population						
All ages, age adjusted	307.2	286.2	253.6	202.0	181.4	176.0	170.8	167.7	157.5	152.0
All ages, crude	355.5	369.0	362.0	336.0	324.1	318.8	313.8	312.9	297.3	289.5
Under 1 year	3.5	6.6	13.1	22.8	25.0	26.5	25.7	23.2	20.1	20.1
1–4 years	1.3	1.3	1.7	2.6	2.2	2.6	2.2	2.4	1.9	1.9
5–14 years	2.1	1.3	0.8	0.9	1.0	0.9	1.0	0.9	0.8	0.9
15–24 years	6.8	4.0	3.0	2.9	2.8	2.8	2.7	2.9	2.5	2.5
25–34 years	19.4	15.6	11.4	8.3	8.3	8.7	8.5	8.3	8.0	7.6
35–44 years	86.4	74.6	66.7	44.6	38.1	37.6	35.7	34.3	32.4	31.4
45–54 years	308.6	271.8	238.4	180.2	153.8	145.6	141.6	132.6	125.5	120.5
55–64 years	808.1	737.9	652.3	494.1	443.0	428.8	413.9	406.8	383.0	367.3
65–74 years	1,839.8	1,740.5	1,558.2	1,218.6	1,089.8	1,054.9	1,021.8	999.2	928.1	894.3
75–84 years	4,310.1	4,089.4	3,683.8	2,993.1	2,693.1	2,617.8	2,539.5	2,518.9	2,378.9	2,295.7
85 years and over	9,150.6	9,317.8	7,891.3	7,777.1	7,384.1	7,267.7	7,184.4	7,253.1	6,868.7	6,739.9
White male										
All ages, age adjusted	381.1	375.4	347.6	277.5	246.2	236.7	228.1	223.0	208.7	202.0
All ages, crude	433.0	454.6	438.3	384.0	360.3	350.2	341.8	338.9	320.5	312.7
Under 1 year	4.1	6.9	12.0	22.5	24.2	26.5	25.4	22.0	19.0	17.5
1–4 years	1.1	1.0	1.5	2.1	1.7	2.1	1.8	2.0	1.7	1.5
5–14 years	1.7	1.1	0.8	0.9	0.8	0.9	0.9	1.0	0.8	0.9
15–24 years	5.8	3.6	3.0	2.9	2.9	3.0	2.9	3.0	2.6	2.6
25–34 years	20.1	17.6	12.3	9.1	9.3	9.6	9.5	9.3	9.1	8.4
35–44 years	110.6	107.5	94.6	61.8	52.7	52.1	49.1	46.6	43.5	42.6
45–54 years	423.6	413.2	365.7	269.8	225.5	209.9	202.9	187.7	176.4	170.6
55–64 years	1,081.7	1,056.0	979.3	730.6	640.1	615.4	588.0	571.2	537.9	516.7
65–74 years	2,308.3	2,297.9	2,177.2	1,729.7	1,522.7	1,467.6	1,408.3	1,381.1	1,278.0	1,230.5
75–84 years	4,907.3	4,839.9	4,617.6	3,883.2	3,527.0	3,401.9	3,291.0	3,255.6	3,067.0	2,983.4
85 years and over	9,950.5	10,135.8	8,818.0	8,958.0	8,481.7	8,161.5	8,052.8	8,160.9	7,660.7	7,558.7
Black male										
All ages, age adjusted	415.5	381.2	375.9	327.3	310.8	306.1	301.0	301.7	289.7	275.9
All ages, crude	348.4	330.6	330.3	301.0	288.6	285.5	280.7	281.6	268.8	256.8
Under 1 year	- - -	13.9	33.5	42.8	48.6	51.4	46.0	43.4	34.3	43.7
1–4 years	- - -	3.8	3.9	6.3	4.5	5.4	5.2	4.6	4.7	4.0
5–14 years	6.4	3.0	1.4	1.3	1.6	1.4	1.7	1.8	1.4	1.3
15–24 years	18.0	8.7	8.3	8.3	7.2	6.7	6.9	7.9	6.3	6.4
25–34 years	51.9	43.1	41.6	30.3	29.5	29.7	27.3	28.1	25.8	24.5
35–44 years	198.1	168.1	189.2	136.6	119.8	120.9	115.8	109.6	104.5	100.0
45–54 years	624.1	514.0	512.8	433.4	385.2	368.5	366.7	357.0	363.4	328.9
55–64 years	1,434.0	1,236.8	1,135.4	987.2	935.3	925.2	881.6	912.1	880.7	824.0
65–74 years	2,140.1	2,281.4	2,237.8	1,847.2	1,839.2	1,792.0	1,801.7	1,772.4	1,700.0	1,632.9
75–84 years	- - -	3,533.6	3,783.4	3,578.8	3,436.6	3,407.3	3,384.3	3,448.3	3,191.6	3,107.1
85 years and over	- - -	6,037.9	5,367.6	6,819.5	6,393.5	6,666.7	6,523.4	6,640.0	6,368.2	6,479.6
White female										
All ages, age adjusted	223.6	197.1	167.8	134.6	121.7	118.9	116.2	114.1	106.6	103.1
All ages, crude	289.4	306.5	313.8	319.2	321.8	320.4	318.7	319.9	305.1	298.4
Under 1 year	2.7	4.3	7.0	15.7	18.6	19.5	19.8	17.4	14.7	14.5
1–4 years	1.1	0.9	1.2	2.1	1.6	2.1	1.7	2.2	1.3	1.6
5–14 years	1.9	0.9	0.7	0.8	0.9	0.7	0.7	0.7	0.7	0.7
15–24 years	5.3	2.8	1.7	1.7	1.7	1.6	1.6	1.7	1.5	1.4
25–34 years	12.2	8.2	5.5	3.9	3.9	4.1	4.2	3.9	3.9	3.7
35–44 years	40.5	28.6	23.9	16.4	14.4	13.9	13.2	12.6	12.1	11.4
45–54 years	141.9	103.4	91.4	71.2	62.5	60.2	59.3	55.0	51.0	50.2
55–64 years	460.2	383.0	317.7	248.1	227.1	223.0	218.9	215.3	198.3	192.4
65–74 years	1,400.9	1,229.8	1,044.0	796.7	713.3	693.9	675.3	656.2	604.7	583.6
75–84 years	3,925.2	3,629.7	3,143.5	2,493.6	2,207.5	2,152.7	2,089.5	2,065.1	1,954.5	1,874.3
85 years and over	9,084.7	9,280.8	7,839.9	7,501.6	7,170.0	7,091.3	7,017.6	7,081.4	6,711.3	6,563.4

See footnotes at end of table.

Table 35 (page 2 of 2). Death rates for diseases of heart, according to sex, race, and age: United States, selected years 1950–90

[Data are based on the National Vital Statistics System]

Sex, race, and age	1950[1]	1960[1]	1970	1980	1985	1986	1987	1988	1989	1990
Black female				Deaths per 100,000 resident population						
All ages, age adjusted.............	349.5	292.6	251.7	201.1	188.3	186.6	182.6	183.3	175.6	168.1
All ages, crude	289.9	268.5	261.0	249.7	250.3	253.4	251.1	254.6	246.2	237.0
Under 1 year	- - -	12.0	31.3	43.6	41.0	44.0	36.7	40.2	39.2	35.8
1–4 years......................	- - -	2.8	4.2	4.4	5.3	4.8	4.4	4.2	3.2	3.8
5–14 years.....................	8.8	3.0	1.8	1.7	1.8	1.5	1.4	1.0	1.7	1.4
15–24 years....................	19.8	10.0	6.0	4.6	4.6	4.6	4.4	4.4	4.2	4.4
25–34 years....................	52.0	35.9	24.7	15.7	13.2	15.4	15.0	13.4	13.3	13.4
35–44 years....................	185.0	125.3	99.8	61.7	50.1	49.7	46.1	50.3	46.6	43.6
45–54 years....................	526.8	360.7	290.9	202.4	176.2	177.0	170.5	173.4	159.6	155.3
55–64 years....................	1,210.7	952.3	710.5	530.1	510.7	490.5	482.8	486.8	470.3	442.0
65–74 years....................	1,659.4	1,680.5	1,553.2	1,210.3	1,149.9	1,126.7	1,111.9	1,087.0	1,054.1	1,017.5
75–84 years....................	- - -	2,926.9	2,964.1	2,707.2	2,533.4	2,529.4	2,465.9	2,514.8	2,380.0	2,250.9
85 years and over...............	- - -	5,650.0	5,003.8	5,796.5	5,686.5	5,987.7	5,940.3	5,989.3	5,898.7	5,766.1

[1]Includes deaths of nonresidents of the United States.

NOTES: For data years shown, the code numbers for cause of death are based on the then current International Classification of Diseases, which are described in Appendix II, tables IV and V. Data for the 1980's have been revised based on intercensal population estimates and differ from previous editions of Health, United States. See Appendix I, Department of Commerce.

SOURCES: Centers for Disease Control and Prevention, National Center for Health Statistics: Vital Statistics of the United States, Vol. II, Mortality, Part A, for data years 1950–90. Public Health Service. Washington. U.S. Government Printing Office; Data computed by the Division of Analysis from data compiled by the Division of Vital Statistics and from table 1.

Table 36 (page 1 of 2). Death rates for cerebrovascular diseases, according to sex, race, and age: United States, selected years 1950–90

[Data are based on the National Vital Statistics System]

Sex, race, and age	1950[1]	1960[1]	1970	1980	1985	1986	1987	1988	1989	1990
All races				Deaths per 100,000 resident population						
All ages, age adjusted	88.6	79.7	66.3	40.8	32.5	31.1	30.4	29.9	28.3	27.7
All ages, crude	104.0	108.0	101.9	75.1	64.3	62.3	61.8	61.6	59.0	57.9
Under 1 year	5.1	4.1	5.0	4.4	3.7	2.9	3.4	4.0	3.3	3.8
1–4 years	0.9	0.8	1.0	0.5	0.3	0.3	0.4	0.4	0.3	0.3
5–14 years	0.5	0.7	0.7	0.3	0.2	0.2	0.2	0.2	0.2	0.2
15–24 years	1.6	1.8	1.6	1.0	0.8	0.7	0.6	0.7	0.6	0.6
25–34 years	4.2	4.7	4.5	2.6	2.2	2.3	2.3	2.2	2.1	2.2
35–44 years	18.7	14.7	15.6	8.5	7.2	7.1	7.0	6.9	6.5	6.5
45–54 years	70.4	49.2	41.6	25.2	21.3	20.5	20.2	19.3	18.6	18.7
55–64 years	195.3	147.3	115.8	65.2	54.8	53.6	52.8	52.0	49.6	48.0
65–74 years	549.7	469.2	384.1	219.5	172.8	166.0	159.3	157.1	147.3	144.4
75–84 years	1,499.6	1,491.3	1,254.2	788.6	601.5	569.5	558.1	548.4	515.1	499.3
85 years and over	2,990.1	3,680.5	3,014.3	2,288.9	1,865.1	1,784.5	1,760.1	1,744.7	1,671.6	1,633.9
White male										
All ages, age adjusted	87.0	80.3	68.8	41.9	33.0	31.2	30.6	30.3	28.4	27.7
All ages, crude	100.5	102.7	93.5	63.3	52.7	50.7	50.2	50.3	47.8	47.0
Under 1 year	5.9	4.3	4.5	3.8	3.7	2.5	3.7	3.2	2.9	3.1
1–4 years	1.1	0.8	1.2	0.4	*0.3	*0.2	0.5	0.3	*0.2	*0.2
5–14 years	0.5	0.7	0.8	0.2	0.2	0.2	0.2	0.2	0.3	0.2
15–24 years	1.6	1.7	1.6	1.0	0.7	0.6	0.6	0.7	0.5	0.6
25–34 years	3.4	3.5	3.2	2.0	1.8	1.8	1.8	1.8	1.7	1.8
35–44 years	13.1	11.3	11.8	6.5	5.5	5.7	5.4	5.5	5.0	4.9
45–54 years	53.7	40.9	35.6	21.7	18.1	16.6	16.8	16.2	15.0	15.4
55–64 years	182.2	139.0	119.9	64.2	54.6	51.8	51.1	50.9	48.0	45.8
65–74 years	569.7	501.0	420.0	240.4	186.4	174.6	169.0	167.4	156.3	153.2
75–84 years	1,556.3	1,564.8	1,361.6	854.8	650.0	616.7	601.2	590.4	554.8	540.7
85 years and over	3,127.1	3,734.8	3,018.1	2,236.9	1,765.6	1,701.8	1,667.7	1,685.4	1,591.3	1,549.8
Black male										
All ages, age adjusted	146.2	141.2	122.5	77.5	62.7	61.1	59.7	60.8	57.3	56.1
All ages, crude	122.0	122.9	108.8	73.1	59.2	58.0	56.6	57.6	54.3	53.1
Under 1 year	- - -	8.5	12.3	11.2	10.1	8.2	*5.9	9.4	7.6	10.2
1–4 years	- - -	1.9	*1.4	*0.6	*0.8	*0.6	*0.5	*0.5	*0.4	*0.8
5–14 years	*0.7	*0.9	0.8	*0.5	*0.1	*0.2	*0.3	*0.2	*0.4	*0.2
15–24 years	3.3	3.7	3.0	2.1	1.3	1.1	0.9	0.9	1.0	0.9
25–34 years	12.0	12.8	14.6	7.7	5.8	6.2	5.5	6.9	4.9	4.6
35–44 years	59.3	47.4	52.7	29.2	25.4	26.6	26.4	25.1	24.0	22.7
45–54 years	211.9	166.1	136.1	82.1	71.1	68.9	68.2	67.4	67.6	68.4
55–64 years	522.8	439.9	343.4	189.8	160.7	154.3	155.7	160.3	150.1	141.8
65–74 years	783.6	899.2	780.1	472.8	379.7	361.8	345.8	357.1	335.0	327.2
75–84 years	- - -	1,475.2	1,445.7	1,067.6	814.4	809.9	780.5	799.3	723.3	723.7
85 years and over	- - -	2,700.0	1,963.1	1,873.2	1,429.0	1,436.5	1,443.8	1,403.1	1,454.5	1,430.5
White female										
All ages, age adjusted	79.7	68.7	56.2	35.2	27.9	27.0	26.3	25.5	24.2	23.8
All ages, crude	103.3	110.1	109.8	88.8	78.4	76.5	76.2	75.4	72.6	71.8
Under 1 year	2.9	2.6	3.2	3.3	2.3	1.8	2.1	2.9	2.6	2.6
1–4 years	0.6	0.5	0.6	0.4	*0.3	*0.2	*0.3	*0.3	*0.3	0.3
5–14 years	0.4	0.6	0.6	0.3	0.3	0.2	0.2	0.2	0.2	0.2
15–24 years	1.2	1.4	1.1	0.7	0.7	0.6	0.6	0.6	0.5	0.5
25–34 years	2.9	3.4	3.4	2.0	1.6	1.7	1.7	1.6	1.6	1.7
35–44 years	13.6	10.1	11.5	6.7	5.3	5.0	5.2	4.6	4.4	4.4
45–54 years	55.0	33.8	30.5	18.7	15.5	15.6	14.6	14.0	13.3	13.5
55–64 years	156.9	103.0	78.1	48.7	40.0	40.4	39.0	37.3	35.9	35.8
65–74 years	498.1	383.3	303.2	172.8	137.9	136.3	129.3	125.3	117.8	116.3
75–84 years	1,471.3	1,444.7	1,176.8	730.3	552.9	524.0	516.3	503.8	471.0	457.6
85 years and over	3,017.9	3,795.7	3,167.6	2,367.8	1,944.9	1,855.6	1,832.1	1,798.5	1,729.6	1,691.4

See footnotes at end of table.

Table 36 (page 2 of 2). Death rates for cerebrovascular diseases, according to sex, race, and age: United States, selected years 1950–90

[Data are based on the National Vital Statistics System]

Sex, race, and age	1950[1]	1960[1]	1970	1980	1985	1986	1987	1988	1989	1990
Black female				Deaths per 100,000 resident population						
All ages, age adjusted..............	155.6	139.5	107.9	61.7	50.6	47.9	47.1	47.1	45.5	42.7
All ages, crude..................	128.3	127.7	112.2	77.9	68.6	65.6	65.1	66.3	64.5	60.7
Under 1 year	- - -	*6.7	9.1	*6.4	*5.5	*5.5	7.8	8.2	*4.5	*6.0
1–4 years.......................	- - -	*1.3	*1.4	*0.5	*0.5	*0.4	*0.6	*0.7	*0.5	*0.1
5–14 years.....................	*0.6	1.0	0.8	*0.3	*0.3	*0.3	*0.2	*0.4	*0.3	*0.3
15–24 years....................	4.2	3.4	3.0	1.7	1.5	1.0	1.1	1.1	1.3	1.1
25–34 years....................	15.9	17.4	14.3	7.0	5.7	6.1	5.9	5.4	5.8	5.5
35–44 years....................	75.0	57.4	49.1	21.6	19.1	18.3	17.4	18.3	16.7	18.6
45–54 years....................	248.9	166.2	119.4	61.9	50.8	47.6	48.6	44.4	45.7	44.1
55–64 years....................	567.7	452.0	272.4	138.7	113.6	112.0	111.7	109.2	103.3	97.0
65–74 years....................	754.4	830.5	673.5	362.2	285.6	273.0	266.4	271.4	255.1	236.8
75–84 years....................	- - -	1,413.1	1,338.3	918.6	753.8	685.2	658.9	671.1	669.3	596.0
85 years and over...............	- - -	2,578.9	2,210.5	1,896.3	1,657.1	1,580.4	1,563.2	1,609.4	1,530.7	1,496.5

[1]Includes deaths of nonresidents of the United States.

*Based on fewer than 20 deaths.

NOTES: For data years shown, the code numbers for cause of death are based on the then current International Classification of Diseases, which are described in Appendix II, tables IV and V. Data for the 1980's have been revised based on intercensal population estimates and differ from previous editions of Health, United States. See Appendix I, Department of Commerce.

SOURCES: Centers for Disease Control and Prevention, National Center for Health Statistics: Vital Statistics of the United States, Vol. II, Mortality, Part A, for data years 1950–90. Public Health Service. Washington. U.S. Government Printing Office; Data computed by the Division of Analysis from data compiled by the Division of Vital Statistics and from table 1.

[Data are based on the National Vital Statistics System]

Sex, race, and age	1950[1]	1960[1]	1970	1980	1985	1986	1987	1988	1989	1990
All races				Deaths per 100,000 resident population						
All ages, age adjusted	125.3	125.8	129.8	132.8	134.4	134.1	134.0	134.0	134.5	135.0
All ages, crude	139.8	149.2	162.8	183.9	194.0	195.5	196.8	198.4	201.0	203.2
Under 1 year	8.7	7.2	4.7	3.2	3.1	2.6	2.7	2.4	2.8	2.3
1–4 years	11.7	10.9	7.5	4.5	3.8	4.0	3.8	3.8	3.5	3.5
5–14 years	6.7	6.8	6.0	4.3	3.5	3.5	3.4	3.2	3.3	3.1
15–24 years	8.6	8.3	8.3	6.3	5.4	5.3	5.0	5.0	5.0	4.9
25–34 years	20.0	19.5	16.5	13.7	13.2	13.2	12.5	12.1	12.3	12.6
35–44 years	62.7	59.7	59.5	48.6	45.9	45.4	43.6	44.3	43.2	43.3
45–54 years	175.1	177.0	182.5	180.0	170.1	166.8	165.6	161.9	158.9	158.9
55–64 years	392.9	396.8	423.0	436.1	454.6	449.2	452.5	453.9	452.5	449.6
65–74 years	692.5	713.9	751.2	817.9	845.5	856.6	855.3	855.7	867.8	872.3
75–84 years	1,153.3	1,127.4	1,169.2	1,232.3	1,271.8	1,277.7	1,288.0	1,301.0	1,326.0	1,348.5
85 years and over	1,451.0	1,450.0	1,320.7	1,594.6	1,615.4	1,632.0	1,643.2	1,674.7	1,703.7	1,752.9
White male										
All ages, age adjusted	130.9	141.6	154.3	160.5	160.4	160.2	160.1	159.6	159.4	160.3
All ages, crude	147.2	166.1	185.1	208.7	218.1	219.8	221.6	222.8	224.9	227.7
Under 1 year	9.6	7.9	4.3	3.5	3.1	3.1	2.8	2.4	2.9	2.2
1–4 years	13.1	13.1	8.5	5.4	4.4	4.7	4.1	4.0	3.9	3.7
5–14 years	7.6	8.0	7.0	5.2	4.0	3.9	4.1	3.8	3.7	3.5
15–24 years	9.9	10.3	10.6	7.8	6.4	6.6	5.8	5.8	5.5	5.7
25–34 years	17.7	18.8	16.2	13.6	13.1	13.7	12.1	11.7	11.6	12.3
35–44 years	44.5	46.3	50.1	41.1	39.8	37.9	37.0	37.2	35.9	35.8
45–54 years	150.8	164.1	172.0	175.4	162.0	159.4	158.1	154.6	151.0	149.9
55–64 years	409.4	450.9	498.1	497.4	512.0	508.5	514.5	514.1	511.8	508.2
65–74 years	798.7	887.3	997.0	1,070.7	1,076.5	1,083.0	1,084.4	1,075.5	1,083.3	1,090.7
75–84 years	1,367.6	1,413.7	1,592.7	1,779.7	1,817.1	1,825.2	1,826.6	1,838.6	1,853.6	1,883.2
85 years and over	1,732.7	1,791.4	1,772.2	2,375.6	2,449.1	2,469.3	2,482.4	2,560.7	2,603.7	2,715.1
Black male										
All ages, age adjusted	126.1	158.5	198.0	229.9	239.9	239.0	240.0	240.4	246.2	248.1
All ages, crude	106.6	136.7	171.6	205.5	214.9	214.5	215.8	215.7	220.6	221.9
Under 1 year	- - -	*6.8	*5.3	*4.5	*2.5	*1.8	*2.1	*2.7	*1.6	*3.4
1–4 years	- - -	7.9	7.6	5.1	3.4	3.2	4.3	3.4	3.0	3.6
5–14 years	5.8	4.4	4.8	3.7	3.7	3.9	2.8	3.2	3.4	3.4
15–24 years	7.9	9.7	9.4	8.1	6.4	6.3	6.5	6.2	6.9	6.1
25–34 years	18.0	18.4	18.8	14.1	14.9	14.4	14.5	14.2	15.2	15.7
35–44 years	55.7	72.9	81.3	73.8	69.9	69.8	63.3	66.0	63.0	64.3
45–54 years	211.7	244.7	311.2	333.0	315.9	306.4	299.9	305.7	308.0	302.6
55–64 years	490.8	579.7	689.2	812.5	851.3	830.1	830.4	821.0	840.5	859.2
65–74 years	636.4	938.5	1,168.9	1,417.2	1,532.8	1,558.5	1,578.0	1,572.6	1,621.3	1,613.9
75–84 years	- - -	1,053.3	1,624.8	2,029.6	2,229.6	2,249.2	2,338.2	2,353.1	2,436.7	2,478.3
85 years and over	- - -	1,155.2	1,387.0	2,393.9	2,629.0	2,787.3	2,867.2	2,929.2	3,040.9	3,238.3
White female										
All ages, age adjusted	119.4	109.5	107.6	107.7	110.5	110.3	110.0	110.4	111.1	111.2
All ages, crude	139.9	139.8	149.4	170.3	184.4	186.4	187.9	190.5	194.2	196.1
Under 1 year	7.8	6.8	5.4	2.7	3.1	2.4	3.0	2.3	3.2	2.2
1–4 years	11.3	9.7	6.9	3.6	3.5	3.4	3.6	3.7	3.0	3.2
5–14 years	6.3	6.2	5.4	3.7	3.1	3.1	2.9	2.7	3.0	2.9
15–24 years	7.5	6.5	6.2	4.7	4.3	4.2	3.9	4.1	4.2	4.0
25–34 years	20.9	18.8	16.3	13.5	12.7	12.2	12.4	11.7	12.2	11.9
35–44 years	74.5	66.6	62.4	50.9	47.3	47.7	45.4	46.6	46.0	46.2
45–54 years	185.8	175.7	177.3	166.4	161.6	156.8	156.3	152.8	149.9	150.9
55–64 years	362.5	329.0	338.6	355.5	376.3	372.0	373.1	376.1	375.0	368.5
65–74 years	616.5	562.1	554.7	605.2	644.9	658.7	654.2	660.0	671.2	675.1
75–84 years	1,026.6	939.3	903.5	905.4	938.2	944.3	954.4	967.4	995.5	1,011.8
85 years and over	1,348.3	1,304.9	1,126.6	1,266.8	1,285.4	1,296.4	1,308.3	1,323.2	1,348.3	1,372.3

See footnotes at end of table.

Table 37 (page 2 of 2). Death rates for malignant neoplasms, according to sex, race, and age: United States, selected years 1950–90

[Data are based on the National Vital Statistics System]

Sex, race, and age	1950[1]	1960[1]	1970	1980	1985	1986	1987	1988	1989	1990
Black female				Deaths per 100,000 resident population						
All ages, age adjusted	131.9	127.8	123.5	129.7	131.8	133.7	133.9	133.5	133.5	137.2
All ages, crude	111.8	113.8	117.3	136.5	145.2	148.3	149.5	150.9	151.8	156.1
Under 1 year.	- - -	*6.7	*3.3	*3.0	*4.4	*2.9	*1.8	*3.4	*3.2	*1.9
1–4 years	- - -	6.9	5.7	3.9	2.5	4.4	2.6	3.8	3.7	3.4
5–14 years	3.9	4.8	4.0	3.4	3.0	3.0	3.1	2.9	2.9	2.4
15–24 years	8.8	6.9	6.4	5.7	4.4	4.7	5.4	4.9	4.9	4.8
25–34 years	34.3	31.0	20.9	18.3	17.2	18.0	16.0	17.8	16.1	18.7
35–44 years	119.8	102.4	94.6	73.5	69.0	71.7	72.3	70.5	66.7	67.4
45–54 years	277.0	254.8	228.6	230.2	212.4	220.9	220.8	202.9	205.3	209.9
55–64 years	484.6	442.7	404.8	450.4	474.9	462.4	469.8	468.9	459.1	482.4
65–74 years	477.3	541.6	615.8	662.4	704.2	729.4	717.4	746.9	769.4	773.2
75–84 years	- - -	696.3	763.3	923.9	986.3	981.4	1,004.6	1,017.7	1,029.8	1,059.9
85 years and over	- - -	728.9	791.5	1,159.9	1,284.2	1,318.1	1,326.4	1,365.8	1,383.0	1,431.3

[1]Includes deaths of nonresidents of the United States.

*Based on fewer than 20 deaths.

NOTES: For data years shown, the code numbers for cause of death are based on the then current International Classification of Diseases, which are described in Appendix II, tables IV and V. Data for the 1980's have been revised based on intercensal population estimates and differ from previous editions of Health, United States. See Appendix I, Department of Commerce.

SOURCES: Centers for Disease Control and Prevention, National Center for Health Statistics: Vital Statistics of the United States, Vol. II, Mortality, Part A, for data years 1950–90. Public Health Service. Washington. U.S. Government Printing Office; Data computed by the Division of Analysis from data compiled by the Division of Vital Statistics and from table 1.

Table 38. Death rates for malignant neoplasms of respiratory system, according to sex, race, and age: United States, selected years 1950–90

[Data are based on the National Vital Statistics System]

Sex, race, and age	1950[1]	1960[1]	1970	1980	1985	1986	1987	1988	1989	1990
All races				Deaths per 100,000 resident population						
All ages, age adjusted	12.8	19.2	28.4	36.4	39.1	39.3	40.0	40.3	40.8	41.4
All ages, crude	14.1	22.2	34.2	47.9	53.5	54.3	55.7	56.5	57.6	58.9
Under 25 years	0.1	0.1	0.1	0.1	0.1	0.1	0.1	0.1	0.1	0.1
25–34 years	0.9	1.1	1.0	0.8	0.8	0.7	0.8	0.7	0.7	0.8
35–44 years	5.1	7.3	11.6	9.6	8.2	7.9	7.7	7.6	7.3	7.2
45–54 years	22.9	32.0	46.2	56.5	53.1	52.1	52.0	50.4	49.3	48.8
55–64 years	55.2	81.5	116.2	144.3	159.8	159.5	162.3	164.6	165.0	166.5
65–74 years	69.3	117.2	174.6	243.1	270.3	274.8	281.9	284.4	292.1	298.1
75–84 years	69.3	102.9	175.1	251.4	292.4	301.6	310.8	321.2	333.5	344.1
85 years and over	64.0	79.1	113.5	184.5	205.0	217.6	225.2	233.4	238.0	252.9
White male										
All ages, age adjusted	21.6	34.6	49.9	58.0	58.7	58.6	59.2	58.8	58.3	59.0
All ages, crude	24.1	39.6	58.3	73.4	77.6	78.1	79.5	79.5	79.6	81.0
Under 25 years	0.1	0.1	0.1	0.1	0.1	0.1	*0.1	0.1	0.1	0.1
25–34 years	1.2	1.6	1.4	0.9	0.7	0.9	0.9	0.8	0.7	0.9
35–44 years	7.9	10.4	15.4	11.2	9.5	8.6	8.6	8.5	7.9	8.0
45–54 years	39.1	53.0	67.6	74.3	65.5	64.1	63.9	61.1	59.0	57.9
55–64 years	95.9	149.8	199.3	215.0	223.3	223.2	225.8	225.4	221.8	222.5
65–74 years	119.4	225.1	344.8	418.4	425.2	424.7	432.2	428.8	430.1	438.2
75–84 years	109.1	191.9	360.7	516.1	561.7	570.2	572.9	578.7	580.6	593.6
85 years and over	102.7	133.9	221.8	391.5	463.8	478.8	496.8	499.3	517.7	540.4
Black male										
All ages, age adjusted	16.9	36.6	60.8	82.0	87.7	87.9	88.9	88.7	90.8	91.0
All ages, crude	14.3	31.1	51.2	70.8	75.5	75.8	76.8	76.7	78.0	77.8
Under 25 years	*0.0	*0.1	*0.2	*0.2	*0.1	*0.1	*0.1	*0.1	*0.2	*0.2
25–34 years	2.1	2.6	2.9	1.9	1.9	1.5	1.8	1.3	1.2	2.1
35–44 years	9.4	20.7	32.6	26.9	22.4	21.9	19.1	20.3	19.4	20.0
45–54 years	41.1	75.0	123.5	142.8	133.1	132.5	128.1	124.2	128.0	125.0
55–64 years	78.8	161.8	250.3	340.3	373.2	360.9	360.7	352.9	364.9	377.5
65–74 years	65.2	184.6	322.2	499.4	565.9	580.9	610.9	610.1	622.8	613.4
75–84 years	- - -	126.3	290.6	499.6	579.0	606.5	632.2	666.8	684.7	669.9
85 years and over	- - -	110.3	154.4	337.7	409.7	485.7	495.3	569.2	507.6	535.7
White female										
All ages, age adjusted	4.6	5.1	10.1	18.2	22.7	23.1	23.9	24.9	25.9	26.5
All ages, crude	5.4	6.4	13.1	26.5	34.8	36.1	37.7	39.7	41.9	43.4
Under 25 years	*0.0	0.1	0.1	0.1	0.1	*0.0	0.1	*0.1	*0.0	*0.0
25–34 years	0.5	0.6	0.6	0.5	0.6	0.5	0.6	0.5	0.5	0.6
35–44 years	2.2	3.4	6.0	6.8	5.7	5.8	5.7	5.7	5.3	5.2
45–54 years	6.5	9.8	22.1	33.9	36.2	35.2	35.3	35.3	34.4	35.2
55–64 years	15.5	16.7	39.3	74.2	94.7	95.5	98.9	104.2	107.4	108.0
65–74 years	27.2	26.5	45.4	108.1	149.0	156.0	161.1	168.1	180.3	185.3
75–84 years	40.0	36.5	56.8	99.3	138.7	147.1	159.3	170.4	188.2	199.0
85 years and over	44.0	45.2	57.4	96.8	103.2	114.9	119.2	129.3	131.5	143.2
Black female										
All ages, age adjusted	4.1	5.5	10.9	19.5	22.8	23.7	24.7	25.2	26.0	27.5
All ages, crude	3.4	4.9	10.1	19.3	23.5	24.5	25.7	26.5	27.8	29.2
Under 25 years	*0.1	*0.1	*0.1	*0.1	*0.1	*0.0	*0.1	*0.1	*0.1	*0.1
25–34 years	*1.2	0.8	*0.5	*0.8	1.0	*0.6	*0.4	*0.6	1.0	0.8
35–44 years	2.7	3.4	10.5	7.9	7.6	8.5	8.9	6.5	7.8	7.9
45–54 years	8.8	12.8	25.3	46.4	41.5	43.9	45.2	42.4	42.7	43.4
55–64 years	15.3	20.7	36.4	83.8	107.8	104.9	110.0	113.9	111.2	122.8
65–74 years	16.4	20.7	49.3	91.7	120.6	133.1	139.2	149.5	161.3	169.9
75–84 years	- - -	33.1	52.6	81.1	105.6	119.1	124.8	139.9	151.2	153.8
85 years and over	- - -	44.7	47.6	90.5	117.3	107.2	116.7	112.1	132.0	138.1

[1]Includes deaths of nonresidents of the United States.

*Based on fewer than 20 deaths.

NOTES: For data years shown, the code numbers for cause of death are based on the then current International Classification of Diseases, which are described in Appendix II, tables IV and V. Data for the 1980's have been revised based on intercensal population estimates and differ from previous editions of Health, United States. See Appendix I, Department of Commerce.

SOURCES: Centers for Disease Control and Prevention, National Center for Health Statistics: Vital Statistics of the United States, Vol. II, Mortality, Part A, for data years 1950–90. Public Health Service. Washington. U.S. Government Printing Office; Data computed by the Division of Analysis from data compiled by the Division of Vital Statistics and from table 1.

Table 39. Death rates for malignant neoplasm of breast for females, according to race and age: United States, selected years 1950–90

[Data are based on the National Vital Statistics System]

Race and age	1950[1]	1960[1]	1970	1980	1985	1986	1987	1988	1989	1990
All races			Deaths per 100,000 resident population							
All ages, age adjusted	22.2	22.3	23.1	22.7	23.3	23.2	23.0	23.3	23.1	23.1
All ages, crude................	24.7	26.1	28.4	30.6	32.8	32.9	32.9	33.6	33.9	34.0
Under 25 years	*0.1	*0.1	*0.0	*0.0	0.0	*0.0	*0.0	*0.0	*0.0	*0.0
25–34 years..................	3.8	3.8	3.9	3.3	3.0	3.1	3.1	3.1	3.0	2.9
35–44 years.................	20.8	20.2	20.4	17.9	17.5	18.3	17.6	17.6	17.8	17.8
45–54 years.................	46.9	51.4	52.6	48.1	47.1	45.8	45.9	45.8	45.3	45.4
55–64 years.................	70.4	70.8	77.6	80.5	84.2	81.6	81.5	82.8	79.7	78.6
65–74 years.................	94.0	90.0	93.8	101.1	107.8	110.1	108.7	109.8	111.6	111.7
75–84 years.................	139.8	129.9	127.4	126.4	136.2	134.5	135.9	140.8	145.1	146.3
85 years and over	195.5	191.9	157.1	169.3	178.5	182.5	179.7	188.2	190.5	196.8
White										
All ages, age adjusted	22.5	22.4	23.4	22.8	23.4	23.1	22.9	23.1	23.1	22.9
All ages, crude................	25.7	27.2	29.9	32.3	34.7	34.8	34.7	35.4	35.8	35.9
Under 25 years	*0.1	*0.0	*0.0	*0.0	*0.0	*0.0	*0.0	*0.0	*0.0	*0.0
25–34 years..................	3.7	3.6	3.7	3.0	2.8	2.8	2.9	2.8	2.8	2.6
35–44 years.................	20.8	19.7	20.2	17.3	16.8	17.4	16.5	16.6	17.2	17.1
45–54 years.................	47.1	51.2	53.0	48.1	46.8	44.8	44.7	44.8	44.1	44.3
55–64 years.................	70.9	71.8	79.3	81.3	84.7	82.4	81.9	83.0	80.4	78.5
65–74 years.................	96.3	91.6	95.9	103.7	109.9	112.4	110.6	111.8	113.2	113.3
75–84 years.................	143.6	132.8	129.6	128.4	138.8	137.9	138.4	142.7	147.7	148.2
85 years and over	204.2	199.7	161.9	171.7	180.9	184.6	181.6	189.9	192.7	198.0
Black										
All ages, age adjusted	19.3	21.3	21.5	23.3	25.5	26.2	26.9	27.5	26.5	27.5
All ages, crude................	16.4	18.7	19.7	22.9	25.9	26.5	27.5	28.5	27.7	29.0
Under 25 years	*0.1	*0.2	*0.1	*0.0	*0.1	*0.1	*0.1	*0.1	*0.1	*0.1
25–34 years..................	4.9	6.1	5.9	5.3	4.5	5.7	4.8	5.4	5.2	5.3
35–44 years.................	21.0	24.8	24.4	24.1	26.1	28.1	28.6	28.8	25.1	25.8
45–54 years.................	46.5	54.4	52.0	52.7	55.5	60.6	61.9	60.5	61.4	60.5
55–64 years.................	64.3	63.2	64.7	79.9	90.4	85.6	90.6	93.4	85.3	93.1
65–74 years.................	67.0	72.3	77.3	84.3	100.7	102.1	103.0	105.1	109.9	112.2
75–84 years.................	- - -	87.5	101.8	114.1	117.6	108.1	120.4	133.1	129.2	140.5
85 years and over	- - -	92.1	112.1	149.9	159.4	170.3	171.5	187.2	184.3	201.5

[1]Includes deaths of nonresidents of the United States.

*Based on fewer than 20 deaths.

NOTES: For data years shown, the code numbers for cause of death are based on the then current International Classification of Diseases, which are described in Appendix II, tables IV and V. Data for the 1980's have been revised based on intercensal population estimates and differ from previous editions of Health, United States. See Appendix I, Department of Commerce.

SOURCES: Centers for Disease Control and Prevention, National Center for Health Statistics: Vital Statistics of the United States, Vol. II, Mortality, Part A, for data years 1950–90. Public Health Service. Washington. U.S. Government Printing Office; Data computed by the Division of Analysis from data compiled by the Division of Vital Statistics and from table 1.

Table 40. Death rates for human immunodeficiency virus (HIV) infection, according to sex, race, and age: United States, 1987–90

[Data are based on the National Vital Statistics System]

Race and age	Both sexes				Male				Female			
	1987	1988	1989	1990	1987	1988	1989	1990	1987	1988	1989	1990
All races	Deaths per 100,000 resident population											
All ages, age adjusted	5.5	6.7	8.7	9.8	10.0	12.1	15.8	17.7	1.1	1.4	1.8	2.1
All ages, crude	5.6	6.8	8.9	10.1	10.2	12.4	16.4	18.5	1.1	1.4	1.8	2.2
Under 1 year	2.3	2.2	3.1	2.7	2.2	2.5	2.7	2.4	2.5	1.7	3.5	3.0
1–4 years	0.7	0.8	0.8	0.8	0.7	0.8	0.7	0.8	0.7	0.7	0.8	0.8
5–14 years	0.1	0.2	0.2	0.2	0.2	0.2	0.2	0.3	*0.1	0.1	0.1	0.2
15–24 years	1.3	1.4	1.6	1.5	2.2	2.3	2.6	2.2	0.3	0.5	0.6	0.7
25–34 years	11.7	14.0	17.9	19.7	20.7	24.5	31.5	34.5	2.8	3.5	4.4	4.9
35–44 years	14.0	17.6	23.5	27.4	26.3	32.6	43.6	50.2	2.1	3.0	3.9	5.2
45–54 years	8.0	9.8	13.3	15.2	15.5	19.0	25.6	29.1	0.8	1.1	1.6	1.9
55–64 years	3.5	4.0	5.4	6.2	6.8	7.8	10.5	12.0	0.5	0.7	0.8	1.1
65–74 years	1.3	1.6	1.8	2.0	2.4	2.9	3.3	3.7	0.5	0.6	0.7	0.8
75–84 years	0.8	0.8	0.7	0.7	1.2	1.5	1.2	1.1	0.5	0.4	0.4	0.4
85 years and over	*0.5	*0.4	*0.4	*0.4	*0.8	*1.0	*1.0	*0.5	*0.3	*0.1	*0.2	*0.4
White												
All ages, age adjusted	4.5	5.3	7.1	8.0	8.4	10.0	13.2	15.0	0.6	0.7	0.9	1.1
All ages, crude	4.6	5.5	7.3	8.3	8.7	10.4	13.9	15.8	0.6	0.7	0.9	1.1
Under 1 year	1.1	1.1	1.7	1.0	1.3	1.5	1.7	*1.1	*0.9	*0.7	1.7	*0.8
1–4 years	0.4	0.4	0.4	0.4	0.4	0.4	*0.2	*0.3	0.4	0.4	0.5	0.5
5–14 years	0.1	0.1	0.1	0.1	0.2	0.2	0.2	*0.1	*0.1	*0.1	*0.1	*0.1
15–24 years	1.0	1.0	1.2	1.0	1.7	1.8	2.0	1.7	0.1	0.3	0.4	0.4
25–34 years	9.3	10.8	14.3	15.7	17.0	19.8	26.2	28.8	1.4	1.7	2.2	2.4
35–44 years	11.4	14.1	18.9	22.4	21.8	26.9	36.1	42.5	1.0	1.4	1.6	2.3
45–54 years	6.9	8.5	11.5	13.2	13.6	16.5	22.5	25.8	0.5	0.6	0.9	1.0
55–64 years	3.1	3.4	4.6	5.1	6.0	6.6	9.1	10.0	0.4	0.5	0.5	0.7
65–74 years	1.3	1.5	1.6	1.7	2.3	2.6	2.8	3.1	0.5	0.6	0.6	0.6
75–84 years	0.8	0.8	0.7	0.6	1.2	1.4	1.2	1.0	0.6	0.4	0.4	*0.3
85 years and over	*0.4	*0.4	*0.4	*0.3	*0.6	*1.0	*0.8	*0.1	*0.3	*0.2	*0.2	*0.3
Black												
All ages, age adjusted	14.3	17.9	23.0	25.7	25.4	31.6	40.3	44.2	4.7	6.2	8.1	9.9
All ages, crude	13.8	17.5	22.5	25.4	23.8	29.9	38.4	42.3	4.8	6.4	8.3	10.2
Under 1 year	9.5	8.2	10.9	11.9	7.3	8.8	8.6	9.3	11.7	7.6	13.3	14.6
1–4 years	2.4	3.0	3.0	3.3	2.4	3.3	3.5	3.6	2.5	2.8	2.5	3.0
5–14 years	*0.3	0.4	0.4	1.0	*0.3	*0.4	*0.4	1.1	*0.3	*0.5	*0.4	0.9
15–24 years	3.3	3.8	4.5	4.2	5.3	5.9	6.8	5.7	1.4	1.7	2.1	2.7
25–34 years	31.4	38.4	46.8	51.0	52.9	64.0	77.4	84.1	12.2	15.6	19.4	21.4
35–44 years	38.4	49.2	65.3	73.1	71.0	89.0	116.9	127.1	10.7	15.3	21.0	26.6
45–54 years	18.0	23.5	31.7	35.9	35.7	45.7	60.6	67.1	3.4	5.1	7.7	10.0
55–64 years	8.3	10.3	13.5	17.5	16.9	20.1	27.1	34.5	*1.6	2.6	2.9	4.4
65–74 years	1.7	3.5	5.1	6.0	*2.5	7.0	10.2	10.6	*1.1	*1.2	*1.6	2.8
75–84 years	*0.4	*1.3	*1.3	*1.8	*0.4	*2.6	*1.5	*2.5	*0.4	*0.6	*1.2	*1.4
85 years and over	*1.4	*0.5	*0.5	*1.8	*3.1	*1.5	*1.5	*4.5	*0.7	*–	*–	*0.6

*Based on fewer than 20 deaths.

NOTES: Categories for the coding and classification of human immunodeficiency virus infection were introduced in the United States beginning with mortality data for 1987. Data for the 1980's have been revised based on intercensal population estimates and differ from previous editions of Health, United States. See Appendix I, Department of Commerce.

SOURCE: Centers for Disease Control and Prevention, National Center for Health Statistics: Vital Statistics of the United States, Vol. II, Mortality, Part A, for data years 1987–90. Public Health Service. Washington. U.S. Government Printing Office.

Table 41. Maternal mortality rates for complications of pregnancy, childbirth, and the puerperium, according to race and age: United States, selected years 1950–90

[Data are based on the National Vital Statistics System]

Race and age	1950[1]	1960[1]	1970	1980	1985	1986	1987	1988	1989	1990
All races				Deaths per 100,000 live births						
All ages, age adjusted	73.7	32.1	21.5	9.4	7.6	7.0	6.1	8.0	7.3	7.6
All ages, crude	83.3	37.1	21.5	9.2	7.8	7.2	6.6	8.4	7.9	8.2
Under 20 years	70.7	22.7	18.9	7.6	6.9	5.9	5.1	7.0	5.8	7.5
20–24 years	47.6	20.7	13.0	5.8	5.4	5.7	4.8	7.2	6.4	6.1
25–29 years	63.5	29.8	17.0	7.7	6.4	5.8	5.3	6.1	6.7	6.0
30–34 years	107.7	50.3	31.6	13.6	8.9	7.8	8.9	9.3	10.0	9.5
35 years and over [2]	222.0	104.3	81.9	36.3	25.0	21.4	15.1	21.9	15.3	20.7
White										
All ages, age adjusted	53.1	22.4	14.4	6.7	4.9	4.6	4.8	5.5	5.4	5.1
All ages, crude	61.1	26.0	14.3	6.6	5.1	4.8	5.0	5.8	5.6	5.4
Under 20 years	44.9	14.8	13.8	5.8	*4.3	*4.0	*5.3	*3.7	*5.2	*5.3
20–24 years	35.7	15.3	8.4	4.2	3.3	3.7	3.8	5.4	4.9	3.9
25–29 years	45.0	20.3	11.1	5.4	4.6	3.6	3.8	4.5	4.8	4.8
30–34 years	75.9	34.3	18.7	9.3	5.1	5.1	5.9	7.0	6.4	5.0
35 years and over [2]	174.1	73.9	59.3	25.5	17.5	15.8	11.6	12.2	9.7	12.6
Black										
All ages, age adjusted	- - -	92.0	65.5	24.9	22.1	20.3	15.2	20.9	18.6	21.7
All ages, crude	- - -	103.6	60.9	22.4	21.3	19.7	14.9	20.5	18.4	22.4
Under 20 years	- - -	54.8	32.3	13.1	*12.4	*10.9	*4.3	*12.3	*7.0	*12.0
20–24 years	- - -	56.9	41.9	13.9	14.6	14.5	9.8	15.2	13.5	14.7
25–29 years	- - -	92.8	65.2	22.4	19.4	20.4	15.1	15.1	17.9	14.9
30–34 years	- - -	150.6	117.8	44.0	38.0	30.9	32.8	28.4	33.8	44.2
35 years and over [2]	- - -	299.5	207.5	100.6	77.2	*62.4	*46.1	90.7	57.5	79.7

[1] Includes deaths of nonresidents of the United States.
[2] Rates computed by relating deaths of women 35 years and over to live births to women 35–49 years.

*Based on fewer than 20 deaths.

NOTE: For data years shown, the code numbers for cause of death are based on the then current International Classification of Diseases, which are described in Appendix II, tables IV and V.

SOURCES: Centers for Disease Control and Prevention, National Center for Health Statistics: Vital Statistics of the United States, Vol. II, Mortality, Part A, for data years 1950–90. Public Health Service. Washington. U.S. Government Printing Office; Vital Statistics of the United States, Vol. I, Natality, for data years 1950–90. Public Health Service. Washington. U.S. Government Printing Office; Data computed by the Division of Analysis from data compiled by the Division of Vital Statistics.

Table 42 (page 1 of 2). Death rates for motor vehicle crashes, according to sex, race, and age: United States, selected years 1950–90

[Data are based on the National Vital Statistics System]

Sex, race, and age	1950[1]	1960[1]	1970	1980	1985	1986	1987	1988	1989	1990
All races				Deaths per 100,000 resident population						
All ages, age adjusted	23.3	22.5	27.4	22.9	18.8	19.4	19.4	19.7	18.9	18.5
All ages, crude	23.1	21.3	26.9	23.5	19.3	19.9	19.9	20.1	19.3	18.8
Under 1 year	8.4	8.1	9.8	7.0	4.9	4.9	5.4	5.7	5.6	4.9
1–4 years	11.5	10.0	11.5	9.2	7.2	7.0	6.9	7.0	6.9	6.3
5–14 years	8.8	7.9	10.2	7.9	6.9	7.0	7.1	7.1	6.5	5.9
15–24 years	34.4	38.0	47.2	44.8	35.7	38.5	37.1	37.8	34.6	34.1
25–34 years	24.6	24.3	30.9	29.1	23.0	24.4	24.4	24.2	23.8	23.6
35–44 years	20.3	19.3	24.9	20.9	17.2	16.6	17.3	17.5	17.3	16.9
45–54 years	22.2	21.4	25.5	18.6	15.2	15.2	15.5	16.0	15.7	15.6
55–64 years	29.2	25.1	27.9	17.4	15.6	15.3	15.8	15.9	16.0	15.9
65–74 years	38.8	31.4	32.8	19.2	17.9	18.1	18.8	19.5	19.4	18.6
75–84 years	52.7	41.8	43.5	28.1	27.4	28.6	29.1	29.9	29.5	29.1
85 years and over	45.1	37.9	34.2	27.6	26.5	25.6	27.6	29.7	29.5	31.2
White male										
All ages, age adjusted	35.9	34.0	40.1	34.8	27.6	28.7	28.3	28.4	26.7	26.3
All ages, crude	35.1	31.5	39.1	35.9	28.3	29.3	29.0	28.9	27.2	26.7
Under 1 year	9.1	8.8	9.1	7.0	4.6	4.2	4.4	6.0	5.1	4.8
1–4 years	13.2	11.3	12.2	9.5	7.7	7.1	7.2	7.0	6.9	6.1
5–14 years	12.0	10.3	12.6	9.8	8.6	8.8	9.2	8.8	7.9	6.8
15–24 years	58.3	62.7	75.2	73.8	56.5	61.4	57.8	58.6	52.5	52.5
25–34 years	39.1	38.6	47.0	46.6	35.8	37.8	37.4	36.7	35.4	35.4
35–44 years	30.9	28.4	35.2	30.7	24.3	23.9	24.6	24.8	23.9	23.7
45–54 years	31.6	29.7	34.6	26.3	21.0	20.9	20.8	21.7	20.9	20.7
55–64 years	41.9	34.4	39.0	23.9	20.7	20.1	21.0	20.7	21.2	20.6
65–74 years	59.1	45.5	46.2	25.8	22.0	22.8	24.5	24.8	24.2	23.5
75–84 years	86.4	66.8	69.2	43.6	41.2	42.9	43.4	43.4	43.1	41.1
85 years and over	79.3	61.9	65.5	57.3	57.0	51.7	58.8	59.9	62.9	65.3
Black male										
All ages, age adjusted	39.8	38.2	50.1	32.9	28.0	29.5	28.9	30.1	29.8	28.9
All ages, crude	37.2	33.1	44.3	31.1	27.1	29.0	28.2	29.4	28.9	28.1
Under 1 year	- - -	*6.8	10.6	7.8	*6.2	8.2	8.4	7.7	7.6	*5.6
1–4 years	- - -	12.7	16.9	13.7	10.9	10.9	10.0	9.3	9.0	10.1
5–14 years	9.7	10.4	16.1	10.5	9.2	9.9	9.5	9.8	9.0	8.4
15–24 years	41.6	46.4	58.1	34.9	32.0	35.2	36.1	37.8	36.4	36.1
25–34 years	57.4	51.0	70.4	44.9	37.7	42.3	38.9	39.1	38.6	39.5
35–44 years	45.9	43.6	59.5	41.2	34.7	34.3	34.3	36.2	36.4	33.5
45–54 years	49.9	48.1	61.4	39.1	30.1	31.7	32.8	32.6	36.2	34.1
55–64 years	58.8	47.3	62.1	40.3	36.3	34.1	32.5	33.1	35.4	32.5
65–74 years	48.5	46.1	54.9	41.8	31.7	29.1	33.9	40.5	33.3	33.2
75–84 years	- - -	51.8	51.6	46.5	42.0	53.1	36.3	45.4	44.4	40.8
85 years and over	- - -	*58.6	45.7	*34.0	38.7	66.7	43.8	70.8	53.0	48.3
White female										
All ages, age adjusted	10.6	11.1	14.4	12.3	10.8	11.0	11.4	11.6	11.6	11.0
All ages, crude	10.9	11.2	14.8	12.8	11.4	11.6	12.0	12.2	12.1	11.6
Under 1 year	7.8	7.5	10.2	7.1	3.9	4.7	5.9	5.5	4.9	4.7
1–4 years	10.1	8.3	9.6	7.7	5.8	6.1	5.9	6.2	6.1	5.2
5–14 years	5.6	5.3	6.9	5.7	5.2	4.9	5.0	5.2	5.1	4.7
15–24 years	12.6	15.6	22.7	23.0	20.0	21.4	21.5	21.6	21.1	19.5
25–34 years	9.0	9.0	12.7	12.2	10.1	10.9	11.7	11.8	12.1	11.6
35–44 years	8.1	8.9	12.3	10.6	9.4	8.5	9.3	9.2	9.6	9.2
45–54 years	10.8	11.4	14.3	10.2	9.0	8.6	9.3	9.6	9.6	9.4
55–64 years	15.0	15.3	16.1	10.5	9.9	9.7	10.4	10.6	10.2	10.5
65–74 years	20.9	19.3	22.1	13.4	14.3	14.4	13.8	14.5	15.3	14.0
75–84 years	25.4	23.8	28.1	19.0	19.7	20.3	21.7	22.4	22.0	22.4
85 years and over	22.3	22.2	18.1	15.3	15.3	14.9	16.1	18.0	17.7	19.1

See footnotes at end of table.

Table 42 (page 2 of 2). Death rates for motor vehicle crashes, according to sex, race, and age: United States, selected years 1950–90

[Data are based on the National Vital Statistics System]

Sex, race, and age	1950[1]	1960[1]	1970	1980	1985	1986	1987	1988	1989	1990
Black female				Deaths per 100,000 resident population						
All ages, age adjusted............	10.3	10.0	13.8	8.4	8.2	8.5	8.8	9.4	9.3	9.3
All ages, crude..................	10.2	9.7	13.4	8.3	8.3	8.6	8.9	9.5	9.4	9.4
Under 1 year	- - -	8.1	11.9	*5.3	8.1	*5.5	*5.3	*5.5	7.8	7.0
1–4 years.......................	- - -	8.8	12.6	9.5	6.8	6.9	7.5	7.5	6.3	7.7
5–14 years.....................	6.2	5.9	9.3	5.2	4.4	4.9	4.8	5.7	4.7	4.3
15–24 years....................	11.5	9.9	13.4	8.0	9.1	9.2	9.6	10.8	10.2	9.9
25–34 years....................	10.7	9.8	13.3	10.6	9.3	10.4	11.2	11.3	12.1	11.1
35–44 years....................	11.1	11.0	16.1	8.3	9.1	8.6	9.2	10.0	10.3	9.4
45–54 years....................	10.6	11.8	16.4	9.1	8.3	8.9	9.3	9.2	8.7	9.6
55–64 years....................	14.0	14.0	17.0	9.3	9.7	11.2	9.0	10.1	10.0	12.2
65–74 years....................	12.7	14.2	16.3	8.5	9.7	9.8	12.1	9.8	12.9	13.7
75–84 years....................	- - -	*8.8	14.4	11.1	14.6	9.6	10.4	13.5	13.0	15.0
85 years and over...............	- - -	*21.1	*15.4	*12.3	*9.8	*11.6	*7.6	*11.4	*6.5	*9.0

[1]Includes deaths of nonresidents of the United States.

*Based on fewer than 20 deaths.

NOTES: For data years shown, the code numbers for cause of death are based on the then current International Classification of Diseases, which are described in Appendix II, tables IV and V. Data for the 1980's have been revised based on intercensal population estimates and differ from previous editions of Health, United States. See Appendix I, Department of Commerce.

SOURCES: Centers for Disease Control and Prevention, National Center for Health Statistics: Vital Statistics of the United States, Vol. II, Mortality, Part A, for data years 1950–90. Public Health Service. Washington. U.S. Government Printing Office; Data computed by the Division of Analysis from data compiled by the Division of Vital Statistics and from table 1.

Table 43 (page 1 of 2). Death rates for homicide and legal intervention, according to sex, race, and age: United States, selected years 1950–90

[Data are based on the National Vital Statistics System]

Sex, race, and age	1950[1]	1960[1]	1970	1980	1985	1986	1987	1988	1989	1990
All races				Deaths per 100,000 resident population						
All ages, age adjusted	5.4	5.2	9.1	10.8	8.3	9.0	8.6	9.0	9.4	10.2
All ages, crude	5.3	4.7	8.3	10.7	8.4	9.0	8.7	9.0	9.3	10.0
Under 1 year	4.4	4.8	4.3	5.9	5.4	7.5	7.4	8.4	8.7	8.4
1–4 years	0.6	0.7	1.9	2.5	2.5	2.7	2.3	2.6	2.7	2.6
5–14 years	0.5	0.5	0.9	1.2	1.2	1.1	1.2	1.3	1.5	1.5
15–24 years	6.3	5.9	11.7	15.6	11.9	14.0	13.8	15.1	16.5	19.9
25–34 years	9.9	9.7	16.6	19.6	14.8	16.3	15.3	16.2	16.5	17.7
35–44 years	8.8	8.1	13.7	15.1	11.3	11.5	10.9	10.9	11.0	11.8
45–54 years	6.1	6.2	10.1	11.1	8.1	8.4	7.8	7.2	7.7	7.6
55–64 years	4.0	4.2	7.1	7.0	5.7	5.4	5.5	5.3	5.1	5.0
65–74 years	3.2	2.8	5.0	5.7	4.3	4.4	4.4	4.3	4.1	3.8
75–84 years	2.6	2.4	4.0	5.2	4.3	4.6	4.8	4.5	4.2	4.3
85 years and over	2.3	2.4	4.2	5.3	4.2	4.7	5.2	4.8	4.4	4.6
White male										
All ages, age adjusted	3.9	3.9	7.3	10.9	8.1	8.4	7.8	7.8	8.1	8.9
All ages, crude	3.9	3.6	6.8	10.9	8.2	8.6	8.0	7.9	8.2	9.0
Under 1 year	4.3	3.8	2.9	4.3	3.8	5.5	6.1	5.8	5.8	6.4
1–4 years	0.4	0.6	1.4	2.0	1.9	1.9	1.8	2.2	1.9	1.8
5–14 years	0.4	0.4	0.5	0.9	1.1	0.9	0.8	1.0	1.0	1.1
15–24 years	3.7	4.4	7.9	15.5	11.0	12.2	11.0	11.2	12.3	15.4
25–34 years	5.4	6.2	13.0	18.9	14.0	14.8	13.4	13.5	14.0	15.1
35–44 years	6.4	5.5	11.0	15.5	11.5	11.7	10.3	10.5	10.6	11.4
45–54 years	5.5	5.0	9.0	11.9	8.6	8.7	8.4	7.7	8.6	8.3
55–64 years	4.4	4.3	7.7	7.8	6.3	6.0	6.4	6.1	5.7	5.5
65–74 years	4.1	3.4	5.6	6.9	4.5	4.4	4.3	4.2	4.0	4.1
75–84 years	3.5	2.7	5.1	6.3	4.5	4.6	4.9	4.3	3.9	3.9
85 years and over	1.8	2.7	6.4	6.4	3.9	4.4	5.4	5.2	5.2	4.9
Black male										
All ages, age adjusted	51.1	44.9	82.1	71.9	50.2	56.3	54.2	58.6	61.9	68.7
All ages, crude	47.3	36.6	67.6	66.6	49.0	55.8	54.2	59.1	62.3	69.2
Under 1 year	- - -	10.3	14.3	18.6	16.7	23.2	19.5	19.5	21.9	21.4
1–4 years	- - -	1.7	5.1	7.2	6.6	9.5	4.9	7.6	8.0	7.6
5–14 years	1.8	1.4	4.2	2.9	3.3	3.3	4.5	4.3	5.1	5.1
15–24 years	58.9	46.4	102.5	84.3	65.9	78.9	85.3	101.4	114.2	138.3
25–34 years	110.5	92.0	158.5	145.1	95.6	109.6	100.6	110.9	114.9	125.4
35–44 years	83.7	77.5	126.2	110.3	74.9	77.7	76.3	76.9	75.9	82.3
45–54 years	54.6	54.8	100.5	83.8	51.4	56.8	46.5	45.8	46.7	47.7
55–64 years	35.7	31.8	59.8	55.6	40.0	37.9	35.5	31.9	33.4	34.0
65–74 years	18.7	19.1	40.6	33.9	29.2	32.1	30.4	28.7	29.2	24.3
75–84 years	- - -	16.1	19.0	27.6	21.4	27.9	29.6	30.6	28.7	29.2
85 years and over	- - -	*10.3	*19.6	*17.0	*17.7	*27.0	31.3	33.8	37.9	*27.2
White female										
All ages, age adjusted	1.4	1.5	2.2	3.2	2.9	2.9	2.9	2.9	2.8	2.8
All ages, crude	1.4	1.4	2.1	3.2	2.9	3.0	3.0	2.9	2.8	2.8
Under 1 year	3.9	3.5	2.9	4.3	4.3	5.2	4.3	6.2	5.8	5.1
1–4 years	0.6	0.5	1.2	1.5	1.7	1.4	1.6	1.6	1.5	1.4
5–14 years	0.4	0.3	0.5	1.0	0.8	0.8	0.8	0.8	0.9	0.8
15–24 years	1.3	1.5	2.7	4.7	3.6	4.3	3.8	3.9	3.8	4.0
25–34 years	1.9	2.0	3.4	4.3	4.4	4.4	4.7	4.5	4.2	4.3
35–44 years	2.2	2.2	3.2	4.1	3.6	3.5	3.6	3.3	3.3	3.2
45–54 years	1.6	1.9	2.2	3.0	2.9	2.8	2.7	2.5	2.6	2.6
55–64 years	1.3	1.5	2.0	2.1	2.3	2.0	1.9	2.0	1.7	1.8
65–74 years	1.1	1.1	1.7	2.5	2.2	2.2	2.4	2.3	2.1	1.8
75–84 years	1.2	1.2	2.5	3.3	3.1	3.0	3.1	2.9	2.6	2.8
85 years and over	1.9	1.5	1.9	4.0	3.2	3.3	3.8	3.0	2.0	2.5

See footnotes at end of table.

Table 43 (page 2 of 2). Death rates for homicide and legal intervention, according to sex, race, and age: United States, selected years 1950–90

[Data are based on the National Vital Statistics System]

Sex, race, and age	1950[1]	1960[1]	1970	1980	1985	1986	1987	1988	1989	1990
Black female				Deaths per 100,000 resident population						
All ages, age adjusted.............	11.7	11.8	15.0	13.7	10.9	11.9	12.5	12.8	12.7	13.0
All ages, crude	11.5	10.4	13.3	13.5	11.1	12.2	12.7	13.3	13.1	13.5
Under 1 year	- - -	13.8	10.7	12.8	10.7	17.5	18.9	23.7	23.6	22.8
1–4 years......................	- - -	*1.7	6.3	6.4	6.3	6.8	7.3	6.3	7.3	7.2
5–14 years.....................	1.2	1.0	2.0	2.2	2.0	2.4	2.0	3.2	3.0	3.6
15–24 years....................	16.5	11.9	17.7	18.4	14.2	16.3	17.8	17.5	17.4	18.9
25–34 years....................	26.6	24.9	25.6	25.8	20.0	22.1	22.7	25.8	23.5	25.3
35–44 years....................	17.8	20.5	25.1	17.7	14.7	14.7	14.3	14.4	14.6	15.6
45–54 years....................	8.5	12.7	17.5	12.5	9.2	8.8	10.9	8.0	8.7	7.3
55–64 years....................	3.6	6.8	8.1	8.9	6.5	6.9	7.9	7.1	8.4	5.6
65–74 years....................	3.4	3.3	7.7	8.6	7.3	8.9	7.0	9.3	8.4	6.8
75–84 years....................	- - -	*2.5	*5.7	6.7	7.4	8.3	10.0	9.5	9.5	11.3
85 years and over...............	- - -	*2.6	*9.8	*8.5	*12.0	*13.8	*11.1	13.4	16.3	19.2

[1]Includes deaths of nonresidents of the United States.

*Based on fewer than 20 deaths.

NOTES: For data years shown, the code numbers for cause of death are based on the then current International Classification of Diseases, which are described in Appendix II, tables IV and V. Data for the 1980's have been revised based on intercensal population estimates and differ from previous editions of Health, United States. See Appendix I, Department of Commerce.

SOURCES: Centers for Disease Control and Prevention, National Center for Health Statistics: Vital Statistics of the United States, Vol. II, Mortality, Part A, for data years 1950–90. Public Health Service. Washington. U.S. Government Printing Office; Data computed by the Division of Analysis from data compiled by the Division of Vital Statistics and from table 1.

Table 44 (page 1 of 2). Death rates for suicide, according to sex, race, and age: United States, selected years 1950–90

[Data are based on the National Vital Statistics System]

Sex, race, and age	1950[1]	1960[1]	1970	1980	1985	1986	1987	1988	1989	1990
All races				Deaths per 100,000 resident population						
All ages, age adjusted	11.0	10.6	11.8	11.4	11.5	11.9	11.7	11.5	11.3	11.5
All ages, crude	11.4	10.6	11.6	11.9	12.4	12.9	12.7	12.4	12.2	12.4
Under 1 year	. . .	. . .	. . .	. . .	. . .	. . .	. . .	. . .	. . .	. . .
1–4 years	. . .	. . .	. . .	. . .	. . .	. . .	. . .	. . .	. . .	. . .
5–14 years	0.2	0.3	0.3	0.4	0.8	0.8	0.7	0.7	0.7	0.8
15–24 years	4.5	5.2	8.8	12.3	12.8	12.9	12.7	12.9	13.0	13.2
25–34 years	9.1	10.0	14.1	16.0	15.3	15.8	15.5	15.6	15.2	15.2
35–44 years	14.3	14.2	16.9	15.4	14.6	15.2	15.0	14.8	14.6	15.3
45–54 years	20.9	20.7	20.0	15.9	15.7	16.5	16.1	14.7	14.8	14.8
55–64 years	27.0	23.7	21.4	15.9	16.8	17.2	16.8	15.8	15.7	16.0
65–74 years	29.3	23.0	20.8	16.9	18.7	19.9	19.7	18.7	18.3	17.9
75–84 years	31.1	27.9	21.2	19.1	23.9	25.0	25.6	25.6	22.9	24.9
85 years and over	28.8	26.0	19.0	19.2	19.4	21.1	22.5	21.0	23.4	22.2
White male										
All ages, age adjusted	18.1	17.5	18.2	18.9	19.9	20.6	20.2	19.9	19.7	20.1
All ages, crude	19.0	17.6	18.0	19.9	21.6	22.4	22.2	21.8	21.5	22.0
Under 1 year	. . .	. . .	. . .	. . .	. . .	. . .	. . .	. . .	. . .	. . .
1–4 years	. . .	. . .	. . .	. . .	. . .	. . .	. . .	. . .	. . .	. . .
5–14 years	0.3	0.5	0.5	0.7	1.3	1.2	1.2	1.1	1.1	1.1
15–24 years	6.6	8.6	13.9	21.4	22.3	23.1	22.2	22.7	22.5	23.2
25–34 years	13.8	14.9	19.9	25.6	25.6	26.8	26.0	26.1	25.5	25.6
35–44 years	22.4	21.9	23.3	23.5	23.7	24.1	24.1	24.3	24.1	25.3
45–54 years	34.1	33.7	29.5	24.2	25.2	26.4	25.6	23.4	24.4	24.8
55–64 years	45.9	40.2	35.0	25.8	28.8	28.9	28.9	27.3	26.9	27.5
65–74 years	53.2	42.0	38.7	32.5	35.8	38.2	37.6	36.2	36.0	34.2
75–84 years	61.9	55.7	45.5	45.5	57.0	58.8	60.9	61.4	55.3	60.2
85 years and over	61.9	61.3	45.8	52.8	60.9	66.5	72.1	66.5	72.9	70.3
Black male										
All ages, age adjusted	7.0	7.8	9.9	11.1	11.5	11.6	12.1	11.9	12.6	12.4
All ages, crude	6.3	6.4	8.0	10.3	11.0	11.2	11.8	11.7	12.4	12.0
Under 1 year	. . .	. . .	. . .	. . .	. . .	. . .	. . .	. . .	. . .	. . .
1–4 years	. . .	. . .	. . .	. . .	. . .	. . .	. . .	. . .	. . .	. . .
5–14 years	*–	*0.1	*0.1	*0.3	*0.7	0.8	0.8	*0.6	0.9	0.8
15–24 years	4.9	4.1	10.5	12.3	13.3	11.4	12.9	14.5	16.6	15.1
25–34 years	9.3	12.4	19.2	21.8	19.9	21.6	21.5	22.5	22.5	21.9
35–44 years	10.4	12.8	12.6	15.6	14.6	17.1	17.4	15.9	17.4	16.9
45–54 years	10.4	10.8	13.8	12.0	13.6	12.9	13.1	11.8	11.1	14.8
55–64 years	16.5	16.2	10.6	11.7	12.2	10.6	11.1	11.6	11.5	10.8
65–74 years	10.0	11.3	8.7	11.1	16.7	17.3	19.1	14.1	17.1	14.7
75–84 years	– – –	6.6	8.9	10.5	15.6	16.0	21.0	17.7	14.9	14.4
85 years and over	– – –	6.9	*8.7	*18.9	*8.1	*19.0	*14.1	*10.8	*24.2	*19.6
White female										
All ages, age adjusted	5.3	5.3	7.2	5.7	5.3	5.5	5.3	5.1	4.8	4.8
All ages, crude	5.5	5.3	7.1	5.9	5.6	5.9	5.8	5.5	5.3	5.3
Under 1 year	. . .	. . .	. . .	. . .	. . .	. . .	. . .	. . .	. . .	. . .
1–4 years	. . .	. . .	. . .	. . .	. . .	. . .	. . .	. . .	. . .	. . .
5–14 years	*0.1	*0.1	0.1	0.2	0.5	0.3	0.3	0.4	0.3	0.4
15–24 years	2.7	2.3	4.2	4.6	4.7	4.7	4.6	4.5	4.3	4.2
25–34 years	5.2	5.8	9.0	7.5	6.4	6.3	6.4	6.2	6.0	6.0
35–44 years	8.2	8.1	13.0	9.1	7.7	8.4	7.9	7.5	7.2	7.4
45–54 years	10.5	10.9	13.5	10.2	9.1	9.7	9.4	8.7	8.1	7.5
55–64 years	10.7	10.9	12.3	9.1	8.4	9.1	8.4	8.0	8.0	8.0
65–74 years	10.6	8.8	9.6	7.0	7.3	7.7	7.6	7.3	6.4	7.2
75–84 years	8.4	9.2	7.2	5.7	7.0	7.9	7.4	7.2	6.1	6.7
85 years and over	8.9	6.1	5.8	5.8	4.8	5.0	4.8	5.4	6.3	5.4

See footnotes at end of table.

Table 44 (page 2 of 2). **Death rates for suicide, according to sex, race, and age: United States, selected years 1950–90**

[Data are based on the National Vital Statistics System]

Sex, race, and age	1950[1]	1960[1]	1970	1980	1985	1986	1987	1988	1989	1990
Black female				Deaths per 100,000 resident population						
All ages, age adjusted............	1.7	1.9	2.9	2.4	2.1	2.4	2.1	2.5	2.4	2.4
All ages, crude..................	1.5	1.6	2.6	2.2	2.1	2.3	2.1	2.4	2.4	2.3
Under 1 year	. . .	. . .	. . .	. . .	. . .	. . .	. . .	. . .	. . .	. . .
1–4 years.......................	. . .	. . .	. . .	. . .	. . .	. . .	. . .	. . .	. . .	. . .
5–14 years.....................	*–	*0.0	0.2	*0.1	*0.2	*0.2	*0.2	*0.5	*0.3	*0.3
15–24 years	*1.8	*1.3	3.8	2.3	2.0	2.3	2.5	2.6	2.9	2.3
25–34 years	2.6	3.0	5.7	4.1	3.0	3.8	4.0	3.9	3.8	3.7
35–44 years	2.0	3.0	3.7	4.6	3.6	2.8	2.8	3.4	3.8	4.0
45–54 years	3.5	3.1	3.7	2.8	3.3	3.3	2.2	4.0	3.2	3.2
55–64 years	*1.1	3.0	*2.0	2.3	2.2	4.3	1.9	2.6	2.6	2.6
65–74 years	*1.9	*2.3	*2.9	*1.7	*2.0	2.8	2.6	*2.1	*2.2	2.6
75–84 years	- - -	*1.3	*1.7	*1.4	*4.4	*2.5	*2.2	*1.3	*1.6	*0.6
85 years and over...............	- - -	*–	*2.8	*–	*1.5	*–	*–	*–	*0.7	*2.6

[1]Includes deaths of nonresidents of the United States.

*Based on fewer than 20 deaths.

NOTES: For data years shown, the code numbers for cause of death are based on the then current International Classification of Diseases, which are described in Appendix II, tables IV and V. Data for the 1980's have been revised based on intercensal population estimates and differ from previous editions of Health, United States. See Appendix I, Department of Commerce.

SOURCES: Centers for Disease Control and Prevention, National Center for Health Statistics: Vital Statistics of the United States, Vol. II, Mortality, Part A, for data years 1950–90. Public Health Service. Washington. U.S. Government Printing Office; Data computed by the Division of Analysis from data compiled by the Division of Vital Statistics and from table 1.

Table 45 (page 1 of 2). Death rates for firearm injuries, according to sex, race, and age: United States, selected years 1970–90

[Data are based on the National Vital Statistics System]

Sex, race, and age	1970	1980	1981	1982	1983	1984	1985	1986	1987	1988	1989	1990
All races												

Sex, race, and age	1970	1980	1981	1982	1983	1984	1985	1986	1987	1988	1989	1990
All races					Deaths per 100,000 resident population							
All ages, age adjusted	14.0	14.8	14.6	13.9	12.9	12.8	13.3	13.3	13.0	13.4	13.7	14.6
All ages, crude	13.1	14.9	14.8	14.2	13.3	13.3	13.3	13.9	13.6	13.9	14.1	14.9
Under 1 year	*0.4	*0.5	*0.4	*0.4	*0.3	*0.4	*0.2	*0.3	*0.2	*0.3	*0.4	*0.4
1–4 years	1.0	0.7	0.7	0.7	0.5	0.6	0.7	0.6	0.5	0.6	0.7	0.6
5–14 years	1.7	1.6	1.6	1.6	1.4	1.8	1.8	1.7	1.8	1.9	2.0	1.9
15–24 years	15.5	20.6	19.9	18.4	16.9	16.9	17.2	18.9	18.7	20.6	22.6	25.8
25–34 years	22.2	24.3	23.7	22.1	20.3	19.5	19.3	20.4	19.4	20.4	20.4	21.8
35–44 years	19.6	20.0	19.7	18.8	16.8	16.4	16.0	16.2	15.6	15.8	15.5	16.3
45–54 years	18.1	16.4	17.3	16.5	15.4	15.1	14.7	15.1	14.3	13.5	13.8	13.9
55–64 years	17.0	13.9	14.8	14.3	14.0	14.2	13.9	13.8	13.8	13.3	13.1	13.3
65–74 years	14.5	13.8	12.8	14.2	14.2	15.1	15.1	15.9	15.5	14.9	15.1	14.4
75–84 years	13.4	13.4	13.4	15.1	15.7	16.2	17.7	18.5	19.2	19.3	17.5	19.4
85 years and over	10.2	11.6	11.6	10.9	11.8	11.4	12.2	12.7	14.1	13.6	14.7	14.7
White male												
All ages, age adjusted	18.2	21.1	21.0	20.5	19.4	19.6	19.4	20.0	19.2	19.3	19.5	20.5
All ages, crude	17.6	21.8	21.7	21.4	20.5	20.8	20.7	21.4	20.7	20.7	20.8	21.8
Under 1 year	*0.3	*0.5	*0.3	*0.4	*0.2	*0.5	*0.1	*0.1	*0.4	*0.2	*0.3	*0.4
1–4 years	0.8	0.7	0.7	0.8	0.6	0.8	0.6	0.5	0.5	0.6	0.7	0.6
5–14 years	2.1	2.3	2.2	2.3	2.1	2.6	2.7	2.5	2.5	2.4	2.7	2.4
15–24 years	16.9	28.4	27.2	25.7	23.4	23.8	24.1	25.6	23.9	25.3	26.5	29.5
25–34 years	24.3	31.1	30.5	29.1	27.8	27.0	26.3	27.0	25.8	26.0	26.2	27.8
35–44 years	24.1	27.1	27.2	26.5	24.3	23.5	23.3	23.2	22.1	22.5	22.2	23.3
45–54 years	25.7	23.8	25.5	24.7	23.5	23.9	23.0	23.6	22.7	21.5	22.4	22.0
55–64 years	29.5	22.7	24.3	24.2	23.6	24.7	24.2	24.5	24.6	23.6	22.7	23.7
65–74 years	29.1	27.8	25.6	28.3	28.3	31.1	30.5	32.0	31.3	30.3	30.7	29.0
75–84 years	32.0	34.0	33.4	38.8	40.4	41.7	45.0	47.6	48.8	49.3	44.7	49.8
85 years and over	27.7	36.1	38.0	36.9	40.6	38.5	40.8	44.6	47.7	46.2	51.6	52.4
Black male												
All ages, age adjusted	73.4	61.8	58.7	51.7	44.6	42.6	42.2	47.1	46.4	51.0	55.0	61.5
All ages, crude	60.8	57.7	55.4	49.3	42.9	41.2	41.3	46.9	46.5	51.7	55.4	61.9
Under 1 year	*2.0	*0.7	*1.1	*1.5	*0.7	*1.1	*0.4	*1.1	*–	*0.7	*1.3	*0.9
1–4 years	3.3	2.1	2.3	2.1	*0.9	*0.8	2.2	1.9	*1.6	1.8	*1.7	*1.2
5–14 years	6.1	3.3	4.0	2.6	2.5	2.6	2.8	3.0	4.3	5.0	5.4	5.8
15–24 years	97.3	77.9	72.0	64.1	59.1	55.8	61.3	72.1	81.3	99.0	115.3	138.0
25–34 years	145.6	128.4	119.7	106.8	86.3	82.8	79.8	93.1	84.8	97.1	98.8	108.6
35–44 years	104.2	92.3	86.7	74.7	65.7	64.0	59.2	62.5	62.1	60.7	60.9	66.1
45–54 years	83.9	63.4	62.7	56.4	46.0	43.0	40.8	45.7	36.7	34.4	36.6	39.1
55–64 years	54.3	46.5	47.6	39.1	37.3	34.4	32.1	27.1	27.0	25.9	27.9	28.4
65–74 years	36.0	31.2	28.5	31.4	27.1	27.0	29.2	31.6	28.0	25.1	29.1	24.8
75–84 years	20.2	26.8	35.3	23.7	26.7	26.3	23.0	25.2	27.7	26.9	24.7	22.4
85 years and over	*15.2	*26.4	*19.6	*20.7	*21.7	*14.8	*12.9	*23.8	*17.2	*13.8	31.8	*22.6
White female												
All ages, age adjusted	4.0	4.2	4.4	4.3	4.0	3.9	3.9	3.9	3.8	3.7	3.6	3.7
All ages, crude	3.7	4.1	4.4	4.3	4.0	4.0	4.0	3.9	3.9	3.8	3.7	3.8
Under 1 year	*0.2	*0.4	*0.3	*0.3	*0.2	*0.1	*0.3	*0.3	*0.1	*0.1	*0.3	*0.3
1–4 years	0.6	0.5	0.5	0.4	0.4	0.4	0.5	0.4	*0.3	0.4	0.4	*0.3
5–14 years	0.6	0.7	0.8	0.9	0.6	0.8	0.7	0.6	0.8	0.7	0.7	0.7
15–24 years	3.4	5.1	5.4	5.1	4.7	5.0	4.4	4.7	4.3	4.1	4.3	4.8
25–34 years	6.7	6.0	6.6	6.2	5.9	5.3	5.7	5.5	5.6	5.5	5.2	5.5
35–44 years	7.1	6.6	6.5	6.6	5.7	5.7	5.5	5.4	5.3	5.2	4.9	5.0
45–54 years	5.7	5.9	6.4	6.1	5.7	5.4	5.4	5.4	5.3	5.1	4.7	4.9
55–64 years	4.0	4.4	4.7	4.7	4.9	4.5	4.7	4.5	4.4	4.3	4.4	4.1
65–74 years	2.7	3.1	2.9	3.5	3.8	3.4	3.7	3.8	3.9	3.7	3.3	3.7
75–84 years	1.7	1.7	1.7	2.0	2.2	2.5	2.7	2.7	3.1	3.1	2.7	3.0
85 years and over	*0.8	*1.3	*1.1	*0.7	*0.9	1.5	1.9	*0.9	1.9	2.1	1.2	1.2

See footnotes at end of table.

Table 45 (page 2 of 2). Death rates for firearm injuries, according to sex, race, and age: United States, selected years 1970–90

[Data are based on the National Vital Statistics System]

Sex, race, and age	1970	1980	1981	1982	1983	1984	1985	1986	1987	1988	1989	1990
Black female					Deaths per 100,000 resident population							
All ages, age adjusted	11.4	9.1	8.7	7.1	6.5	6.5	6.6	7.0	7.3	7.6	7.4	7.8
All ages, crude	10.0	8.8	8.5	6.9	6.4	6.4	6.5	7.1	7.3	7.7	7.4	7.8
Under 1 year.	*0.8	*0.8	*1.5	*0.4	*0.4	*0.8	*0.7	*0.4	*0.4	*1.0	*0.6	*1.0
1–4 years	2.5	*0.9	*1.1	*0.5	*0.8	*0.8	*0.9	*0.9	*0.8	*0.9	*1.2	*1.1
5–14 years	1.6	1.1	1.4	0.9	1.0	1.4	1.0	1.5	1.0	2.2	1.6	2.4
15–24 years	15.2	12.3	12.2	9.1	9.2	8.8	8.3	10.0	11.6	11.2	12.6	13.3
25–34 years	21.2	18.3	15.4	13.5	12.4	12.0	12.8	13.8	14.0	14.7	13.2	14.6
35–44 years	17.4	12.8	12.2	11.6	10.0	9.7	9.4	9.6	9.1	10.9	9.5	9.7
45–54 years	13.2	9.1	8.6	7.0	7.1	5.5	7.4	5.9	7.0	5.8	5.7	5.5
55–64 years	6.2	7.1	8.3	5.0	3.2	5.2	3.9	4.8	4.4	4.4	5.2	3.9
65–74 years	4.6	3.9	5.0	3.6	2.5	3.9	2.9	4.0	3.9	3.7	3.2	3.2
75–84 years	*2.6	*1.9	*2.1	*2.8	*1.7	*1.7	6.0	*3.4	*3.5	*1.3	*2.7	*3.2
85 years and over	*7.0	*1.9	*1.8	*1.7	*0.8	*1.6	*1.5	*1.4	*2.8	*2.7	*2.6	*2.6

*Based on fewer than 20 deaths.

NOTES: International Classification of Diseases code numbers for causes of death included in firearm injuries are described in Appendix II, tables IV and V. Data for the 1980's are based on intercensal population estimates. See Appendix I, Department of Commerce.

SOURCE: Centers for Disease Control and Prevention, National Center for Health Statistics: Data computed by the Division of Analysis from data compiled by the Division of Vital Statistics and from table 1.

Table 46. Deaths for selected occupational diseases for males, according to age: United States, selected years 1970–90

[Data are based on the National Vital Statistics System]

Age and cause of death	1970	1975	1979	1980	1981	1982	1983	1984	1985	1986	1987	1988	1989	1990
25 years and over						Number of deaths [1]								
Malignant neoplasm of peritoneum and pleura (mesothelioma)	602	591	559	552	556	576	584	584	571	564	575	556	565	629
Coalworkers' pneumoconiosis.	1,155	973	918	977	1,053	954	926	923	947	882	823	757	725	727
Asbestosis	25	43	86	96	98	99	128	131	130	180	195	206	261	282
Silicosis	351	243	220	202	165	176	149	160	138	135	153	128	130	146
25–64 years														
Malignant neoplasm of peritoneum and pleura (mesothelioma)	308	280	246	241	229	234	211	211	210	200	196	187	179	199
Coalworkers' pneumoconiosis.	294	188	130	136	116	116	88	97	89	71	71	56	50	49
Asbestosis	17	22	29	30	21	26	30	25	29	37	32	38	31	50
Silicosis	90	64	51	49	44	42	37	34	30	22	32	26	21	35
65 years and over														
Malignant neoplasm of peritoneum and pleura (mesothelioma)	294	311	313	311	327	342	373	373	361	364	379	369	386	430
Coalworkers' pneumoconiosis.	861	785	788	841	937	838	838	826	858	811	752	701	675	678
Asbestosis	8	21	57	66	77	73	98	106	101	143	163	168	230	232
Silicosis	261	179	169	153	121	134	112	126	108	113	121	102	109	111

[1]This table classifies deaths according to underlying cause. Additional deaths for which occupational disease are classified as nonunderlying causes can be identified from multiple cause of death data from the National Vital Statistics System. The numbers of such deaths are shown below for men 25 years of age and over.

Nonunderlying cause of death	1980	1983	1984	1985	1986	1987	1988	1989	1990
Malignant neoplasm of peritoneum and pleura (mesothelioma)	135	115	124	102	106	111	104	83	105
Coalworkers' pneumoconiosis	1,587	1,758	1,742	1,652	1,536	1,419	1,445	1,402	1,248
Asbestosis.	228	321	298	382	494	488	536	588	619
Silicosis	232	205	210	187	175	173	162	156	152

NOTES: Selection of occupational diseases based on definitions in D. Rutstein et al.: Sentinel health events (occupational): A basis for physician recognition and public health surveillance, Am. J. Public Health 73(9): 1054–1062, Sept. 1983. For data years shown, the code numbers for cause of death are based on the then current International Classification of Diseases, which are described in Appendix II, tables IV and V.

SOURCES: Data computed by the Centers for Disease Control and Prevention, National Institute for Occupational Safety and Health from data compiled by National Center for Health Statistics, Division of Vital Statistics; Data computed by the Division of Epidemiology and Health Promotion from data compiled by the Division of Vital Statistics.

Table 47. Occupational injury deaths, according to industry: United States, 1980–89

[Data are based on the National Vital Statistics System]

Industry	1980	1981	1982	1983	1984	1985	1986	1987	1988	1989
	Deaths per 100,000 workers [1]									
Total civilian work force	8.9	8.6	7.8	7.2	7.1	7.0	6.1	6.2	5.9	5.6
Agriculture, forestry, and fishing	26.9	25.1	21.9	19.1	19.2	19.3	15.8	15.5	13.9	13.3
Mining	41.4	44.4	28.8	27.0	37.7	29.9	26.0	26.2	23.9	27.0
Construction	28.9	28.9	27.7	28.3	25.7	25.9	23.4	24.3	22.9	21.8
Manufacturing	4.8	4.6	4.5	4.3	4.5	4.3	4.2	4.4	4.2	4.1
Transportation, communication, and public utilities	29.3	27.8	25.0	22.6	24.7	24.6	21.1	19.8	20.3	19.3
Wholesale trade.	3.2	3.0	2.5	2.7	2.2	2.2	2.0	2.1	2.3	1.7
Retail trade	4.0	3.8	3.6	3.2	2.6	2.9	2.3	2.4	2.4	2.2
Finance, insurance, and real estate	1.6	1.7	1.4	1.5	1.6	1.1	1.2	1.4	1.1	1.2
Services	3.9	3.3	3.4	3.1	2.8	2.8	2.4	2.3	2.6	2.2
Public administration	7.7	7.5	6.9	7.6	6.9	6.4	6.2	6.8	6.1	5.3
Not classified.	- - -	- - -	- - -	- - -	- - -	- - -	- - -	- - -	- - -	- - -
	Number of deaths									
Total civilian work force	7,405	7,136	6,459	5,856	6,162	6,250	5,672	5,884	5,751	5,714
Agriculture, forestry, and fishing	848	835	765	682	746	791	701	730	687	695
Mining	412	492	342	263	367	282	220	190	176	192
Construction	1,294	1,240	1,091	1,066	1,074	1,160	1,091	1,188	1,130	1,096
Manufacturing	1,014	940	882	780	878	834	802	831	810	791
Transportation, communication, and public utilities	1,355	1,281	1,159	1,027	1,155	1,184	1,032	1,013	1,068	1,046
Wholesale trade.	167	159	131	140	118	122	113	120	135	107
Retail trade	595	576	544	481	423	489	407	449	443	429
Finance, insurance, and real estate	84	91	78	81	93	69	79	94	72	81
Services	663	593	629	588	561	603	554	563	642	607
Public administration	401	386	361	360	329	319	318	359	333	292
Not classified.	572	543	477	388	418	397	355	347	255	378

[1]Denominators for death rates are average annual employment (U.S. Bureau of Labor Statistics. Employment and Earnings, annual average supplements; Vol. 28–37:1, 1981–90).

NOTES: Includes deaths to United States residents, 16 years of age and over, that resulted from an "external" cause and the item "injury at work" was checked on the death certificate. Industry is coded based on Standard Industrial Classification Manual, 1987 Edition (see Appendix II, table VI). Some numbers in this table have been revised and differ from previous editions of Health, United States.

SOURCE: Centers for Disease Control and Prevention, National Institute for Occupational Safety and Health, Division of Safety Research: National Traumatic Occupational Fatalities (NTOF) surveillance system. Morgantown, WV. 1992.

Table 48. Provisional death rates for all causes, according to race, sex, and age: United States, 1989–91

[Data are based on a 10-percent sample of death certificates from the National Vital Statistics System]

Sex and age	All races			White			Black		
	1989	1990	1991	1989	1990	1991	1989	1990	1991
Both sexes	Deaths per 100,000 resident population								
All ages, age adjusted.	524.1	515.1	507.9	500.0	494.3	483.7	761.2	729.6	742.8
All ages, crude.	868.1	861.9	853.9	893.3	891.6	880.1	848.1	820.4	835.4
Under 1 year	986.0	936.6	901.8	819.2	814.4	747.9	1,899.8	1,652.5	1,725.2
1–4 years.	43.8	44.2	46.7	39.0	40.0	40.3	69.6	66.9	81.1
5–14 years.	26.6	24.1	24.0	24.5	23.1	21.8	38.5	30.8	35.8
15–24 years.	103.5	104.1	107.1	95.8	95.1	96.1	150.1	161.8	176.2
25–34 years.	139.7	139.6	137.4	119.1	120.6	117.6	286.5	276.1	273.1
35–44 years.	221.0	221.1	222.7	191.1	192.4	191.7	485.4	471.4	484.9
45–54 years.	479.1	463.1	458.2	434.1	425.3	416.6	904.1	832.3	861.9
55–64 years.	1,210.0	1,175.6	1,162.4	1,153.3	1,125.2	1,105.1	1,825.2	1,767.5	1,779.5
65–74 years.	2,628.2	2,607.4	2,568.7	2,573.2	2,565.7	2,512.5	3,504.1	3,319.7	3,413.4
75–84 years.	6,167.5	6,084.5	5,932.3	6,155.4	6,081.0	5,929.6	6,970.4	6,873.2	6,736.1
85 years and over.	15,083.2	14,784.4	14,395.6	15,362.5	15,087.7	14,673.0	13,110.2	12,707.3	12,593.0
Male									
All ages, age adjusted.	679.6	668.9	660.1	647.9	642.7	629.1	1,010.0	956.9	977.7
All ages, crude.	922.0	917.2	909.1	934.6	937.2	924.3	984.5	941.5	961.5
Under 1 year	1,076.7	1,037.5	1,007.2	910.0	908.8	845.5	1,993.6	1,796.4	1,899.4
1–4 years.	46.6	48.7	48.9	42.0	43.9	43.1	73.6	71.7	82.1
5–14 years.	32.3	29.1	28.8	30.3	27.7	26.2	44.5	38.4	43.5
15–24 years.	152.0	156.1	160.8	139.0	140.7	142.7	235.7	258.6	277.1
25–34 years.	203.3	205.6	201.1	173.4	178.9	171.6	432.9	414.8	413.5
35–44 years.	301.7	306.1	311.3	260.4	265.6	268.7	701.2	688.0	706.7
45–54 years.	628.2	600.9	598.2	563.8	547.1	541.4	1,288.9	1,181.1	1,202.8
55–64 years.	1,569.8	1,507.5	1,503.6	1,497.5	1,454.8	1,431.0	2,371.3	2,180.2	2,323.2
65–74 years.	3,414.6	3,358.5	3,307.3	3,348.0	3,316.2	3,246.4	4,516.3	4,172.9	4,285.5
75–84 years.	7,950.4	7,950.2	7,663.1	7,943.6	7,976.4	7,688.8	8,902.9	8,731.4	8,358.6
85 years and over.	17,695.3	17,521.6	17,150.9	18,110.4	17,973.3	17,620.4	14,958.3	14,743.2	14,324.7
Female									
All ages, age adjusted.	396.4	389.0	382.1	378.8	372.8	363.8	564.6	549.4	554.5
All ages, crude.	816.9	809.3	801.6	853.8	847.9	837.6	725.0	711.0	721.3
Under 1 year	890.9	831.2	790.5	722.9	715.0	645.0	1,803.3	1,504.6	1,545.7
1–4 years.	40.8	39.4	44.5	35.9	35.9	37.4	65.4	62.0	80.0
5–14 years.	20.6	18.9	19.0	18.3	18.2	17.1	32.3	23.0	27.9
15–24 years.	53.9	50.8	52.2	51.4	48.2	48.2	66.5	67.0	77.3
25–34 years.	75.9	73.4	73.6	63.8	61.1	62.5	155.4	152.0	147.3
35–44 years.	142.2	138.1	135.8	122.0	119.2	114.5	304.6	289.5	297.9
45–54 years.	337.9	332.6	325.6	308.7	307.5	295.9	593.2	550.8	587.3
55–64 years.	887.8	877.5	854.7	841.2	825.1	807.1	1,373.6	1,424.2	1,327.5
65–74 years.	1,997.1	2,002.1	1,971.7	1,946.8	1,956.9	1,915.4	2,744.7	2,673.9	2,749.5
75–84 years.	5,083.4	4,941.7	4,862.2	5,072.3	4,921.1	4,841.9	5,812.5	5,763.7	5,761.9
85 years and over.	14,070.3	13,727.5	13,328.4	14,317.0	13,993.7	13,552.9	12,224.2	11,831.4	11,856.4

NOTES: Before 1991 data include deaths of nonresidents of the United States. Starting in 1991 data exclude deaths of nonresidents of the United States. Provisional data for 1989–91 were calculated using 1980's-based postcensal population estimates. See Appendix I, National Center for Health Statistics and Department of Commerce.

SOURCES: Centers for Disease Control and Prevention, National Center for Health Statistics: Annual summary of births, marriages, divorces, and deaths, United States, 1990 and 1991. Monthly Vital Statistics Report. Vols. 39 and 40, No. 13. DHHS Pub. Nos. (PHS) 91-1120 and 92-1120. 1991 and 1992. Public Health Service. Hyattsville, Md.

Table 49. Provisional death rates for selected causes of death: United States, 1989–91

[Data are based on a 10-percent sample of death certificates from the National Vital Statistics System]

Cause of death	Age-adjusted death rate			Crude death rate			Rank		
	1989	1990	1991	1989	1990	1991	1989	1990	1991
	Deaths per 100,000 resident population								
All causes	524.1	515.1	507.9	868.1	861.9	853.9	. . .	. . .	. . .
Diseases of heart	155.9	150.3	146.1	296.3	289.0	283.3	1	1	1
Ischemic heart disease	104.9	101.0	97.0	200.6	195.1	188.8	. . .	. . .	. . .
Cerebrovascular diseases	28.5	27.6	26.5	59.4	57.9	56.8	3	3	3
Malignant neoplasms	133.7	133.0	132.6	200.3	201.7	202.9	2	2	2
Respiratory system	40.1	39.9	40.3	57.0	57.3	58.7	. . .	. . .	. . .
Breast [1]	23.4	23.6	22.8	34.1	34.9	34.1	. . .	. . .	. . .
Chronic obstructive pulmonary diseases	19.4	19.7	19.4	34.0	35.5	35.2	5	5	5
Pneumonia and influenza	13.3	13.5	12.6	30.3	31.3	29.6	6	6	6
Chronic liver disease and cirrhosis	8.7	8.3	8.0	10.6	10.2	9.8	9	10	11
Diabetes mellitus	11.3	11.7	12.0	18.8	19.5	19.7	7	7	7
Nephritis, nephrotic syndrome, and nephrosis	4.4	4.2	4.3	8.6	8.3	8.7	12	12	12
Septicemia	4.1	4.2	4.1	7.7	7.9	7.7	14	13	13
Atherosclerosis	3.0	2.4	2.5	7.7	6.6	6.7	13	15	14
Human immunodeficiency virus infection	8.3	9.1	11.2	8.6	9.6	11.8	11	11	9
Unintentional injuries	33.5	32.7	31.7	38.2	37.3	36.2	4	4	4
Motor vehicle crashes	19.4	18.9	17.7	19.7	19.1	17.8	. . .	. . .	. . .
Suicide	11.7	11.3	11.0	12.6	12.3	11.9	8	8	8
Homicide and legal intervention	9.4	10.6	11.3	9.3	10.2	10.8	10	9	10

[1]Female only.

NOTES: Before 1991 data include deaths of nonresidents of the United States. Starting in 1991 data exclude deaths of nonresidents of the United States. Code numbers for cause of death are based on the International Classification of Diseases, Ninth Revision, described in Appendix II, table V. Categories for the coding and classification of human immunodeficiency virus infection were introduced in the United States beginning with data year 1987. Provisional data for 1989–91 were calculated using 1980's-based postcensal population estimates. See Appendix I, National Center for Health Statistics and Department of Commerce.

SOURCES: Centers for Disease Control and Prevention, National Center for Health Statistics: Annual summary of births, marriages, divorces, and deaths, United States, 1990 and 1991. Monthly Vital Statistics Report. Vols. 39 and 40, No. 13. DHHS Pub. Nos. (PHS) 91-1120 and 92-1120. 1991 and 1992. Public Health Service. Hyattsville, Md.

Table 50. Provisional death rates for the three leading causes of death, according to age: United States, 1989–91

[Data are based on a 10-percent sample of death certificates from the National Vital Statistics System]

Cause of death and age	1989	1990	1991
Diseases of heart	Deaths per 100,000 resident population		
All ages, age adjusted	155.9	150.3	146.1
All ages, crude	296.3	289.0	283.3
Under 1 year	18.8	17.9	20.3
1–14 years	1.1	1.1	1.1
15–24 years	2.1	2.4	3.0
25–34 years	7.5	7.6	7.3
35–44 years	30.8	30.2	30.1
45–54 years	124.6	117.9	118.7
55–64 years	377.8	357.2	354.3
65–74 years	910.1	885.8	850.5
75–84 years	2,412.5	2,344.3	2,229.2
85 years and over	6,742.6	6,451.4	6,306.5
Malignant neoplasms			
All ages, age adjusted	133.7	133.0	132.6
All ages, crude	200.3	201.7	202.9
Under 1 year	*	*	*
1–14 years	3.2	3.0	3.3
15–24 years	5.3	4.8	5.8
25–34 years	13.3	12.7	12.3
35–44 years	45.0	43.2	43.2
45–54 years	158.5	155.7	154.2
55–64 years	451.4	440.7	433.2
65–74 years	843.5	857.3	855.0
75–84 years	1,338.4	1,348.7	1,367.3
85 years and over	1,655.2	1,702.1	1,716.6
Cerebrovascular diseases			
All ages, age adjusted	28.5	27.6	26.5
All ages, crude	59.4	57.9	56.8
Under 1 year	2.8	*	*
1–14 years	0.3	0.3	0.3
15–24 years	0.4	0.8	0.5
25–34 years	1.9	1.9	1.8
35–44 years	6.7	6.6	6.7
45–54 years	18.1	19.7	16.7
55–64 years	50.6	46.5	46.8
65–74 years	147.6	144.5	139.0
75–84 years	530.2	501.5	486.6
85 years and over	1,632.8	1,573.9	1,525.9

*Rates based on 100 or fewer estimated deaths have relative standard errors of 30 percent or more and are not shown.

NOTES: Before 1991 data include deaths of nonresidents of the United States. Starting in 1991 data exclude deaths of nonresidents of the United States. Code numbers for cause of death are based on the International Classification of Diseases, Ninth Revision, described in Appendix II, table V. Provisional data for 1989–91 were calculated using 1980's-based postcensal population estimates. See Appendix I, National Center for Health Statistics and Department of Commerce.

SOURCES: Centers for Disease Control and Prevention, National Center for Health Statistics: Annual summary of births, marriages, divorces, and deaths, United States, 1990 and 1991. Monthly Vital Statistics Report. Vols. 39 and 40, No. 13. DHHS Pub. Nos. (PHS) 91-1120 and 92-1120. 1991 and 1992. Public Health Service. Hyattsville, Md.

Table 51. Vaccinations of children 1–4 years of age for selected diseases, according to race and residence in metropolitan statistical area (MSA): United States, 1970, 1976, 1983–85, and 1991

[Data are based on household interviews of a sample of the civilian noninstitutionalized population]

Vaccination and year	Total	Race		Inside MSA		Outside MSA
		White	All other	Central city	Remaining areas	
All respondents	Percent of population					
DTP [1,2]:						
1970	76.1	79.7	58.8	68.9	80.7	77.1
1976	71.4	75.3	53.2	64.1	75.7	72.9
1983	65.7	70.1	47.7	55.4	69.4	69.4
1984	65.7	69.1	51.3	57.9	66.6	69.8
1985	64.9	68.7	48.7	55.5	68.4	67.9
1991	65.8	68.6	54.6	60.1	68.7	68.2
Polio [2]:						
1970	65.9	69.2	50.1	61.0	70.8	64.7
1976	61.6	66.2	39.9	53.8	65.3	63.9
1983	57.0	61.9	36.7	47.7	60.3	60.3
1984	54.8	58.4	39.9	48.7	55.2	58.5
1985	55.3	58.9	40.1	47.1	58.4	58.0
1991	50.6	52.7	42.1	47.3	52.2	52.1
MMR [3]:						
Measles:						
1970.	57.2	60.4	41.9	55.2	61.7	54.3
1976.	65.9	68.3	54.8	62.5	67.2	67.3
1983.	64.9	66.8	57.2	60.4	66.3	66.7
1984.	62.8	65.4	52.0	56.6	63.3	66.4
1985.	60.8	63.6	48.8	55.5	63.3	61.9
Mumps:						
1970.	- - -	- - -	- - -	- - -	- - -	- - -
1976.	48.3	50.3	38.7	45.6	50.7	47.9
1983.	59.5	61.8	50.0	52.6	60.2	63.6
1984.	58.7	61.3	47.7	51.8	58.3	63.6
1985.	58.9	61.8	47.0	52.4	61.0	61.4
Rubella:						
1970.	37.2	38.3	31.8	38.3	39.2	34.3
1976.	61.7	63.8	51.5	59.5	63.5	61.5
1983.	64.0	66.3	54.7	59.5	65.2	66.0
1984:	60.9	63.9	48.3	56.1	60.4	64.6
1985.	58.9	61.6	47.7	53.9	61.0	60.3
MMR [3]:						
1991.	77.6	77.9	76.4	75.6	78.8	77.9
Respondents consulting vaccination records, 1991 [4]						
DTP [1,2]	84.2	86.2	74.1	78.9	86.3	86.7
Polio [2]	68.9	70.6	60.3	65.5	70.9	69.2
MMR [3]	79.5	80.2	75.7	76.6	80.9	80.3

[1]Diphtheria-tetanus-pertussis.
[2]Three doses or more.
[3]Measles-mumps-rubella.
[4]The data in this panel are based only on 49.3 percent of white respondents and 40.7 percent of all other respondents who either consulted records for all of the vaccination questions or reported no vaccinations.

NOTES: Beginning in 1976, the category "don't know" was added to response categories. In 1970, the lack of this option resulted in some forced positive answers, particularly for vaccinations requiring multiple dose schedules, that is, polio and DTP. In 1991, refusals and unknowns (2 percent of sample) were coded as not vaccinated.

SOURCES: Centers for Disease Control and Prevention: Data computed by the Division of Immunization, Center for Prevention Services from data compiled by the Division of Health Interview Statistics, National Center for Health Statistics; Unpublished data from the United States Immunization Survey.

Table 52. Selected notifiable disease rates, according to disease: United States, selected years 1950-91

[Data are based on reporting by State health departments]

Disease	1950	1960	1970	1980	1985	1988	1989	1990	1991
	Cases per 100,000 population								
Diphtheria	3.83	0.51	0.21	0.00	0.00	0.00	0.00	0.00	0.00
Hepatitis A	- - -	- - -	27.87	12.84	10.03	11.60	14.43	12.64	9.67
Hepatitis B	- - -	- - -	4.08	8.39	11.50	9.43	9.43	8.48	7.14
Mumps	- - -	- - -	55.55	3.86	1.30	2.05	2.34	2.17	1.72
Pertussis (whooping cough)	79.82	8.23	2.08	0.76	1.50	1.40	1.67	1.84	1.08
Poliomyelitis, total	22.02	1.77	0.02	0.00	0.00	0.00	0.00	0.00	0.00
Paralytic [1]	- - -	1.40	0.02	0.00	0.00	0.00	0.00	0.00	0.00
Rubella (German measles)	- - -	- - -	27.75	1.72	0.26	0.09	0.16	0.45	0.56
Rubeola (measles)	211.01	245.42	23.23	5.96	1.18	1.38	7.33	11.17	3.82
Salmonellosis, excluding typhoid fever	- - -	3.85	10.84	14.88	27.37	19.91	19.26	19.54	19.10
Shigellosis	15.45	6.94	6.79	8.41	7.14	12.46	10.07	10.89	9.34
Tuberculosis [2]	80.45	30.83	18.28	12.25	9.30	9.13	9.46	10.33	10.42
Varicella (chickenpox)	- - -	- - -	- - -	96.69	123.23	122.43	121.77	120.06	135.82
Sexually transmitted diseases [3]:									
Syphilis [4]	146.02	68.78	45.26	30.51	28.50	42.53	46.37	53.80	51.69
Primary and secondary	16.73	9.06	10.89	12.06	11.45	16.47	18.47	20.10	17.26
Early latent	39.71	10.11	8.08	9.00	9.15	14.63	18.29	22.10	21.66
Late and late latent	70.22	45.91	24.94	9.30	7.77	11.13	8.88	10.30	11.05
Congenital [5]	8.97	2.48	0.97	0.12	0.14	0.30	0.73	1.30	1.74
Gonorrhea	192.45	145.33	297.22	444.99	384.28	300.30	295.70	276.60	249.48
Chancroid	3.34	0.94	0.70	0.35	0.87	2.04	1.90	1.70	1.40
Granuloma inguinale	1.19	0.17	0.06	0.02	0.02	0.00	0.00	0.00	0.01
Lymphogranuloma venereum	0.95	0.47	0.30	0.09	0.10	0.08	0.07	0.10	0.19
	Number of cases								
Diphtheria	5,796	918	435	3	3	2	3	4	5
Hepatitis A	- - -	- - -	56,797	29,087	23,210	28,507	35,821	31,441	24,378
Hepatitis B	- - -	- - -	8,310	19,015	26,611	23,177	23,419	21,102	18,003
Mumps	- - -	- - -	104,953	8,576	2,982	4,866	5,712	5,292	4,264
Pertussis (whooping cough)	120,718	14,809	4,249	1,730	3,589	3,450	4,157	4,570	2,719
Poliomyelitis, total	33,300	3,190	33	9	7	9	5	7	6
Paralytic [1]	- - -	2,525	31	8	7	9	5	7	6
Rubella (German measles)	- - -	- - -	56,552	3,904	630	225	396	1,125	1,401
Rubeola (measles)	319,124	441,703	47,351	13,506	2,822	3,396	18,193	27,786	9,643
Salmonellosis, excluding typhoid fever	- - -	6,929	22,096	33,715	65,347	48,948	47,812	48,603	48,154
Shigellosis	23,367	12,487	13,845	19,041	17,057	30,617	25,010	27,077	23,548
Tuberculosis [2]	121,742	55,494	37,137	27,749	22,201	22,436	23,495	25,701	26,283
Varicella (chickenpox)	- - -	- - -	- - -	190,894	178,162	192,857	185,441	173,099	147,076
Sexually transmitted diseases [3]:									
Syphilis [4]	217,558	122,538	91,382	68,832	67,563	104,546	115,113	134,255	128,569
Primary and secondary	23,939	16,145	21,982	27,204	27,131	40,474	45,854	50,233	42,935
Early latent	59,256	18,017	16,311	20,297	21,689	35,968	45,409	55,132	53,870
Late and late latent	113,569	81,798	50,348	20,979	18,414	27,363	22,035	25,612	27,500
Congenital [5]	13,377	4,416	1,953	277	329	741	1,809	3,288	4,352
Gonorrhea	286,746	258,933	600,072	1,004,029	911,419	738,160	734,127	690,169	620,478
Chancroid	4,977	1,680	1,416	788	2,067	4,891	4,697	4,212	3,476
Granuloma inguinale	1,783	296	124	51	44	11	7	97	29
Lymphogranuloma venereum	1,427	835	612	199	226	194	182	277	471

[1]Data beginning in 1986 may be updated due to late reports.

[2]Data after 1974 are not comparable to prior years because of changes in reporting criteria effective in 1975.

[3]Newly reported civilian cases prior to 1991; includes military cases beginning in 1991.

[4]Includes stage of syphilis not stated.

[5]Data reported for 1990 and later years reflect change in case definition introduced in 1989.

NOTES: Rates greater than 0 but less than 0.005 are shown as 0.00. The total resident population was used to calculate all rates except sexually transmitted diseases, for which the civilian resident population was used prior to 1991. Population data from those States where diseases were not notifiable or not available were excluded from rate calculation. See Appendix I for information on underreporting of notifiable diseases.

SOURCES: Centers for Disease Control and Prevention: Final 1991 reports of notifiable diseases, Morbidity and Mortality Weekly Report 40(53). Public Health Service, Atlanta, Ga., Oct. 1992; Division of Sexually Transmitted Diseases, Center for Prevention Services, Centers for Disease Control and Prevention: Selected data.

Table 53. Acquired immunodeficiency syndrome (AIDS) cases, according to age at diagnosis, sex, detailed race, and Hispanic origin: United States, 1985–92

[Data are based on reporting by State health departments]

Age at diagnosis, sex, race, and Hispanic origin	All years [1]	All years [1]	1985	1986	1987	1988	1989	1990	1991	1992	1992
	Percent distribution	Number, by year of report									Cases per 100,000 population [2]
All races	. . .	244,939	8,210	13,147	21,088	30,719	33,595	41,653	43,701	45,472	18.1
Male											
All males, 13 years and over . . .	100.0	214,981	7,555	12,002	19,082	27,108	29,625	36,378	37,656	38,789	39.5
White, not Hispanic	58.0	124,778	4,798	7,527	12,332	16,060	17,509	20,935	20,686	20,740	27.5
Black, not Hispanic	27.5	59,083	1,712	2,760	4,321	7,159	8,055	10,292	11,105	12,031	115.3
Hispanic.	13.4	28,809	987	1,608	2,242	3,648	3,729	4,749	5,431	5,498	63.0
American Indian [3]	0.2	374	7	19	24	33	57	68	68	94	14.1
Asian or Pacific Islander [4]	0.7	1,435	48	78	130	163	213	254	252	276	9.8
13–19 years	0.3	635	31	44	68	85	89	100	99	95	. . .
20–29 years	18.6	39,959	1,470	2,490	3,798	5,464	5,719	6,845	6,478	6,292	. . .
30–39 years	46.5	99,956	3,620	5,654	8,868	12,612	13,904	16,844	17,414	17,795	. . .
40–49 years	24.1	51,837	1,663	2,576	4,290	6,112	6,823	8,914	9,642	10,317	. . .
50–59 years	7.6	16,367	605	917	1,471	1,995	2,241	2,657	2,904	3,059	. . .
60 years and over	2.9	6,227	166	321	587	840	849	1,018	1,119	1,231	. . .
Female											
All females, 13 years and over . .	100.0	25,928	526	962	1,684	3,040	3,374	4,552	5,378	5,940	5.6
White, not Hispanic	26.7	6,924	143	268	545	853	949	1,228	1,362	1,457	1.8
Black, not Hispanic	56.1	14,538	286	523	896	1,655	1,896	2,543	3,101	3,391	27.8
Hispanic.	16.2	4,207	93	160	229	500	493	741	862	1,026	12.2
American Indian [3]	0.2	61	3	2	3	5	9	10	12	16	2.3
Asian or Pacific Islander [4]	0.5	141	1	8	11	22	17	19	25	36	1.2
13–19 years	1.0	259	4	12	11	23	29	63	53	57	. . .
20–29 years	24.9	6,454	175	275	482	771	889	1,106	1,222	1,359	. . .
30–39 years	46.8	12,128	236	446	749	1,506	1,620	2,100	2,540	2,730	. . .
40–49 years	17.0	4,398	46	127	229	412	506	787	1,001	1,240	. . .
50–59 years	5.7	1,468	26	47	91	151	172	277	342	344	. . .
60 years and over	4.7	1,221	39	55	122	177	158	219	220	210	. . .
Children											
All children, under 13 years	100.0	4,030	129	183	322	571	596	723	667	743	1.6
White, not Hispanic	21.6	871	27	42	85	150	111	162	145	128	0.4
Black, not Hispanic	57.3	2,308	83	105	162	304	342	385	403	468	6.7
Hispanic.	20.1	811	19	35	72	112	136	168	112	138	2.3
American Indian [3]	0.3	13	–	–	2	–	2	4	2	3	0.6
Asian or Pacific Islander [4]	0.5	19	–	1	1	4	3	4	4	2	0.1
Under 1 year.	39.7	1,601	54	78	141	193	239	284	248	305	. . .
1–12 years	60.3	2,429	75	105	181	378	357	439	419	438	. . .

[1] Includes cases prior to 1985.
[2] Resident population estimates for 1991 based on extrapolation from 1990 census counts from the U.S. Bureau of the Census.
[3] Includes Aleut and Eskimo.
[4] Includes Chinese, Japanese, Filipino, Hawaiian and part Hawaiian, and other Asian or Pacific Islander.

NOTES: The AIDS case definition was changed in September 1987 to allow for the presumptive diagnosis of AIDS-associated diseases and conditions and to expand the spectrum of human immunodeficiency virus-associated diseases reportable as AIDS. Excludes residents of U.S. territories. Data are updated periodically because of reporting delays. Data for all years have been updated through December 31, 1992.

SOURCE: Centers for Disease Control and Prevention, National Center for Infectious Diseases, Division of HIV/AIDS.

Table 54. Deaths among acquired immunodeficiency syndrome (AIDS) cases, according to age at death, sex, detailed race, and Hispanic origin: United States, 1985–92

[Data are based on reporting by State health departments]

Age at death, sex, race, and Hispanic origin	All years [1]	All years [1]	1985	1986	1987	1988	1989	1990	1991	1992
	Percent distribution	Number, by year of death								
All races	. . .	166,211	6,681	11,535	15,451	19,656	26,151	28,053	30,579	22,660
Male										
All males, 13 years and over at diagnosis	100.0	147,497	6,117	10,479	13,768	17,393	23,224	24,749	26,870	19,962
White, not Hispanic	58.9	86,930	3,805	6,575	8,204	10,075	13,463	14,544	15,664	11,667
Black, not Hispanic.	26.8	39,554	1,493	2,475	3,616	4,780	6,336	6,670	7,365	5,521
Hispanic	13.3	19,577	784	1,355	1,837	2,375	3,191	3,296	3,519	2,544
American Indian [2]	0.2	232	4	12	24	22	31	37	63	36
Asian or Pacific Islander [3]	0.7	962	29	52	76	109	156	164	202	154
Age at death:										
13–19 years	0.2	339	21	37	41	37	53	48	54	30
20–29 years	15.5	22,859	1,131	1,881	2,496	3,003	3,641	3,603	3,583	2,569
30–39 years	45.4	67,001	2,800	4,860	6,301	7,827	10,577	11,229	12,170	8,973
40–49 years	26.3	38,841	1,382	2,424	3,174	4,227	6,021	6,820	7,713	5,929
50–59 years	8.9	13,168	577	898	1,193	1,600	2,119	2,199	2,362	1,776
60 years and over	3.6	5,289	206	379	563	699	813	850	988	685
Female										
All females, 13 years and over at diagnosis	100.0	16,545	458	905	1,410	1,971	2,592	2,946	3,387	2,470
White, not Hispanic	26.8	4,436	147	258	443	551	663	771	864	643
Black, not Hispanic.	56.1	9,284	224	486	776	1,076	1,461	1,696	1,914	1,428
Hispanic	16.2	2,677	84	150	183	326	439	454	576	381
American Indian [2]	0.2	31	3	1	2	1	5	5	10	3
Asian or Pacific Islander [3]	0.6	95	–	7	6	16	19	12	21	12
Age at death:										
13–19 years	0.7	113	5	10	10	12	13	24	22	12
20–29 years	22.2	3,672	129	236	354	450	554	624	714	459
30–39 years	46.7	7,732	208	423	627	941	1,286	1,402	1,513	1,167
40–49 years	17.8	2,946	53	106	194	295	443	543	712	560
50–59 years	6.3	1,048	22	43	93	114	152	188	261	155
60 years and over	6.2	1,034	41	87	132	159	144	165	165	117
Children										
All children, under 13 years at diagnosis	100.0	2,169	106	151	273	292	335	358	322	228
White, not Hispanic	23.0	498	28	37	70	68	90	63	74	47
Black, not Hispanic.	55.3	1,200	60	82	133	159	169	217	184	136
Hispanic	20.7	448	16	30	67	62	73	73	60	44
American Indian [2]	0.4	8	–	–	2	–	1	2	3	–
Asian or Pacific Islander [3]	0.6	13	2	2	1	3	1	2	1	1
Age at death:										
Under 1 year	30.9	670	35	51	84	93	110	108	75	55
1 year and over	69.1	1,499	71	100	189	199	225	250	247	173

[1] Includes cases prior to 1985.
[2] Includes Aleut and Eskimo.
[3] Includes Chinese, Japanese, Filipino, Hawaiian and part Hawaiian, and other Asian or Pacific Islander.

NOTES: The AIDS case definition was changed in September 1987 to allow for the presumptive diagnosis of AIDS-associated diseases and conditions and to expand the spectrum of human immunodeficiency virus-associated diseases reportable as AIDS. The number of deaths among AIDS cases reported to the CDC AIDS Surveillance System differs from the number of HIV infection deaths based on the National Vital Statistics System. See Appendix I. Excludes residents of U.S. territories. Data are updated periodically because of reporting delays. Data for all years have been updated through December 31, 1992.

SOURCE: Centers for Disease Control and Prevention, National Center for Infectious Diseases, Division of HIV/AIDS.

Table 55 (page 1 of 2). Acquired immunodeficiency syndrome (AIDS) cases, according to race, Hispanic origin, sex, and transmission category for persons 13 years of age and over at diagnosis: United States, 1985–92

[Data are based on reporting by State health departments]

Race, Hispanic origin, sex, and transmission category	All years [1] Percent distribution	All years [1]	1985	1986	1987	1988	1989	1990	1991	1992
		Number, by year of report								
All races	100.0	240,909	8,081	12,964	20,766	30,148	32,999	40,930	43,034	44,729
Men who have sex with men.	58.6	141,137	5,429	8,542	13,550	17,860	19,688	23,890	23,872	23,653
Injecting drug use	21.9	52,790	1,395	2,244	3,548	6,926	7,212	9,252	10,347	10,580
Men who have sex with men and injecting drug use.	6.3	15,244	592	989	1,551	2,037	2,189	2,389	2,454	2,355
Hemophilia/coagulation disorder . . .	0.8	2,001	74	122	206	297	285	337	311	313
Born in Caribbean/African countries.	1.2	2,960	140	216	261	370	366	415	492	453
Heterosexual contact [2]	5.1	12,178	144	341	647	1,187	1,507	2,220	2,707	3,335
Sex with injecting drug user.	3.2	7,787	107	237	444	862	1,063	1,481	1,681	1,846
Transfusion [3]	2.0	4,800	171	298	616	810	722	791	663	650
Undetermined [4]	4.1	9,799	136	212	387	661	1,030	1,636	2,188	3,390
Race and Hispanic origin										
White, not Hispanic	100.0	131,702	4,941	7,795	12,877	16,913	18,458	22,163	22,048	22,197
Men who have sex with men.	75.2	98,979	4,038	6,223	10,018	12,783	13,858	16,691	16,184	15,728
Injecting drug use	9.0	11,790	252	406	820	1,485	1,694	2,061	2,333	2,494
Men who have sex with men and injecting drug use.	6.9	9,040	377	647	1,007	1,180	1,303	1,358	1,423	1,322
Hemophilia/coagulation disorder . . .	1.3	1,651	63	113	180	242	236	277	253	242
Born in Caribbean/African countries.	0.0	10	–	1	1	1	–	1	4	1
Heterosexual contact [2]	2.6	3,384	33	97	209	368	448	653	723	833
Sex with injecting drug user.	1.3	1,754	18	48	103	211	262	348	367	386
Transfusion [3]	2.6	3,370	133	229	471	603	531	520	418	403
Undetermined [4]	2.6	3,478	45	79	171	251	388	602	710	1,174
Black, not Hispanic.	100.0	73,621	1,998	3,283	5,217	8,814	9,951	12,835	14,206	15,422
Men who have sex with men.	34.7	25,523	795	1,327	2,124	3,088	3,598	4,464	4,604	4,831
Injecting drug use	39.3	28,950	748	1,207	1,891	3,757	4,014	5,144	5,722	5,805
Men who have sex with men and injecting drug use.	6.0	4,405	143	239	386	607	657	766	726	713
Hemophilia/coagulation disorder . . .	0.2	167	4	3	11	28	18	28	35	35
Born in Caribbean/African countries.	4.0	2,925	140	215	258	365	361	410	483	447
Heterosexual contact [2]	9.0	6,652	82	164	325	575	799	1,182	1,548	1,938
Sex with injecting drug user.	6.1	4,498	64	121	252	456	600	841	1,014	1,122
Transfusion [3]	1.2	907	26	43	93	135	126	168	148	157
Undetermined [4]	5.6	4,092	60	85	129	259	378	673	940	1,496
Hispanic	100.0	33,016	1,080	1,768	2,471	4,148	4,222	5,490	6,293	6,524
Men who have sex with men.	45.2	14,920	551	907	1,258	1,797	1,992	2,434	2,763	2,735
Injecting drug use	35.7	11,793	387	619	828	1,658	1,459	2,006	2,236	2,224
Men who have sex with men and injecting drug use.	5.1	1,686	70	99	146	242	212	244	290	288
Hemophilia/coagulation disorder . . .	0.4	145	7	5	10	22	22	27	18	29
Born in Caribbean/African countries.	0.0	16	–	–	2	2	2	4	3	3
Heterosexual contact [2]	6.2	2,039	29	77	110	231	241	371	414	535
Sex with injecting drug user.	4.5	1,483	25	68	88	187	189	283	287	329
Transfusion [3]	1.2	403	7	20	38	54	54	79	75	72
Undetermined [4]	6.1	2,014	29	41	79	142	240	325	494	638

See footnotes at end of table.

Table 55 (page 2 of 2). **Acquired immunodeficiency syndrome (AIDS) cases, according to race, Hispanic origin, sex, and transmission category for persons 13 years of age and over at diagnosis: United States, 1985–92**

[Data are based on reporting by State health departments]

Race, Hispanic origin, sex, and transmission category	All years [1]	All years [1]	1985	1986	1987	1988	1989	1990	1991	1992
Sex	Percent distribution	Number, by year of report								
Male	100.0	214,981	7,555	12,002	19,082	27,108	29,625	36,378	37,656	38,789
Men who have sex with men	65.7	141,137	5,429	8,542	13,550	17,860	19,688	23,890	23,872	23,653
Injecting drug use	18.5	39,865	1,111	1,767	2,708	5,296	5,441	6,992	7,664	7,879
Men who have sex with men and injecting drug use	7.1	15,244	592	989	1,551	2,037	2,189	2,389	2,454	2,355
Hemophilia/coagulation disorder	0.9	1,958	73	118	202	293	279	328	303	310
Born in Caribbean/African countries	1.0	2,075	109	160	187	262	236	304	325	283
Heterosexual contact [2]	1.8	3,942	28	65	161	326	504	721	881	1,243
Sex with injecting drug user	1.1	2,413	25	44	114	228	369	462	521	639
Transfusion [3]	1.4	2,952	111	193	399	488	438	467	424	387
Undetermined [4]	3.6	7,808	102	168	324	546	850	1,287	1,733	2,679
Female	100.0	25,928	526	962	1,684	3,040	3,374	4,552	5,378	5,940
Injecting drug use	49.8	12,925	284	477	840	1,630	1,771	2,260	2,683	2,701
Hemophilia/coagulation disorder	0.2	43	1	4	4	4	6	9	8	3
Born in Caribbean/African countries	3.4	885	31	56	74	108	130	111	167	170
Heterosexual contact [2]	31.8	8,236	116	276	486	861	1,003	1,499	1,826	2,092
Sex with injecting drug user	20.7	5,374	82	193	330	634	694	1,019	1,160	1,207
Transfusion [3]	7.1	1,848	60	105	217	322	284	324	239	263
Undetermined [4]	7.7	1,991	34	44	63	115	180	349	455	711

[1] Includes cases prior to 1985.
[2] Includes persons who have had heterosexual contact with a person with human immunodeficiency virus (HIV) infection or at risk of HIV infection.
[3] Receipt of blood transfusion, blood components, or tissue.
[4] Includes persons for whom risk information is incomplete (because of death, refusal to be interviewed, or loss to followup), persons still under investigation, men reported only to have had heterosexual contact with prostitutes, and interviewed persons for whom no specific risk is identified.

NOTES: The AIDS case definition was changed in September 1987 to allow for the presumptive diagnosis of AIDS-associated diseases and conditions and to expand the spectrum of HIV-associated diseases reportable as AIDS. Excludes residents of U.S. territories. Data are updated periodically because of reporting delays. Data for all years have been updated through December 31, 1992.

SOURCE: Centers for Disease Control and Prevention, National Center for Infectious Diseases, Division of HIV/AIDS.

Table 56 (page 1 of 2). **Deaths among acquired immunodeficiency syndrome (AIDS) cases, according to race, Hispanic origin, sex, and transmission category for persons 13 years of age and over at diagnosis: United States, 1985–92**

[Data are based on reporting by State health departments]

Race, Hispanic origin, sex, and transmission category	All years[1]	All years[1]	1985	1986	1987	1988	1989	1990	1991	1992
	Percent distribution	Number, by year of death								
All races	100.0	164,042	6,575	11,384	15,178	19,364	25,816	27,695	30,257	22,432
Men who have sex with men	60.0	98,432	4,227	7,314	9,131	11,476	15,388	16,394	17,858	13,390
Injecting drug use	21.4	35,152	1,214	2,051	3,172	4,366	5,827	6,162	6,752	4,571
Men who have sex with men and injecting drug use	6.4	10,474	496	857	1,136	1,265	1,564	1,655	1,715	1,275
Hemophilia/coagulation disorder	0.9	1,441	76	108	159	193	216	248	231	168
Born in Caribbean/African countries	1.1	1,724	114	155	196	194	249	202	220	193
Heterosexual contact[2]	4.4	7,239	128	275	463	730	1,074	1,420	1,688	1,394
Sex with injecting drug user	2.9	4,763	89	189	325	518	772	940	1,062	816
Transfusion[3]	2.3	3,828	196	369	535	608	616	546	523	344
Undetermined[4]	3.5	5,752	124	255	386	532	882	1,068	1,270	1,097
Race and Hispanic origin										
White, not Hispanic	100.0	91,366	3,952	6,833	8,647	10,626	14,126	15,315	16,528	12,310
Men who have sex with men	76.2	69,627	3,125	5,361	6,480	7,985	10,811	11,632	12,571	9,308
Injecting drug use	8.2	7,483	222	364	646	876	1,232	1,337	1,482	1,125
Men who have sex with men and injecting drug use	6.7	6,134	310	546	685	719	869	954	1,012	743
Hemophilia/coagulation disorder	1.3	1,212	62	97	137	170	172	207	195	134
Born in Caribbean/African countries	0.0	2	–	–	–	–	–	–	–	2
Heterosexual contact[2]	2.2	2,037	32	83	127	211	305	399	468	401
Sex with injecting drug user	1.2	1,056	12	40	69	108	178	201	241	201
Transfusion[3]	3.0	2,771	152	288	415	463	424	395	354	206
Undetermined[4]	2.3	2,100	49	94	157	202	313	391	446	391
Black, not Hispanic	100.0	48,838	1,717	2,961	4,392	5,856	7,797	8,366	9,279	6,949
Men who have sex with men	35.7	17,454	656	1,161	1,626	2,174	2,798	2,865	3,156	2,487
Injecting drug use	39.9	19,488	669	1,148	1,737	2,409	3,215	3,452	3,794	2,516
Men who have sex with men and injecting drug use	6.3	3,101	129	222	321	387	485	528	515	378
Hemophilia/coagulation disorder	0.2	115	7	3	13	11	21	18	21	20
Born in Caribbean/African countries	3.5	1,709	113	155	195	194	244	202	217	188
Heterosexual contact[2]	8.1	3,945	68	123	269	379	566	777	936	793
Sex with injecting drug user	5.6	2,751	54	90	205	292	429	554	628	473
Transfusion[3]	1.4	667	27	45	79	94	127	100	97	87
Undetermined[4]	4.8	2,359	48	104	152	208	341	424	543	480
Hispanic	100.0	22,254	868	1,505	2,020	2,701	3,630	3,750	4,095	2,925
Men who have sex with men	46.1	10,259	423	736	934	1,187	1,610	1,714	1,887	1,422
Injecting drug use	36.1	8,034	319	530	783	1,064	1,350	1,349	1,440	911
Men who have sex with men and injecting drug use	5.3	1,170	56	86	126	153	198	159	173	142
Hemophilia/coagulation disorder	0.4	97	5	8	7	10	19	19	13	13
Born in Caribbean/African countries	0.0	11	1	–	1	–	3	–	3	3
Heterosexual contact[2]	5.4	1,202	28	66	66	135	190	234	266	195
Sex with injecting drug user	4.2	931	23	58	51	115	158	178	187	141
Transfusion[3]	1.4	302	11	28	30	41	50	41	55	42
Undetermined[4]	5.3	1,179	25	51	73	111	210	234	258	197

See footnotes at end of table.

Table 56 (page 2 of 2). Deaths among acquired immunodeficiency syndrome (AIDS) cases, according to race, Hispanic origin, sex, and transmission category for persons 13 years of age and over at diagnosis: United States, 1985–92

[Data are based on reporting by State health departments]

Race, Hispanic origin, sex, and transmission category	All years [1]	All years [1]	1985	1986	1987	1988	1989	1990	1991	1992
Sex	Percent distribution	Number, by year of death								
Male	100.0	147,497	6,117	10,479	13,768	17,393	23,224	24,749	26,870	19,962
Men who have sex with men	66.7	98,432	4,227	7,314	9,131	11,476	15,388	16,394	17,858	13,390
Injecting drug use	18.2	26,846	973	1,599	2,453	3,336	4,497	4,688	5,072	3,424
Men who have sex with men and injecting drug use	7.1	10,474	496	857	1,136	1,265	1,564	1,655	1,715	1,275
Hemophilia/coagulation disorder . . .	1.0	1,410	71	105	157	188	213	242	228	165
Born in Caribbean/African countries	0.8	1,209	91	104	142	131	163	142	142	129
Heterosexual contact [2]	1.5	2,179	30	52	121	186	309	443	530	500
Sex with injecting drug user	0.9	1,357	26	36	82	137	205	284	319	261
Transfusion [3]	1.6	2,371	126	254	317	371	379	343	315	213
Undetermined [4]	3.1	4,576	103	194	311	440	711	842	1,010	866
Female	100.0	16,545	458	905	1,410	1,971	2,592	2,946	3,387	2,470
Injecting drug use	50.2	8,306	241	452	719	1,030	1,330	1,474	1,680	1,147
Hemophilia/coagulation disorder . . .	0.2	31	5	3	2	5	3	6	3	3
Born in Caribbean/African countries	3.1	515	23	51	54	63	86	60	78	64
Heterosexual contact [2]	30.6	5,060	98	223	342	544	765	977	1,158	894
Sex with injecting drug user	20.6	3,406	63	153	243	381	567	656	743	555
Transfusion [3]	8.8	1,457	70	115	218	237	237	203	208	131
Undetermined [4]	7.1	1,176	21	61	75	92	171	226	260	231

[1]Includes cases prior to 1985.
[2]Includes persons who have had heterosexual contact with a person with human immunodeficiency virus (HIV) infection or at risk of HIV infection.
[3]Receipt of blood transfusion, blood components, or tissue.
[4]Includes persons for whom risk information is incomplete (because of death, refusal to be interviewed, or loss to followup), persons still under investigation, men reported only to have had heterosexual contact with prostitutes, and interviewed persons for whom no specific risk is identified.

NOTES: The AIDS case definition was changed in September 1987 to allow for the presumptive diagnosis of AIDS-associated diseases and conditions and to expand the spectrum of human immunodeficiency virus-associated diseases reportable as AIDS. The number of deaths among AIDS cases reported to the CDC AIDS Surveillance System differs from the number of HIV infection deaths based on the National Vital Statistics System. See Appendix I. Excludes residents of U.S. territories. Data are updated periodically because of reporting delays. Data for all years have been updated through December 31, 1992.

SOURCE: Centers for Disease Control and Prevention, National Center for Infectious Diseases, Division of HIV/AIDS.

Table 57. Acquired immunodeficiency syndrome (AIDS) cases, according to geographic division and State: United States, 1985–92

[Data are based on reporting by State health departments]

Geographic division and State	All years [1]	1985	1986	1987	1988	1989	1990	1991	1992	1992
					Number, by year of report					Cases per 100,000 population [2]
United States	244,939	8,210	13,147	21,088	30,719	33,595	41,653	43,701	45,472	18.12
New England	9,561	279	528	847	1,282	1,394	1,507	1,745	1,743	13.11
Maine	313	11	22	28	27	66	65	50	44	3.55
New Hampshire	292	4	13	32	38	37	65	52	46	4.08
Vermont	121	2	6	15	11	20	22	17	26	4.58
Massachusetts	5,177	164	282	452	710	752	842	967	875	14.48
Rhode Island	579	12	30	68	84	88	88	92	106	10.50
Connecticut	3,079	86	175	252	412	431	425	567	646	19.55
Middle Atlantic	72,654	3,147	4,843	6,110	10,269	9,289	12,040	11,673	11,764	31.22
New York	50,985	2,479	3,768	3,948	6,965	5,993	8,389	8,152	8,398	46.57
New Jersey	14,702	467	766	1,509	2,452	2,225	2,459	2,303	2,040	26.27
Pennsylvania	6,967	201	309	653	852	1,071	1,192	1,218	1,326	11.16
East North Central	18,060	353	822	1,405	2,139	2,655	3,035	3,369	3,994	9.50
Ohio	3,674	54	213	336	506	488	679	619	733	6.75
Indiana	1,744	26	71	132	78	399	292	315	402	7.24
Illinois	8,229	188	346	629	987	1,132	1,276	1,602	1,912	16.73
Michigan	3,343	61	150	211	455	506	579	619	718	7.72
Wisconsin	1,070	24	42	97	113	130	209	214	229	4.66
West North Central	5,989	128	241	476	769	831	1,056	1,123	1,302	7.35
Minnesota	1,264	41	96	130	166	176	203	216	218	4.95
Iowa	423	12	21	30	42	56	68	81	111	4.02
Missouri	3,192	50	74	238	411	442	580	654	708	13.78
North Dakota	29	1	4	2	3	8	1	5	5	0.78
South Dakota	37	1	2	2	7	4	9	4	8	1.15
Nebraska	309	7	10	24	51	32	58	63	61	3.86
Kansas	735	16	34	50	89	113	137	100	191	7.67
South Atlantic	49,961	1,299	2,076	3,667	5,421	7,046	8,808	10,409	10,288	23.26
Delaware	539	12	22	39	62	80	93	87	140	20.79
Maryland	5,307	150	188	457	544	713	996	969	1,204	24.89
District of Columbia	4,118	178	227	464	494	493	734	709	706	116.93
Virginia	3,525	109	160	242	348	392	744	679	784	12.50
West Virginia	297	6	8	23	20	55	64	62	54	3.04
North Carolina	2,854	66	81	209	276	444	571	600	584	8.71
South Carolina	1,785	38	58	84	174	327	360	335	391	11.10
Georgia	7,044	191	304	517	838	1,093	1,228	1,454	1,324	20.12
Florida	24,492	549	1,028	1,632	2,665	3,449	4,018	5,514	5,101	38.48
East South Central	5,566	73	165	324	756	761	1,044	1,089	1,318	8.66
Kentucky	885	18	32	48	90	115	190	165	213	5.78
Tennessee	1,864	18	72	72	329	266	341	351	408	8.32
Alabama	1,702	29	33	153	211	214	239	375	437	10.78
Mississippi	1,115	8	28	51	126	166	274	198	260	10.08
West South Central	23,260	617	1,181	2,158	2,845	3,137	4,448	4,245	4,182	15.49
Arkansas	930	10	29	48	80	79	208	195	280	11.88
Louisiana	3,794	104	165	336	401	508	703	794	710	16.82
Oklahoma	1,173	20	50	107	149	169	203	189	272	8.61
Texas	17,363	483	937	1,667	2,215	2,381	3,334	3,067	2,920	16.92
Mountain	7,006	160	332	633	892	1,106	1,116	1,304	1,349	9.71
Montana	108	1	3	6	16	13	17	30	22	2.75
Idaho	147	4	3	10	11	23	28	33	35	3.45
Wyoming	58	1	4	3	6	16	5	17	5	1.11
Colorado	2,433	62	166	226	324	386	362	433	410	12.29
New Mexico	567	14	21	47	60	94	108	112	107	6.96
Arizona	1,943	49	78	214	275	321	309	282	386	10.27
Utah	609	17	21	39	81	73	99	135	135	7.72
Nevada	1,141	12	36	88	119	180	188	262	249	20.05
Pacific	52,882	2,154	2,959	5,468	6,346	7,376	8,599	8,744	9,532	23.91
Washington	3,404	109	168	324	342	526	746	572	551	11.15
Oregon	1,565	35	63	160	177	228	336	257	289	10.09
California	46,818	1,977	2,656	4,885	5,703	6,426	7,337	7,700	8,539	28.12
Alaska	132	5	16	16	19	17	24	18	15	2.66
Hawaii	963	28	56	83	105	179	156	197	138	12.29

[1] Includes cases prior to 1985.

[2] Resident population estimates for 1991 based on extrapolation from 1990 census counts from the U.S. Bureau of the Census.

NOTES: The AIDS case definition was changed in September 1987 to allow for the presumptive diagnosis of AIDS-associated diseases and conditions and to expand the spectrum of human immunodeficiency virus-associated diseases reportable as AIDS. Excludes residents of U.S. territories. Data are updated periodically because of reporting delays. Data for all years have been updated through December 31, 1992.

SOURCE: Centers for Disease Control and Prevention, National Center for Infectious Diseases, Division of HIV/AIDS.

Table 58. Deaths among acquired immunodeficiency syndrome (AIDS) cases, according to geographic division and State: United States, 1985–92

[Data are based on reporting by State health departments]

Geographic division and State	All years[1]	1985	1986	1987	1988	1989	1990	1991	1992
					Number, by year of death				
United States	166,211	6,681	11,535	15,451	19,656	26,151	28,053	30,579	22,660
New England	6,058	225	394	591	745	961	1,051	1,168	749
Maine	172	7	16	10	19	28	41	35	16
New Hampshire	171	7	14	17	25	23	29	30	23
Vermont	68	1	6	6	5	10	13	11	14
Massachusetts	3,368	115	193	324	416	552	578	682	412
Rhode Island	402	9	24	44	46	56	74	82	60
Connecticut	1,877	86	141	190	234	292	316	328	224
Middle Atlantic	52,056	2,641	4,181	5,395	6,592	8,596	8,283	8,668	5,070
New York	37,363	2,052	3,036	3,769	4,700	6,263	5,915	6,086	3,430
New Jersey	9,926	429	830	1,180	1,320	1,609	1,541	1,714	914
Pennsylvania	4,767	160	315	446	572	724	827	868	726
East North Central	11,770	322	605	898	1,285	1,827	2,055	2,366	2,203
Ohio	2,439	62	127	186	261	386	433	499	438
Indiana	1,098	22	61	81	113	151	194	228	223
Illinois	5,468	160	285	402	606	849	913	1,096	1,054
Michigan	2,125	60	97	169	244	351	404	417	360
Wisconsin	640	18	35	60	61	90	111	126	128
West North Central	3,796	100	221	315	403	550	641	796	719
Minnesota	865	26	61	78	84	105	164	183	151
Iowa	254	7	16	20	22	35	36	69	44
Missouri	1,894	48	94	144	211	307	316	373	375
North Dakota	23	2	4	2	3	6	1	3	2
South Dakota	26	1	3	1	3	1	2	9	6
Nebraska	212	4	13	16	30	26	33	42	45
Kansas	522	12	30	54	50	70	89	117	96
South Atlantic	32,412	1,041	1,826	2,712	3,622	4,980	5,761	6,533	5,206
Delaware	338	7	21	30	30	47	68	60	72
Maryland	3,375	120	181	276	355	544	627	717	485
District of Columbia	2,649	134	203	241	315	401	474	467	352
Virginia	2,354	80	141	208	284	334	406	478	376
West Virginia	203	6	8	12	12	36	46	48	30
North Carolina	1,841	44	92	134	193	323	307	442	277
South Carolina	1,201	30	46	81	119	161	244	273	230
Georgia	4,458	128	229	356	519	668	825	955	697
Florida	15,993	492	905	1,374	1,795	2,466	2,764	3,093	2,687
East South Central	3,461	85	153	262	382	526	621	749	641
Kentucky	621	21	26	42	62	104	117	120	111
Tennessee	1,127	27	65	84	118	151	205	260	208
Alabama	1,038	27	34	80	111	150	170	233	223
Mississippi	675	10	28	56	91	121	129	136	99
West South Central	15,292	522	1,001	1,521	1,895	2,403	2,739	2,974	1,913
Arkansas	472	10	24	37	64	83	74	104	74
Louisiana	2,486	98	143	222	270	385	397	474	445
Oklahoma	770	12	40	68	92	131	116	170	129
Texas	11,564	402	794	1,194	1,469	1,804	2,152	2,226	1,265
Mountain	4,609	136	284	408	539	663	824	915	748
Montana	68	1	3	5	7	10	9	20	13
Idaho	91	1	3	7	12	7	20	14	27
Wyoming	38	2	1	4	2	6	4	7	11
Colorado	1,721	57	112	149	181	214	302	357	295
New Mexico	357	8	23	26	33	59	57	75	73
Arizona	1,223	41	90	124	186	219	252	200	92
Utah	377	12	25	32	44	40	63	78	78
Nevada	734	14	27	61	74	108	117	164	159
Pacific	36,757	1,609	2,870	3,349	4,193	5,645	6,078	6,410	5,411
Washington	2,221	80	129	186	239	313	366	451	419
Oregon	1,030	24	67	74	112	140	204	221	177
California	32,821	1,466	2,632	3,032	3,753	5,101	5,396	5,590	4,720
Alaska	64	6	7	5	9	9	7	12	8
Hawaii	621	33	35	52	80	82	105	136	87

[1]Includes cases prior to 1985.

NOTES: The AIDS case definition was changed in September 1987 to allow for the presumptive diagnosis of AIDS-associated diseases and conditions and to expand the spectrum of human immunodeficiency virus-associated diseases reportable as AIDS. The number of deaths among AIDS cases reported to the CDC AIDS Surveillance System differs from the number of HIV infection deaths based on the National Vital Statistics System. See Appendix I. Excludes residents of U.S. territories. Data are updated periodically because of reporting delays. Data for all years have been updated through December 31, 1992.

SOURCE: Centers for Disease Control and Prevention, National Center for Infectious Diseases, Division of HIV/AIDS.

Table 59. Age-adjusted cancer incidence rates for selected cancer sites, according to sex and race: Selected geographic areas, selected years 1973–90

[Data are based on the Surveillance, Epidemiology, and End Results Program's population-based registries in Atlanta, Detroit, Seattle-Puget Sound, San Francisco-Oakland, Connecticut, Iowa, New Mexico, Utah, and Hawaii]

Race, sex, and site	1973	1975	1980	1985	1986	1987	1988	1989	1990	Estimated annual percent change [1]
White male	Number of new cases per 100,000 population [2]									
All sites	363.0	378.5	405.7	428.1	434.3	452.5	448.0	451.8	464.9	1.3
Oral cavity and pharynx	17.5	18.3	16.9	16.7	16.2	17.2	15.4	15.1	15.8	−0.8
Esophagus	4.8	4.8	4.9	5.3	5.2	5.4	5.4	5.1	6.0	0.9
Stomach	13.9	12.5	12.3	10.5	10.8	10.5	10.7	10.7	9.2	−1.7
Colon and rectum	54.1	55.0	58.5	63.4	62.0	61.1	59.3	58.6	58.0	0.5
Colon	34.7	36.1	39.2	43.3	42.8	41.9	40.9	40.0	39.6	0.8
Rectum	19.4	19.0	19.3	20.0	19.2	19.2	18.4	18.6	18.4	−0.3
Pancreas	12.7	12.4	11.0	10.6	10.8	10.5	10.5	10.0	9.8	−1.0
Lung and bronchus	72.2	75.7	82.0	81.9	81.7	83.9	81.6	80.1	78.6	0.5
Prostate gland	62.3	68.8	78.4	86.4	90.1	101.9	104.9	110.2	128.5	3.5
Urinary bladder	27.2	28.6	31.3	31.0	32.1	33.5	32.7	31.9	31.6	1.0
Non-Hodgkin's lymphoma	10.2	11.4	12.6	15.9	16.6	18.2	17.9	18.1	19.0	3.9
Leukemia	14.3	14.1	14.5	14.2	14.2	13.8	13.5	13.5	12.3	−0.5
Black male										
All sites	441.2	437.3	509.1	529.3	529.8	544.2	535.3	533.3	556.3	1.5
Oral cavity and pharynx	16.6	17.3	23.1	22.5	24.5	26.2	22.6	24.3	24.8	2.2
Esophagus	13.0	17.4	16.4	19.5	21.8	18.2	16.7	15.7	19.9	0.7
Stomach	26.1	19.9	21.4	18.4	18.4	20.7	20.0	18.4	17.6	−1.0
Colon and rectum	42.6	47.2	63.6	60.2	59.4	60.9	57.2	63.9	59.0	1.7
Colon	31.5	34.2	45.8	46.5	43.9	47.1	42.3	49.0	45.8	2.1
Rectum	11.1	13.0	17.7	13.7	15.5	13.8	14.9	14.9	13.1	0.8
Pancreas	15.8	15.4	17.6	19.8	16.2	16.0	16.9	12.7	15.0	−0.6
Lung and bronchus	105.1	101.2	131.2	131.7	134.3	123.7	125.8	121.0	116.0	1.3
Prostate gland	106.4	111.2	125.7	131.8	130.8	144.9	144.3	144.2	163.6	2.2
Urinary bladder	10.7	13.7	14.5	16.0	17.4	17.4	14.1	13.9	14.8	1.1
Non-Hodgkin's lymphoma	9.0	7.1	9.3	9.9	10.9	9.3	13.0	11.3	13.6	3.4
Leukemia	12.0	12.5	13.0	12.9	10.5	13.7	10.7	12.9	10.4	−0.2
White female										
All sites	293.7	309.7	309.9	341.4	339.5	350.2	346.5	344.3	348.1	0.9
Colon and rectum	41.6	42.9	44.6	45.8	42.9	41.0	40.0	40.7	39.7	−0.3
Colon	30.2	30.8	32.9	33.8	32.1	30.1	29.3	29.9	29.7	−0.2
Rectum	11.4	12.0	11.8	11.9	10.8	10.9	10.7	10.8	10.0	−0.6
Pancreas	7.4	7.1	7.3	8.1	7.8	7.5	7.6	7.4	7.6	0.2
Lung and bronchus	17.8	21.9	28.3	35.9	37.7	39.6	41.4	40.6	41.5	4.9
Melanoma of skin	5.8	6.9	9.1	10.2	10.6	11.0	10.3	10.7	10.4	3.5
Breast	83.9	89.5	87.1	106.1	108.7	116.7	113.3	109.1	112.7	1.8
Cervix uteri	12.8	11.1	9.1	7.6	8.0	7.4	7.9	8.2	8.3	−2.6
Corpus uteri	29.4	33.7	25.3	23.1	22.3	22.6	21.3	22.0	22.7	−2.5
Ovary	14.6	14.4	13.9	15.0	13.5	14.6	15.5	16.0	15.7	0.4
Non-Hodgkin's lymphoma	7.5	8.4	9.2	11.3	11.1	11.4	12.1	11.7	12.4	2.8
Black female										
All sites	282.8	296.0	304.3	322.7	328.2	326.2	334.4	320.5	334.4	1.0
Colon and rectum	41.1	43.4	49.4	45.8	47.2	47.8	45.9	44.4	48.8	0.9
Colon	29.5	32.8	40.9	36.0	36.7	37.1	36.4	34.1	38.3	1.3
Rectum	11.6	10.6	8.5	9.9	10.5	10.7	9.5	10.2	10.5	−0.0
Pancreas	11.6	11.8	13.0	11.3	13.0	14.8	14.2	11.1	10.6	0.5
Lung and bronchus	20.9	20.6	34.0	40.8	43.3	38.9	42.6	45.0	45.3	4.9
Breast	68.8	78.3	74.0	92.2	93.8	90.3	97.7	87.8	95.8	1.9
Cervix uteri	29.7	27.9	19.0	15.9	15.2	15.0	15.3	12.9	13.3	−4.5
Corpus uteri	15.0	17.2	14.1	15.1	14.2	13.8	14.0	16.5	14.5	−0.2
Ovary	10.5	10.1	10.0	10.0	9.1	10.0	10.6	10.7	10.4	0.2
Non-Hodgkin's lymphoma	5.5	4.1	6.2	6.8	6.8	8.0	7.2	7.8	8.5	3.9

[1]The estimated annual percent change has been calculated by fitting a linear regression model to the natural logarithm of the yearly rates from 1973–90.
[2]Age adjusted by the direct method to the 1970 U.S. population.

SOURCE: National Cancer Institute, National Institutes of Health, Cancer Statistics Review, 1973–1990. NIH Pub. No. 93–2789. U.S. Department of Health and Human Services. Public Health Service. Bethesda, Md., 1993.

Table 60. Five-year relative cancer survival rates for selected sites, according to race and sex: Selected geographic areas, 1974–76, 1977–79, 1980–82, and 1983–89

[Data are based on the Surveillance, Epidemiology, and End Results Program's population-based registries in Atlanta, Detroit, Seattle-Puget Sound, San Francisco-Oakland, Connecticut, Iowa, New Mexico, Utah, and Hawaii]

Sex and site	All races				White				Black			
	1974–76	1977–79	1980–82	1983–89	1974–76	1977–79	1980–82	1983–89	1974–76	1977–79	1980–82	1983–89
Male					Percent of patients							
All sites	40.9	43.0	44.9	47.8	42.0	44.3	46.3	49.6	31.2	32.1	33.9	34.4
Oral cavity and pharynx.	52.3	51.1	50.7	49.5	54.5	53.4	54.0	52.4	30.8	30.8	25.5	27.4
Esophagus.	3.5	4.7	6.0	8.2	4.2	5.6	6.7	9.2	2.1	2.4	4.6	6.3
Stomach	13.9	15.3	16.2	16.2	13.1	14.4	15.1	15.4	15.6	14.6	18.3	15.5
Colon	49.5	51.4	55.3	60.1	49.9	51.8	55.7	61.2	43.8	45.1	46.7	47.9
Rectum	47.4	48.7	50.1	56.3	47.8	49.8	51.2	57.3	34.1	38.0	36.1	42.8
Pancreas	2.9	2.2	2.8	2.6	3.2	2.2	2.7	2.3	1.2	2.8	3.7	4.4
Lung and bronchus	11.1	11.8	12.0	11.8	11.1	12.0	12.1	11.9	11.0	9.0	10.9	10.4
Prostate gland	66.7	70.8	73.1	77.6	67.7	71.9	74.2	79.4	57.8	62.1	64.2	64.4
Urinary bladder.	73.7	76.3	79.1	81.0	74.5	76.7	79.8	81.5	54.5	62.4	62.3	66.9
Non-Hodgkin's lymphoma. . .	46.9	45.5	50.0	49.8	47.7	46.1	50.7	50.4	43.1	42.1	47.1	41.7
Leukemia.	33.0	35.8	36.8	37.5	33.5	36.7	38.0	38.9	31.9	29.4	29.3	29.6
Female												
All sites	56.7	56.0	55.9	57.9	57.5	56.8	56.7	59.1	46.7	46.2	45.5	44.7
Colon	50.6	53.6	55.0	58.1	50.7	53.7	55.2	59.1	46.9	49.5	50.5	49.2
Rectum	49.4	50.8	53.9	57.0	49.7	51.4	54.6	57.7	49.3	38.5	40.3	47.5
Pancreas	2.1	2.6	3.4	3.9	2.1	2.3	3.0	3.7	3.1	4.8	5.9	5.1
Lung and bronchus	15.6	17.0	15.9	15.7	15.8	17.0	16.0	16.0	12.9	16.9	15.4	13.0
Melanoma of skin	84.7	85.8	87.5	88.4	84.8	86.1	87.5	88.5	- - -	- - -	- - -	73.3
Breast	74.3	74.5	76.1	79.3	74.9	75.2	76.9	80.5	62.8	62.5	65.6	64.1
Cervix uteri.	68.5	67.8	66.8	66.8	69.3	68.9	67.5	69.1	63.4	61.9	60.3	57.0
Corpus uteri.	87.8	84.9	81.4	82.9	88.7	86.2	82.7	84.6	60.6	57.8	53.8	55.5
Ovary	36.5	38.1	38.8	40.6	36.3	37.5	38.7	40.2	40.1	39.8	37.3	40.2
Non-Hodgkin's lymphoma. . .	47.3	50.5	52.5	53.9	47.4	50.4	52.6	54.5	54.1	58.9	54.7	46.5

NOTES: Rates are based on followup of patients through 1990. The rate is the ratio of the observed survival rate for the patient group to the expected survival rate for persons in the general population similar to the patient group with respect to age, sex, race, and calendar year of observation. It estimates the chance of surviving the effects of cancer.

SOURCES: National Cancer Institute, National Institutes of Health, Cancer Statistics Review, 1973–1989. NIH Pub. No. 92-2789. U.S. Department of Health and Human Services. Public Health Service. Bethesda, Md., 1992; National Cancer Institute, Division of Cancer Prevention and Control: Unpublished data.

Table 61. Limitation of activity caused by chronic conditions, according to selected characteristics: United States, 1986 and 1991

[Data are based on household interviews of a sample of the civilian noninstitutionalized population]

Characteristic	Total with limitation of activity		Limited but not in major activity		Limited in amount or kind of major activity		Unable to carry on major activity	
	1986	1991	1986	1991	1986	1991	1986	1991
	Percent of population							
Total [1,2]	13.3	13.5	4.2	4.3	5.4	5.2	3.7	4.0
Age								
Under 15 years	4.8	5.4	1.2	1.3	3.2	3.7	0.4	0.5
Under 5 years	2.5	2.4	0.6	0.7	1.3	1.2	0.6	0.5
5–14 years	6.1	7.1	1.6	1.6	4.2	5.0	0.3	0.4
15–44 years	8.4	9.1	2.8	2.9	3.5	3.6	2.0	2.6
45–64 years	23.2	22.2	5.4	5.9	9.1	7.6	8.6	8.7
65 years and over	38.8	37.9	16.1	15.6	12.1	11.7	10.7	10.6
65–74 years	35.5	33.7	14.2	13.9	10.5	9.6	10.7	10.2
75 years and over	44.3	44.2	19.1	18.1	14.5	14.9	10.6	11.2
Sex [1]								
Male	13.4	13.7	3.8	4.1	5.2	5.0	4.4	4.6
Female	13.2	13.3	4.5	4.5	5.5	5.3	3.2	3.5
Race [1]								
White	13.2	13.4	4.3	4.4	5.5	5.2	3.4	3.8
Black	16.1	15.8	3.8	3.7	5.8	5.9	6.6	6.3
Family income [1,3]								
Less than $14,000	23.0	24.0	5.5	5.5	8.5	8.6	9.0	10.0
$14,000–$24,999	15.5	15.3	4.4	4.5	6.2	6.2	4.9	4.7
$25,000–$34,999	11.2	11.7	3.6	3.9	5.0	4.8	2.6	3.1
$35,000–$49,999	10.2	10.3	3.2	3.9	4.6	4.0	2.4	2.4
$50,000 or more	9.6	9.0	3.9	3.5	3.9	3.7	1.7	1.9
Geographic region [1]								
Northeast	11.5	11.6	3.7	3.6	4.3	4.4	3.5	3.6
Midwest	13.7	13.6	4.3	4.3	6.1	5.8	3.4	3.5
South	14.8	14.7	4.4	4.4	5.9	5.7	4.5	4.7
West	12.5	13.6	4.2	4.8	5.1	4.8	3.3	4.0
Location of residence [1]								
Within MSA	12.8	13.1	4.0	4.1	5.2	5.1	3.6	3.9
Outside MSA	15.1	15.1	4.6	4.7	6.3	5.7	4.3	4.7

[1] Age adjusted.
[2] Includes all other races not shown separately and unknown family income.
[3] Family income categories for 1991. Income categories for 1986 are: less than $11,000; $11,000–$19,999; $20,000–$29,999; $30,000–$39,999; and $40,000 or more.

SOURCE: Centers for Disease Control and Prevention, National Center for Health Statistics, Division of Health Interview Statistics: Data from the National Health Interview Survey.

Table 62. Disability days associated with acute conditions and incidence of acute conditions, according to age: United States, 1983–91

[Data are based on household interviews of a sample of the civilian noninstitutionalized population]

Age	1983	1984	1985	1986	1987	1988	1989	1990	1991
Restricted-activity days	Number per person								
All ages [1]	7.2	7.4	6.8	7.7	6.8	7.1	7.5	7.0	7.4
Under 15 years	8.2	7.9	6.9	8.2	7.5	8.1	8.4	7.6	8.4
Under 5 years	9.5	8.8	7.5	9.0	9.4	9.7	9.6	9.5	10.0
5–14 years	7.5	7.4	6.7	7.8	6.6	7.2	7.8	6.5	7.5
15–44 years	6.6	7.1	6.5	7.0	6.5	6.7	7.3	6.9	6.8
45–64 years	6.3	6.6	6.0	7.0	6.1	5.8	5.9	5.8	6.4
65 years and over	9.2	9.1	9.6	10.2	8.0	8.2	9.1	8.7	8.8
65–74 years	8.7	8.3	8.9	10.2	8.2	7.3	8.2	7.6	8.2
75 years and over	10.1	10.2	10.9	10.1	7.7	9.6	10.4	10.3	9.6
Bed-disability days [2]									
All ages [1]	3.4	3.3	3.1	3.4	3.0	3.1	3.5	3.1	3.2
Under 15 years	4.0	3.6	3.4	3.8	3.4	3.9	4.2	3.5	3.7
Under 5 years	4.7	3.8	3.5	3.9	4.4	4.9	4.5	4.5	4.2
5–14 years	3.6	3.5	3.3	3.8	2.8	3.4	4.0	3.0	3.4
15–44 years	3.0	3.2	2.8	3.1	2.8	2.8	3.2	3.0	2.9
45–64 years	2.8	2.6	2.7	3.1	2.6	2.4	2.8	2.7	2.7
65 years and over	4.5	3.9	3.9	4.6	3.4	3.4	4.2	3.2	3.6
65–74 years	4.4	3.7	2.8	3.9	3.7	3.1	3.6	2.6	3.5
75 years and over	4.7	4.3	5.7	5.5	3.0	4.0	5.0	4.0	3.8
Incidence of acute conditions [3]	Number per 100 persons								
All ages [1]	182.9	184.9	183.1	189.5	180.8	184.8	190.5	181.2	201.7
Under 15 years	288.1	289.3	280.0	302.7	281.7	296.5	299.7	288.1	318.3
Under 5 years	354.5	345.1	334.6	360.4	358.9	362.8	369.5	365.0	390.7
5–14 years	252.8	259.2	250.9	271.7	240.4	261.3	262.3	246.9	279.6
15–44 years	165.1	172.2	170.1	180.5	168.7	162.6	173.5	157.0	176.6
45–64 years	109.3	104.4	112.9	125.1	101.4	107.9	113.6	114.4	128.4
65 years and over	100.9	98.8	98.4	119.5	100.4	108.9	100.2	105.8	115.7
65–74 years	103.1	97.4	98.9	118.2	94.8	107.8	97.4	108.2	113.6
75 years and over	97.3	101.0	97.7	121.5	109.4	110.6	104.6	102.1	118.9

[1] Age adjusted.
[2] A subset of restricted-activity days.
[3] Excludes conditions involving neither medical attention nor activity restriction.

SOURCE: Centers for Disease Control and Prevention, National Center for Health Statistics, Division of Health Interview Statistics: Data from the National Health Interview Survey.

Table 63. Self-assessment of health, according to selected characteristics: United States, 1986 and 1991

[Data are based on household interviews of a sample of the civilian noninstitutionalized population]

Characteristic	Total	Excellent		Very good		Good		Fair or poor	
		1986	1991	1986	1991	1986	1991	1986	1991
		Percent distribution [1]							
Total [2,3]	100.0	40.2	39.7	27.3	28.5	22.9	22.6	9.6	9.3
Age									
Under 15 years......................	100.0	52.7	52.3	27.3	28.0	17.5	17.3	2.6	2.5
Under 5 years	100.0	53.8	52.8	26.5	27.7	16.9	16.8	2.8	2.6
5–14 years	100.0	52.0	52.0	27.7	28.1	17.9	17.5	2.4	2.4
15–44 years	100.0	43.9	42.0	29.4	31.0	21.2	21.2	5.5	5.8
45–64 years	100.0	26.6	28.5	26.1	26.7	29.2	28.1	18.2	16.7
65 years and over....................	100.0	16.4	15.7	20.8	22.8	32.9	32.4	29.9	29.0
65–74 years.......................	100.0	17.2	17.1	21.5	24.5	33.8	32.3	27.5	26.0
75 years and over	100.0	15.1	13.7	19.7	20.2	31.5	32.6	33.7	33.6
Sex [2]									
Male...............................	100.0	42.8	41.7	26.6	28.1	21.5	21.3	9.1	8.9
Female.............................	100.0	37.7	37.7	28.0	28.7	24.3	23.8	10.1	9.7
Race [2]									
White................................	100.0	41.8	41.2	28.0	28.9	21.6	21.3	8.7	8.6
Black................................	100.0	29.6	30.4	22.7	25.3	30.5	29.2	17.2	15.1
Family income [2,4]									
Less than $14,000....................	100.0	28.4	25.9	22.7	25.3	29.0	28.9	19.9	19.9
$14,000–$24,999.....................	100.0	33.6	34.0	27.6	28.5	26.5	26.7	12.3	10.8
$25,000–$34,999.....................	100.0	42.1	40.8	27.9	29.2	22.7	22.8	7.4	7.1
$35,000–$49,999.....................	100.0	44.2	43.7	29.9	31.4	19.8	19.5	6.1	5.5
$50,000 or more	100.0	52.2	52.1	27.6	28.2	16.3	15.8	3.9	3.9
Geographic region [2]									
Northeast............................	100.0	39.1	42.2	29.9	28.5	22.3	21.8	8.8	7.4
Midwest.............................	100.0	41.2	40.9	27.6	29.9	22.8	21.1	8.4	8.1
South...............................	100.0	37.0	36.2	26.5	27.5	24.5	24.5	12.0	11.7
West	100.0	45.7	41.3	25.7	28.1	20.8	22.0	7.8	8.8
Location of residence [2]									
Within MSA...........................	100.0	41.2	40.6	27.6	28.4	22.1	22.1	9.0	8.9
Outside MSA..........................	100.0	36.9	36.3	26.0	28.7	25.6	24.2	11.4	10.7

[1]Denominator excludes unknown health status.
[2]Age adjusted.
[3]Includes all other races not shown separately and unknown family income.
[4]Family income categories for 1991. Income categories for 1986 are: less than $11,000; $11,000–$19,999; $20,000–$29,999; $30,000–$39,999; and $40,000 or more.

SOURCE: Centers for Disease Control and Prevention, National Center for Health Statistics, Division of Health Interview Statistics: Data from the National Health Interview Survey.

Table 64. Current cigarette smoking by persons 18 years of age and over, according to sex, race, and age: United States, selected years 1965–91

[Data are based on household interviews of a sample of the civilian noninstitutionalized population]

Sex, race, and age	1965	1974	1979	1983	1985	1987	1988	1990	1991
All persons	Percent of persons 18 years of age and over								
18 years and over, age adjusted	42.3	37.2	33.5	32.2	30.0	28.7	27.9	25.4	25.4
18 years and over, crude	42.4	37.1	33.5	32.1	30.1	28.8	28.1	25.5	25.6
All males									
18 years and over, age adjusted	51.6	42.9	37.2	34.7	32.1	31.0	30.1	28.0	27.5
18 years and over, crude	51.9	43.1	37.5	35.1	32.6	31.2	30.8	28.4	28.1
18–24 years	54.1	42.1	35.0	32.9	28.0	28.2	25.5	26.6	23.5
25–34 years	60.7	50.5	43.9	38.8	38.2	34.8	36.2	31.6	32.8
35–44 years	58.2	51.0	41.8	41.0	37.6	36.6	36.5	34.5	33.1
45–64 years	51.9	42.6	39.3	35.9	33.4	33.5	31.3	29.3	29.3
65 years and over	28.5	24.8	20.9	22.0	19.6	17.2	18.0	14.6	15.1
White:									
18 years and over, age adjusted	50.8	41.7	36.5	34.1	31.3	30.4	29.5	27.6	27.0
18 years and over, crude	51.1	41.9	36.8	34.5	31.7	30.5	30.1	28.0	27.4
18–24 years	53.0	40.8	34.3	32.5	28.4	29.2	26.7	27.4	25.1
25–34 years	60.1	49.5	43.6	38.6	37.3	33.8	35.4	31.6	32.1
35–44 years	57.3	50.1	41.3	40.8	36.6	36.2	35.8	33.5	32.1
45–64 years	51.3	41.2	38.3	35.0	32.1	32.4	30.0	28.7	28.0
65 years and over	27.7	24.3	20.5	20.6	18.9	16.0	16.9	13.7	14.2
Black:									
18 years and over, age adjusted	59.2	54.0	44.1	41.3	39.9	39.0	36.5	32.2	34.7
18 years and over, crude	60.4	54.3	44.1	40.6	39.9	39.0	36.5	32.5	35.0
18–24 years	62.8	54.9	40.2	34.2	27.2	24.9	18.6	21.3	15.0
25–34 years	68.4	58.5	47.5	39.9	45.6	44.9	41.6	33.8	39.4
35–44 years	67.3	61.5	48.6	45.5	45.0	44.0	42.5	42.0	44.4
45–64 years	57.9	57.8	50.0	44.8	46.1	44.3	43.2	36.7	42.0
65 years and over	36.4	29.7	26.2	38.9	27.7	30.3	29.8	21.5	24.3
All females									
18 years and over, age adjusted	34.0	32.5	30.3	29.9	28.2	26.7	26.0	23.1	23.6
18 years and over, crude	33.9	32.1	29.9	29.5	27.9	26.5	25.7	22.8	23.5
18–24 years	38.1	34.1	33.8	35.5	30.4	26.1	26.3	22.5	22.4
25–34 years	43.7	38.8	33.7	32.6	32.0	31.8	31.3	28.2	28.4
35–44 years	43.7	39.8	37.0	33.8	31.5	29.6	27.8	24.8	27.6
45–64 years	32.0	33.4	30.7	31.0	29.9	28.6	27.7	24.8	24.6
65 years and over	9.6	12.0	13.2	13.1	13.5	13.7	12.8	11.5	12.0
White:									
18 years and over, age adjusted	34.3	32.3	30.6	30.1	28.3	27.2	26.2	23.9	24.2
18 years and over, crude	34.0	31.7	30.1	29.4	27.7	26.7	25.7	23.4	23.7
18–24 years	38.4	34.0	34.5	36.5	31.8	27.8	27.5	25.4	25.1
25–34 years	43.4	38.6	34.1	32.2	32.0	31.9	31.0	28.5	28.4
35–44 years	43.9	39.3	37.2	34.8	31.0	29.2	28.3	25.0	27.0
45–64 years	32.7	33.0	30.6	30.6	29.7	29.0	27.7	25.4	25.3
65 years and over	9.8	12.3	13.8	13.2	13.3	13.9	12.6	11.5	12.1
Black:									
18 years and over, age adjusted	32.1	35.9	30.8	31.8	30.7	27.2	27.1	20.4	23.1
18 years and over, crude	33.7	36.4	31.1	32.2	31.0	28.0	27.8	21.2	24.4
18–24 years	37.1	35.6	31.8	32.0	23.7	20.4	21.8	10.0	11.8
25–34 years	47.8	42.2	35.2	38.0	36.2	35.8	37.2	29.1	32.4
35–44 years	42.8	46.4	37.7	32.7	40.2	35.3	27.6	25.5	35.3
45–64 years	25.7	38.9	34.2	36.3	33.4	28.4	29.5	22.6	23.4
65 years and over	7.1	8.9	8.5	13.1	14.5	11.7	14.8	11.1	9.6

NOTES: A current smoker is a person who has ever smoked at least 100 cigarettes in their lifetime and who now smokes; includes occasional smokers. Excludes unknown smoking status.

SOURCE: Centers for Disease Control and Prevention, National Center for Health Statistics, Division of Health Interview Statistics: Data from the National Health Interview Survey; Data computed by the Division of Epidemiology and Health Promotion from data compiled by the Division of Health Interview Statistics.

Table 65. Age-adjusted prevalence of current cigarette smoking by persons 25 years of age and over, according to sex, race, and education: United States, selected years 1974–91

[Data are based on household interviews of a sample of the civilian noninstitutionalized population]

Sex, race, and education	1974	1979	1983	1985	1987	1988	1990	1991
	Percent of persons 25 years of age and over, age adjusted							
All persons [1]	37.1	33.3	31.7	30.2	29.1	28.4	25.6	26.0
Less than 12 years	43.8	41.1	40.8	41.0	40.6	39.4	36.7	37.4
12 years	36.4	33.7	33.6	32.1	31.8	31.8	29.3	29.7
13–15 years	35.8	33.2	30.3	29.7	27.2	26.4	23.5	24.7
16 or more years	27.5	22.8	20.7	18.6	16.7	16.3	14.1	13.9
All males [1]	43.0	37.6	35.1	32.9	31.5	31.1	28.3	28.4
Less than 12 years	52.4	48.1	47.2	46.0	45.7	44.9	41.8	42.4
12 years	42.6	39.1	37.4	35.6	35.2	35.2	33.2	32.9
13–15 years	41.6	36.5	33.0	33.0	28.4	29.0	25.9	27.2
16 or more years	28.6	23.1	21.8	19.7	17.3	17.2	14.6	14.8
White males [1]	41.9	36.9	34.5	31.9	30.6	30.1	27.7	27.3
Less than 12 years	51.6	48.0	47.9	45.2	45.3	44.8	41.7	41.8
12 years	42.2	38.6	37.1	34.8	34.6	34.2	33.0	32.4
13–15 years	41.4	36.4	32.6	32.3	28.0	28.2	25.4	26.0
16 or more years	28.1	22.8	21.1	19.2	17.4	17.1	14.5	14.7
Black males [1]	53.8	44.9	42.8	42.5	41.9	40.3	34.5	38.8
Less than 12 years	58.3	50.1	46.0	51.1	49.4	45.3	41.4	47.8
12 years	*51.2	48.4	47.2	41.9	43.6	48.3	37.4	39.6
13–15 years	*45.7	39.3	44.7	42.3	32.4	34.8	28.3	32.7
16 or more years	*41.8	*37.9	*31.3	*32.0	20.9	21.5	20.6	18.3
All females [1]	32.2	29.6	28.8	27.8	26.9	25.9	23.2	23.9
Less than 12 years	36.8	35.0	35.3	36.7	36.1	34.5	32.1	33.0
12 years	32.5	29.9	30.9	29.6	29.2	29.1	26.3	27.1
13–15 years	30.2	30.0	27.5	26.7	26.0	24.1	21.1	22.5
16 or more years	26.1	22.5	19.2	17.4	16.1	15.3	13.6	12.8
White females [1]	31.9	29.8	28.8	27.6	27.0	25.9	23.6	24.0
Less than 12 years	37.0	36.1	35.5	37.1	37.0	35.2	33.6	33.7
12 years	32.1	29.9	30.9	29.4	29.4	29.3	26.8	27.5
13–15 years	30.5	30.6	28.0	27.1	26.2	23.8	21.4	22.3
16 or more years	25.8	21.9	18.9	16.8	16.4	15.1	13.7	13.3
Black females [1]	35.9	30.6	31.8	32.1	28.6	28.2	22.6	25.5
Less than 12 years	36.4	31.9	36.9	39.2	35.0	33.9	26.8	33.3
12 years	41.9	33.0	35.2	32.3	28.1	30.1	24.0	26.0
13–15 years	33.2	*28.8	26.5	23.7	27.2	26.8	23.1	24.8
16 or more years	*35.2	*43.4	*38.7	27.5	19.5	22.2	16.9	14.4

[1]Includes unknown education.

*For age groups where percent smoking was 0 or 100 the age-adjustment procedure was modified to substitute the percent from the next lower education group. These age-adjusted percents should be considered unreliable because of small sample size.

NOTES: A current smoker is a person who has ever smoked at least 100 cigarettes in their lifetime and who now smokes; includes occasional smokers. Excludes unknown smoking status.

SOURCE: Data computed by the Centers for Disease Control and Prevention, National Center for Health Statistics, Division of Epidemiology and Health Promotion from data compiled by the Division of Health Interview Statistics.

Table 66 (page 1 of 2). Use of selected substances in the past month by youths 12–17 years of age and young adults 18–25 years of age, according to age, sex, race, and Hispanic origin: United States, selected years 1974–91

[Data are based on household interviews of a sample of the population 12 years of age and over in the coterminous United States]

Substance, age, sex, race, and Hispanic origin	1974	1976	1977	1979	1982	1985	1988	1990	1991
Cigarettes					Percent of population				
12–17 years	25	23	22	(1)	15	15	12	12	11
12–13 years	13	11	10	(1)	*3	6	3	2	3
14–15 years	25	20	22	(1)	10	14	11	14	9
16–17 years	38	39	35	(1)	30	25	20	18	21
Male	27	21	23	(1)	16	16	12	12	12
Female	24	26	22	(1)	13	15	11	11	10
White, non-Hispanic	- - -	- - -	- - -	- - -	- - -	17	14	14	13
Black, non-Hispanic	- - -	- - -	- - -	- - -	- - -	9	5	4	4
Hispanic	- - -	- - -	- - -	- - -	- - -	11	8	11	9
18–25 years	49	49	47	(1)	40	37	35	32	32
Male	50	52	49	(1)	37	38	36	36	32
Female	47	46	46	(1)	42	35	35	27	32
White, non-Hispanic	- - -	- - -	- - -	- - -	- - -	38	37	35	36
Black, non-Hispanic	- - -	- - -	- - -	- - -	- - -	34	30	21	22
Hispanic	- - -	- - -	- - -	- - -	- - -	30	28	25	25
Alcohol [2]									
12–17 years	34	32	31	37	27	31	25	25	20
12–13 years	19	19	13	20	10	11	7	8	7
14–15 years	32	31	28	36	23	35	23	26	19
16–17 years	51	47	52	55	45	46	42	38	35
Male	39	36	37	39	27	34	27	25	22
Female	29	29	25	36	27	28	23	24	18
White, non-Hispanic	- - -	- - -	- - -	- - -	- - -	34	27	28	20
Black, non-Hispanic	- - -	- - -	- - -	- - -	- - -	21	16	15	20
Hispanic	- - -	- - -	- - -	- - -	- - -	22	25	19	23
18–25 years	69	69	70	76	68	71	65	63	64
Male	- - -	79	82	84	75	78	75	74	70
Female	- - -	58	59	68	61	64	57	53	58
White, non-Hispanic	- - -	- - -	- - -	- - -	- - -	76	69	66	67
Black, non-Hispanic	- - -	- - -	- - -	- - -	- - -	57	50	59	56
Hispanic	- - -	- - -	- - -	- - -	- - -	58	61	57	53
Marijuana									
12–17 years	12	12	17	17	12	12	6	5	4
12–13 years	*2	*3	*4	4	*2	*4	1	*	*
14–15 years	12	13	16	17	8	11	5	5	4
16–17 years	20	21	30	28	23	21	12	10	9
Male	12	14	20	19	13	13	6	6	5
Female	11	11	13	14	10	11	7	4	4
White, non-Hispanic	- - -	- - -	- - -	- - -	- - -	13	7	6	4
Black, non-Hispanic	- - -	- - -	- - -	- - -	- - -	8	4	3	5
Hispanic	- - -	- - -	- - -	- - -	- - -	9	5	4	5
18–25 years	25	25	27	35	27	22	15	13	13
Male	- - -	31	35	45	36	27	20	17	16
Female	- - -	19	20	26	19	17	11	9	11
White, non-Hispanic	- - -	- - -	- - -	- - -	- - -	22	16	14	14
Black, non-Hispanic	- - -	- - -	- - -	- - -	- - -	24	15	13	15
Hispanic	- - -	- - -	- - -	- - -	- - -	15	14	8	9
Cocaine									
12–17 years	*1.0	*1.0	*0.8	1.4	1.6	1.5	1.1	0.6	0.4
Male	- - -	- - -	- - -	- - -	1.8	2.0	0.9	0.7	0.5
Female	- - -	- - -	- - -	- - -	*1.5	*1.0	1.4	*	0.3
White, non-Hispanic	- - -	- - -	- - -	- - -	- - -	1.5	1.3	0.4	*0.3
Black, non-Hispanic	- - -	- - -	- - -	- - -	- - -	1.0	*	*	*0.5
Hispanic	- - -	- - -	- - -	- - -	- - -	2.5	1.3	*	1.3

See footnotes at end of table.

Table 66 (page 2 of 2). Use of selected substances in the past month by youths 12–17 years of age and young adults 18–25 years of age, according to age, sex, race, and Hispanic origin: United States, selected years 1974–91

[Data are based on household interviews of a sample of the population 12 years of age and over in the coterminous United States]

Substance, age, sex, race, and Hispanic origin	1974	1976	1977	1979	1982	1985	1988	1990	1991
Cocaine—Con.					Percent of population				
18–25 years.	3.1	2.0	3.7	9.3	6.8	7.6	4.5	2.2	2.0
Male	- - -	- - -	- - -	- - -	9.1	9.0	6.0	2.8	2.8
Female.	- - -	- - -	- - -	- - -	4.7	6.3	3.0	1.6	1.3
White, non-Hispanic	- - -	- - -	- - -	- - -	- - -	8.1	4.1	1.9	1.7
Black, non-Hispanic	- - -	- - -	- - -	- - -	- - -	6.4	4.3	3.6	3.1
Hispanic.	- - -	- - -	- - -	- - -	- - -	6.6	6.7	3.1	2.7

[1]Data not comparable because definitions differ.

[2]In surveys conducted in 1979 and later years, private answer sheets were used for alcohol questions; prior to 1979, respondents answered questions aloud.

*Relative standard error greater than 30 percent. Estimates with relative standard error greater than 50 percent are not shown.

SOURCES: National Institute on Drug Abuse: National Household Survey on Drug Abuse: Main Findings, 1979, by P. M. Fishburne, H. I. Abelson, and I. Cisin. DHHS Pub. No. (ADM) 80-976. Alcohol, Drug Abuse, and Mental Health Administration. Washington. U.S. Government Printing Office, 1980; National Household Survey on Drug Abuse: Main Findings, 1982, by J. D. Miller et al. DHHS Pub. No. (ADM) 83-1263. Alcohol, Drug Abuse, and Mental Health Administration. Washington. U.S. Government Printing Office, 1983; National Household Survey on Drug Abuse: Main Findings, 1985. DHHS Pub. No. (ADM) 88-1586. National Household Survey on Drug Abuse: Main Findings, 1988; National Household Survey on Drug Abuse: Main Findings, 1990; and National Household Survey on Drug Abuse: Main Findings, 1991.

Table 67. Use of selected substances in the past month by high school seniors, according to sex, race, and average parental education: United States, 1980–91

[Data are based on a survey of high school seniors in the coterminous United States]

Substance, sex, race, and average parental education	Class of											
	1980	1981	1982	1983	1984	1985	1986	1987	1988	1989	1990	1991
Cigarettes	Percent using substance in the past month											
All seniors	30.5	29.4	30.0	30.3	29.3	30.1	29.6	29.4	28.7	28.6	29.4	28.3
Male	26.8	26.5	26.8	28.0	25.9	28.2	27.9	27.0	28.0	27.7	29.1	29.0
Female	33.4	31.6	32.6	31.6	31.9	31.4	30.6	31.4	28.9	29.0	29.2	27.5
White	31.0	30.1	31.3	31.3	31.0	31.7	32.0	32.2	32.3	32.1	32.5	31.8
Black	25.2	22.3	21.2	21.2	17.6	18.7	14.6	13.9	12.8	12.4	12.0	9.4
Average parental education [1]:												
Less than high school	32.7	32.5	32.6	32.7	33.6	32.3	28.6	28.8	28.1	25.4	26.3	31.3
High school graduate	34.2	31.7	32.0	32.2	31.8	32.3	32.3	31.4	29.9	30.8	30.8	28.7
Some college	28.0	28.2	29.0	28.0	28.1	29.7	29.7	28.8	27.8	29.4	29.3	28.4
College graduate	25.7	26.0	25.5	27.8	25.2	27.7	26.4	27.6	28.6	27.0	29.1	26.9
Some postgraduate	24.0	22.5	25.1	25.5	23.7	22.6	26.7	29.3	27.8	26.3	28.6	27.1
Alcohol												
All seniors	72.0	70.7	69.7	69.4	67.2	65.9	65.3	66.4	63.9	60.0	57.1	54.0
Male	77.4	75.7	74.1	74.4	71.4	69.8	69.0	69.9	68.0	65.1	61.3	58.4
Female	66.8	65.7	65.4	64.3	62.8	62.1	61.9	63.1	59.9	54.9	52.3	49.0
White	75.8	75.0	74.2	73.5	72.1	70.2	70.2	71.8	69.5	65.3	62.2	57.7
Black	47.7	45.8	46.2	49.3	42.1	43.6	40.4	38.5	40.9	38.1	32.9	34.4
Average parental education [1]:												
Less than high school	65.9	62.1	61.3	61.2	58.1	58.7	56.1	56.3	54.5	47.8	47.2	49.9
High school graduate	72.0	70.7	69.4	69.2	67.4	65.9	65.3	67.0	64.6	59.7	57.2	53.3
Some college	73.3	71.5	72.7	70.4	69.6	66.9	66.7	67.2	64.3	62.9	57.7	54.3
College graduate	74.4	73.1	74.5	73.1	69.3	68.9	68.0	68.8	66.0	62.1	60.8	54.8
Some postgraduate	77.2	77.4	74.1	75.0	70.3	67.9	69.9	70.5	67.3	62.2	60.8	58.0
Marijuana												
All seniors	33.7	31.6	28.5	27.0	25.2	25.7	23.4	21.0	18.0	16.7	14.0	13.8
Male	37.8	35.3	31.4	31.0	28.2	28.7	26.8	23.1	20.7	19.5	16.1	16.1
Female	29.1	27.3	24.9	22.2	21.1	22.4	20.0	18.6	15.2	13.8	11.5	11.2
White	34.2	32.4	29.1	26.6	25.3	26.4	24.6	22.3	19.9	18.6	15.6	15.0
Black	26.5	24.9	24.8	26.9	22.8	21.7	16.6	12.4	9.8	9.4	5.2	6.5
Average parental education [1]:												
Less than high school	29.9	29.7	24.9	26.2	23.8	23.4	21.0	19.9	15.6	13.9	11.4	11.7
High school graduate	34.6	31.5	28.4	27.3	25.4	25.9	24.1	20.9	16.8	16.3	14.3	12.9
Some college	33.6	31.4	29.3	26.1	25.8	26.5	24.1	21.1	17.7	17.9	13.5	13.8
College graduate	33.7	31.9	30.1	26.9	23.3	27.1	23.1	21.1	19.3	17.1	15.0	13.7
Some postgraduate	36.2	31.9	27.7	25.5	23.4	20.6	21.7	21.2	20.6	16.2	15.0	17.6
Cocaine												
All seniors	5.2	5.8	5.0	4.9	5.8	6.7	6.2	4.3	3.4	2.8	1.9	1.4
Male	6.0	6.3	5.9	5.7	7.0	7.7	7.2	4.9	4.2	3.6	2.3	1.7
Female	4.3	5.0	3.8	4.1	4.4	5.6	5.1	3.7	2.6	2.0	1.3	0.9
White	5.4	6.1	4.9	4.9	6.0	7.0	6.4	4.4	3.7	2.9	1.8	1.3
Black	2.0	2.1	3.2	3.0	2.4	2.7	2.7	1.8	1.4	1.2	0.5	0.8
Average parental education [1]:												
Less than high school	3.8	3.9	3.6	4.6	4.5	6.5	5.8	3.4	3.2	3.5	2.0	1.8
High school graduate	4.5	4.9	4.6	4.2	5.9	6.7	6.1	4.1	3.3	2.7	1.8	1.3
Some college	5.8	6.0	5.2	4.7	5.6	6.7	6.7	4.9	3.0	2.6	2.0	1.4
College graduate	5.9	7.6	5.9	6.0	6.2	6.8	6.1	4.2	4.0	3.1	1.2	1.2
Some postgraduate	7.0	7.4	5.4	6.0	6.6	6.4	5.3	4.0	3.6	2.4	2.0	0.9

[1]Average parental education is calculated by averaging the following respondent-reported parental educational categories: (1) completed grade school or less, (2) some high school, (3) completed high school, (4) some college, (5) completed college, and (6) graduate or professional school after college.

NOTES: The Nation's High School Seniors survey excludes high school dropouts (about 15 percent of the age group during the 1980's) and absentees (about 16–19 percent of high school students). High school dropouts and absentees have higher drug usage than those included in the survey.

SOURCE: National Institute on Drug Abuse: Monitoring the Future Study: Annual surveys.

Table 68. Cocaine-related emergency room episodes, according to age, sex, race, and Hispanic origin: Selected metropolitan areas, 1985–89 and United States 1989–91

[Data are based on a sample of emergency rooms]

Age, sex, race, and Hispanic origin	Data from 21 metropolitan areas				Data from national sample				
	1985–86	1986–87	1987–88	1988–89	1989–90	1990–91	1989	1990	1991
All races, both sexes [1]	Annual percent change						Number of episodes		
All ages [2]	81.3	72.7	32.7	–2.1	–27.0	27.8	110,013	80,355	102,727
12–17 years	94.9	34.4	33.8	–10.4	–26.9	16.6	2,544	1,859	2,167
18–24 years	81.1	67.1	32.5	–10.8	–39.7	14.0	25,996	15,665	17,857
25–34 years	82.8	73.0	29.5	–1.5	–28.6	29.0	55,422	39,589	51,077
35–44 years	74.8	87.1	40.8	6.2	–10.9	35.4	21,529	19,186	25,974
45–64 years	71.8	73.2	43.6	9.4	–5.4	32.6	3,965	3,749	4,973
White, non-Hispanic male									
All ages [2]	74.2	55.0	28.5	–9.2	–37.4	26.9	24,789	15,512	19,678
12–17 years	46.8	37.2	20.6	4.3	–40.8	–5.6	880	521	492
18–24 years	65.0	48.0	25.6	–13.7	–48.8	48.2	6,138	3,143	4,657
25–34 years	74.3	60.9	24.0	–12.7	–41.9	30.1	12,714	7,392	9,614
35–44 years	102.1	52.1	49.0	2.3	–14.1	8.5	4,369	3,755	4,073
45–64 years	76.4	47.4	48.3	13.7	2.7	20.8	594	610	737
Black, non-Hispanic male									
All ages [2]	82.4	85.3	40.5	–0.1	–16.1	33.9	33,070	27,745	37,162
12–17 years	127.0	67.9	41.1	–4.0	–35.3	1.7	363	235	239
18–24 years	104.9	85.3	41.2	–7.6	–37.5	17.0	6,098	3,811	4,460
25–34 years	86.0	80.2	37.6	–0.1	–16.9	32.8	16,193	13,453	17,861
35–44 years	56.6	107.0	45.0	4.5	–0.2	42.0	8,271	8,253	11,723
45–64 years	69.3	66.4	51.5	8.0	–3.6	32.4	1,989	1,917	2,539
Hispanic male									
All ages [2]	76.8	41.1	27.8	–2.2	–31.8	38.4	7,067	4,821	6,673
12–17 years	*	24.0	41.9	–20.5	–52.2	43.0	297	142	203
18–24 years	75.8	32.0	44.9	–11.2	–31.7	2.7	2,088	1,426	1,465
25–34 years	78.9	40.3	18.6	–1.8	–30.0	50.0	3,009	2,106	3,160
35–44 years	52.5	67.6	17.4	10.8	–32.8	55.8	1,367	918	1,430
45–64 years	*	35.7	59.2	15.7	–30.9	94.5	291	201	391
White, non-Hispanic female									
All ages [2]	62.7	52.4	27.1	–5.0	–37.0	16.3	13,226	8,331	9,690
12–17 years	98.5	–9.9	36.4	–16.1	–4.0	–2.5	505	485	473
18–24 years	48.0	49.2	29.6	–17.7	–44.2	9.7	3,908	2,179	2,390
25–34 years	67.6	58.6	21.2	–0.8	–38.9	19.2	6,740	4,120	4,912
35–44 years	84.5	72.1	45.1	11.9	–21.9	20.4	1,782	1,391	1,675
45–64 years	*	*	34.3	55.3	*	*	220	*	162
Black, non-Hispanic female									
All ages [2]	103.9	85.0	29.5	0.8	–16.0	30.8	17,657	14,833	19,406
12–17 years	*	112.2	17.3	–18.9	*	*	248	*	*
18–24 years	125.9	88.4	26.1	–9.7	–24.4	1.6	3,944	2,981	3,029
25–34 years	97.0	80.6	29.2	4.4	–15.0	27.4	9,714	8,257	10,520
35–44 years	105.8	84.5	38.1	7.6	–8.4	67.3	3,181	2,914	4,876
45–64 years	45.7	139.2	33.6	2.5	–4.3	58.2	465	445	704
Hispanic female									
All ages [2]	79.6	39.1	26.7	–6.1	–32.7	39.0	2,556	1,719	2,389
12–17 years	*	*	*	–30.8	–31.2	190.6	93	64	186
18–24 years	75.5	34.2	30.5	–16.3	–29.0	–13.5	730	518	448
25–34 years	82.3	53.4	7.1	–5.5	–30.1	58.5	1,115	779	1,235
35–44 years	48.8	32.8	76.5	16.7	–42.7	42.3	557	319	454
45–64 years	*	*	*	*	–27.5	75.7	51	37	65

[1]Includes unknown race/ethnicity and/or sex.

[2]Includes ages under 12 years, over 64 years, and unknown.

*Annual percent change based on fewer than 30 episodes in any year 1985–88 from the 21 metropolitan areas is considered unreliable and is not shown. National estimates with relative standard error 50 percent or greater and annual percent change based on these estimates are considered unreliable and are not shown.

NOTES: Prior to 1989, data from the Drug Abuse Warning Network (DAWN) were derived from a nonrandom sample of emergency rooms primarily located in 21 metropolitan areas. Starting in 1989, estimates are based on weighted data from a nationally representative sample of emergency rooms.

SOURCE: Substance Abuse and Mental Health Services Administration, Drug Abuse Warning Network.

Table 69. Alcohol consumption by persons 18 years of age and over, according to sex, race, Hispanic origin, and age: United States, 1985 and 1990

[Data are based on household interviews of a sample of the civilian noninstitutionalized population]

Alcohol consumption, race, Hispanic origin, and age	Both sexes		Male		Female	
	1985	1990	1985	1990	1985	1990
Drinking status	Percent distribution					
All	100.0	100.0	100.0	100.0	100.0	100.0
Abstainer	26.9	29.7	14.4	16.6	38.0	41.5
Former drinker	7.5	9.6	9.2	11.6	6.1	7.8
Current drinker	65.6	60.7	76.4	71.8	55.9	50.7
All races:	Percent current drinkers among all persons					
18–44 years.	72.8	67.5	82.4	77.1	63.8	58.3
18–24 years	71.8	63.7	79.5	71.7	64.5	56.1
25–44 years	73.2	68.8	83.5	78.9	63.5	59.0
45 years and over	55.5	51.3	67.4	63.8	45.6	40.8
45–64 years	62.2	57.6	72.2	68.4	53.0	47.6
65 years and over.	44.3	41.4	58.2	55.6	34.7	31.3
White, non-Hispanic:						
18–44 years.	76.9	72.7	85.0	80.4	68.9	65.1
18–24 years	77.9	71.5	84.9	77.5	71.0	65.7
25–44 years	76.5	73.1	85.0	81.2	68.2	65.0
45 years and over	57.6	53.8	69.0	65.5	48.2	44.0
45–64 years	65.2	61.0	74.1	70.6	56.9	52.2
65 years and over.	45.8	43.3	59.6	57.1	36.2	33.3
Black, non-Hispanic:						
18–44 years.	59.0	51.5	72.2	68.1	48.2	37.9
45 years and over	41.5	36.0	57.1	51.3	29.9	24.5
Hispanic:						
18–44 years.	58.7	55.7	73.2	71.3	45.6	42.0
45 years and over	48.5	43.4	64.3	63.3	35.4	27.8
Level of alcohol consumption in past 2 weeks for current drinkers	Percent distribution of current drinkers					
All drinking levels	100.0	100.0	100.0	100.0	100.0	100.0
None	21.6	24.1	18.0	20.3	26.1	29.1
Light.	37.1	39.4	30.9	33.9	44.7	46.4
Moderate	29.5	27.4	34.0	32.3	24.0	21.1
Heavier.	11.8	9.1	17.2	13.6	5.3	3.4
All races:	Percent heavier drinkers among current drinkers					
18–44 years.	11.0	8.5	16.6	13.0	4.2	2.8
18–24 years	12.2	8.8	18.3	13.8	5.0	2.7
25–44 years	10.6	8.4	16.0	12.7	3.8	2.9
45 years and over	13.3	10.3	18.2	14.7	7.4	4.6
45–64 years	13.2	9.9	18.1	14.4	7.2	4.1
65 years and over.	13.6	11.0	18.4	15.3	7.9	5.5
White, non-Hispanic:						
18–44 years.	11.2	8.5	17.1	13.2	4.0	2.8
18–24 years	13.3	9.9	20.4	16.0	5.2	3.0
25–44 years	10.4	8.1	16.0	12.4	3.6	2.7
45 years and over	13.4	10.4	18.2	15.0	7.6	4.7
45–64 years	13.2	10.0	18.0	14.6	7.3	4.2
65 years and over.	13.9	11.3	18.7	15.8	8.3	5.7
Black, non-Hispanic:						
18–44 years.	9.6	10.3	13.4	14.7	5.1	3.9
45 years and over	10.3	7.7	16.2	10.1	*	*
Hispanic:						
18–44 years.	10.6	7.9	15.2	11.3	*	*
45 years and over	15.7	12.1	*	17.2	*	*

*Estimates based on fewer than 30 subjects are not shown.

NOTES: Abstainers consumed less than 12 drinks in any single year. Former drinkers consumed 12 or more drinks in any single year, but no drinks in the past year. Current drinkers consumed 12 or more drinks in a single year and at least 1 drink in the past year. For current drinkers, drinking levels are classified according to the average daily consumption of absolute alcohol (ethanol), in ounces, in the previous 2-week period, assuming 0.5 ounce ethanol per drink, as follows: none; light, .01–.21; moderate, .22–.99; and heavier, 1.00 or more. This corresponds to up to 3, 4–13, and 14 or more drinks per week for light, moderate, and heavier drinkers. Because of differences in the methods used to collect alcohol consumption, data from this table should not be compared with data in previous editions of Health, United States.

SOURCE: Data computed by the Alcohol Epidemiologic Data System of the National Institute on Alcohol Abuse and Alcoholism from data in the National Health Interview Survey compiled by the Division of Health Interview Statistics, National Center for Health Statistics, Centers for Disease Control and Prevention.

Table 70. Elevated blood pressure among persons 20–74 years of age, according to race, sex, and age: United States, 1960–62, 1971–74, and 1976–80

[Data are based on physical examinations of a sample of the civilian noninstitutionalized population]

Sex and age	All races			White			Black		
	1960–62	1971–74	1976–80	1960–62	1971–74	1976–80	1960–62	1971–74	1976–80
	Percent of population with systolic pressure at least 140 mmHg or diastolic pressure at least 90 mmHg								
Both sexes [1]									
20–74 years, age adjusted	37.4	38.4	38.0	36.2	37.3	37.0	48.8	49.6	46.6
20–74 years, crude	38.1	38.1	37.2	37.1	37.3	36.5	48.7	47.3	43.2
20–24 years	12.9	13.5	16.1	13.1	13.7	16.0	13.1	13.7	16.9
25–34 years	16.2	20.0	21.3	15.3	19.2	21.2	23.4	28.2	22.8
35–44 years	30.0	32.3	33.1	28.3	29.7	31.0	44.0	54.5	47.6
45–54 years	44.4	46.9	47.0	42.4	45.8	45.8	60.6	57.4	58.2
55–64 years	62.3	59.4	56.7	60.9	58.4	55.2	78.9	71.8	70.5
65–74 years	73.8	70.3	63.1	73.1	69.3	61.9	85.2	80.0	71.9
Male									
20–74 years, age adjusted	40.8	42.7	43.6	40.0	42.1	43.1	48.9	51.0	48.5
20–74 years, crude	41.0	42.0	42.5	40.4	41.6	42.3	49.6	48.9	45.7
20–24 years	21.7	20.2	24.7	22.1	20.7	25.6	*18.4	18.6	22.2
25–34 years	23.3	27.5	31.1	22.3	27.2	31.3	31.9	33.6	31.7
35–44 years	37.4	38.1	39.5	37.0	36.0	37.7	44.2	60.5	52.8
45–54 years	47.2	52.8	51.8	46.0	53.0	51.8	56.3	53.3	49.8
55–64 years	59.3	59.3	58.7	58.2	58.9	57.6	75.1	67.5	71.8
65–74 years	65.9	65.4	62.0	65.0	64.0	60.6	*76.8	79.3	69.2
Female [1]									
20–74 years, age adjusted	34.0	34.3	32.6	32.3	32.6	31.0	49.0	48.5	45.2
20–74 years, crude	35.3	34.6	32.3	34.0	33.3	31.0	47.9	46.1	41.2
20–24 years	4.2	7.1	7.8	3.8	6.9	6.5	8.7	9.3	12.2
25–34 years	9.2	12.7	11.7	8.2	11.2	11.0	17.3	24.0	15.6
35–44 years	22.9	26.9	27.1	19.9	23.8	24.6	43.8	49.9	43.7
45–54 years	41.8	41.5	42.4	39.0	39.1	40.1	64.8	61.0	65.6
55–64 years	65.0	59.5	54.9	63.3	57.9	53.0	82.8	75.3	69.4
65–74 years	80.3	74.1	63.9	79.8	73.4	62.9	*92.1	80.6	74.0
	Percent of population with systolic pressure at least 160 mmHg or diastolic pressure at least 95 mmHg								
Both sexes [1]									
20–74 years, age adjusted	18.8	19.3	18.1	17.2	18.0	17.4	32.9	32.4	24.6
20–74 years, crude	19.2	19.2	17.6	17.8	18.0	17.0	32.6	30.5	22.3
20–24 years	4.3	3.7	4.9	4.3	3.7	5.0	5.1	4.5	4.3
25–34 years	5.6	6.8	8.0	4.3	6.1	7.8	14.8	13.3	9.3
35–44 years	13.4	15.5	13.9	11.5	13.5	12.4	29.0	31.9	24.7
45–54 years	21.4	24.3	25.1	19.1	22.2	24.1	39.5	43.7	36.1
55–64 years	31.8	33.2	28.1	30.1	31.6	26.9	50.4	52.1	39.3
65–74 years	48.7	40.9	34.5	46.9	39.5	33.9	71.9	55.7	36.7
Male									
20–74 years, age adjusted	18.8	20.7	20.9	17.4	19.6	20.4	32.9	31.8	26.1
20–74 years, crude	19.0	20.2	20.1	17.6	19.3	19.8	32.9	30.1	23.9
20–24 years	6.7	5.7	7.4	6.5	5.8	8.0	*9.7	5.6	4.3
25–34 years	7.8	8.9	12.2	6.1	8.3	12.2	21.8	16.1	13.4
35–44 years	16.2	19.1	17.0	14.9	17.2	15.2	28.1	36.8	33.9
45–54 years	21.4	26.8	28.2	19.6	25.8	28.4	34.6	37.0	27.8
55–64 years	29.3	32.5	31.2	27.4	31.2	29.8	50.3	49.5	45.5
65–74 years	40.5	36.4	33.3	38.6	35.1	32.6	*63.3	50.3	32.3
Female [1]									
20–74 years, age adjusted	18.6	18.0	15.4	16.9	16.3	14.4	33.2	33.0	23.5
20–74 years, crude	19.3	18.3	15.2	18.0	16.8	14.5	32.3	30.9	21.0
20–24 years	1.9	1.9	2.5	2.1	1.7	2.0	1.3	3.5	4.4
25–34 years	3.4	4.8	3.8	2.5	4.0	3.4	9.7	11.2	6.0
35–44 years	10.8	12.2	11.0	8.3	10.0	9.7	29.8	28.2	17.5
45–54 years	21.5	21.9	22.3	18.7	18.8	20.0	44.3	49.4	43.4
55–64 years	34.1	33.9	25.2	32.5	32.0	24.3	50.5	54.2	34.2
65–74 years	55.4	44.4	35.4	53.8	42.9	34.9	*79.0	59.8	40.0

[1]Excludes pregnant women.

*Percents based on fewer than 45 persons are considered unreliable. Percents based on fewer than 25 persons are considered highly unreliable and are not shown.

NOTE: Percents are based on a single measurement of blood pressure to provide comparable data across the 3 time periods.

SOURCE: Centers for Disease Control and Prevention, National Center for Health Statistics, Division of Health Examination Statistics: Unpublished data.

Table 71. Hypertension among persons 20–74 years of age, according to race, sex, and age: United States, 1960–62, 1971–74, and 1976–80

[Data are based on physical examinations of a sample of the civilian noninstitutionalized population]

Sex and age	All races			White			Black		
	1960–62	1971–74	1976–80	1960–62	1971–74	1976–80	1960–62	1971–74	1976–80
Both sexes [1]	Percent of population								
20–74 years, age adjusted	38.5	40.0	40.6	37.1	38.7	39.4	51.4	53.5	50.5
20–74 years, crude	39.0	39.7	39.7	37.9	38.7	38.9	51.3	51.0	46.7
20–24 years	13.4	13.6	16.4	13.3	13.8	16.2	15.6	13.7	18.2
25–34 years	17.3	20.6	22.0	16.1	19.5	21.9	26.5	31.3	24.2
35–44 years	30.7	33.4	34.5	28.6	30.6	32.3	47.0	58.0	49.6
45–54 years	45.5	49.1	50.2	43.4	47.5	48.9	62.2	63.5	64.3
55–64 years	63.5	62.5	61.4	61.9	61.2	59.8	82.0	77.7	76.0
65–74 years	75.7	73.5	69.7	74.9	72.5	68.5	88.1	83.8	80.7
Male									
20–74 years, age adjusted	41.4	44.0	45.3	40.6	43.3	44.8	49.7	54.2	50.5
20–74 years, crude	41.7	43.3	44.0	41.0	42.8	43.8	50.5	52.1	47.4
20–24 years	21.6	20.4	24.7	22.0	20.9	25.6	*18.4	18.4	22.2
25–34 years	23.5	27.6	31.4	22.5	27.3	31.7	32.4	33.6	32.1
35–44 years	37.7	39.1	40.5	37.1	36.6	38.6	46.6	64.7	54.3
45–54 years	47.6	55.0	53.6	46.5	54.6	53.5	56.3	61.1	53.3
55–64 years	60.3	62.5	61.8	59.1	62.1	60.8	76.2	72.0	73.8
65–74 years	68.8	67.2	67.1	68.1	65.8	65.8	*76.8	81.5	75.1
Female [1]									
20–74 years, age adjusted	35.5	36.1	36.0	33.4	34.1	34.2	53.4	52.9	50.6
20–74 years, crude	36.6	36.5	35.6	34.9	34.9	34.2	52.0	50.2	46.1
20–24 years	5.3	7.2	8.3	4.4	6.9	6.8	13.3	9.5	14.6
25–34 years	11.2	13.7	12.8	9.7	11.7	12.0	22.2	29.6	17.7
35–44 years	24.0	28.2	28.8	20.6	24.9	26.2	47.3	52.8	46.0
45–54 years	43.4	43.6	47.1	40.6	40.9	44.5	68.1	65.6	73.9
55–64 years	66.4	62.5	61.1	64.4	60.5	59.0	87.8	82.5	77.9
65–74 years	81.5	78.3	71.8	80.7	77.5	70.6	*97.5	85.6	85.0

[1]Excludes pregnant women.

*Percents based on fewer than 45 persons are considered unreliable. Percents based on fewer than 25 persons are considered highly unreliable and are not shown.

NOTE: A person with hypertension is defined by either having elevated blood pressure (systolic pressure of at least 140 mmHg or diastolic pressure of at least 90 mmHg) or taking antihypertensive medication. Percents are based on a single measurement of blood pressure to provide comparable data across the 3 time periods. In 1976–80, 31.3 percent of persons 20–74 years of age had hypertension, based on the average of 3 blood pressure measurements, in contrast to 39.7 percent when a single measurement is used.

SOURCE: Centers for Disease Control and Prevention, National Center for Health Statistics, Division of Health Examination Statistics: Unpublished data.

Table 72. Persons 20 years of age and over with high serum cholesterol levels and mean serum cholesterol levels, according to sex, age, race, and Hispanic origin: United States, 1960–62, 1971–74, 1976–80, and 1988–91

[Data are based on physical examinations of a sample of the civilian noninstitutionalized population]

Sex, age, race, and Hispanic origin [1]	Percent of population with high serum cholesterol				Mean serum cholesterol level, mg/dL			
	1960–62	1971–74	1976–80 [2]	1988–91	1960–62	1971–74	1976–80 [2]	1988–91
20–74 years, age adjusted [3]								
Both sexes	31.8	27.2	26.3	19.7	220	214	213	205
Male	28.7	25.8	24.6	19.0	217	213	211	205
Female	34.5	28.2	27.6	20.2	222	215	214	205
White male	29.4	25.9	24.6	19.3	218	213	211	205
White female	35.1	28.1	28.0	20.3	223	215	214	205
Black male	24.5	25.1	24.1	16.5	210	212	208	200
Black female	30.7	29.2	24.9	20.7	216	217	213	205
White, non-Hispanic male	- - -	- - -	24.7	19.1	- - -	- - -	211	205
White, non-Hispanic female	- - -	- - -	28.3	20.0	- - -	- - -	214	205
Black, non-Hispanic male	- - -	- - -	24.0	16.6	- - -	- - -	208	201
Black, non-Hispanic female	- - -	- - -	24.9	20.7	- - -	- - -	214	205
Mexican-American male	- - -	- - -	18.8	20.3	- - -	- - -	207	207
Mexican-American female	- - -	- - -	20.0	19.4	- - -	- - -	207	205
20–74 years, crude								
Both sexes	33.6	28.2	26.8	19.7	222	216	213	205
Male	30.7	26.8	24.9	19.0	220	214	211	205
Female	36.3	29.6	28.5	20.3	225	217	215	205
White male	31.4	26.9	25.0	19.6	221	215	211	206
White female	37.5	29.8	29.2	20.8	227	217	216	206
Black male	26.7	25.1	23.9	15.3	214	212	208	198
Black female	29.9	28.8	23.7	18.1	216	216	212	201
White, non-Hispanic male	- - -	- - -	25.1	19.6	- - -	- - -	211	206
White, non-Hispanic female	- - -	- - -	29.8	20.9	- - -	- - -	216	206
Black, non-Hispanic male	- - -	- - -	23.7	15.4	- - -	- - -	208	199
Black, non-Hispanic female	- - -	- - -	23.7	18.2	- - -	- - -	212	202
Mexican-American male	- - -	- - -	16.6	17.6	- - -	- - -	203	202
Mexican-American female	- - -	- - -	16.5	15.6	- - -	- - -	202	200
Male								
20–34 years	15.1	12.4	11.9	9.3	198	194	192	189
35–44 years	33.9	31.8	27.9	19.3	227	221	217	207
45–54 years	39.2	37.5	36.9	26.1	231	229	227	218
55–64 years	41.6	36.2	36.8	31.4	233	229	229	221
65–74 years	38.0	34.7	31.7	27.7	230	226	221	218
75 years and over	- - -	- - -	- - -	19.9	- - -	- - -	- - -	205
Female								
20–34 years	12.4	10.9	9.8	8.3	194	191	189	185
35–44 years	23.1	19.3	20.7	11.7	214	207	207	195
45–54 years	46.9	38.7	40.5	25.2	237	232	232	217
55–64 years	70.1	53.1	52.9	40.4	262	245	249	237
65–74 years	68.5	57.7	51.6	43.2	266	250	246	234
75 years and over	- - -	- - -	- - -	39.2	- - -	- - -	- - -	230

[1] The race groups, white and black, include persons of both Hispanic and non-Hispanic origin. Conversely, persons of Hispanic origin may be of any race.
[2] Data for Mexican-Americans are for 1982–84. See Appendix I.
[3] Age-adjusted by the direct method to the 1980 U.S. resident population using the following 5 age groups: 20–34 years, 35–44 years, 45–54 years, 55–64 years, and 65–74 years. Other Health, U.S. tables based on data from the NHES and NHANES are age-adjusted using a 1970 standard population as described in Appendix II.

NOTES: High serum cholesterol is defined as greater than or equal to 240 mg/dL (6.20 mmol/L). Risk levels have been defined by the National Cholesterol Education Program Expert Panel on Detection, Evaluation and Treatment of High Blood Cholesterol in Adults, Nov. 1987. (Archives of Internal Medicine: January 1988, 148: 36–69.)

SOURCE: Centers for Disease Control and Prevention, National Center for Health Statistics, Division of Health Examination Statistics.

Table 73. Overweight persons 20–74 years of age, according to race, sex, and age: United States, 1960–62, 1971–74, and 1976–80

[Data are based on physical examinations of a sample of the civilian noninstitutionalized population]

Sex and age	All races			White			Black		
	1960–62	1971–74	1976–80	1960–62	1971–74	1976–80	1960–62	1971–74	1976–80
Both sexes			Percent of population						
20–74 years, age adjusted	25.0	25.7	26.2	24.1	24.8	25.1	32.6	35.7	37.7
20–74 years, crude	25.5	25.5	25.7	24.6	24.7	24.8	33.4	34.9	35.7
20–24 years	11.6	11.3	11.7	11.5	10.9	11.2	11.6	15.8	15.3
25–34 years	18.7	20.5	20.2	17.5	19.7	19.4	31.1	29.1	26.3
35–44 years	23.5	28.4	27.9	21.4	26.6	26.4	38.0	45.3	40.8
45–54 years	29.4	30.0	31.7	28.6	29.1	30.2	34.3	39.4	52.1
55–64 years	35.4	32.0	32.8	34.6	31.0	31.9	44.0	43.9	44.2
65–74 years	33.5	31.5	32.7	33.8	31.0	31.9	31.5	37.3	46.0
Male									
20–74 years, age adjusted	23.2	24.1	24.8	23.5	24.3	24.9	21.7	25.0	27.5
20–74 years, crude	23.4	24.0	24.2	23.7	24.1	24.4	22.5	24.5	25.7
20–24 years	15.5	12.1	12.1	16.1	12.8	12.7	*8.5	8.2	5.5
25–34 years	21.6	23.6	20.4	21.2	23.6	20.9	33.0	26.1	17.5
35–44 years	22.8	29.4	28.9	22.0	28.9	28.2	28.6	39.3	40.9
45–54 years	28.1	27.6	31.0	29.0	28.2	30.5	20.6	22.4	41.4
55–64 years	26.9	24.8	28.1	28.5	24.9	28.6	17.1	25.6	26.0
65–74 years	21.8	23.0	25.2	22.6	23.1	25.8	*11.7	21.6	26.4
Female									
20–74 years, age adjusted	26.5	26.9	27.4	24.4	25.0	25.2	42.9	44.5	46.1
20–74 years, crude	27.4	27.0	27.1	25.4	25.2	25.1	43.0	43.2	43.8
20–24 years	7.9	10.5	11.4	6.7	9.1	9.6	14.2	22.5	23.7
25–34 years	15.9	17.6	20.0	13.9	15.9	17.9	29.6	31.5	33.5
35–44 years	24.1	27.3	27.0	20.9	24.5	24.8	46.1	49.9	40.8
45–54 years	30.7	32.3	32.5	28.2	29.9	29.9	47.8	53.5	61.2
55–64 years	43.2	38.5	37.0	40.1	36.6	34.8	71.4	58.7	59.4
65–74 years	42.9	38.0	38.5	42.8	37.0	36.5	*47.8	49.2	60.8

*Based on fewer than 45 persons.

NOTES: Overweight is defined for men as body mass index greater than or equal to 27.8 kilograms/meter ^{2}, and for women as body mass index greater than or equal to 27.3 kilograms/meter ^{2}. These cut points were used because they represent the sex-specific 85th percentiles for persons 20–29 years of age in the 1976–80 National Health and Nutrition Examination Survey. Excludes pregnant women. Height was measured without shoes; two pounds are deducted from data for 1960–62 to allow for weight of clothing.

SOURCE: Centers for Disease Control and Prevention, National Center for Health Statistics, Division of Health Examination Statistics: Unpublished data.

Table 74. Air pollution, according to source and type of pollutant: United States, selected years 1970–91

[Data are calculated emissions estimates]

Type of pollutant and year	All sources	Transportation	Stationary fuel combustion	Industrial processes	Solid waste	Other
Particulate matter		Emissions in 10^6 metric tons per year				
1970	19.0	1.2	5.1	10.5	1.1	1.1
1975	11.0	1.3	3.3	5.2	0.4	0.8
1980	9.1	1.3	3.0	3.3	0.3	1.1
1986	7.3	1.4	2.5	2.4	0.3	0.8
1987	7.4	1.4	2.4	2.4	0.3	0.9
1988	7.9	1.5	2.4	2.5	0.3	1.3
1989	7.6	1.5	2.4	2.5	0.3	0.9
1990	7.4	1.5	1.9	2.5	0.3	1.2
1991 [1]	7.4	1.6	1.9	2.6	0.3	1.0
Sulfur oxides						
1970	28.4	0.6	21.3	6.4	0.0	0.1
1975	25.5	0.6	20.2	4.6	0.0	0.0
1980	23.8	0.9	19.1	3.7	0.0	0.0
1986	21.2	0.9	17.1	3.2	0.0	0.0
1987	21.0	0.9	17.0	3.0	0.0	0.0
1988	21.3	0.9	17.3	3.1	0.0	0.0
1989	21.5	1.0	17.4	3.1	0.0	0.0
1990	21.1	1.0	17.0	3.1	0.0	0.0
1991 [1]	20.7	1.0	16.6	3.2	0.0	0.0
Nitrogen oxides						
1970	19.0	8.5	9.1	0.7	0.4	0.3
1975	20.3	10.0	9.3	0.7	0.1	0.2
1980	23.6	12.5	10.1	0.7	0.1	0.2
1986	18.8	8.5	9.6	0.6	0.1	0.2
1987	19.0	8.1	10.1	0.6	0.1	0.2
1988	19.7	8.2	10.5	0.6	0.1	0.3
1989	19.3	7.9	10.6	0.6	0.1	0.2
1990	19.4	7.8	10.6	0.6	0.1	0.3
1991 [1]	18.8	7.3	10.6	0.6	0.1	0.2
Volatile organic compounds						
1970	27.4	12.8	0.6	8.9	1.8	3.3
1975	22.5	10.3	0.6	8.2	0.9	2.5
1980	21.8	8.1	1.0	9.1	0.7	2.9
1986	18.5	6.9	0.9	7.9	0.6	2.2
1987	18.6	6.6	0.9	8.2	0.6	2.4
1988	18.6	6.3	0.9	8.0	0.6	2.9
1989	17.4	5.5	0.9	8.0	0.6	2.4
1990	17.6	5.5	0.6	8.0	0.6	2.8
1991 [1]	16.9	5.1	0.7	7.9	0.7	2.6
Carbon monoxide						
1970	123.6	96.9	4.2	9.0	6.4	7.2
1975	104.8	86.2	4.0	6.9	2.9	4.8
1980	100.0	77.4	6.6	6.3	2.1	7.6
1986	76.0	58.7	6.3	4.2	1.7	5.1
1987	75.1	56.2	6.3	4.3	1.7	6.4
1988	75.5	53.5	6.3	4.6	1.7	9.5
1989	68.3	49.3	6.4	4.6	1.7	6.3
1990	67.7	48.5	4.3	4.6	1.7	8.6
1991 [1]	62.1	43.5	4.7	4.7	2.1	7.2
Lead		Emissions in 10^3 metric tons per year				
1970	199.1	163.6	9.6	23.9	2.0	0.0
1975	143.8	122.7	9.4	10.3	1.5	0.0
1980	68.0	59.4	3.9	3.6	1.1	0.0
1986	6.6	3.5	0.5	1.9	0.8	0.0
1987	6.2	3.0	0.5	1.9	0.8	0.0
1988	5.9	2.6	0.5	2.0	0.7	0.0
1989	5.5	2.2	0.5	2.2	0.7	0.0
1990	5.1	1.7	0.5	2.2	0.7	0.0
1991 [1]	5.0	1.6	0.5	2.2	0.7	0.0

[1] Preliminary data.

NOTE: Because of ongoing improvements in methods for estimating emissions and changes in emission factors used to calculate emissions, data from this table should not be compared with data in previous editions of Health, United States.

SOURCE: Office of Air Quality Planning and Standards, Technical Support Division, Emission Inventory Branch: National Air Pollutant Emission Estimates, 1940–1991. EPA-454/R-92-013. U.S. Environmental Protection Agency. Research Triangle Park, N.C., Oct. 1992.

Table 75. Occupational injuries with lost workdays in the private sector, according to industry: United States, 1980–90

[Data are based on employer records from a sample of business establishments]

Industry	1980	1981	1982	1983	1984	1985	1986	1987	1988	1989	1990
	Number of injuries with lost workdays in thousands										
Total private sector [1]	2,491.0	2,408.9	2,141.3	2,140.3	2,449.7	2,484.7	2,533.2	2,721.3	2,880.4	2,955.5	2,987.3
Agriculture, fishing, and forestry [1]	39.3	42.2	42.0	44.1	46.3	45.2	43.7	49.3	51.3	52.2	57.2
Mining	66.2	70.8	57.1	41.7	51.4	43.9	31.6	34.6	37.1	33.9	35.6
Construction	242.6	222.1	195.8	207.9	256.5	272.8	290.4	292.3	304.4	301.2	296.3
Manufacturing	1,009.5	951.0	760.1	738.6	841.8	825.1	825.4	923.2	1,007.3	1,007.4	975.0
Transportation, communication, and public utilities	263.0	252.3	230.0	215.7	249.3	243.5	235.7	247.5	261.3	273.9	293.3
Wholesale trade	191.1	177.1	166.7	159.0	179.3	188.4	195.8	203.3	214.7	230.3	211.5
Retail trade	330.2	328.3	322.1	343.5	395.0	399.9	421.0	445.0	461.6	480.6	483.9
Finance, insurance, and real estate	38.1	37.5	41.1	41.2	44.3	45.5	49.1	49.9	54.0	52.6	63.7
Services	311.1	327.5	326.3	348.5	385.8	420.6	440.4	476.0	488.6	523.4	570.8
	Injuries with lost workdays per 100 full-time employees										
Total private sector [1]	3.9	3.7	3.4	3.4	3.6	3.6	3.6	3.7	3.8	3.9	3.9
Agriculture, fishing, and forestry [1]	5.6	5.8	5.7	6.0	5.9	5.6	5.4	5.5	5.5	5.6	5.7
Mining	6.4	6.2	5.4	4.4	5.3	4.7	4.1	4.8	5.1	4.8	4.9
Construction	6.5	6.3	6.0	6.2	6.9	6.8	6.8	6.7	6.8	6.7	6.6
Manufacturing	5.2	4.9	4.3	4.2	4.5	4.4	4.5	5.0	5.3	5.3	5.3
Transportation, communication, and public utilities	5.4	5.2	4.8	4.7	5.1	4.9	4.8	4.9	5.0	5.2	5.4
Wholesale trade	3.8	3.5	3.4	3.2	3.4	3.5	3.6	3.7	3.8	3.9	3.6
Retail trade	2.9	2.9	2.9	3.0	3.2	3.1	3.2	3.3	3.3	3.4	3.4
Finance, insurance, and real estate	0.8	0.8	0.9	0.8	0.9	0.9	0.9	0.9	0.9	0.9	1.1
Services	2.3	2.3	2.3	2.3	2.4	2.5	2.5	2.6	2.6	2.6	2.7
	Total lost workdays per 100 full-time employees										
Total private sector [1]	63.7	60.4	57.5	57.2	61.8	63.3	63.9	67.3	72.6	74.2	78.3
Agriculture, fishing, and forestry [1]	81.3	81.4	84.2	89.5	89.4	90.1	92.4	92.5	99.8	99.4	108.9
Mining	162.8	145.7	136.7	124.1	159.3	144.3	124.4	142.5	150.3	134.7	117.7
Construction	116.1	112.1	114.6	117.3	126.7	128.1	133.3	134.9	141.1	141.6	146.1
Manufacturing	84.0	79.4	72.4	70.4	74.2	76.2	80.2	87.9	96.4	98.7	103.0
Transportation, communication, and public utilities	103.3	100.0	95.8	94.4	104.2	106.3	101.0	107.1	117.5	120.0	131.6
Wholesale trade	57.1	53.5	51.6	50.1	54.8	59.1	62.0	63.2	68.4	70.7	69.5
Retail trade	44.1	40.8	42.1	46.3	47.9	46.2	50.0	52.2	56.2	59.0	61.4
Finance, insurance, and real estate	11.6	11.3	12.8	12.4	13.2	14.6	16.0	13.8	16.3	16.5	24.8
Services	34.5	34.7	35.1	36.2	40.3	44.7	42.2	44.8	47.1	49.9	54.6

[1]Excludes farms with fewer than 11 employees.

NOTES: Industry is coded based on various editions of the Standard Industrial Classification Manual as follows: data for 1980–87 are based on the 1972 Edition, 1977 Supplement; and data for 1988–90 are based on the 1987 Edition (See Appendix II).

SOURCE: Bureau of Labor Statistics, U.S. Department of Labor: Occupational Injuries and Illnesses in the United States by Industry, 1980–90 Editions, 1981–1992.

Table 76. Production employees with potential exposure to elemental lead or to continuous noise, according to industry and size of facility: United States, 1972–74 and 1981–83

[Data are based on interviews of a sample of nonagricultural businesses]

Industry	All facilities 1972–74	All facilities 1981–83	8–99 employees 1972–74	8–99 employees 1981–83	100–499 employees 1972–74	100–499 employees 1981–83	500 or more employees 1972–74	500 or more employees 1981–83
	Number of employees in thousands							
All production employees [1]	28,379	19,546	9,957	7,303	8,331	6,091	10,091	6,151
Textile mill products	246	546	94	82	109	261	*43	203
Apparel and other textile mill products	920	991	515	345	367	482	*38	*164
Lumber and wood products	217	442	105	230	85	143	*27	*70
Printing and publishing	1,248	636	365	283	306	218	578	135
Chemicals and allied products	964	462	193	106	192	132	579	224
Rubber and miscellaneous plastics	508	473	132	165	171	204	205	104
Stone, clay, and glass products	687	382	173	175	300	124	*214	*83
Primary metals industries	1,322	556	112	96	215	212	995	248
Fabricated metal products	1,441	967	515	393	522	379	404	194
Machinery, except electrical	1,529	1,270	271	418	359	338	900	513
Electrical and electronic machinery, equipment, and supplies	1,493	964	97	143	326	327	1,070	494
Transportation equipment	1,160	837	95	95	131	155	935	587
Measuring, analyzing, and controlling instruments; photographic, medical, and optical goods; watches and clocks	392	328	91	66	74	92	227	170
Miscellaneous manufacturing industries	393	360	140	109	159	104	*93	*147
	Percent of employees with any potential exposure to elemental lead							
All production employees [1]	0.6	3.6	0.4	3.4	0.4	4.0	0.9	3.6
Textile mill products	–	0.1	–	0.1	–	0.2	*–	0.3
Apparel and other textile mill products	0.1	0.6	0.0	0.1	–	0.7	*–	*1.1
Lumber and wood products	–	0.6	–	0.7	–	0.4	*–	*0.5
Printing and publishing	1.7	2.0	3.1	2.9	1.0	1.0	1.2	1.6
Chemicals and allied products	1.1	4.4	0.4	1.9	2.6	5.2	0.8	5.1
Rubber and miscellaneous plastics	0.2	2.0	0.1	3.7	0.2	0.6	0.5	2.1
Stone, clay, and glass products	1.7	4.0	0.3	2.7	1.2	0.5	*3.5	*12.3
Primary metals industries	0.5	3.0	0.3	3.6	0.2	4.9	0.7	1.1
Fabricated metal products	0.2	4.8	0.1	0.8	0.4	9.8	0.1	3.2
Machinery, except electrical	0.7	6.1	0.3	3.8	1.2	8.8	0.6	6.1
Electrical and electronic machinery, equipment, and supplies	1.2	18.5	0.4	23.4	2.1	15.8	1.0	18.9
Transportation equipment	1.1	1.1	0.9	–	0.5	0.3	1.2	1.5
Measuring, analyzing, and controlling instruments; photographic, medical, and optical goods; watches and clocks	1.0	–	2.9	–	0.7	–	0.4	–
Miscellaneous manufacturing industries	0.5	4.8	1.1	6.2	0.1	3.0	*0.2	*5.0
	Percent of employees with potential exposure to continuous noise at 85 dBA or greater							
All production employees [1]	22.4	21.2	14.7	17.3	24.4	24.9	28.3	22.0
Textile mill products	36.2	48.0	29.1	36.4	43.0	51.6	*34.2	48.2
Apparel and other textile mill products	21.4	15.2	20.5	5.8	23.2	16.5	*14.9	*31.4
Lumber and wood products	42.8	44.4	48.9	45.0	28.9	53.3	*63.1	*24.4
Printing and publishing	24.0	24.4	20.4	19.5	12.0	26.0	32.7	32.0
Chemicals and allied products	13.1	22.2	15.3	14.8	22.8	19.7	9.1	27.2
Rubber and miscellaneous plastics	52.9	28.7	48.9	20.0	55.4	33.7	53.4	32.4
Stone, clay, and glass products	32.6	24.7	28.1	22.2	38.9	29.6	*27.3	*27.3
Primary metals industries	53.5	48.4	45.2	33.4	68.0	53.2	51.3	50.2
Fabricated metal products	49.5	34.9	40.6	33.0	55.6	34.8	53.0	38.5
Machinery, except electrical	31.1	18.1	28.2	17.3	29.0	19.7	32.8	17.6
Electrical and electronic machinery, equipment, and supplies	13.1	10.8	6.7	9.9	17.4	7.2	12.3	13.6
Transportation equipment	48.3	28.5	24.2	32.4	48.9	32.5	50.6	26.8
Measuring, analyzing, and controlling instruments; photographic, medical, and optical goods; watches and clocks	14.5	14.5	2.2	7.6	16.9	6.1	18.6	22.0
Miscellaneous manufacturing industries	31.0	10.9	22.7	16.3	34.6	19.3	*37.1	*1.0

[1] Production employees work in locations where production or service work is conducted.

*Based on fewer than 10 facilities.

NOTES: Data are displayed for elemental lead (Chemical Abstract Number 7439921) only. These data do not include potential exposures to lead in approximately 150 compounds also measured in the surveys. Industry categories are based on the Standard Industrial Classification (SIC) Manual. For a listing of the code numbers, see Appendix II, table VI.

SOURCE: Centers for Disease Control and Prevention: National Institute for Occupational Safety and Health: Unpublished data from the 1972–74 National Occupational Hazard Survey and 1981–83 National Occupational Exposure Survey.

Table 77. Health and safety services available in nonagricultural industries, according to size of facility: United States, 1972–74 and 1981–83

[Data are based on interviews of a sample of nonagricultural businesses]

Health and safety services available in facility	All facilities		8–99 employees		100–499 employees		500 or more employees	
	1972–74	1981–83	1972–74[1]	1981–83	1972–74	1981–83	1972–74	1981–83
	Number of employees in thousands							
All employees	38,263	33,413	15,394	11,083	10,883	9,870	11,985	12,460
Occupational health and safety practices	Percent of employees							
Regularly monitor environmental conditions[2]	21.7	48.5	2.5	11.2	12.1	43.6	55.2	85.7
Personal protective devices in some work areas[3]	39.2	53.4	32.5	45.9	46.1	59.1	41.4	55.5
Employer provides protective devices	52.5	80.2	41.9	70.4	60.1	82.9	59.4	86.8
Medical facilities and practices								
Health unit at facility	31.5	43.0	3.3	3.8	18.4	31.7	79.6	86.9
Access to physician or clinic	70.7	77.2	49.0	53.2	76.2	79.1	93.5	96.9
Physician available on-site	18.8	26.6	1.2	1.3	4.3	8.2	52.7	63.7
Physician available off-site	17.0	52.7	17.5	50.5	25.2	67.1	8.8	43.2
Preemployment medical exams	38.5	49.9	12.8	20.0	35.2	47.1	74.5	78.4
Periodic tests available	14.4	30.5	6.0	8.4	13.5	26.7	25.9	53.1
Audiometric tests available	5.1	16.7	1.4	5.0	3.7	16.8	11.1	26.6
Blood tests available	3.0	14.5	1.3	4.0	3.7	9.9	4.7	27.4
Records of employee absenteeism showing type of illness	14.2	17.6	4.7	9.5	9.5	18.3	30.8	24.1

[1]Includes facilities with fewer than eight employees.
[2]Monitoring environmental conditions such as presence of fumes, gases, dust, noise, vibration, and radiation.
[3]Includes respirators, protective clothing, etc.

SOURCE: Centers for Disease Control and Prevention: National Institute for Occupational Safety and Health, National Occupational Exposure Survey: Analysis of Management Interview Responses. DHHS Pub. No. (NIOSH) 89–103. Public Health Service. Washington. U.S. Government Printing Office, 1989.

Table 78. Physician contacts, according to place of contact and selected patient characteristics: United States, 1986 and 1991

[Data are based on household interviews of a sample of the civilian noninstitutionalized population]

Characteristic	Physician contacts 1986	Physician contacts 1991	Total	Doctor's office 1986	Doctor's office 1991	Hospital outpatient department [1] 1986	Hospital outpatient department [1] 1991	Telephone 1986	Telephone 1991	Home 1986	Home 1991	Other [2] 1986	Other [2] 1991
	Number per person		Percent distribution										
Total [3,4]	5.3	5.6	100.0	56.0	58.9	15.1	14.2	13.3	12.2	2.2	2.7	13.4	11.9
Age													
Under 15 years	4.4	4.7	100.0	57.7	61.4	12.2	13.6	17.7	14.2	*0.3	*0.6	12.1	10.1
Under 5 years	6.3	7.1	100.0	59.4	61.2	10.8	13.5	18.0	16.5	*0.2	*0.8	11.5	8.1
5–14 years	3.4	3.4	100.0	56.0	61.7	13.6	13.7	17.3	11.7	*0.4	*0.5	12.7	12.4
15–44 years	4.5	4.7	100.0	55.5	58.0	16.1	14.6	11.5	12.2	0.9	1.1	16.0	14.2
45–64 years	6.6	6.6	100.0	55.5	58.2	18.8	15.6	11.7	11.3	2.3	3.1	11.6	11.8
65 years and over	9.1	10.4	100.0	54.2	56.9	11.8	11.5	10.8	8.4	12.9	14.9	10.3	8.3
65–74 years	8.1	9.2	100.0	56.6	61.1	12.9	12.9	11.6	9.2	8.1	7.5	10.8	9.3
75 years and over	10.6	12.3	100.0	51.2	52.1	10.4	9.8	9.9	7.5	18.8	23.4	9.7	7.2
Sex [3]													
Male	4.6	4.9	100.0	54.9	57.8	18.5	16.0	11.1	11.1	1.6	2.4	14.0	12.7
Female	6.0	6.3	100.0	56.6	59.5	12.7	12.9	14.9	12.9	2.6	2.9	13.2	11.7
Race [3]													
White	5.4	5.8	100.0	57.5	60.1	13.8	13.0	14.2	12.8	2.2	2.6	12.4	11.5
Black	4.8	5.2	100.0	44.2	52.0	24.4	21.2	7.4	7.3	2.4	3.6	21.7	15.8
Family income [3,5]													
Less than $14,000	6.4	6.8	100.0	45.6	48.7	20.7	20.2	11.1	10.1	2.9	3.8	19.7	17.2
$14,000–$24,999	5.3	5.6	100.0	54.8	55.9	18.8	16.6	13.1	12.4	0.9	1.7	12.5	13.4
$25,000–$34,999	5.3	5.5	100.0	56.9	60.7	13.0	13.6	15.2	12.8	1.6	1.7	13.4	11.3
$35,000–$49,999	5.3	5.8	100.0	60.1	61.4	13.3	12.4	13.6	13.5	1.0	1.7	12.0	11.0
$50,000 or more	5.5	5.8	100.0	59.9	64.2	11.3	10.6	14.3	14.4	3.9	1.5	10.6	9.3
Geographic region [3]													
Northeast	4.9	5.4	100.0	54.5	61.6	16.9	14.2	13.1	10.6	2.7	1.5	12.8	12.1
Midwest	5.5	5.8	100.0	51.7	57.5	14.9	13.6	15.3	13.8	2.5	4.3	15.6	10.7
South	5.2	5.5	100.0	59.5	61.0	13.9	13.4	12.6	12.1	2.0	2.9	12.1	10.6
West	5.9	5.9	100.0	57.0	55.2	15.7	16.2	12.0	12.0	1.8	1.6	13.5	15.0
Location of residence [3]													
Within MSA	5.4	5.8	100.0	56.0	58.5	14.9	13.8	13.6	12.6	1.9	2.7	13.6	12.4
Outside MSA	5.2	5.1	100.0	56.1	60.7	15.8	16.1	12.3	10.6	3.1	2.5	12.7	10.2

[1]Includes hospital outpatient clinic, emergency room, and other hospital contacts.
[2]Includes clinics or other places outside a hospital.
[3]Age adjusted.
[4]Includes all other races not shown separately and unknown family income.
[5]Family income categories for 1991. Income categories for 1986 are: less than $11,000; $11,000–$19,999; $20,000–$29,999; $30,000–$39,999; and $40,000 or more.

*Relative standard error greater than 30 percent.

SOURCE: Centers for Disease Control and Prevention, National Center for Health Statistics, Division of Health Interview Statistics: Data from the National Health Interview Survey.

Table 79. Interval since last physician contact, according to selected patient characteristics: United States, 1964, 1986, and 1991

[Data are based on household interviews of a sample of the civilian noninstitutionalized population]

Characteristic	Total	Less than 1 year			1 year–less than 2 years			2 years or more [1]		
		1964	1986	1991	1964	1986	1991	1964	1986	1991
		Percent distribution [2]								
Total [3,4].	100.0	66.9	76.5	78.9	14.0	10.1	9.9	19.1	13.4	11.2
Age										
Under 15 years	100.0	68.4	81.6	84.1	14.8	10.8	10.0	16.7	7.6	5.9
Under 5 years	100.0	80.7	92.4	94.4	11.1	5.5	4.5	8.2	2.1	1.2
5–14 years	100.0	61.7	75.8	78.6	16.9	13.6	12.9	21.4	10.6	8.5
15–44 years	100.0	66.3	71.9	73.7	15.0	11.6	11.7	18.7	16.5	14.6
45–64 years	100.0	64.5	75.0	78.0	13.0	8.6	8.7	22.5	16.4	13.3
65 years and over	100.0	69.7	84.1	87.6	9.3	5.1	4.6	21.0	10.8	7.9
65–74 years.	100.0	68.8	82.2	86.2	9.4	5.5	4.9	21.8	12.3	9.0
75 years and over	100.0	71.3	87.2	89.8	9.3	4.4	4.0	19.5	8.3	6.2
Sex [3]										
Male.	100.0	63.5	71.4	74.0	15.0	11.3	11.1	21.5	17.3	14.8
Female.	100.0	69.9	81.3	83.5	13.1	9.0	8.7	17.0	9.7	7.7
Race [3]										
White	100.0	68.1	77.1	79.3	13.8	9.9	9.6	18.1	13.0	11.0
Black [5]	100.0	58.3	74.7	78.3	15.1	11.3	11.0	26.6	14.0	10.7
Family income [3,6]										
Less than $14,000.	100.0	58.6	75.8	78.1	13.2	9.6	9.1	28.2	14.5	12.8
$14,000–$24,999.	100.0	62.5	74.2	76.4	14.2	10.7	10.5	23.3	15.1	13.1
$25,000–$34,999.	100.0	66.8	76.8	78.5	14.5	9.6	10.0	18.7	13.6	11.6
$35,000–$49,999.	100.0	70.2	78.6	80.8	14.0	9.2	9.8	15.7	12.2	9.5
$50,000 or more	100.0	73.6	80.4	83.2	12.9	9.0	8.3	13.5	10.6	8.5
Geographic region [3]										
Northeast	100.0	68.0	78.1	81.9	14.1	9.7	8.7	17.9	12.2	9.4
Midwest	100.0	66.6	77.6	79.9	14.2	10.0	9.6	19.2	12.4	10.5
South.	100.0	65.2	75.4	77.0	13.9	10.9	11.1	20.9	13.6	11.9
West	100.0	69.0	75.6	78.2	13.7	9.2	9.5	17.3	15.2	12.3
Location of residence [3]										
Within MSA.	100.0	68.2	77.1	79.6	14.0	9.8	9.7	17.8	13.1	10.7
Outside MSA.	100.0	64.0	74.4	76.5	14.1	11.3	10.7	21.9	14.3	12.8

[1]Includes persons who never visited a physician.
[2]Denominator excludes persons with unknown interval.
[3]Age adjusted.
[4]Includes all other races not shown separately and unknown family income.
[5]1964 data include all other races.
[6]Family income categories for 1991. Income categories in 1964 are: less than $2,000; $2,000–$3,999; $4,000–$6,999; $7,000–$9,999; and $10,000 or more; and, in 1986 are: less than $11,000; $11,000–$19,999; $20,000–$29,999; $30,000–$39,999; and $40,000 or more.

SOURCE: Centers for Disease Control and Prevention, National Center for Health Statistics, Division of Health Interview Statistics: Data from the National Health Interview Survey.

Table 80. Office visits to physicians, according to physician specialty and selected patient characteristics: United States, 1985 and 1990

[Data are based on reporting by a sample of office-based physicians]

Characteristic	All specialties	General and family practice 1985	General and family practice 1990	Internal medicine 1985	Internal medicine 1990	Pediatrics 1985	Pediatrics 1990	Obstetrics and gynecology 1985	Obstetrics and gynecology 1990
					Percent distribution				
Total	100.0	30.5	29.8	11.6	13.7	11.4	11.5	8.9	8.7
Age									
Under 15 years.	100.0	25.0	25.2	2.2	2.3	55.2	54.4	0.5	0.5
15–44 years	100.0	33.0	32.0	8.3	11.4	2.6	2.0	19.1	19.7
45–64 years	100.0	32.0	32.0	15.7	18.5	*	*	4.7	4.6
65 years and over.	100.0	29.1	28.0	22.1	23.3	*	*	1.4	1.1
65–74 years	100.0	28.8	28.0	22.1	22.9	*	*	2.0	2.0
75 years and over	100.0	29.4	28.0	22.1	23.7	*	*	*	*
Male									
15–44 years	100.0	36.4	35.1	9.9	14.5	2.5	2.8	*	*
45–64 years	100.0	31.0	30.9	16.0	19.1	*	*	*	*
65 years and over.	100.0	28.1	27.7	20.8	23.3	*	*	*	*
Female									
15–44 years	100.0	31.3	30.5	7.5	9.9	2.6	1.7	28.4	29.2
45–64 years	100.0	32.7	32.7	15.5	18.1	*	*	7.7	7.7
65 years and over.	100.0	29.7	28.2	23.0	23.3	*	*	2.3	1.8
Race									
White.	100.0	30.0	29.7	11.8	13.1	11.4	11.2	8.7	8.7
Black.	100.0	35.4	28.6	10.4	20.0	11.3	12.1	9.9	8.5

Characteristic	General surgery 1985	General surgery 1990	Ophthalmology 1985	Ophthalmology 1990	Orthopedic surgery 1985	Orthopedic surgery 1990	Dermatology 1985	Dermatology 1990	All others 1985	All others 1990
				Percent distribution						
Total	4.7	3.2	6.3	6.2	5.0	4.7	3.8	3.4	17.9	18.8
Age										
Under 15 years.	1.4	0.7	2.6	1.6	2.9	2.4	1.4	1.5	9.0	11.5
15–44 years	4.4	3.2	3.9	3.1	6.1	6.0	5.1	4.5	17.4	18.2
45–64 years	6.6	4.1	7.1	7.2	6.1	5.2	3.8	3.7	23.6	24.5
65 years and over.	6.2	4.4	13.5	14.9	3.4	4.0	3.4	3.0	20.8	21.1
65–74 years	6.4	4.3	11.2	12.2	3.6	4.2	3.5	3.5	22.4	23.2
75 years and over	6.0	4.6	16.6	18.5	3.1	3.9	3.3	2.4	18.7	18.3
Male										
15–44 years	5.0	3.8	5.2	4.2	11.0	10.9	6.7	5.5	23.1	23.3
45–64 years	6.2	3.6	7.2	7.6	7.0	5.7	4.8	4.3	27.5	28.4
65 years and over.	6.7	4.1	11.8	13.4	2.6	3.0	4.0	3.7	25.8	24.8
Female										
15–44 years	4.1	2.9	3.3	2.5	3.8	3.6	4.4	4.0	14.6	15.7
45–64 years	6.9	4.5	7.0	6.8	5.5	4.8	3.2	3.3	21.0	21.9
65 years and over.	5.9	4.7	14.5	15.9	3.8	4.7	3.0	2.6	17.7	18.8
Race										
White.	4.6	3.1	6.4	6.4	5.0	4.8	3.9	3.6	18.4	19.6
Black.	6.2	5.4	4.7	4.7	4.8	3.2	3.2	1.3	14.0	16.3

*Relative standard error greater than 30 percent.

NOTES: Rates are based on the civilian noninstitutionalized population. In 1985 the survey excluded Alaska and Hawaii. Beginning in 1989, the survey included all 50 States.

SOURCE: Centers for Disease Control and Prevention, National Center for Health Statistics, Division of Health Care Statistics: Data from the National Ambulatory Medical Care Survey.

Table 81. Office visits to physicians, according to selected patient and visit characteristics and physician specialty: United States, 1985 and 1990

[Data are based on reporting by a sample of office-based physicians]

Characteristic	All specialties		All specialties		Patient's first visit		Visit lasted 10 minutes or less [1]		Return visit scheduled	
	1985	1990	1985	1990	1985	1990	1985	1990	1985	1990
	Visits per person		Number of visits in thousands		Percent of visits					
Total.	2.7	2.9	636,386	704,604	16.9	16.2	41.0	38.4	61.5	62.1
Age										
Under 15 years	2.3	2.5	118,768	138,427	17.8	16.5	50.9	53.9	49.2	47.9
15–44 years	2.3	2.3	249,688	263,113	20.9	20.5	41.7	38.8	59.0	59.2
45–64 years	3.1	3.2	137,391	149,786	14.9	14.6	36.4	32.3	65.7	67.1
65 years and over	4.8	5.1	130,538	153,278	10.6	10.0	35.6	29.9	72.9	75.0
65–74 years.	4.5	4.8	75,427	86,422	11.3	11.0	34.7	29.9	72.7	74.6
75 years and over	5.4	5.7	55,111	66,856	9.7	8.8	36.9	29.9	73.2	75.5
Sex										
Male.	2.2	2.3	248,905	277,452	18.3	18.5	42.2	39.6	59.2	59.6
Female.	3.2	3.4	387,481	427,151	16.0	14.7	40.2	37.7	62.9	63.7
Race										
White	2.9	2.9	572,507	597,306	16.6	15.9	40.6	37.7	61.2	61.5
Black	1.9	2.1	52,143	62,317	18.2	17.9	44.4	41.3	65.5	67.3

Characteristic	All specialties		General and family practice		Internal medicine		Pediatrics		General surgery	
	1985	1990	1985	1990	1985	1990	1985	1990	1985	1990
	Percent of visits with drug administered or prescribed									
Total.	61.2	60.3	72.7	68.7	77.4	74.5	66.8	66.9	38.5	31.1
Age										
Under 15 years	62.0	62.0	68.1	62.5	68.1	86.0	67.0	66.3	37.9	28.0
15–44 years	55.9	55.4	68.6	65.7	70.6	67.4	63.1	72.7	35.6	27.6
45–64 years	63.4	62.1	76.1	73.3	79.3	74.9	*	*	35.3	29.6
65 years and over	68.2	65.2	81.2	74.2	81.7	79.1	*	*	46.1	37.1
65–74 years.	67.1	64.7	80.2	74.1	81.0	78.8	*	*	43.5	35.4
75 years and over	69.7	65.9	82.5	74.3	82.7	79.4	*	*	49.9	39.1
Sex										
Male.	60.2	59.5	70.5	67.5	74.1	72.4	65.7	66.6	41.3	29.7
Female.	61.8	60.8	74.1	69.4	79.5	75.9	67.7	67.1	36.7	31.9
Race										
White	60.6	59.9	71.8	69.5	77.3	74.1	66.3	65.8	37.9	28.2
Black	67.2	67.9	78.6	71.5	80.2	80.2	70.3	74.3	44.6	*

[1]Time spent in face-to-face contact between physician and patient.

*Relative standard error greater than 30 percent.

NOTES: Rates are based on the civilian noninstitutionalized population. In 1985 the survey excluded Alaska and Hawaii. Beginning in 1989, the survey included all 50 States.

SOURCE: Centers for Disease Control and Prevention, National Center for Health Statistics, Division of Health Care Statistics: Data from the National Ambulatory Medical Care Survey.

Table 82. Dental visits and interval since last visit, according to selected patient characteristics: United States, 1964, 1983, and 1989

[Data are based on household interviews of a sample of the civilian noninstitutionalized population]

| | | | | Interval since last dental visit [1] | | | | | | | | |
| | Dental visits | | | Less than 1 year | | | 2 years or more | | | Never visited dentist | | |
Characteristic	1964	1983	1989	1964	1983	1989	1964	1983	1989	1964	1983	1989
	Number per person			Percent of population								
Total [2,3,4]	1.6	1.9	2.1	42.7	55.3	57.7	28.7	24.1	21.4	15.5	7.7	6.4
Age												
2–14 years [4]	1.3	2.0	2.1	39.6	57.9	60.5	5.4	7.6	6.6	46.6	23.5	19.7
2–4 years [4]	0.3	0.7	0.9	11.1	28.4	32.1	0.3	1.0	1.0	87.0	64.2	55.0
5–14 years	1.9	2.5	2.5	55.1	67.3	69.5	8.2	9.7	8.4	24.6	10.5	8.6
15–44 years	1.9	1.9	2.0	51.8	58.5	59.7	26.9	24.3	22.8	4.0	1.7	1.4
45–64 years	1.7	2.0	2.4	39.1	53.1	56.8	46.3	34.3	28.9	1.3	0.6	0.4
65 years and over	0.8	1.5	2.0	21.5	38.6	43.2	69.0	51.3	43.7	1.5	0.9	0.5
65–74 years	0.9	1.8	2.2	24.9	43.2	47.6	65.2	46.9	39.7	1.1	0.8	0.4
75 years and over.	0.6	1.1	1.8	14.9	31.1	36.3	76.3	58.4	50.0	2.4	1.0	0.6
Sex [2]												
Male.	1.4	1.7	2.0	40.9	53.3	55.4	29.6	25.7	23.2	16.1	7.9	6.7
Female	1.7	2.1	2.3	44.4	57.2	60.0	28.0	22.7	19.6	15.0	7.6	6.1
Race [2]												
White	1.7	2.0	2.3	45.3	57.5	60.0	27.8	23.0	20.2	13.8	7.2	6.1
Black [5]	0.8	1.2	1.2	22.3	41.1	44.0	37.6	32.2	29.5	28.0	10.3	7.7
Family income [2,6]												
Less than $14,000	0.9	1.2	1.3	26.4	40.4	41.9	35.4	35.2	33.7	27.4	11.2	9.6
$14,000–$24,999	0.9	1.5	1.6	30.0	46.7	49.5	35.2	29.7	27.5	22.0	9.8	7.8
$25,000–$34,999	1.4	2.2	2.2	39.7	58.4	60.3	30.6	22.2	20.3	15.8	7.2	6.3
$35,000–$49,999	1.9	2.5	2.7	50.1	68.2	69.7	25.3	16.2	15.1	10.9	4.5	4.5
$50,000 or more	2.7	2.9	3.1	63.9	75.3	76.1	16.8	12.2	10.6	7.2	3.6	3.4
Geographic region [2]												
Northeast	2.1	2.4	2.2	48.5	61.5	61.4	26.1	20.9	17.9	12.5	5.7	4.8
Midwest	1.6	1.9	2.1	44.6	58.0	62.2	29.3	23.4	20.1	12.9	6.1	5.0
South	1.2	1.6	1.8	35.8	49.2	52.5	30.9	27.3	25.4	20.9	10.0	8.0
West.	1.7	2.0	2.4	43.8	55.9	58.0	27.9	23.3	19.7	14.3	8.0	6.7
Location of residence [2]												
Within MSA.	1.8	2.1	2.2	44.9	57.4	58.8	27.5	22.4	20.2	14.4	7.2	6.2
Outside MSA.	1.2	1.6	1.7	37.8	51.0	54.2	31.8	27.6	25.5	17.9	8.6	6.8

[1]Percent not shown for an interval of 1 year–less than 2 years. Denominators exclude persons with unknown interval (5.2 percent in 1989).
[2]Age adjusted.
[3]Includes all other races not shown separately and unknown family income.
[4]Data for 1983 and 1989 are shown for ages 2 years and over because children under 2 years of age rarely visit a dentist. For 1964, data for children under 2 years of age are included.
[5]1964 data are for all other races.
[6]Family income categories for 1989. Income categories in 1964 are: less than $2,000; $2,000–$3,999; $4,000–$6,999; $7,000–$9,999; and $10,000 or more; and, in 1983 are: less than $10,000; $10,000–$18,999; $19,000–$29,999; $30,000–$39,999; and $40,000 or more.

SOURCE: Centers for Disease Control and Prevention, National Center for Health Statistics, Division of Health Interview Statistics: Data from the National Health Interview Survey.

Table 83. Discharges, days of care, and average length of stay in short-stay hospitals, according to selected characteristics: United States, 1964, 1986, and 1991

[Data are based on household interviews of a sample of the civilian noninstitutionalized population]

Characteristic	Discharges			Days of care			Average length of stay		
	1964	1986	1991	1964	1986	1991	1964	1986	1991
	Number per 1,000 population						Number of days		
Total [1,2].	109.1	98.3	88.7	970.9	685.1	586.6	8.9	7.0	6.6
Age									
Under 15 years	67.6	48.1	44.2	405.7	289.2	236.5	6.0	6.0	5.4
Under 5 years	94.3	73.8	73.3	731.1	562.5	424.7	7.8	7.6	5.8
5–14 years	53.1	34.2	28.7	229.1	142.2	135.8	4.3	4.2	4.7
15–44 years	100.6	70.0	62.8	760.7	432.8	365.2	7.6	6.2	5.8
45–64 years	146.2	142.0	116.7	1,559.3	963.9	816.4	10.7	6.8	7.0
65 years and over	190.0	275.3	272.8	2,292.7	2,347.5	2,085.7	12.1	8.5	7.6
65–74 years.	181.2	236.8	240.3	2,150.4	2,065.0	1,837.2	11.9	8.7	7.6
75 years and over	206.7	337.3	322.5	2,560.4	2,802.4	2,464.8	12.4	8.3	7.6
Sex [1]									
Male.	103.8	102.0	89.2	1,010.2	726.4	599.6	9.7	7.1	6.7
Female.	113.7	95.4	89.1	933.4	653.0	580.3	8.2	6.8	6.5
Race [1]									
White	112.4	98.4	88.6	961.4	662.1	565.5	8.6	6.7	6.4
Black [3]	84.0	103.3	96.3	1,062.9	913.8	764.0	12.7	8.8	7.9
Family income [1,4]									
Less than $14,000.	102.4	128.4	131.7	1,051.2	894.8	948.7	10.3	7.0	7.2
$14,000–$24,999.	116.4	116.9	94.4	1,213.9	863.0	673.7	10.4	7.4	7.1
$25,000–$34,999.	110.7	89.5	79.1	939.8	584.7	532.2	8.5	6.5	6.7
$35,000–$49,999.	109.2	100.7	71.8	882.6	686.3	387.3	8.1	6.8	5.4
$50,000 or more	110.7	77.6	64.0	918.9	430.2	366.7	8.3	5.5	5.7
Geographic region [1]									
Northeast	98.5	87.9	79.5	993.8	674.6	626.8	10.1	7.7	7.9
Midwest	109.2	100.2	92.9	944.9	706.9	577.0	8.7	7.1	6.2
South.	117.8	115.0	103.4	968.0	762.9	670.3	8.2	6.6	6.5
West	110.5	78.8	69.4	985.9	522.9	414.2	8.9	6.6	6.0
Location of residence [1]									
Within MSA.	107.5	95.0	84.5	1,015.4	678.1	570.4	9.4	7.1	6.8
Outside MSA.	113.3	108.8	103.7	871.9	705.6	650.6	7.7	6.5	6.3

[1]Age adjusted.

[2]Includes all other races not shown separately and unknown family income.

[3]1964 data include all other races.

[4]Family income categories for 1991. Income categories in 1964 are: less than $2,000; $2,000–$3,999; $4,000–$6,999; $7,000–$9,999; and $10,000 or more; and, in 1986 are: less than $11,000; $11,000–$19,999; $20,000–$29,999; $30,000–$39,999; and $40,000 or more.

NOTE: Excludes deliveries.

SOURCE: Centers for Disease Control and Prevention, National Center for Health Statistics, Division of Health Interview Statistics: Data from the National Health Interview Survey.

Table 84. Discharges, days of care, and average length of stay in nonfederal short-stay hospitals, according to selected characteristics: United States, selected years 1980–91

[Data are based on a sample of hospital records]

Characteristic	1980[1]	1982	1983	1984	1985	1986	1987	1988[2]	1989[2]	1990[2]	1991[2]
	Discharges per 1,000 population										
Total[3]	159.1	158.5	157.1	148.2	138.0	132.8	127.9	117.8	115.5	113.1	113.6
Sex[3]											
Male	140.1	140.5	139.9	131.8	123.5	119.8	115.0	105.8	103.9	99.6	101.3
Female	178.1	176.5	174.4	164.7	152.7	146.2	141.2	130.2	127.4	126.9	126.5
Age											
Under 15 years	71.6	71.2	70.8	62.0	57.2	53.5	51.3	49.2	48.2	43.9	45.3
15–44 years	150.2	145.0	140.3	132.2	125.1	118.9	115.1	104.0	102.8	101.7	99.3
45–64 years	194.8	195.5	192.2	183.3	169.5	162.2	156.9	140.5	135.0	133.1	132.2
65 years and over	383.7	398.8	412.7	400.4	368.3	367.3	350.5	334.1	330.2	327.1	340.3
65–74 years	315.9	324.2	334.2	319.6	294.9	296.8	280.9	262.8	257.3	253.9	264.2
75 years and over	489.1	511.4	529.3	520.1	476.5	470.5	451.6	436.5	433.6	430.0	443.5
Geographic region[3]											
Northeast	148.4	145.9	144.2	135.1	129.7	124.1	118.9	126.5	125.1	121.5	126.7
Midwest	176.4	176.0	167.9	156.7	143.5	139.8	135.3	120.2	116.8	114.7	110.3
South	166.2	165.2	167.7	159.5	143.4	136.3	127.9	118.9	119.0	119.1	119.4
West	138.0	138.2	139.6	132.3	131.0	127.8	128.6	103.6	98.3	92.6	94.7
	Days of care per 1,000 population										
Total[3]	1,136.5	1,101.7	1,068.8	960.1	877.1	833.1	808.7	754.8	732.2	709.5	710.0
Sex[3]											
Male	1,072.6	1,047.6	1,025.7	917.6	841.2	803.4	789.2	739.6	720.8	681.0	696.1
Female	1,201.7	1,157.7	1,115.7	1,005.8	914.7	865.0	831.1	772.6	746.6	738.7	727.5
Age											
Under 15 years	315.8	326.4	323.4	277.7	260.8	244.7	240.6	245.3	234.3	212.4	218.3
15–44 years	787.0	742.0	707.5	647.3	603.6	575.7	556.9	493.1	481.1	466.2	461.8
45–64 years	1,597.6	1,536.7	1,460.6	1,316.8	1,192.8	1,101.4	1,068.6	955.3	903.7	898.2	858.5
65 years and over	4,098.3	4,026.2	4,004.3	3,574.8	3,215.1	3,120.7	3,029.9	2,970.0	2,930.4	2,834.6	2,927.0
65–74 years	3,147.6	3,101.1	3,069.5	2,711.0	2,417.8	2,363.8	2,294.4	2,214.8	2,115.5	2,026.3	2,130.8
75 years and over	5,576.5	5,423.5	5,392.7	4,855.5	4,389.4	4,227.9	4,097.8	4,054.3	4,087.4	3,972.2	4,007.2
Geographic region[3]											
Northeast	1,217.3	1,149.8	1,115.6	1,012.3	963.1	877.6	847.1	928.7	918.1	887.2	887.5
Midwest	1,309.4	1,283.0	1,184.4	1,059.9	955.7	914.2	885.3	749.3	727.7	715.7	695.4
South	1,114.5	1,083.3	1,087.1	962.9	851.4	817.6	781.5	729.0	731.5	707.2	726.6
West	844.6	825.7	821.9	756.5	717.9	703.0	712.5	606.7	537.0	513.3	513.1
	Average length of stay in days										
Total[3]	7.1	7.0	6.8	6.5	6.4	6.3	6.3	6.4	6.3	6.3	6.3
Sex[3]											
Male	7.7	7.5	7.3	7.0	6.8	6.7	6.9	7.0	6.9	6.8	6.9
Female	6.7	6.6	6.4	6.1	6.0	5.9	5.9	5.9	5.9	5.8	5.8
Age											
Under 15 years	4.4	4.6	4.6	4.5	4.6	4.6	4.7	5.0	4.9	4.8	4.8
15–44 years	5.2	5.1	5.0	4.9	4.8	4.8	4.8	4.7	4.7	4.6	4.7
45–64 years	8.2	7.9	7.6	7.2	7.0	6.8	6.8	6.8	6.7	6.7	6.5
65 years and over	10.7	10.1	9.7	8.9	8.7	8.5	8.6	8.9	8.9	8.7	8.6
65–74 years	10.0	9.6	9.2	8.5	8.2	8.0	8.2	8.4	8.2	8.0	8.1
75 years and over	11.4	10.6	10.2	9.3	9.2	9.0	9.1	9.3	9.4	9.2	9.0
Geographic region[3]											
Northeast	8.2	7.9	7.7	7.5	7.4	7.1	7.1	7.3	7.3	7.3	7.0
Midwest	7.4	7.3	7.1	6.8	6.7	6.5	6.5	6.2	6.2	6.2	6.3
South	6.7	6.6	6.5	6.0	5.9	6.0	6.1	6.1	6.1	5.9	6.1
West	6.1	6.0	5.9	5.7	5.5	5.5	5.5	5.9	5.5	5.5	5.4

[1]Geographic data for 1980 are based on the civilian population as of April 1, 1980.
[2]Comparisons of data from 1988 through 1991 with data from earlier years should be made with caution as estimates of change may reflect improvements in the design (see Appendix I) rather than true changes in hospital use.
[3]Age adjusted.

NOTES: Excludes newborn infants. Rates are based on the civilian population as of July 1.

SOURCE: Centers for Disease Control and Prevention, National Center for Health Statistics, Division of Health Care Statistics: Data from the National Hospital Discharge Survey.

Table 85. Discharges, days of care, and average length of stay in nonfederal short-stay hospitals for discharges with the diagnosis of human immunodeficiency virus (HIV) and for all discharges: United States, 1984–91

[Data are based on a sample of hospital records]

Type of discharge, sex, age, and year	Discharges Number in thousands	Discharges Number per 1,000 population	Days of care Number in thousands	Days of care Number per 1,000 population	Average length of stay in days
Discharges with diagnosis of HIV					
Total:					
1984 [1]	10	0.04	123	0.52	12.1
1985 [1]	23	0.10	387	1.63	17.1
1986	44	0.18	714	2.98	16.4
1987	67	0.28	936	3.87	14.1
1988 [2]	95	0.39	1,277	5.23	13.4
1989 [2]	140	0.57	1,731	7.02	12.4
1990 [2]	146	0.59	2,188	8.77	14.9
1991 [2]	165	0.66	2,108	8.41	12.8
Male, 20–49 years:					
1984 [1]	*9	*0.17	*114	*2.26	*13.2
1985 [1]	21	0.41	355	6.90	16.8
1986	35	0.67	573	10.96	16.4
1987	51	0.97	724	13.64	14.1
1988 [2]	73	1.36	914	16.97	12.5
1989 [2]	102	1.87	1,235	22.64	12.1
1990 [2]	102	1.84	1,645	29.71	16.2
1991 [2]	111	1.97	1,407	25.01	12.7
Female, 20–49 years:					
1988	13	0.23	233	4.18	18.0
1989	19	0.34	201	3.56	10.6
1990	27	0.47	341	5.96	12.6
1991	33	0.56	454	7.86	14.0
All discharges					
Total:					
1984	37,162	158.5	244,652	1,043.6	6.6
1985	35,056	147.9	226,217	954.4	6.5
1986	34,256	143.1	218,496	912.8	6.4
1987	33,387	138.2	214,942	889.4	6.4
1988 [2]	31,146	127.6	203,678	834.3	6.5
1989 [2]	30,947	125.5	200,827	814.5	6.5
1990 [2]	30,788	123.5	197,422	791.7	6.4
1991 [2]	31,098	124.1	199,099	794.6	6.4
Male, 20–49 years:					
1984	4,497	89.5	27,725	551.5	6.2
1985	4,393	85.4	27,117	527.4	6.2
1986	4,300	82.2	26,488	506.4	6.2
1987	4,075	76.8	26,295	495.3	6.5
1988 [2]	3,670	68.2	22,697	421.6	6.2
1989 [2]	3,676	67.4	22,967	421.0	6.2
1990 [2]	3,649	65.9	22,539	407.0	6.2
1991 [2]	3,547	63.1	22,258	395.7	6.3
Female, 20–49 years:					
1988	8,169	146.5	34,800	623.9	4.3
1989	8,196	145.2	35,007	620.0	4.3
1990	8,228	143.8	34,473	602.3	4.2
1991	8,146	141.1	34,127	591.0	4.2

[1]During these years, only data for AIDS (ICD-9-CM 279.19) were reported.

[2]Comparisons of data from 1988 through 1991 with data from earlier years should be made with caution as estimates of change may reflect improvements in the design (see Appendix I) rather than true changes in hospital use.

*Statistics based on 5,000–9,000 estimated discharges are to be used with caution.

NOTES: Excludes newborn infants. Rates are based on the civilian population as of July 1. Data for years 1986–91 are tabulated for discharges with the diagnosis human immunodeficiency virus (HIV) (ICD-9-CM 042–044, 279.19, and 795.8) and differ from previous editions of Health, United States in which data for years 1986–89 were tabulated for discharges with the diagnosis acquired immunodeficiency syndrome (AIDS) (ICD-9-CM 042.0–042.2, 042.9, 279.19). Data for years 1984–85 are tabulated for discharges with diagnosis ICD-9-CM 279.19, as in previous editions.

SOURCES: Centers for Disease Control and Prevention, National Center for Health Statistics, Division of Health Care Statistics: Data from the National Hospital Discharge Survey; Utilization of short-stay hospitals by patients with AIDS: United States, 1984–1986, by E. J. Graves. Advance Data From Vital and Health Statistics. No. 156. DHHS Pub. No. (PHS) 88-1250. Public Health Service. Hyattsville, Md., 1988; Unpublished data.

Table 86 (page 1 of 2). Rates of discharges and days of care in nonfederal short-stay hospitals, according to sex, age, and selected first-listed diagnosis: United States, 1980, 1985, 1990, and 1991

[Data are based on a sample of hospital records]

Sex, age, and first-listed diagnosis	Discharges				Days of care			
	1980	1985	1990[1]	1991[1]	1980	1985	1990[1]	1991[1]
Both sexes	Number per 1,000 population							
Total[2,3]	159.1	138.0	113.1	113.6	1,136.5	877.1	709.5	710.0
Females with delivery	14.7	14.1	14.2	13.9	55.5	46.1	39.5	38.4
Diseases of heart	13.1	13.7	12.5	12.9	123.5	98.4	84.5	87.2
Malignant neoplasms	7.6	7.4	5.7	5.7	90.5	65.2	52.6	51.2
Pneumonia, all forms	3.5	3.6	4.0	4.0	27.7	26.5	30.8	31.1
Fracture, all sites	4.9	4.4	3.7	3.7	51.2	37.1	28.9	30.1
Male								
All ages[2,3]	140.1	123.5	99.6	101.3	1,072.6	841.2	681.0	696.1
Diseases of heart	15.9	16.8	15.4	16.0	145.0	116.9	102.6	106.3
Malignant neoplasms	8.2	7.8	5.9	6.3	98.7	71.1	55.8	60.2
Pneumonia, all forms	4.1	3.9	4.4	4.5	32.5	29.8	34.7	34.6
Fracture, all sites	5.2	4.7	3.7	3.8	46.9	35.3	24.2	27.7
Cerebrovascular diseases	3.5	3.6	2.8	2.9	41.9	36.0	26.2	26.3
Inguinal hernia	4.3	3.0	1.2	1.0	20.0	9.3	2.7	2.4
Under 15 years[3]	78.7	63.8	48.5	50.8	341.5	287.5	230.7	247.3
Pneumonia, all forms	5.2	4.3	4.3	4.2	25.2	18.1	18.9	17.7
Bronchitis, emphysema, and asthma	4.0	4.1	4.1	4.5	16.3	13.7	11.6	13.7
Acute respiratory infection	5.9	5.2	3.9	4.9	22.0	17.2	12.7	14.7
Congenital anomalies	4.0	3.8	2.6	2.7	22.2	20.5	14.8	16.6
Noninfectious enteritis and colitis	4.0	2.8	1.9	1.8	16.1	8.3	5.2	5.5
Otitis media and eustachian tube disorders	4.5	2.2	1.5	1.3	11.3	4.7	3.6	3.6
Chronic disease of tonsils and adenoids	5.4	3.5	1.0	0.9	9.2	5.1	1.3	1.1
15–44 years[3]	91.5	75.4	58.0	55.9	581.0	458.9	355.4	356.5
Fracture, all sites	6.3	5.3	4.2	4.0	50.1	34.7	23.0	24.2
Psychoses	3.0	3.7	3.8	4.3	39.2	47.4	52.4	55.1
Diseases of heart	2.9	3.0	2.9	2.5	21.7	16.6	15.5	13.9
Intervertebral disc disorders	2.3	2.9	2.4	2.3	20.7	18.7	10.0	9.5
Lacerations and open wounds	3.4	2.6	2.3	1.8	17.9	11.0	9.6	6.4
Alcohol dependence syndrome	3.5	3.5	2.1	2.0	33.4	38.8	20.1	19.0
45–64 years[3]	195.4	176.2	138.3	137.5	1,590.3	1,219.9	930.3	897.4
Diseases of heart	33.7	36.6	31.2	31.9	288.1	237.4	182.3	198.9
Malignant neoplasms	14.4	13.1	10.5	10.7	167.2	119.8	97.9	90.7
Cerebrovascular diseases	4.7	5.0	4.0	3.8	49.6	50.7	40.1	29.8
Intervertebral disc disorders	3.7	4.6	3.6	3.0	34.5	32.8	18.3	14.0
Psychoses	2.6	3.2	3.4	3.5	31.6	42.4	41.7	44.4
Alcohol dependence syndrome	6.4	4.5	2.3	2.2	67.8	43.4	21.5	16.8
Inguinal hernia	6.9	5.1	1.9	1.7	36.5	15.3	4.3	3.0
65 years and over[3]	411.8	393.2	346.2	368.1	4,244.0	3,315.0	2,882.8	3,056.5
Diseases of heart	78.5	82.6	80.2	86.5	786.3	626.9	602.4	611.2
Malignant neoplasms	46.2	44.4	31.8	35.6	587.9	418.4	316.0	369.9
Pneumonia, all forms	15.0	17.3	20.4	22.4	166.1	172.6	204.7	215.4
Cerebrovascular diseases	24.4	25.1	19.1	20.6	301.2	249.7	176.4	195.5
Hyperplasia of prostate	18.1	15.5	15.1	14.1	176.7	103.5	78.6	67.0
Female								
All ages[2,3]	178.1	152.7	126.9	126.5	1,201.7	914.7	738.7	727.5
Delivery	29.0	27.7	28.0	27.5	109.4	91.0	78.1	76.3
Diseases of heart	10.7	11.0	10.0	10.3	105.1	82.5	69.4	71.4
Malignant neoplasms	7.3	7.3	5.7	5.4	85.8	61.7	51.0	44.9
Pneumonia, all forms	3.0	3.2	3.6	3.7	24.0	24.3	27.9	28.4
Fracture, all sites	4.4	4.0	3.4	3.4	52.1	36.6	31.4	30.3
Pregnancy with abortive outcome	4.1	2.8	1.5	1.2	8.7	5.9	3.1	3.0
Under 15 years[3]	64.2	50.2	39.2	39.5	288.9	232.9	193.1	187.9
Pneumonia, all forms	3.6	3.6	3.4	3.6	17.7	16.4	15.8	14.3
Acute respiratory infection	4.6	3.6	2.8	3.0	16.0	11.3	9.4	9.8
Bronchitis, emphysema, and asthma	2.5	2.6	2.5	2.6	9.6	9.0	7.8	7.4
Congenital anomalies	3.2	1.9	1.7	1.8	19.4	11.3	9.9	13.9
Noninfectious enteritis and colitis	3.7	2.3	1.6	1.5	16.8	6.8	4.7	5.0
Chronic disease of tonsils and adenoids	6.4	3.7	1.4	1.0	11.2	6.0	1.8	1.1

See footnotes at end of table.

Table 86 (page 2 of 2). Rates of discharges and days of care in nonfederal short-stay hospitals, according to sex, age, and selected first-listed diagnosis: United States, 1980, 1985, 1990, and 1991

[Data are based on a sample of hospital records]

Sex, age, and first-listed diagnosis	Discharges				Days of care			
	1980	1985	1990[1]	1991[1]	1980	1985	1990[1]	1991[1]
Female — Con.	Number per 1,000 population							
15–44 years [3]	206.9	173.4	144.5	142.1	986.4	744.3	574.7	565.6
Delivery	70.7	67.8	68.4	67.2	264.5	222.4	190.8	186.5
Psychoses	2.4	3.4	3.9	4.0	36.7	52.3	56.9	54.0
Pregnancy with abortive outcome	9.9	6.7	3.5	3.0	21.2	14.4	7.4	7.3
Cholelithiasis	2.6	2.4	2.9	2.7	19.5	14.4	11.9	13.0
Benign neoplasms	4.8	3.4	2.8	2.9	25.7	17.2	11.2	11.0
Inflammatory disease of female pelvic organs	5.1	3.7	2.2	2.0	25.7	17.7	9.0	7.8
Disorders of menstruation	6.6	2.6	1.2	1.3	21.6	9.7	3.9	4.3
45–64 years [3]	194.3	163.4	128.2	127.2	1,604.1	1,168.1	868.5	822.4
Diseases of heart	17.8	17.9	16.3	15.6	152.9	120.5	98.9	98.3
Malignant neoplasms	16.6	15.6	12.7	10.7	190.8	129.6	106.3	85.4
Cholelithiasis	4.7	4.4	4.7	5.2	42.9	30.9	26.5	20.5
Benign neoplasms	6.7	5.1	4.4	4.1	44.8	32.0	21.6	18.9
Psychoses	3.1	4.1	4.2	4.5	50.6	70.5	62.0	62.9
Diabetes	6.3	3.8	2.9	2.9	63.5	31.4	25.3	22.6
65 years and over [3]	364.7	351.4	313.8	321.6	3,999.8	3,147.1	2,801.4	2,839.6
Diseases of heart	64.8	68.1	62.3	66.1	701.1	551.3	472.9	480.0
Malignant neoplasms	28.5	28.1	21.5	22.6	383.8	280.6	219.1	221.8
Cerebrovascular diseases	21.6	23.3	19.4	19.9	287.9	249.3	187.4	196.0
Fracture, all sites	19.2	19.3	18.7	18.2	309.5	232.5	211.0	208.5
Pneumonia, all forms	9.7	11.8	15.1	16.0	109.2	116.9	157.8	171.3
Eye diseases and conditions	16.4	8.2	3.1	4.0	67.3	21.0	6.3	7.2

[1]Comparisons of data from 1988 through 1991 with data from earlier years should be made with caution as estimates of change may reflect improvements in the design (see Appendix I) rather than true changes in hospital use.
[2]Age adjusted.
[3]Includes discharges with first-listed diagnoses not shown in table.

NOTES: Excludes newborn infants. Rates are based on the civilian population as of July 1. In each sex and age group, data are shown for diagnoses with the five highest discharge rates in 1980 and 1990. Diagnostic categories are based on the International Classification of Diseases, 9th Revision, Clinical Modification. For a listing of the code numbers, see Appendix II, table VII.

SOURCE: Centers for Disease Control and Prevention, National Center for Health Statistics, Division of Health Care Statistics: Data from the National Hospital Discharge Survey.

Table 87 (page 1 of 2). Discharges and average length of stay in nonfederal short-stay hospitals, according to sex, age, and selected first-listed diagnosis: United States, 1980, 1985, 1990, and 1991

[Data are based on a sample of hospital records]

Sex, age, and first-listed diagnosis	Discharges				Average length of stay			
	1980	1985	1990 [1]	1991 [1]	1980	1985	1990 [1]	1991 [1]
Both sexes	Number in thousands				Number of days			
Total [2]	37,832	35,056	30,788	31,098	7.3	6.5	6.4	6.4
Females with delivery	3,762	3,854	4,025	3,973	3.8	3.3	2.8	2.8
Diseases of heart	3,201	3,584	3,556	3,704	9.5	7.3	6.9	6.8
Malignant neoplasms	1,829	1,911	1,571	1,594	12.0	8.9	9.4	9.2
Pneumonia, all forms	782	854	1,052	1,088	8.3	7.9	8.3	8.2
Fracture, all sites	1,163	1,129	1,017	1,034	10.8	8.7	8.3	8.4
Male								
All ages [2]	15,145	14,160	12,280	12,478	7.7	6.9	6.9	7.0
Diseases of heart	1,688	1,910	1,913	1,977	9.1	7.0	6.7	6.7
Malignant neoplasms	875	892	730	781	12.0	9.1	9.5	9.7
Pneumonia, all forms	414	433	530	545	8.2	7.8	8.2	7.9
Fracture, all sites	582	550	466	481	9.0	7.7	6.7	7.3
Cerebrovascular diseases	371	416	359	370	12.1	10.0	9.2	9.1
Inguinal hernia	458	343	149	120	4.7	3.1	2.2	2.4
Under 15 years [2]	2,063	1,698	1,362	1,435	4.3	4.5	4.8	4.9
Pneumonia, all forms	136	115	119	118	4.9	4.2	4.4	4.2
Bronchitis, emphysema, and asthma	105	110	115	128	4.0	3.3	2.8	3.0
Acute respiratory infection	154	138	111	138	3.8	3.3	3.2	3.0
Congenital anomalies	106	101	74	76	5.5	5.4	5.6	6.2
Noninfectious enteritis and colitis	106	74	52	50	4.0	3.0	2.8	3.1
Otitis media and eustachian tube disorders	118	59	41	38	2.5	2.1	2.5	2.7
Chronic disease of tonsils and adenoids	141	92	29	25	1.7	1.5	1.3	1.3
15–44 years [2]	4,687	4,153	3,330	3,248	6.3	6.1	6.1	6.4
Fracture, all sites	320	290	238	230	8.0	6.6	5.5	6.1
Psychoses	155	204	220	252	12.9	12.8	13.6	12.7
Diseases of heart	149	165	166	145	7.5	5.5	5.3	5.5
Intervertebral disc disorders	120	161	138	135	8.8	6.4	4.2	4.1
Lacerations and open wounds	176	143	134	102	5.2	4.2	4.1	3.7
Alcohol dependence syndrome	180	195	118	114	9.5	11.0	9.8	9.7
45–64 years [2]	4,127	3,776	3,115	3,088	8.1	6.9	6.7	6.5
Diseases of heart	712	784	704	716	8.5	6.5	5.8	6.2
Malignant neoplasms	304	281	236	239	11.6	9.1	9.3	8.5
Cerebrovascular diseases	99	107	91	86	10.6	10.2	10.0	7.8
Intervertebral disc disorders	78	98	82	67	9.4	7.2	5.0	4.7
Psychoses	55	69	76	80	12.1	13.1	12.4	12.5
Alcohol dependence syndrome	134	97	51	49	10.7	9.6	9.5	7.8
Inguinal hernia	146	110	42	38	5.3	3.0	2.3	1.7
65 years and over [2]	4,268	4,533	4,472	4,708	10.3	8.4	8.3	8.3
Diseases of heart	814	953	1,036	1,107	10.0	7.6	7.5	7.1
Malignant neoplasms	479	512	411	455	12.7	9.4	9.9	10.4
Pneumonia, all forms	156	199	264	286	11.1	10.0	10.0	9.6
Cerebrovascular diseases	253	289	247	263	12.3	9.9	9.2	9.5
Hyperplasia of prostate	188	179	195	180	9.8	6.7	5.2	4.8
Female								
All ages [2]	22,686	20,896	18,508	18,620	7.0	6.2	6.1	6.0
Delivery	3,762	3,854	4,025	3,973	3.8	3.3	2.8	2.8
Diseases of heart	1,513	1,674	1,643	1,727	10.0	7.6	7.1	7.0
Malignant neoplasms	954	1,019	841	812	12.0	8.7	9.2	8.7
Pneumonia, all forms	368	421	522	543	8.4	8.1	8.4	8.5
Fracture, all sites	580	579	551	553	12.6	9.8	9.7	9.4
Pregnancy with abortive outcome	531	382	208	180	2.1	2.1	2.1	2.4

See footnotes at end of table.

Table 87 (page 2 of 2). Discharges and average length of stay in nonfederal short-stay hospitals, according to sex, age, and selected first-listed diagnosis: United States, 1980, 1985, 1990, and 1991

[Data are based on a sample of hospital records]

Sex, age, and first-listed diagnosis	Discharges				Average length of stay			
	1980	1985	1990[1]	1991[1]	1980	1985	1990[1]	1991[1]
Female—Con.	Number in thousands				Number of days			
Under 15 years[2]	1,609	1,274	1,049	1,064	4.5	4.6	4.9	4.8
Pneumonia, all forms	91	91	92	96	4.9	4.6	4.6	4.0
Acute respiratory infection	115	91	75	82	3.5	3.2	3.4	3.2
Bronchitis, emphysema, and asthma	63	65	68	69	3.8	3.5	3.1	2.9
Congenital anomalies	80	49	46	48	6.1	5.9	5.8	7.8
Noninfectious enteritis and colitis	92	59	43	41	4.6	2.9	3.0	3.3
Chronic disease of tonsils and adenoids	160	94	38	28	1.8	1.6	1.2	1.1
15–44 years[2]	10,949	9,813	8,469	8,372	4.8	4.3	4.0	4.0
Delivery	3,741	3,838	4,008	3,956	3.7	3.3	2.8	2.8
Psychoses	129	192	228	236	15.1	15.4	14.6	13.5
Pregnancy with abortive outcome	525	378	205	178	2.1	2.2	2.1	2.4
Cholelithiasis	138	133	169	159	7.5	6.1	4.1	4.8
Benign neoplasms	253	194	163	173	5.4	5.0	4.0	3.8
Inflammatory disease of female pelvic organs	268	210	130	115	5.1	4.8	4.1	4.0
Disorders of menstruation	347	148	70	74	3.3	3.7	3.3	3.4
45–64 years[2]	4,533	3,834	3,129	3,085	8.3	7.1	6.8	6.5
Diseases of heart	415	420	397	379	8.6	6.7	6.1	6.3
Malignant neoplasms	387	367	309	260	11.5	8.3	8.4	8.0
Cholelithiasis	109	103	114	127	9.2	7.1	5.7	3.9
Benign neoplasms	156	120	107	100	6.7	6.3	4.9	4.6
Psychoses	72	95	103	109	16.3	17.4	14.6	13.9
Diabetes	148	88	70	70	10.0	8.3	8.9	7.8
65 years and over[2]	5,596	5,975	5,861	6,098	11.0	9.0	8.9	8.8
Diseases of heart	995	1,158	1,164	1,254	10.8	8.1	7.6	7.3
Malignant neoplasms	437	478	401	428	13.5	10.0	10.2	9.8
Cerebrovascular diseases	331	396	362	377	13.3	10.7	9.7	9.9
Fracture, all sites	295	328	350	346	16.1	12.1	11.3	11.4
Pneumonia, all forms	150	201	283	303	11.2	9.9	10.4	10.7
Eye diseases and conditions	251	140	58	75	4.1	2.5	2.0	1.8

[1]Comparisons of data from 1988 through 1991 with data from earlier years should be made with caution as estimates of change may reflect improvements in the design (see Appendix I) rather than true changes in hospital use.
[2]Includes discharges with first-listed diagnoses not shown in table.

NOTES: Excludes newborn infants. In each sex and age group, data are shown for diagnoses with the five highest discharge rates in 1980 and 1990. Diagnostic categories are based on the International Classification of Diseases, 9th Revision, Clinical Modification. For a listing of the code numbers, see Appendix II, table VII.

SOURCE: Centers for Disease Control and Prevention, National Center for Health Statistics, Division of Health Care Statistics: Data from the National Hospital Discharge Survey.

Table 88 (page 1 of 2). Operations for inpatients discharged from nonfederal short-stay hospitals, according to sex, age, and surgical category: United States, 1980, 1985, 1990, and 1991

[Data are based on a sample of hospital records]

Sex, age, and surgical category	Operations in thousands				Operations per 1,000 population			
	1980	1985	1990[1]	1991[1]	1980	1985	1990[1]	1991[1]
Male								
All ages [2,3,4]	8,505	8,805	8,538	8,692	78.1	76.3	68.8	70.1
Cardiac catheterization	228	439	620	603	2.2	3.9	5.2	5.1
Prostatectomy	335	367	364	363	3.1	3.2	2.8	2.8
Reduction of fracture (excluding skull, nose, and jaw)	325	339	300	337	2.9	2.8	2.4	2.7
Direct heart revascularization (coronary bypass)	108	172	286	296	1.0	1.6	2.4	2.5
Excision or destruction of intervertebral disc and spinal fusion	118	191	248	258	1.1	1.6	2.0	2.0
Repair of inguinal hernia	483	370	181	155	4.6	3.3	1.5	1.3
Operations on muscles, tendons, fascia, and bursa	210	194	175	175	1.9	1.7	1.4	1.4
Under 15 years [2,4]	1,068	831	598	617	40.7	31.3	21.3	21.9
Reduction of fracture (excluding skull, nose, and jaw)	55	57	42	58	2.1	2.1	1.5	2.1
Appendectomy, excluding incidental [5]	43	41	40	33	1.6	1.5	1.4	1.2
Tonsillectomy, with or without adenoidectomy	138	97	33	27	5.3	3.6	1.2	1.0
Myringotomy	115	53	30	25	4.4	2.0	1.1	0.9
Circumcision	43	31	24	21	1.6	1.2	0.8	0.7
Repair of inguinal hernia	86	46	19	23	3.3	1.7	0.7	0.8
15–44 years [2,4]	2,900	2,717	2,257	2,241	56.6	49.4	39.3	38.6
Reduction of fracture (excluding skull, nose, and jaw)	188	187	159	167	3.7	3.4	2.8	2.9
Excision or destruction of intervertebral disc and spinal fusion	67	119	147	147	1.3	2.2	2.6	2.5
Operations on muscles, tendons, fascia, and bursa	110	100	93	81	2.2	1.8	1.6	1.4
Debridement of wound, infection, or burn	75	75	82	80	1.5	1.4	1.4	1.4
Appendectomy, excluding incidental [5]	85	88	80	82	1.7	1.6	1.4	1.4
Repair of inguinal hernia	127	91	37	28	2.5	1.7	0.7	0.5
Excision of semilunar cartilage of knee	94	48	25	29	1.8	0.9	0.4	0.5
45–64 years [2,4]	2,313	2,494	2,499	2,486	109.5	116.4	110.9	110.7
Cardiac catheterization	129	241	306	296	6.1	11.3	13.6	13.2
Direct heart revascularization (coronary bypass)	72	102	132	135	3.4	4.8	5.9	6.0
Excision or destruction of intervertebral disc and spinal fusion	43	60	80	79	2.1	2.8	3.6	3.5
Prostatectomy	83	81	80	68	3.9	3.8	3.5	3.0
Repair of inguinal hernia	152	116	50	47	7.2	5.4	2.2	2.1
Operations on muscles, tendons, fascia, and bursa	58	50	44	47	2.8	2.3	2.0	2.1
65 years and over [2,4]	2,224	2,762	3,184	3,348	214.6	239.5	246.5	261.8
Prostatectomy	251	284	284	295	24.2	24.7	22.0	23.1
Cardiac catheterization	52	126	236	235	5.0	10.9	18.3	18.4
Direct heart revascularization (coronary bypass)	27	57	137	144	2.6	5.0	10.6	11.3
Pacemaker insertion or replacement	75	82	100	117	7.3	7.1	7.7	9.1
Biopsies on the digestive system	61	107	76	89	5.9	9.3	5.9	6.9
Repair of inguinal hernia	119	116	74	57	11.4	10.1	5.8	4.5
Extraction of lens	124	53	18	20	12.0	4.6	1.4	1.6
Female								
All ages [2,3,4]	15,989	15,994	14,513	14,711	126.1	117.2	100.3	100.7
Procedures to assist delivery [2]	2,391	2,494	2,491	2,558	18.4	18.0	17.3	17.7
Cesarean section [6]	619	877	945	933	4.8	6.3	6.6	6.5
Repair of current obstetrical laceration	355	548	795	795	2.8	3.9	5.5	5.5
Hysterectomy	649	670	591	546	5.2	5.0	4.3	3.9
Oophorectomy and salpingo-oophorectomy	483	525	476	458	3.9	4.0	3.4	3.3
Bilateral destruction or occlusion of fallopian tubes	641	466	419	401	4.9	3.3	2.9	2.8
Diagnostic dilation and curettage of uterus	923	349	109	100	7.3	2.6	0.8	0.7
Under 15 years [2,4]	771	553	413	414	30.8	21.8	15.4	15.4
Tonsillectomy, with or without adenoidectomy	156	100	41	27	6.2	3.9	1.5	1.0
Appendectomy, excluding incidental [5]	34	28	26	24	1.4	1.1	1.0	0.9
Myringotomy	87	36	22	18	3.5	1.4	0.8	0.7
Reduction of fracture (excluding skull, nose, and jaw)	32	33	18	26	1.3	1.3	0.7	1.0
Operations on muscles, tendons, fascia, and bursa	23	11	11	14	0.9	0.5	0.4	0.5
Adenoidectomy without tonsillectomy	31	*7	*	*	1.2	*0.3	*	*

See footnotes at end of table.

Table 88 (page 2 of 2). **Operations for inpatients discharged from nonfederal short-stay hospitals, according to sex, age, and surgical category: United States, 1980, 1985, 1990, and 1991**

[Data are based on a sample of hospital records]

Sex, age, and surgical category	Operations in thousands				Operations per 1,000 population			
	1980	1985	1990 [1]	1991 [1]	1980	1985	1990 [1]	1991 [1]
Female—Con.								
15–44 years [2,4]	9,625	9,340	8,129	8,159	181.9	165.0	138.7	138.5
Procedures to assist delivery [2]	2,381	2,483	2,480	2,546	45.0	43.9	42.3	43.2
Cesarean section [6]	614	875	940	931	11.6	15.5	16.0	15.8
Repair of current obstetrical laceration	352	546	793	792	6.7	9.6	13.5	13.4
Bilateral destruction or occlusion of fallopian tubes	632	461	418	400	11.9	8.1	7.1	6.8
Hysterectomy	402	421	349	322	7.6	7.4	6.0	5.5
Diagnostic dilation and curettage of uterus	625	232	67	64	11.8	4.1	1.1	1.1
45–64 years [2,4]	3,113	2,893	2,586	2,526	133.4	123.3	106.0	104.2
Hysterectomy	203	190	184	161	8.7	8.1	7.5	6.6
Oophorectomy and salpingo-oophorectomy	162	165	160	150	7.0	7.0	6.5	6.2
Cardiac catheterization	58	108	151	151	2.5	4.6	6.2	6.2
Cholecystectomy	107	104	118	132	4.6	4.4	4.8	5.4
Excision or destruction of intervertebral disc and spinal fusion	33	48	67	66	1.4	2.0	2.8	2.7
Diagnostic dilation and curettage of uterus	241	83	31	21	10.3	3.5	1.3	0.9
Biopsies on the integumentary system (breast, skin, and subcutaneous tissue)	69	48	25	18	2.9	2.1	1.0	0.7
65 years and over [2,4]	2,480	3,208	3,385	3,612	161.6	188.7	181.3	190.5
Cardiac catheterization	32	101	185	211	2.1	6.0	9.9	11.1
Reduction of fracture (excluding skull, nose, and jaw)	127	163	171	174	8.3	9.6	9.1	9.2
Arthroplasty and replacement of hip	72	108	128	124	4.7	6.4	6.9	6.5
Biopsies on the digestive system	72	140	99	107	4.7	8.2	5.3	5.6
Pacemaker insertion or replacement	70	86	99	128	4.6	5.0	5.3	6.7
Cholecystectomy	83	89	83	115	5.4	5.2	4.5	6.1
Extraction of lens	211	104	33	48	13.8	6.1	1.8	2.5
Insertion of prosthetic lens (pseudophakos)	93	92	31	45	6.1	5.4	1.7	2.4

[1]Comparisons of data from 1988 through 1991 with data from earlier years should be made with caution as estimates of change may reflect improvements in the design (see Appendix I) rather than true changes in hospital use.

[2]Beginning in 1989, the definition of some surgical and diagnostic and other nonsurgical procedures was revised, thus causing a discontinuity in the trends for the totals and selected surgical procedures. See Appendix II.

[3]Rates are age adjusted.

[4]Includes operations not listed in table.

[5]Limited to estimated number of appendectomies, excluding those performed incidental to other abdominal surgery.

[6]Cesarean sections accounted for 16.5 percent of all deliveries in 1980, 22.7 percent in 1985, and 23.5 percent in 1990 and 1991.

*Statistics based on fewer than 5,000 estimated discharges are not shown; those based on 5,000–9,000 estimated discharges are to be used with caution.

NOTES: Excludes newborn infants. Data do not reflect total use of operations because operations for outpatients are not included in the National Hospital Discharge Survey. In recent years, for example, lens extractions and myringotomies are frequently performed on outpatients. Rates are based on the civilian population as of July 1. In each sex and age group, data are shown for the five most common operations in 1980 and 1990. Surgical categories are based on the International Classification of Diseases, 9th Revision, Clinical Modification. For a listing of the code numbers, see Appendix II, table VIII.

SOURCE: Centers for Disease Control and Prevention, National Center for Health Statistics, Division of Health Care Statistics: Data from the National Hospital Discharge Survey.

Table 89 (page 1 of 2). Diagnostic and other nonsurgical procedures for inpatients discharged from nonfederal short-stay hospitals, according to sex, age, and procedure category: United States, 1980, 1985, 1990, and 1991

[Data are based on a sample of hospital records]

Sex, age, and procedure category	Procedures in thousands				Procedures per 1,000 population			
	1980	1985	1990[1]	1991[1]	1980	1985	1990[1]	1991[1]
Male								
All ages [2,3,4]	3,386	5,889	7,378	8,572	31.3	51.1	59.6	69.4
Angiocardiography using contrast material	174	431	833	804	1.6	3.9	6.9	6.7
Computerized axial tomography (CAT scan)	152	671	736	702	1.4	5.8	5.8	5.6
Diagnostic ultrasound	114	478	667	652	1.0	4.1	5.4	5.3
Cystoscopy	543	461	350	314	5.1	4.0	2.7	2.5
Radioisotope scan	236	375	268	228	2.1	3.3	2.1	1.8
Arteriography using contrast material	180	262	217	185	1.7	2.3	1.7	1.5
Endoscopy of large intestine without biopsy	228	259	148	153	2.1	2.2	1.2	1.2
Under 15 years [2,4]	217	297	546	687	8.3	11.1	19.4	24.3
Spinal tap	39	62	94	106	1.5	2.3	3.4	3.7
Diagnostic ultrasound	*6	23	47	40	*0.2	0.9	1.7	1.4
Computerized axial tomography (CAT scan)	17	35	41	43	0.7	1.3	1.5	1.5
Electroencephalogram	*5	19	17	20	*0.2	0.7	0.6	0.7
Radioisotope scan	*8	*9	11	*8	*0.3	*0.4	0.4	*0.3
Application of cast or splint	21	16	10	13	0.8	0.6	0.4	0.5
Cystoscopy	23	11	*	*6	0.9	0.4	*	*0.2
15–44 years [2,4]	884	1,294	1,584	1,880	17.3	23.5	27.6	32.4
Computerized axial tomography (CAT scan)	37	174	215	208	0.7	3.2	3.8	3.6
Diagnostic ultrasound	25	96	118	114	0.5	1.7	2.1	2.0
Angiocardiography using contrast material	30	55	102	93	0.6	1.0	1.8	1.6
Contrast myelogram	88	130	58	42	1.7	2.4	1.0	0.7
Endoscopy of small intestine without biopsy	38	61	57	54	0.7	1.1	1.0	0.9
Arthroscopy of knee	94	75	43	44	1.8	1.4	0.7	0.8
Cystoscopy	80	47	35	31	1.6	0.9	0.6	0.5
Application of cast or splint	54	30	22	15	1.1	0.6	0.4	0.3
Endoscopy of large intestine without biopsy	52	54	21	23	1.0	1.0	0.4	0.4
45–64 years [2,4]	1,128	1,866	2,106	2,359	53.4	87.1	93.5	105.0
Angiocardiography using contrast material	106	251	428	392	5.0	11.7	19.0	17.4
Diagnostic ultrasound	41	146	184	171	1.9	6.8	8.1	7.6
Computerized axial tomography (CAT scan)	43	182	170	156	2.0	8.5	7.5	7.0
Radioisotope scan	75	121	81	66	3.5	5.7	3.6	2.9
Cystoscopy	153	114	80	69	7.3	5.3	3.6	3.1
Arteriography using contrast material	76	94	65	63	3.6	4.4	2.9	2.8
Endoscopy of large intestine without biopsy	86	76	42	36	4.0	3.5	1.9	1.6
65 years and over [2,4]	1,158	2,432	3,143	3,646	111.8	211.0	243.3	285.1
Diagnostic ultrasound	42	213	319	327	4.0	18.4	24.7	25.6
Computerized axial tomography (CAT scan)	54	280	309	294	5.2	24.3	23.9	23.0
Angiocardiography using contrast material	35	123	297	312	3.4	10.7	23.0	24.4
Cystoscopy	287	288	232	209	27.7	25.0	18.0	16.3
Radioisotope scan	105	177	129	104	10.1	15.4	10.0	8.1
Arteriography using contrast material	72	135	109	89	7.0	11.7	8.4	7.0
Endoscopy of large intestine without biopsy	86	126	84	94	8.3	10.9	6.5	7.3
Female								
All ages [2,3,4]	3,532	6,072	10,077	11,947	27.5	43.3	68.0	79.8
Diagnostic ultrasound	204	756	941	940	1.6	5.4	6.2	6.2
Computerized axial tomography (CAT scan)	154	707	770	757	1.2	4.9	4.9	4.9
Angiocardiography using contrast material	84	219	510	562	0.7	1.6	3.5	3.7
Radioisotope scan	289	463	335	311	2.1	3.2	2.1	2.0
Endoscopy of small intestine without biopsy	164	281	294	270	1.3	2.0	1.9	1.7
Endoscopy of large intestine without biopsy	307	331	250	243	2.3	2.3	1.5	1.5
Laparoscopy (excluding that for ligation and division of fallopian tubes)	235	209	147	292	1.8	1.5	1.0	2.1
Cystoscopy	324	184	135	113	2.6	1.3	0.9	0.7

See footnotes at end of table.

Table 89 (page 2 of 2). Diagnostic and other nonsurgical procedures for inpatients discharged from nonfederal short-stay hospitals, according to sex, age, and procedure category: United States, 1980, 1985, 1990, and 1991

[Data are based on a sample of hospital records]

Sex, age, and procedure category	Procedures in thousands				Procedures per 1,000 population			
	1980	1985	1990[1]	1991[1]	1980	1985	1990[1]	1991[1]
Female—Con.								
Under 15 years [2,4]	191	256	403	517	7.6	10.1	15.0	19.2
Spinal tap	26	50	71	77	1.0	2.0	2.7	2.9
Diagnostic ultrasound	*5	25	43	34	*0.2	1.0	1.6	1.2
Computerized axial tomography (CAT scan)	10	33	27	26	0.4	1.3	1.0	1.0
Electroencephalogram	*	15	14	14	*	0.6	0.5	0.5
Radioisotope scan	*6	*8	*9	*8	*0.2	*0.3	*0.3	*0.3
Application of cast or splint	13	*6	*6	*7	0.5	*0.2	*0.2	*0.3
Cystoscopy	38	*8	*	*	1.5	*0.3	*	*
15–44 years [2,4]	1,203	1,606	4,217	4,811	22.7	28.4	72.0	81.7
Diagnostic ultrasound	94	283	309	311	1.8	5.0	5.3	5.3
Computerized axial tomography (CAT scan)	36	137	144	152	0.7	2.4	2.5	2.6
Laparoscopy (excluding that for ligation and division of fallopian tubes)	214	197	120	181	4.1	3.5	2.0	3.1
Biliary tract x ray	60	90	102	61	1.1	1.6	1.7	1.0
Radioisotope scan	49	83	58	54	0.9	1.5	1.0	0.9
Cystoscopy	97	51	39	32	1.8	0.9	0.7	0.5
Contrast myelogram	66	96	36	30	1.2	1.7	0.6	0.5
Endoscopy of large intestine without biopsy	77	58	34	34	1.5	1.0	0.6	0.6
45–64 years [2,4]	1,030	1,584	1,861	2,153	44.2	67.5	76.3	88.8
Angiocardiography using contrast material	49	105	214	224	2.1	4.5	8.8	9.2
Diagnostic ultrasound	44	154	174	184	1.9	6.6	7.1	7.6
Computerized axial tomography (CAT scan)	42	167	163	171	1.8	7.1	6.7	7.1
Radioisotope scan	92	128	79	82	3.9	5.5	3.2	3.4
Endoscopy of small intestine without biopsy	55	78	71	66	2.3	3.3	2.9	2.7
Endoscopy of large intestine without biopsy	94	89	59	54	4.0	3.8	2.4	2.2
Cystoscopy	93	48	37	27	4.0	2.1	1.5	1.1
65 years and over [2,4]	1,107	2,626	3,596	4,466	72.1	154.4	192.6	235.5
Computerized axial tomography (CAT scan)	66	370	436	408	4.3	21.8	23.3	21.5
Diagnostic ultrasound	62	294	415	412	4.0	17.3	22.2	21.7
Angiocardiography using contrast material	21	90	245	292	1.4	5.3	13.1	15.4
Radioisotope scan	143	244	189	167	9.3	14.4	10.1	8.8
Endoscopy of small intestine without biopsy	55	133	168	153	3.6	7.8	9.0	8.1
Endoscopy of large intestine without biopsy	131	181	156	153	8.5	10.7	8.4	8.1
Cystoscopy	96	77	56	51	6.2	4.5	3.0	2.7

[1]Comparisons of data from 1988 through 1991 with data from earlier years should be made with caution as estimates of change may reflect improvements in the design (see Appendix I) rather than true changes in hospital use.
[2]Beginning in 1989, the definition of some surgical and diagnostic and other nonsurgical procedures was revised, thus causing a discontinuity in the trends for the totals. See Appendix II.
[3]Rates are age adjusted.
[4]Includes nonsurgical procedures not shown.

*Statistics based on fewer than 5,000 estimated discharges are not shown; those based on 5,000–9,000 estimated discharges are to be used with caution.

NOTES: Excludes newborn infants. Data do not reflect total use of procedures because procedures for outpatients are not included in the National Hospital Discharge Survey. For example, CAT scans are frequently performed on outpatients. Rates are based on the civilian population as of July 1. In each sex and age group, data are shown for the five most common procedures in 1980 and 1990. Procedure categories are based on the International Classification of Diseases, 9th Revision, Clinical Modification. For a listing of the code numbers, see Appendix II, table IX.

SOURCE: Centers for Disease Control and Prevention, National Center for Health Statistics, Division of Health Care Statistics: Data from the National Hospital Discharge Survey.

Table 90. Admissions, average length of stay, outpatient visits, and percent outpatient surgery in short-stay hospitals, according to type of ownership and size of hospital: United States, selected years 1960–91

[Data are based on reporting by a census of hospitals]

Type of ownership and size of hospital	1960	1970	1975	1980	1985	1987	1988	1989	1990	1991
Admissions					Number in thousands					
All ownerships	24,324	30,706	35,270	38,140	35,478	33,592	33,233	32,842	32,849	32,634
Federal	1,354	1,454	1,751	1,942	1,977	1,959	1,753	1,701	1,646	1,551
Nonfederal	22,970	29,252	33,519	36,198	33,501	31,633	31,480	31,141	31,203	31,084
Nonprofit	16,788	20,948	23,735	25,576	24,188	22,946	22,946	22,798	22,883	22,968
Proprietary	1,550	2,031	2,646	3,165	3,242	3,157	3,090	3,071	3,066	3,016
State-local government	4,632	6,273	7,138	7,458	6,071	5,530	5,444	5,271	5,254	5,100
Size of hospital:										
6–99 beds	- - -	- - -	5,639	5,436	4,311	3,968	3,871	3,784	3,704	3,598
100–199 beds	- - -	- - -	7,276	7,452	6,713	6,244	6,196	6,232	6,135	6,099
200–299 beds	- - -	- - -	6,287	6,789	6,484	6,403	6,480	6,472	6,601	6,463
300–499 beds	- - -	- - -	8,795	10,137	9,620	9,016	8,885	8,845	8,944	9,102
500 beds or more	- - -	- - -	7,274	8,327	8,348	7,961	7,802	7,509	7,465	7,374
Average length of stay					Number of days					
All ownerships	8.4	8.7	8.0	7.8	7.3	7.4	7.5	7.5	7.5	7.4
Federal	21.4	17.0	14.4	12.9	11.6	11.3	12.5	12.1	12.3	12.7
Nonfederal	7.6	8.2	7.7	7.6	7.1	7.2	7.2	7.3	7.3	7.2
Nonprofit	7.4	8.2	7.8	7.7	7.2	7.2	7.2	7.3	7.3	7.2
Proprietary	5.7	6.8	6.6	6.5	6.1	6.3	6.2	6.3	6.4	6.3
State-local government	8.8	8.7	7.6	7.4	7.2	7.6	7.6	7.7	7.8	7.8
Size of hospital:										
6–99 beds	- - -	- - -	6.5	6.3	6.0	6.4	6.5	6.6	6.7	6.8
100–199 beds	- - -	- - -	7.2	7.1	6.7	6.9	6.9	7.0	7.1	7.0
200–299 beds	- - -	- - -	7.6	7.5	6.9	7.0	7.1	7.0	7.0	7.0
300–499 beds	- - -	- - -	8.2	8.0	7.3	7.3	7.4	7.4	7.3	7.2
500 beds or more	- - -	- - -	10.2	9.6	8.8	8.8	9.0	8.9	8.9	8.9
Outpatient visits [1]					Number in thousands					
All ownerships	- - -	173,058	245,938	255,320	272,833	300,960	326,575	342,618	358,833	377,922
Federal	- - -	39,514	49,627	48,568	50,059	53,256	55,139	54,709	56,142	54,720
Nonfederal	- - -	133,545	196,311	206,752	222,773	247,704	271,436	287,909	302,691	323,202
Nonprofit	- - -	90,992	132,368	142,864	160,002	178,089	195,864	209,641	221,175	238,305
Proprietary	- - -	4,698	7,713	9,696	12,378	16,566	17,926	19,341	20,110	21,174
State-local government	- - -	37,854	56,230	54,192	50,394	53,049	57,646	58,926	61,407	63,723
Size of hospital:										
6–99 beds	- - -	- - -	41,346	41,875	41,813	48,273	52,294	53,875	55,780	57,303
100–199 beds	- - -	- - -	40,433	45,686	50,542	57,267	63,663	67,736	70,229	75,187
200–299 beds	- - -	- - -	38,122	41,119	45,805	50,626	56,570	62,975	67,529	71,250
300–499 beds	- - -	- - -	63,019	65,550	68,664	73,369	78,569	82,532	87,585	92,250
500 beds or more	- - -	- - -	63,019	61,089	66,008	71,426	75,480	75,499	77,709	81,934
Outpatient surgery					Percent of total surgeries [2]					
All ownerships	- - -	- - -	- - -	16.4	34.5	44.2	46.9	48.7	50.6	52.1
Federal	- - -	- - -	- - -	18.9	34.0	49.3	49.0	51.3	51.8	47.8
Nonfederal	- - -	- - -	- - -	16.3	34.5	43.9	46.8	48.5	50.5	52.3
Nonprofit	- - -	- - -	- - -	17.1	35.5	44.3	47.0	48.6	50.7	52.5
Proprietary	- - -	- - -	- - -	14.3	34.1	47.3	50.5	52.5	54.7	55.1
State-local government	- - -	- - -	- - -	13.6	29.7	39.3	43.1	45.0	46.5	48.7
Size of hospital:										
6–99 beds	- - -	- - -	- - -	17.8	36.5	49.4	52.8	54.1	56.4	58.7
100–199 beds	- - -	- - -	- - -	15.4	36.4	47.1	50.2	52.4	54.9	56.5
200–299 beds	- - -	- - -	- - -	16.7	36.5	45.7	49.3	50.6	52.8	54.6
300–499 beds	- - -	- - -	- - -	17.1	34.5	43.1	46.6	48.0	48.8	50.5
500 beds or more	- - -	- - -	- - -	15.3	30.5	39.1	39.5	41.5	44.1	44.5

[1]Because of modifications in 1977 and 1982 in the collection of outpatient data, there are discontinuities in the trends for this item.

[2]The American Hospital Association defines surgery as a surgical episode in the operating or procedure room. During a single episode, multiple surgical procedures may be performed.

NOTE: Excludes psychiatric and tuberculosis and other respiratory disease hospitals.

SOURCES: American Hospital Association: Hospitals. JAHA 35(15):396–401 and 45(15):463–467, Aug. 1961 and Aug. 1971; Hospital Statistics, 1976, 1981, 1985–92 Editions. Chicago, 1976, 1981, 1985–92. (Copyrights 1961, 1971, 1976, 1981, 1985–92: Used with the permission of the American Hospital Association.)

Table 91. Nursing home and personal care home residents 65 years of age and over and rate per 1,000 population, according to age, sex, and race: United States, 1963, 1973–74, 1977, and 1985

[Data are based on a sample of nursing homes]

Age, sex, and race	Residents				Residents per 1,000 population[1]			
	1963	1973–74[2]	1977[3]	1985	1963	1973–74[2]	1977[3]	1985
Age								
All ages.	445,600	961,500	1,126,000	1,318,300	25.4	44.7	47.1	46.2
65–74 years	89,600	163,100	211,400	212,100	7.9	12.3	14.4	12.5
75–84 years	207,200	384,900	464,700	509,000	39.6	57.7	64.0	57.7
85 years and over	148,700	413,600	449,900	597,300	148.4	257.3	225.9	220.3
Sex								
Male.	141,000	265,700	294,000	334,400	18.1	30.0	30.3	29.0
65–74 years	35,100	65,100	80,200	80,600	6.8	11.3	12.6	10.8
75–84 years	65,200	102,300	122,100	141,300	29.1	39.9	44.9	43.0
85 years and over	40,700	98,300	91,700	112,600	105.6	182.7	146.3	145.7
Female.	304,500	695,800	832,000	983,900	31.1	54.9	58.6	57.9
65–74 years	54,500	98,000	131,200	131,500	8.8	13.1	15.8	13.8
75–84 years	142,000	282,600	342,600	367,700	47.5	68.9	75.4	66.4
85 years and over	108,000	315,300	358,200	484,700	175.1	294.9	262.4	250.1
Race[4]								
White	431,700	920,600	1,059,900	1,227,400	26.6	46.9	48.9	47.7
65–74 years	84,400	150,100	187,500	187,800	8.1	12.5	14.2	12.3
75–84 years	202,000	369,700	443,200	473,600	41.7	60.3	67.0	59.1
85 years and over	145,400	400,800	429,100	566,000	157.7	270.8	234.2	228.7
Black	13,800	37,700	60,800	82,000	10.3	22.0	30.7	35.0
65–74 years	5,200	12,200	22,000	22,500	5.9	11.1	17.6	15.4
75–84 years	5,300	13,400	19,700	30,600	13.8	26.7	33.4	45.3
85 years and over	3,300	12,100	19,100	29,000	41.8	105.7	133.6	141.5

[1]Residents per 1,000 population for 1973–74 and 1977 will differ from those presented in the sources because the rates have been recomputed using revised census estimates for these years (see source note).
[2]Excludes residents in personal care or domiciliary care homes.
[3]Includes residents in domiciliary care homes.
[4]For data years 1973–74 and 1977, all Hispanics were included in the white category. For 1963, black includes all other races.

SOURCES: Centers for Disease Control and Prevention, National Center for Health Statistics: Characteristics of residents in institutions for the aged and chronically ill, United States, April–June 1963, by G. S. Wunderlich. Vital and Health Statistics. Series 12, No. 2. DHEW Pub. No. (PHS) 1000. Public Health Service. Washington. U.S. Government Printing Office, Sept. 1965; Characteristics, social contacts, and activities of nursing home residents, United States: 1973–74 National Nursing Home Survey, by A. Zappolo. Vital and Health Statistics. Series 13, No. 27. DHEW Pub. No. (HRA) 77-1778. Health Resources Administration. Washington. U.S. Government Printing Office, May 1977; Characteristics of nursing home residents, health status, and care received: National Nursing Home Survey, United States, May–December 1977, by E. Hing. Vital and Health Statistics. Series 13, No. 51. DHHS Pub. No. (PHS) 81-1712. Public Health Service. Washington. U.S. Government Printing Office, April 1981; The National Nursing Home Survey: 1985 summary for the United States, by E. Hing, E. Sekscenski, and G. Strahan. Vital and Health Statistics. Series 13, No. 97. DHHS Pub. No. (PHS) 89-1758. Public Health Service. Washington. U.S. Government Printing Office, Jan. 1989. U.S. Bureau of the Census: Preliminary estimates of the population of the United States by age, sex, and race: 1970–1981. Current Population Reports. Series P-25, No. 917. Washington. U.S. Government Printing Office, July 1982.

Table 92. Nursing home residents, according to selected functional status and age: United States, 1977 and 1985

[Data are based on a sample of nursing homes]

Functional status	1977					1985				
	All ages	Under 65 years	65–74 years	75–84 years	85 years and over	All ages	Under 65 years	65–74 years	75–84 years	85 years and over
	Number of residents									
All residents	1,303,100	177,100	211,400	464,700	449,900	1,491,400	173,100	212,100	509,000	597,300
	Percent distribution									
Total	100.0	100.0	100.0	100.0	100.0	100.0	100.0	100.0	100.0	100.0
Dressing										
Independent.	30.6	44.8	38.8	27.5	24.2	24.6	41.1	29.8	24.1	18.3
Requires assistance [1]	69.4	55.2	61.2	72.5	75.8	75.4	58.9	70.2	75.9	81.7
Using toilet room										
Independent.	47.5	61.8	53.1	45.7	41.0	39.1	57.1	43.4	39.7	32.0
Requires assistance	42.5	28.1	37.8	44.7	48.0	48.9	31.5	45.8	47.8	55.9
Does not use	10.1	10.1	9.1	9.6	11.0	12.0	11.4	10.8	12.6	12.1
Mobility										
Walks independently.	33.9	53.6	43.2	33.2	22.5	29.3	51.0	39.6	30.4	18.4
Walks with assistance	28.8	15.7	21.4	30.5	35.6	24.8	13.5	20.4	24.7	29.6
Chairfast	32.0	25.5	30.5	31.5	35.9	39.5	29.3	33.7	38.7	45.1
Bedfast	5.3	5.2	5.0	4.9	6.1	6.5	6.2	6.3	6.1	6.9
Continence										
No difficulty controlling bowel or bladder	54.7	68.0	62.4	52.9	47.8	48.1	67.7	57.1	45.0	41.9
Difficulty controlling—										
Bowel	3.7	3.0	3.7	4.0	3.8	1.9	*1.5	*2.0	1.7	2.2
Bladder.	9.0	5.8	6.5	9.4	11.1	10.3	6.4	6.8	11.0	12.0
Bowel and bladder.	25.9	16.8	20.6	26.9	30.8	31.7	16.8	27.5	33.6	35.8
Ostomy in either bowel or bladder	6.7	6.4	6.8	6.9	6.5	8.1	7.5	6.6	8.7	8.1
Eating										
Independent.	67.4	73.8	72.9	66.2	63.5	60.7	68.5	66.6	60.9	56.1
Requires assistance [2]	32.6	26.2	27.1	33.8	36.5	39.3	31.5	33.4	39.1	43.9
Vision										
Not impaired	67.2	81.0	75.4	67.9	57.2	75.9	88.5	83.3	77.8	68.1
Partially impaired	19.0	10.9	13.4	19.6	24.1	14.6	5.9	10.0	14.2	19.1
Severely impaired.	6.6	2.2	3.3	6.1	10.4	5.6	*1.9	4.3	4.1	8.4
Completely lost	2.9	2.2	2.6	2.6	3.8	2.5	*2.5	*1.3	2.1	3.2
Unknown	4.3	3.8	5.3	3.9	4.5	1.4	*1.2	*1.0	1.8	1.2
Hearing										
Not impaired	69.5	87.6	81.0	71.6	54.9	78.5	96.1	90.4	82.6	65.7
Partially impaired	21.7	6.6	11.4	21.2	33.1	16.7	*3.1	7.4	14.8	25.5
Severely impaired.	4.3	*0.4	1.9	3.0	8.4	3.4	*0.1	*1.1	1.5	6.8
Completely lost	0.7	*1.1	*0.7	*0.6	*0.7	0.6	*0.1	*0.4	*0.6	*0.8
Unknown	3.7	4.4	5.0	3.6	3.0	0.8	*0.5	*0.7	*0.5	1.1

[1]Includes those who do not dress.
[2]Includes those who are tube or intravenously fed.

*Relative standard error greater than 30 percent.

SOURCES: Centers for Disease Control and Prevention, National Center for Health Statistics, Division of Health Care Statistics: Characteristics of nursing home residents, health status, and care received: National Nursing Home Survey, United States, May–December 1977, by E. Hing. Vital and Health Statistics. Series 13, No. 51. DHHS Pub. No. (PHS) 81-1712. Public Health Service. Washington. U.S. Government Printing Office, April 1981; The National Nursing Home Survey: 1985 summary for the United States, by E. Hing, E. Sekscenski, and G. Strahan. Vital and Health Statistics. Series 13, No. 97. DHHS Pub. No. (PHS) 89-1758. Public Health Service. Washington. U.S. Government Printing Office, Jan. 1989.

Table 93. Additions to mental health organizations and rate per 100,000 civilian population, according to type of service and organization: United States, selected years 1975–88

[Data are based on inventories of mental health organizations]

Service and organization	Additions in thousands				Rate per 100,000 civilian population			
	1975	1983	1986	1988	1975	1983	1986	1988
Inpatient and residential treatment								
All organizations	1,558	1,633	1,817	1,999	736.5	701.4	759.9	819.1
State and county mental hospitals	434	339	330	304	205.1	146.0	139.1	124.5
Private psychiatric hospitals	126	165	235	381	59.4	70.9	98.0	156.2
Nonfederal general hospital psychiatric services	544	786	849	877	257.2	336.8	354.8	359.4
Veterans Administration psychiatric services [1]	181	149	180	246	85.5	64.3	75.1	100.7
Federally funded community mental health centers	236	. . .	. . .	. . .	111.7	. . .	. . .	. . .
Residential treatment centers for emotionally								
disturbed children	12	17	25	23	5.7	7.1	10.2	9.6
All other [2,3]	25	177	198	168	11.9	76.3	82.7	68.7
Outpatient treatment								
All organizations	2,291	2,665	2,765	2,988	1,083.2	1,147.5	1,155.7	1,223.8
State and county mental hospitals	146	84	62	94	69.1	36.3	26.0	38.5
Private psychiatric hospitals	33	78	123	125	15.6	33.4	51.5	51.2
Nonfederal general hospital psychiatric services	255	469	494	466	120.5	202.1	206.3	190.8
Veterans Administration psychiatric services [1]	94	103	125	214	44.4	44.5	52.3	87.7
Federally funded community mental health centers	785	. . .	. . .	. . .	371.2	. . .	. . .	. . .
Residential treatment centers for emotionally								
disturbed children	20	33	62	56	9.4	14.1	25.8	22.8
Freestanding psychiatric outpatient clinics [3]	871	538	391	554	411.8	231.7	163.2	226.8
All other [2,3]	87	1,360	1,508	1,479	41.2	585.4	630.6	606.0
Partial care treatment								
All organizations	163	177	189	276	77.2	76.3	78.9	113.1
State and county mental hospitals	14	4	6	6	6.7	1.6	2.4	2.3
Private psychiatric hospitals	3	6	9	39	1.5	2.4	3.7	16.1
Nonfederal general hospital psychiatric services	14	46	39	39	6.7	19.8	16.4	16.1
Veterans Administration psychiatric services [1]	8	10	7	16	3.7	4.4	3.1	6.5
Federally funded community mental health centers	94	. . .	. . .	. . .	44.5	. . .	. . .	. . .
Residential treatment centers for emotionally								
disturbed children	3	3	5	9	1.6	1.5	2.3	3.5
Freestanding psychiatric outpatient clinics [3,4]	22	5	. . .	. . .	10.4	2.3	. . .	. . .
All other [2,3,5]	5	103	123	167	2.1	44.3	51.0	68.6

[1]Includes Veterans Administration neuropsychiatric hospitals, Veterans Administration general hospitals with separate psychiatric services, and freestanding psychiatric outpatient clinics.
[2]Includes other multiservice mental health organizations with inpatient and residential treatment services that are not elsewhere classified.
[3]Beginning in 1983 a definitional change sharply increased the number of multiservice mental health organizations while decreasing the number of freestanding psychiatric outpatient clinics. See Appendix I.
[4]Beginning in 1986 outpatient psychiatric clinics providing partial care are counted as multiservice mental health organizations in the "all other" category.
[5]Includes freestanding psychiatric partial care organizations.

NOTES: Changes in reporting procedures in 1981 affect the comparability of data from 1981 and later years with those from previous years. Some numbers in this table have been revised and differ from previous editions of Health, United States.

SOURCES: Statistical Research Branch, Division of Applied and Services Research, National Institute of Mental Health: R. W. Manderscheid and S. A. Barrett: Mental Health, United States, 1987. DHHS Pub. No. (ADM) 87-1518. U.S. Government Printing Office, 1987; R. W. Manderscheid and M. A. Sonnenschein: Mental Health, United States, 1990. DHHS Pub. No. (ADM) 90-1708. U.S. Government Printing Office, 1990; Unpublished data.

Table 94. Inpatient and residential treatment episodes in mental health organizations, rate per 100,000 civilian population, and inpatient days, according to type of organization: United States, selected years 1975–88

[Data are based on inventories of mental health organizations]

Organization	1975	1981 [1]	1983	1986	1988
	Episodes in thousands				
All organizations	1,817	1,720	1,861	2,055	2,229
State and county mental hospitals	599	499	459	445	407
Private psychiatric hospitals	137	177	181	258	410
Nonfederal general hospital psychiatric services	566	677	820	883	912
Veterans Administration psychiatric services [2]	214	206	171	204	266
Federally funded community mental health centers	247	. . .	. . .	. . .	. . .
Residential treatment centers for emotionally disturbed children	28	34	33	47	47
All other [3,4]	26	127	197	218	187
	Episodes per 100,000 civilian population				
All organizations	859.6	755.6	799.1	858.9	913.9
State and county mental hospitals	283.3	219.3	197.7	186.0	166.7
Private psychiatric hospitals	64.8	77.5	77.8	107.9	167.9
Nonfederal general hospital psychiatric services	267.6	297.3	351.3	369.0	374.4
Veterans Administration psychiatric services [2]	101.4	90.3	73.4	85.2	109.0
Federally funded community mental health centers	116.8	. . .	. . .	. . .	. . .
Residential treatment centers for emotionally disturbed children	13.4	15.1	14.0	19.7	19.3
All other [3,4]	12.3	56.1	84.9	91.1	76.6
	Inpatient days in thousands				
All organizations	104,970	77,053	81,821	83,413	83,161
State and county mental hospitals	70,584	44,558	42,427	39,075	36,452
Private psychiatric hospitals	4,401	5,578	6,010	8,568	10,840
Nonfederal general hospital psychiatric services	8,349	10,727	12,529	12,570	13,104
Veterans Administration psychiatric services [2]	11,725	7,591	7,425	7,753	7,155
Federally funded community mental health centers	3,718	. . .	. . .	. . .	. . .
Residential treatment centers for emotionally disturbed children	5,900	6,127	5,776	8,267	8,429
All other [3,4]	293	2,472	7,654	7,180	7,181

[1]In 1981, some organizations were reclassified and data for some organization types were not available, resulting in a particularly large increase for the "all other" category in 1981.
[2]Includes Veterans Administration neuropsychiatric hospitals and Veterans Administration general hospitals with separate psychiatric services.
[3]Includes other multiservice mental health organizations with inpatient and residential treatment services that are not elsewhere classified.
[4]Beginning in 1983 a definitional change sharply increased the number of multiservice mental health organizations. See Appendix I.

NOTES: Changes in reporting procedures in 1981 affect the comparability of data from 1981 and later years with those from previous years. Some numbers in this table have been revised and differ from previous editions of Health, United States.

SOURCES: Statistical Research Branch, Division of Applied and Services Research, National Institute of Mental Health: R. W. Manderscheid and S. A. Barrett: Mental Health, United States, 1987. DHHS Pub. No. (ADM) 87-1518. U.S. Government Printing Office, 1987; R. W. Manderscheid and M. A. Sonnenschein: Mental Health, United States, 1990. DHHS Pub. No. (ADM) 90-1708. U.S. Government Printing Office, 1990; Unpublished data.

Table 95. Additions to selected inpatient psychiatric organizations and rate per 100,000 civilian population, according to sex, age, and race: United States, 1975, 1980, and 1986

[Data are based on a sample survey of patients]

Sex, age, and race	State and county mental hospitals			Private psychiatric hospitals			Nonfederal general hospitals [1]		
	1975	1980	1986	1975	1980	1986	1975	1980	1986
Both sexes				Number in thousands					
Total	385	369	326	130	141	207	516	564	794
Under 18 years	25	17	16	15	17	42	43	44	46
18–24 years	72	77	58	19	23	22	93	98	120
25–44 years	166	177	189	47	56	91	220	249	405
45–64 years	102	78	48	35	32	34	121	123	142
65 years and over	21	20	15	13	14	18	38	50	82
White	296	265	217	119	123	177	451	469	607
All other	89	104	109	10	18	30	65	95	187
Male									
Total	249	239	205	56	67	107	212	255	379
Under 18 years	16	11	10	8	9	23	20	20	21
18–24 years	52	56	39	10	13	14	45	52	57
25–44 years	107	119	125	20	27	50	85	115	215
45–64 years	61	43	25	14	13	14	48	46	60
65 years and over	13	11	7	5	5	6	14	21	26
White	191	171	135	51	58	89	184	213	274
All other	58	68	69	5	9	18	27	42	105
Female									
Total	136	130	121	74	74	101	304	309	415
Under 18 years	9	5	6	8	7	20	23	23	25
18–24 years	20	22	19	9	10	8	48	45	63
25–44 years	59	58	64	28	29	41	135	135	190
45–64 years	41	35	24	21	18	20	74	77	81
65 years and over	8	9	8	8	9	12	24	29	56
White	105	94	82	69	65	88	267	256	333
All other	31	36	40	5	9	13	37	53	82
Both sexes				Rate per 100,000 civilian population					
Total	182.2	163.6	136.1	61.4	62.6	86.7	243.8	250.0	331.7
Under 18 years	38.1	26.1	25.2	23.3	26.3	67.1	64.4	68.5	72.0
18–24 years	271.8	264.6	215.5	73.7	79.6	81.3	352.8	334.2	443.7
25–44 years	314.1	282.9	251.9	89.3	89.1	121.6	416.8	399.0	540.4
45–64 years	233.5	175.7	107.0	80.1	71.0	75.2	278.5	276.4	314.9
65 years and over	91.8	78.0	50.9	57.7	54.1	61.9	170.3	195.4	281.5
White	161.1	136.8	106.7	64.9	63.4	87.3	245.4	241.8	299.0
All other	321.9	328.0	299.8	37.9	57.5	83.1	233.3	300.0	514.3
Male									
Total	243.7	219.8	176.6	54.5	61.9	92.1	207.1	233.8	327.6
Under 18 years	48.3	35.4	30.1	22.5	28.9	69.8	59.1	62.6	63.7
18–24 years	409.0	387.9	292.6	78.0	92.2	103.2	350.8	365.3	428.5
25–44 years	418.4	388.1	338.4	76.6	86.8	136.1	332.8	374.7	584.2
45–64 years	291.5	202.3	114.4	66.8	63.2	65.5	228.6	219.1	281.1
65 years and over	136.4	105.3	57.1	50.3	47.3	52.1	152.0	203.4	223.1
White	214.2	182.2	137.1	57.0	61.7	90.3	206.9	226.3	278.3
All other	444.5	457.8	403.0	38.1	62.7	102.8	209.1	281.1	610.3
Female									
Total	124.7	111.1	98.1	67.8	63.3	81.5	278.1	265.1	335.5
Under 18 years	27.5	16.4	20.0	24.1	23.6	64.3	70.0	74.6	80.7
18–24 years	143.1	145.8	141.0	69.6	67.4	60.2	354.6	304.4	458.3
25–44 years	215.9	182.3	168.1	101.2	91.2	107.6	495.8	422.2	498.1
45–64 years	180.5	151.7	100.2	92.3	78.1	84.0	324.3	328.2	345.8
65 years and over	60.8	59.6	46.7	62.8	58.8	68.6	182.9	190.0	321.3
White	111.2	94.1	78.1	72.5	65.0	84.5	281.7	256.4	318.6
All other	212.0	212.6	207.2	37.7	52.8	65.5	254.9	316.7	428.0

[1] Nonfederal general hospitals include public and nonpublic facilities.

SOURCES: National Institute of Mental Health: C. A. Taube and S. A. Barrett: Mental Health, United States, 1985. DHHS Pub. No. (ADM) 85-1378. U.S. Government Printing Office, 1985; R. W. Manderscheid and M. A. Sonnenschein: Mental Health, United States, 1990. DHHS Pub. No. (ADM) 90-1708. U.S. Government Printing Office, 1990; Unpublished data.

Table 96. Additions to selected inpatient psychiatric organizations, according to selected primary diagnoses and age: United States, 1975, 1980, and 1986

[Data are based on a sample survey of patients]

Primary diagnosis and age	State and county mental hospitals			Private psychiatric hospitals			Nonfederal general hospitals [1]		
	1975	1980	1986	1975	1980	1986	1975	1980	1986
All diagnoses [2]	Rate per 100,000 civilian population								
All ages.	182.2	163.6	136.1	61.4	62.6	86.7	243.8	250.0	331.7
Under 25 years	104.8	101.2	82.1	37.7	43.1	71.4	146.7	152.2	183.1
25–44 years	314.1	282.9	251.9	89.3	89.1	121.6	416.8	399.0	540.4
45–64 years	233.5	175.7	107.0	80.1	71.0	75.2	278.5	276.4	314.9
65 years and over	91.8	78.0	50.9	57.7	54.1	61.9	170.3	195.4	281.5
Alcohol related									
All ages.	50.4	35.5	22.5	5.1	5.8	6.6	17.0	18.8	41.4
Under 25 years	10.7	12.4	15.5	0.4	1.4	2.2	2.4	4.4	13.4
25–44 years	86.2	64.0	42.6	7.6	9.3	10.0	31.0	34.3	92.6
45–64 years	110.0	57.7	15.3	12.5	10.9	11.0	34.5	30.6	31.8
65 years and over	14.8	11.5	*3.2	4.3	4.4	4.5	10.2	12.8	11.3
Drug related									
All ages.	6.8	7.8	8.7	1.5	1.8	6.1	8.4	7.4	20.2
Under 25 years	7.2	9.4	5.8	1.5	1.8	7.5	7.7	7.8	18.4
25–44 years	12.6	12.9	14.2	2.3	3.0	9.3	13.8	9.3	41.2
45–64 years	*0.6	1.4	10.5	0.1	1.0	*1.8	6.5	7.1	*2.1
65 years and over	*3.5	*0.7	*0.8	0.4	0.6	- - -	*2.6	*2.0	*0.1
Organic disorders [3]									
All ages.	9.6	6.8	4.3	2.5	2.2	2.0	9.0	7.4	9.8
Under 25 years	2.2	1.2	*0.2	0.7	0.5	*0.5	1.1	*0.8	1.7
25–44 years	6.4	4.7	2.6	1.1	0.9	*0.3	5.4	5.6	6.1
45–64 years	12.2	8.1	7.3	1.7	2.7	*1.5	9.3	6.9	5.7
65 years and over	43.3	30.0	17.2	14.5	10.8	11.7	49.3	36.4	50.7
Affective disorders									
All ages.	21.3	22.0	22.8	26.0	26.8	41.9	91.9	79.2	121.9
Under 25 years	7.5	9.1	9.6	9.5	13.5	28.5	35.3	32.2	49.2
25–44 years	40.6	36.9	43.2	39.4	38.9	63.4	160.9	123.7	176.8
45–64 years	29.4	32.4	25.0	43.3	36.3	38.5	135.6	113.8	147.3
65 years and over	16.8	14.3	7.9	29.6	29.2	33.4	78.5	81.0	166.3
Schizophrenia									
All ages.	61.2	62.1	49.7	13.4	13.3	9.9	58.9	59.9	63.3
Under 25 years	35.9	36.6	18.6	11.1	10.6	5.7	42.0	38.3	30.4
25–44 years	125.8	125.0	107.5	23.8	22.5	18.9	118.0	114.5	118.6
45–64 years	63.5	54.8	35.9	11.3	11.6	8.5	50.3	53.6	68.9
65 years and over	9.3	13.9	18.3	2.7	3.6	*1.8	5.6	16.3	14.0

[1]Nonfederal general hospitals include public and nonpublic facilities.
[2]Includes all other diagnoses not listed separately.
[3]Excludes alcohol and drug-related diagnoses.

*Based on five or fewer sample additions.

NOTES: Primary diagnosis categories are based on the then current International Classification of Diseases and Diagnostic and Statistical Manual of Mental Disorders. For a listing of the code numbers, see Appendix II, table X.

SOURCES: National Institute of Mental Health: C. A. Taube and S. A. Barrett: Mental Health, United States, 1985. DHHS Pub. No. (ADM) 85-1378. U.S. Government Printing Office, 1985; R. W. Manderscheid and M. A. Sonnenschein: Mental Health, United States, 1990. DHHS Pub. No. (ADM) 90-1708. U.S. Government Printing Office, 1990; Unpublished data.

Table 97. Persons employed in health service sites: United States, selected years 1970–91

[Data are based on household interviews of a sample of the civilian noninstitutionalized population]

Site	1970[1]	1975	1980	1983	1984	1985	1986	1987	1988	1989	1990	1991
	Number of persons in thousands											
All employed civilians	76,805	85,846	99,303	100,834	105,005	107,150	109,597	112,440	114,968	117,342	117,914	116,877
All health service sites	4,246	5,945	7,339	7,874	7,934	7,910	8,129	8,478	8,781	9,110	9,447	9,817
Offices of physicians	477	618	777	888	896	894	896	950	985	1,039	1,098	1,128
Offices of dentists	222	331	415	441	468	480	497	552	521	560	580	574
Offices of chiropractors [2]	19	30	40	54	61	59	66	72	77	97	90	105
Hospitals	2,690	3,441	4,036	4,348	4,288	4,269	4,368	4,444	4,520	4,568	4,690	4,839
Nursing and personal care facilities	509	891	1,199	1,342	1,362	1,309	1,339	1,337	1,467	1,521	1,543	1,626
Other health service sites	330	634	872	801	859	899	963	1,123	1,211	1,325	1,446	1,545
	Percent of employed civilians											
All health service sites	5.5	6.9	7.4	7.8	7.6	7.4	7.4	7.5	7.6	7.8	8.0	8.4
	Percent distribution											
All health service sites	100.0	100.0	100.0	100.0	100.0	100.0	100.0	100.0	100.0	100.0	100.0	100.0
Offices of physicians	11.2	10.4	10.6	11.3	11.3	11.3	11.0	11.2	11.2	11.4	11.6	11.5
Offices of dentists	5.2	5.6	5.7	5.6	5.9	6.1	6.1	6.5	5.9	6.1	6.1	5.8
Offices of chiropractors [2]	0.4	0.5	0.5	0.7	0.8	0.7	0.8	0.8	0.9	1.1	1.0	1.1
Hospitals	63.4	57.9	55.0	55.2	54.0	54.0	53.7	52.4	51.5	50.1	49.6	49.3
Nursing and personal care facilities	12.0	15.0	16.3	17.0	17.2	16.5	16.5	15.8	16.7	16.7	16.3	16.6
Other health service sites	7.8	10.7	11.9	10.2	10.8	11.4	11.8	13.2	13.8	14.5	15.3	15.7

[1]April 1, derived from decennial census; all other data years are annual averages from the Current Population Survey.
[2]Data for 1980 are from the American Chiropractic Association; data for all other years are from the U.S. Bureau of Labor Statistics.

NOTES: Totals exclude persons in health-related occupations who are working in nonhealth industries, as classified by the U.S. Bureau of the Census, such as pharmacists employed in drugstores, school nurses, and nurses working in private households. Totals include Federal, State, and county health workers. In 1970–82, employed persons were classified according to the industry groups used in the 1970 Census of Population. Beginning in 1983, persons were classified according to the system used in the 1980 Census of Population.

SOURCES: U.S. Bureau of the Census: 1970 Census of Population, occupation by industry. Subject Reports. Final Report PC(2)-7C. Washington. U.S. Government Printing Office, Oct. 1972; U.S. Bureau of Labor Statistics: Labor Force Statistics Derived from the Current Population Survey: A Databook, Vol. I. Washington. U.S. Government Printing Office, Sept. 1982; Employment and Earnings, January 1983–92. Vol. 30, No. 1, Vol. 31, No. 1, Vol. 32, No. 1, Vol. 33, No. 1, Vol. 34, No. 1, Vol. 35, No. 1, Vol. 36, No. 1, Vol. 37, No. 1, Vol. 38, No. 1, and Vol. 39, No. 1. Washington. U.S. Government Printing Office, Jan. 1983–92; American Chiropractic Association: Unpublished data.

Table 98 (page 1 of 2). Active nonfederal physicians per 10,000 civilian population, according to geographic division, State, and primary specialty: United States, 1975, 1985, 1987, and 1990

[Data based on reporting by physicians]

	Total physicians [1]				Doctors of medicine [2]							
					Patient care [3]				Primary care [4]			
Geographic division and State	1975	1985	1987	1990	1975	1985	1987	1990	1975	1985	1987	1990
	Number per 10,000 civilian population											
United States	15.3	20.7	21.4	22.2	13.5	18.0	18.9	19.5	4.1	5.4	5.5	5.7
New England	19.1	26.7	27.7	29.0	16.9	22.9	24.2	25.5	4.6	6.2	6.2	6.6
Maine.	12.8	18.7	19.3	20.1	10.7	15.6	16.0	16.6	3.8	5.4	5.4	5.6
New Hampshire.	14.3	18.1	18.5	20.1	13.1	16.7	17.2	18.6	4.6	5.6	5.7	6.2
Vermont	18.2	23.8	24.5	25.4	15.5	20.3	21.5	22.4	5.2	6.5	6.6	7.1
Massachusetts	20.8	30.2	31.2	32.8	18.3	25.4	27.0	28.6	4.7	6.4	6.4	6.7
Rhode Island.	17.8	23.3	24.9	26.0	16.1	20.2	21.8	22.6	4.4	5.5	5.6	5.8
Connecticut.	19.8	27.6	29.0	30.1	17.7	24.3	25.7	26.8	4.7	6.4	6.5	6.9
Middle Atlantic	19.5	26.1	27.3	28.4	17.0	22.2	23.6	24.5	4.5	5.9	6.0	6.3
New York	22.7	29.0	30.1	31.1	20.2	25.2	26.9	27.6	5.1	6.3	6.3	6.7
New Jersey	16.2	23.4	24.5	25.9	14.0	19.8	21.1	22.2	4.1	5.5	5.8	6.1
Pennsylvania.	16.6	23.6	24.8	26.0	13.9	19.2	20.4	21.3	4.0	5.4	5.5	5.8
East North Central	13.9	19.3	19.9	20.6	12.0	16.4	17.1	17.6	3.7	5.0	5.1	5.2
Ohio.	14.1	19.9	20.6	21.4	12.2	16.8	17.5	18.0	3.7	4.8	4.8	5.0
Indiana	10.6	14.7	15.4	16.0	9.6	13.2	14.0	14.6	3.8	4.6	4.7	5.0
Illinois	14.5	20.5	21.1	21.6	13.1	18.2	18.9	19.3	4.1	5.5	5.7	5.7
Michigan.	15.4	20.8	21.3	22.1	12.0	16.0	16.4	16.9	3.2	4.5	4.4	4.5
Wisconsin.	12.5	17.7	18.4	19.1	11.4	15.9	16.7	17.4	4.0	5.4	5.6	5.9
West North Central	13.3	18.3	19.1	19.8	11.4	15.6	16.4	17.1	3.8	5.2	5.3	5.5
Minnesota.	14.9	20.5	21.1	22.0	13.7	18.5	19.3	20.1	4.6	6.5	6.5	6.9
Iowa.	11.4	15.6	16.5	17.2	9.4	12.4	13.1	13.8	3.5	4.3	4.4	4.5
Missouri	15.0	20.5	21.3	22.0	11.6	16.3	17.1	17.7	3.3	4.7	4.6	4.8
North Dakota.	9.7	15.8	16.7	17.0	9.2	14.9	15.8	16.0	4.1	5.8	6.0	6.1
South Dakota	8.2	13.4	14.0	14.2	7.7	12.3	13.0	13.2	3.4	5.0	5.6	5.8
Nebraska	12.1	15.7	16.7	17.0	10.9	14.4	15.5	15.9	4.2	5.3	5.4	5.7
Kansas	12.8	17.3	17.8	18.6	11.2	15.1	15.7	16.3	3.9	5.2	5.1	5.3
South Atlantic	14.0	19.7	20.8	21.7	12.6	17.6	18.6	19.3	3.7	5.2	5.4	5.6
Delaware.	14.3	19.7	20.2	21.3	12.7	17.1	17.7	18.3	3.8	4.7	4.7	5.0
Maryland.	18.6	30.4	31.5	32.5	16.5	24.9	26.7	27.8	4.2	6.5	6.8	7.2
District of Columbia	39.6	55.3	57.2	60.0	34.6	45.6	47.5	50.1	7.2	10.3	10.6	11.1
Virginia.	12.9	19.5	20.1	21.2	11.9	17.8	18.6	19.5	3.8	5.4	5.6	5.8
West Virginia.	11.0	16.3	17.2	17.7	10.0	14.6	15.2	15.4	3.3	4.4	4.6	4.8
North Carolina.	11.7	16.9	17.7	18.9	10.6	15.0	16.1	17.2	3.5	4.7	4.9	5.2
South Carolina	10.0	14.7	15.5	16.0	9.3	13.6	14.5	15.0	3.3	4.5	4.7	4.8
Georgia	11.5	16.2	16.8	17.6	10.6	14.7	15.4	16.2	3.3	4.3	4.4	4.7
Florida	15.2	20.2	21.1	21.6	13.4	17.8	18.7	19.2	3.9	5.3	5.6	5.7
East South Central	10.5	15.0	15.9	16.8	9.7	14.0	14.9	15.7	3.2	4.5	4.7	4.9
Kentucky.	10.9	15.1	16.0	16.8	10.1	13.9	15.1	15.7	3.6	4.8	5.0	5.2
Tennessee	12.4	17.7	18.6	19.5	11.3	16.2	17.3	18.1	3.2	4.7	4.9	5.2
Alabama.	9.2	14.2	15.0	15.7	8.6	13.1	14.0	14.6	3.0	4.2	4.4	4.7
Mississippi	8.4	11.8	12.5	13.3	8.0	11.1	11.9	12.6	3.1	4.2	4.3	4.4
West South Central	11.9	16.4	17.1	17.8	10.5	14.5	15.2	15.8	3.5	4.5	4.5	4.7
Arkansas.	9.1	13.8	14.4	15.1	8.5	12.8	13.5	14.1	3.4	4.8	4.9	5.1
Louisiana	11.4	17.3	17.9	18.6	10.5	16.1	16.8	17.4	3.3	4.5	4.5	4.8
Oklahoma.	11.6	16.1	16.7	17.1	9.4	12.9	13.4	13.6	3.2	4.0	4.4	4.5
Texas	12.5	16.8	17.3	18.1	11.0	14.7	15.3	16.0	3.6	4.5	4.5	4.7
Mountain	14.3	17.8	18.5	19.3	12.6	15.7	16.3	17.0	4.1	5.0	5.2	5.3
Montana	10.6	14.0	15.2	16.0	10.1	13.2	14.4	15.2	4.5	5.4	5.7	6.0
Idaho	9.5	12.1	12.2	12.7	8.9	11.4	11.5	12.0	4.0	4.8	4.8	4.9
Wyoming	9.5	12.9	13.3	13.9	8.9	12.0	12.6	13.1	4.1	4.6	5.1	5.2
Colorado.	17.3	20.7	21.0	22.1	15.0	17.7	18.3	19.2	4.6	5.6	5.6	5.9
New Mexico	12.2	17.0	17.7	18.9	10.1	14.7	15.5	16.7	3.4	4.8	5.2	5.4
Arizona.	16.7	20.2	20.9	21.5	14.1	17.1	17.8	18.4	4.2	5.1	5.2	5.4
Utah.	14.1	17.2	17.7	18.5	13.0	15.5	16.1	16.9	3.8	4.4	4.5	4.6
Nevada.	11.9	16.0	16.1	16.6	10.9	14.5	14.7	14.9	3.6	4.6	4.7	4.7

See footnotes at end of table.

Table 98 (page 2 of 2). Active nonfederal physicians per 10,000 civilian population, according to geographic division, State, and primary specialty: United States, 1975, 1985, 1987, and 1990

[Data based on reporting by physicians]

Geographic division and State	Total physicians [1]				Doctors of medicine [2]							
					Patient care [3]				Primary care [4]			
	1975	1985	1987	1990	1975	1985	1987	1990	1975	1985	1987	1990
	Number per 10,000 civilian population											
Pacific	17.9	22.5	22.9	23.4	16.3	20.5	20.9	21.3	5.2	6.6	6.5	6.5
Washington.	15.3	20.2	20.8	21.5	13.6	17.9	18.5	19.3	4.7	6.3	6.4	6.6
Oregon.	15.6	19.7	20.0	21.1	13.8	17.6	18.1	19.1	4.6	6.1	6.0	6.3
California	18.8	23.7	23.8	24.1	17.3	21.5	21.7	21.9	5.5	6.7	6.6	6.5
Alaska	8.4	13.0	13.8	14.8	7.8	12.1	12.7	13.7	3.5	5.6	5.7	5.7
Hawaii	16.2	21.5	22.5	23.8	14.7	19.8	20.7	21.9	4.9	7.0	7.1	7.5

[1]Includes active nonfederal doctors of medicine and doctors of osteopathy in all other specialties not shown separately.

[2]Excludes doctors of osteopathy; States with large numbers are Florida, Michigan, Missouri, New Jersey, Ohio, Pennsylvania, and Texas. Specialty information based on the physician's self-designated primary area of practice.

[3]Excludes doctors of medicine in medical teaching, administration, research, and other nonpatient care activities.

[4]Includes doctors of medicine in patient care office-based general practice and family practice, internal medicine, and pediatrics.

NOTES: Starting in 1989 data for doctors of medicine are as of January 1; in earlier years these data are as of December 31. See Appendix II for physician definitions.

SOURCES: Compiled by Health Resources and Services Administration, Bureau of Health Professions based on data from the American Medical Association Physician Distribution and Licensure in the U.S., 1975, Physician Characteristics and Distribution in the U.S., 1986, 1989, and 1992 Editions; American Osteopathic Association: 1975–76 Yearbook and Directory of Osteopathic Physicians, 1985–86 Yearbook and Directory of Osteopathic Physicians, and 1987–88 Yearbook and Directory of Osteopathic Physicians; American Association of Colleges of Osteopathic Medicine: Annual Statistical Report, 1988 and 1990.

Table 99. Active physicians, according to type of physician, and number per 10,000 population: United States and outlying U.S. areas, selected years 1950–90 and projections for year 2000

[Data are based on reporting by physicians and medical schools]

Year	All active physicians	Doctors of medicine	Doctors of osteopathy	Active physicians per 10,000 population
	Number of physicians			
1950...	219,900	209,000	10,900	14.1
1960...	259,500	247,300	12,200	14.0
1970...	326,500	314,200	12,300	15.6
1971...	337,400	325,000	12,400	16.1
1972...	348,300	335,500	12,800	16.4
1973...	355,700	342,500	13,200	16.4
1974...	370,000	356,400	13,600	16.9
1975...	384,500	370,400	14,100	17.4
1976...	399,500	385,000	14,500	17.9
1977...	405,900	390,800	15,100	18.0
1978...	424,000	408,300	15,700	18.6
1979...	440,400	424,000	16,400	19.1
1980...	457,500	440,400	17,100	19.7
1981...	466,700	448,700	18,000	20.0
1982...	483,700	465,000	18,700	20.5
1983...	501,200	481,500	19,700	21.0
1984...	- - -	- - -	20,800	- - -
1985...	534,800	512,900	21,900	22.0
1986...	544,100	520,900	23,200	22.2
1987...	560,300	536,200	24,100	22.6
1988...	- - -	- - -	25,300	- - -
1989...	577,200	550,700	26,500	23.3
1990...	589,500	561,400	28,100	23.4
Projections				
2000...	725,900	684,900	41,000	27.1

NOTES: Starting in 1989 data for doctors of medicine are as of January 1; in earlier years these data are as of December 31. Population estimates include residents in the United States, Puerto Rico, and other U.S. outlying areas; U.S. citizens in foreign countries; and the Armed Forces in the United States and abroad. For the year 2000, the Series II projections of the total population from the U.S. Bureau of the Census are used. Estimation and projection methods are from the Bureau of Health Professions. See Appendix II for physician definitions. The numbers for doctors of medicine differ from American Medical Association figures because physicians not classified by activity status and whose addresses are unknown are included in this table.

SOURCES: Bureau of Health Professions: Sixth Report to the President and Congress on the Status of Health Personnel in the United States. Health Resources and Services Administration. DHHS Pub. No. HRS-P-OD-88-1, Rockville, Md., 1988, and unpublished data; American Medical Association: data from annual surveys and unpublished data.

Table 100. Physicians, according to activity and place of medical education: United States and outlying U.S. areas, selected years 1970–90

[Data are based on reporting by physicians]

Activity and place of medical education	1970	1975	1980	1985	1987	1989	1990
	Number of physicians						
Doctors of medicine	334,028	393,742	467,679	552,716	585,597	600,789	615,421
Professionally active	310,845	340,280	414,916	497,140	521,328	536,755	547,310
Place of medical education:							
U.S. medical graduates	256,427	- - -	333,325	392,007	410,300	423,172	432,884
International medical graduates [1]	54,418	- - -	81,591	105,133	111,028	113,583	114,426
Activity [2]:							
Nonfederal	281,344	312,089	397,129	475,573	499,582	516,396	526,835
Patient care	255,027	287,837	361,915	431,527	453,230	468,902	479,547
Office-based practice	188,924	213,334	271,268	329,041	337,507	350,066	359,932
General and family practice	50,816	46,347	47,772	53,862	55,117	56,318	57,571
Cardiovascular diseases	3,882	5,046	6,725	9,054	9,925	10,235	10,670
Dermatology	2,932	3,442	4,372	5,325	5,532	5,721	5,996
Gastroenterology	1,112	1,696	2,735	4,135	4,764	4,942	5,200
Internal medicine	22,950	28,188	40,514	52,712	55,452	56,946	57,799
Pediatrics	10,310	12,687	17,436	22,392	23,370	24,692	26,494
Pulmonary diseases	785	1,166	2,040	3,035	3,474	3,578	3,659
General surgery	18,068	19,710	22,409	24,708	23,689	24,737	24,498
Obstetrics and gynecology	13,847	15,613	19,503	23,525	24,271	25,161	25,475
Ophthalmology	7,627	8,795	10,598	12,212	12,538	12,847	13,055
Orthopedic surgery	6,533	8,148	10,719	13,033	13,520	14,071	14,187
Otolaryngology	3,914	4,297	5,262	5,751	6,022	6,223	6,360
Plastic surgery	1,166	1,706	2,437	3,299	3,520	3,648	3,835
Urological surgery	4,273	5,025	6,222	7,081	7,182	7,338	7,392
Anesthesiology	7,369	8,970	11,336	15,285	15,986	16,720	17,789
Diagnostic radiology	896	1,978	4,190	7,735	8,557	9,012	9,806
Emergency medicine	- - -	- - -	- - -		7,564	8,041	8,402
Neurology	1,192	1,862	3,245	4,691	5,087	5,374	5,587
Pathology, anatomical/clinical	2,993	4,195	5,952	6,877	6,747	7,022	7,269
Psychiatry	10,078	12,173	15,946	18,521	18,695	19,625	20,048
Radiology	5,781	6,970	7,791	7,355	6,149	6,164	6,056
Other specialty	12,400	15,320	24,064	28,453	20,346	21,651	22,784
Hospital-based practice	66,103	74,503	90,647	102,486	115,723	118,836	119,615
Residents and interns	45,840	53,527	59,615	72,159	79,483	80,019	81,664
Full-time hospital staff	20,263	20,976	31,032	30,327	36,240	38,817	37,951
Other professional activity [3]	26,317	24,252	35,214	44,046	46,352	47,494	47,288
Federal	29,501	28,191	17,787	21,567	21,746	20,359	20,475
Patient care	23,508	24,100	14,597	17,293	16,902	15,570	15,632
Office-based practice	3,515	2,095	732	1,156	1,149	1,135	1,063
Hospital-based practice	19,993	22,005	13,865	16,137	15,753	14,435	14,569
Residents and interns	5,388	4,275	2,427	3,252	2,717	2,084	1,725
Full-time hospital staff	14,605	17,730	11,438	12,885	13,036	12,351	12,844
Other professional activity [3]	5,993	4,091	3,190	4,274	4,844	4,789	4,843
Inactive	19,621	21,449	25,744	38,646	48,042	48,804	52,653
Not classified [4]	358	26,145	20,629	13,950	13,364	12,405	12,678
Unknown address	3,204	5,868	6,390	2,980	2,863	2,825	2,780

[1] International medical graduates received their medical education in schools outside the United States and Canada.
[2] Specialty information based on the physician's self-designated primary area of practice.
[3] Includes medical teaching, administration, research, clinical fellows, and other.
[4] Not classified established in 1970; however, complete data not available until 1972.

NOTES: Starting in 1989 data for doctors of medicine are as of January 1; in earlier years these data are as of December 31. See Appendix II for physician definitions.

SOURCES: Haug, J. N., Roback, G. A., and Martin, B. C.: Distribution of Physicians in the United States, 1970. Chicago. American Medical Association, 1971; Goodman, L. J., and Mason, H. R.: Physician Distribution and Medical Licensure in the U.S., 1975. Chicago. American Medical Association, 1976; Bidese, C. M., and Danais, D. G.: Physician Characteristics and Distribution in the U.S., 1981. Chicago. American Medical Association, 1982; Roback, G. A., Mead, D., and Randolph, L. L.: Physician Characteristics and Distribution in the U.S., 1986. Chicago. American Medical Association, 1986; Roback, G. A., Randolph, L. L., and Seidman, B.: Physician Characteristics and Distribution in the U.S., 1989; 1990; 1992. Chicago. American Medical Association, 1989; 1990; 1992. (Copyrights 1971, 1976, 1982, 1986, 1989, 1990, and 1992: Used with the permission of the American Medical Association.)

Table 101. Active health personnel and number per 100,000 population, according to occupation and geographic region: United States, 1970, 1980, and 1990

[Data are compiled by the Bureau of Health Professions]

Year and occupation	Number of active health personnel	United States	Geographic region			
			Northeast	Midwest	South	West
1970		Number per 100,000 population [1]				
Physicians	- - -	- - -	- - -	- - -	- - -	- - -
Federal [2]	- - -	- - -	- - -	- - -	- - -	- - -
Nonfederal.	290,862	142.7	185.0	127.5	114.8	158.2
Doctors of medicine [2,3]	279,212	137.0	178.7	118.2	111.5	154.8
Doctors of osteopathy	11,650	5.7	6.3	9.3	3.3	3.4
Dentists [4]	95,700	47.0	58.9	46.3	35.3	54.9
Optometrists	18,400	9.0	9.7	10.3	6.6	10.5
Pharmacists	112,570	55.4	60.1	57.5	50.6	52.9
Podiatrists.	7,110	3.5	6.0	3.6	1.6	3.0
Registered nurses	750,000	368.9	491.2	367.5	281.8	355.9
Veterinarians	25,900	12.7	8.3	16.1	11.8	15.0
1980						
Physicians	427,122	189.8	- - -	- - -	- - -	- - -
Federal [2]	17,642	7.8	- - -	- - -	- - -	- - -
Doctors of medicine [2,3]	16,585	7.4	- - -	- - -	- - -	- - -
Doctors of osteopathy	1,057	0.5	- - -	- - -	- - -	- - -
Nonfederal.	409,480	182.0	224.5	165.2	157.0	200.0
Doctors of medicine [2,3]	393,407	174.9	216.1	153.3	152.8	195.8
Doctors of osteopathy	16,073	7.1	8.4	11.9	4.2	4.2
Dentists [4]	121,240	53.5	66.2	52.7	42.6	59.2
Optometrists	22,330	9.8	9.9	10.9	7.7	11.6
Pharmacists	142,780	62.5	66.5	67.8	62.1	51.8
Podiatrists.	8,880	4.0	6.3	3.9	2.5	4.1
Registered nurses	1,272,900	560.0	736.0	583.6	443.4	533.7
Associate and diploma	908,300	399.9	536.0	429.2	316.5	351.1
Baccalaureate	297,300	130.9	161.0	127.8	103.8	148.1
Masters and doctorate	67,300	29.6	39.0	26.7	23.0	34.6
Veterinarians	36,000	16.3	10.8	19.9	16.0	18.5
1990						
Physicians	567,611	230.2	- - -	- - -	- - -	- - -
Federal [2]	20,784	8.4	- - -	- - -	- - -	- - -
Doctors of medicine [2,3]	19,166	7.7	- - -	- - -	- - -	- - -
Doctors of osteopathy	1,618	0.7	- - -	- - -	- - -	- - -
Nonfederal.	546,827	221.8	285.5	203.9	195.5	223.3
Doctors of medicine [2,3]	520,451	211.1	271.6	186.8	188.6	216.9
Doctors of osteopathy	26,376	10.7	13.9	17.1	6.9	6.3
Dentists [4]	145,500	58.4	70.9	58.0	48.5	62.7
Optometrists	26,000	10.4	- - -	- - -	- - -	- - -
Pharmacists	161,900	64.4	- - -	- - -	- - -	- - -
Podiatrists.	12,000	4.8	- - -	- - -	- - -	- - -
Registered nurses	1,715,600	690.0	859.1	738.7	583.7	622.3
Associate and diploma	1,077,800	433.4	536.7	464.4	379.5	367.4
Baccalaureate	517,800	208.2	256.6	223.4	166.1	208.8
Masters and doctorate	120,000	48.3	65.7	51.0	38.0	45.9
Veterinarians	51,000	20.4	- - -	- - -	- - -	- - -

[1]Ratios for physicians and dentists are based on civilian population; ratios for all other health occupations are based on resident population.
[2]Starting in 1989 data for doctors of medicine are as of January 1; in earlier years these data are as of December 31.
[3]Excludes physicians not classified according to activity status from the number of active health personnel.
[4]Excludes dentists in military service.

NOTE: See Appendix II for physician definitions.

SOURCES: Division of Health Professions Analysis, Bureau of Health Professions: Supply and Characteristics of Selected Health Personnel. DHHS Pub. No. (HRA) 81–20. Health Resources Administration. Hyattsville, Md., June 1981 and Eighth Report to the President and Congress on the Status of Health Personnel in the United States. Health Resources and Services Administration. DHHS Pub. No. HRS-P-OD-92-1, Rockville, Md., 1991; American Medical Association: Physician Characteristics and Distribution in the U.S., 1981 edition; 1992 edition. Chicago 1981; 1992; unpublished data; American Osteopathic Association: 1980–81 Yearbook and Directory of Osteopathic Physicians. Chicago, 1980. American Association of Colleges of Osteopathic Medicine: Annual Statistical Report 1990. Rockville, Md., 1990; unpublished data.

Table 102. Full-time equivalent employment in selected occupations for community hospitals: United States, 1981 and 1986–90

[Data are based on reporting by a census of registered hospitals]

Occupation	1981	1986	1988	1989	1990	Average annual percent change	
						1981–86	1986–90
All hospital personnel [1]	3,069,955	3,055,071	3,231,745	3,328,509	3,439,820	−0.1	3.0
Administrators and assistant administrators	26,734	32,990	35,715	37,269	37,015	4.3	2.9
Registered nurses	629,354	736,253	770,613	791,521	809,920	3.2	2.4
Licensed practical nurses	234,226	174,154	170,637	172,143	167,945	−5.8	−0.9
Ancillary nursing personnel	280,614	226,821	244,297	252,500	268,113	−4.2	4.3
Medical record administrators and technicians	38,186	44,057	46,937	47,834	50,723	2.9	3.6
Licensed pharmacists and pharmacy technicians	47,053	54,679	58,759	60,984	64,004	3.0	4.0
Medical technologists and other laboratory personnel	147,451	145,622	148,635	152,122	157,880	−0.2	2.0
Dietitians and dietetic technicians	40,192	34,241	35,126	34,416	35,553	−3.2	0.9
Radiologic service personnel	90,738	94,683	101,098	104,494	111,298	0.9	4.1
Occupational therapists and recreational therapists	8,481	11,210	13,133	13,604	15,144	5.7	7.8
Physical therapists and physical therapy assistants and aides	27,675	30,216	32,680	33,104	35,455	1.8	4.1
Speech pathologists and audiologists	2,463	3,776	4,346	4,608	4,909	8.9	6.8
Respiratory therapists and respiratory therapy technicians	47,312	52,751	55,690	57,355	60,403	2.2	3.4
Medical social workers	13,915	16,042	18,685	19,698	21,389	2.9	7.5
Total trainee personnel [2]	66,906	67,366	67,587	68,641	69,111	0.1	0.6

[1]Includes occupational categories not shown.
[2]This category is primarily composed of medical residents.

SOURCE: Compiled by the Office of Data Analysis and Management, Bureau of Health Professions, Health Resources and Services Administration, from the American Hospital Association's 1981, 1986, 1988, 1989, and 1990 Annual Survey of Hospitals.

Table 103 (page 1 of 2). Full-time equivalent patient care staff in mental health organizations, according to type of organization and staff discipline: United States, selected years 1984–88

[Data are based on inventories of mental health organizations]

Organization and discipline	1984	1986	1988	1984	1986	1988
All organizations	Number			Percent distribution		
All patient care staff	313,243	346,630	381,216	100.0	100.0	100.0
Professional patient care staff	202,474	232,481	248,430	64.6	67.1	65.2
Psychiatrists	18,482	17,874	18,132	5.9	5.2	4.8
Psychologists	21,052	20,210	23,131	6.7	5.8	6.1
Social workers	36,397	40,951	46,218	11.6	11.8	12.1
Registered nurses	54,406	66,180	73,387	17.4	19.1	19.3
Other professional staff [1]	72,137	87,266	87,562	23.0	25.2	23.0
Other mental health workers	110,769	114,149	132,786	35.4	32.9	34.8
State and county mental hospitals						
All patient care staff	117,630	119,073	116,527	100.0	100.0	100.0
Professional patient care staff	51,290	54,853	49,184	43.6	46.1	42.2
Psychiatrists	4,108	3,762	3,830	3.5	3.2	3.3
Psychologists	3,239	3,412	3,536	2.8	2.9	3.0
Social workers	6,175	6,238	7,164	5.2	5.2	6.1
Registered nurses	16,051	19,425	20,292	13.6	16.3	17.4
Other professional staff [1]	21,717	22,016	14,362	18.5	18.5	12.3
Other mental health workers	66,340	64,220	67,343	56.4	53.9	57.8
Private psychiatric hospitals						
All patient care staff	26,359	35,480	55,658	100.0	100.0	100.0
Professional patient care staff	19,524	27,246	42,965	74.1	76.8	77.2
Psychiatrists	1,447	1,554	1,843	5.5	4.4	3.3
Psychologists	1,461	1,557	1,833	5.5	4.4	3.3
Social workers	2,179	2,893	4,067	8.3	8.2	7.3
Registered nurses	6,818	10,147	14,710	25.9	28.6	26.4
Other professional staff [1]	7,619	11,095	20,512	28.9	31.3	36.9
Other mental health workers	6,835	8,234	12,693	25.9	23.2	22.8
Nonfederal general hospitals' psychiatric services						
All patient care staff	59,848	61,148	62,066	100.0	100.0	100.0
Professional patient care staff	46,335	50,233	48,490	77.4	82.1	78.1
Psychiatrists	6,679	6,009	5,276	11.2	9.8	8.5
Psychologists	3,283	2,983	3,707	5.5	4.9	6.0
Social workers	4,898	5,634	5,568	8.2	9.2	9.0
Registered nurses	20,454	23,454	24,490	34.2	38.4	39.5
Other professional staff [1]	11,021	12,153	9,449	18.4	19.9	15.2
Other mental health workers	13,513	10,915	13,576	22.6	17.9	21.9
Veterans Administration psychiatric services						
All patient care staff	22,948	23,559	22,074	100.0	100.0	100.0
Professional patient care staff	16,265	17,782	15,061	70.9	75.5	68.2
Psychiatrists	2,463	2,245	2,132	10.7	9.5	9.7
Psychologists	1,247	1,439	1,340	5.4	6.1	6.1
Social workers	1,545	1,680	1,424	6.7	7.1	6.5
Registered nurses	5,699	6,761	6,514	24.8	28.7	29.5
Other professional staff [1]	5,311	5,657	3,651	23.1	24.0	16.5
Other mental health workers	6,683	5,777	7,013	29.1	24.5	31.8
Residential treatment centers for emotionally disturbed children						
All patient care staff	15,297	25,146	30,139	100.0	100.0	100.0
Professional patient care staff	10,551	17,599	19,688	69.0	70.0	65.3
Psychiatrists	240	335	449	1.6	1.3	1.5
Psychologists	820	911	1,274	5.4	3.6	4.2
Social workers	2,283	4,585	4,211	14.9	18.2	14.0
Registered nurses	485	746	821	3.2	3.0	2.7
Other professional staff [1]	6,723	11,022	12,933	43.9	43.8	42.9
Other mental health workers	4,746	7,547	10,451	31.0	30.0	34.7

See footnotes at end of table.

Table 103 (page 2 of 2). Full-time equivalent patient care staff in mental health organizations, according to type of organization and staff discipline: United States, selected years 1984–88

[Data are based on inventories of mental health organizations]

Organization and discipline	1984	1986	1988	1984	1986	1988
All other organizations [2]		Number			Percent distribution	
All patient care staff	71,161	82,224	94,749	100.0	100.0	100.0
Professional patient care staff	58,509	64,768	73,039	82.2	78.8	77.1
Psychiatrists	3,545	3,969	4,601	5.0	4.8	4.9
Psychologists	11,002	9,908	11,444	15.5	12.1	12.1
Social workers	19,317	19,921	23,784	27.1	24.2	25.1
Registered nurses	4,899	5,647	6,559	6.9	6.9	6.9
Other professional staff [1]	19,746	25,323	26,651	27.7	30.8	28.1
Other mental health workers	12,652	17,456	21,710	17.8	21.2	22.9

[1] Includes occupational therapists, recreation therapists, vocational rehabilitation counselors, and teachers.
[2] Includes freestanding outpatient, partial care, and multiservice organizations.

SOURCES: Statistical Research Branch, Division of Applied and Services Research, National Institute of Mental Health: R. W. Manderscheid and S. A. Barrett: Mental Health, United States, 1987. DHHS Pub. No. (ADM) 87-1518. U.S. Government Printing Office, 1987; R. W. Manderscheid and M. A. Sonnenschein: Mental Health, United States, 1990. DHHS Pub. No. (ADM) 90-1708. U.S. Government Printing Office, 1990; Unpublished data.

Table 104. First-year enrollment and graduates of health professions schools and number of schools, according to profession: United States, selected years 1950–91 and projections for year 2000

[Data are based on reporting by health professions schools]

Year	Medicine	Osteopathy	Registered nursing Total	Baccalaureate	Associate degree	Diploma	Licensed practical nursing	Dentistry	Optometry	Pharmacy	Chiropractic
First-year enrollment [1]											
1980	16,930	1,426	105,952	35,414	53,633	16,905	56,316	6,066	1,185	7,905	- - -
1981	17,186	1,496	110,201	35,808	56,899	17,494	58,479	5,964	1,174	7,442	- - -
1982	17,268	1,582	115,279	35,928	60,423	18,928	60,426	5,789	1,162	6,617	- - -
1983	17,254	1,682	120,579	37,264	63,947	19,368	61,453	5,498	1,120	6,280	- - -
1984	17,150	1,746	123,824	39,400	66,576	17,848	57,865	5,207	1,187	6,598	- - -
1985	16,997	1,750	118,224	39,573	63,776	14,875	47,034	4,983	1,177	6,749	- - -
1986 [2]	16,963	1,737	100,791	34,310	56,635	9,846	44,477	4,777	1,154	6,584	- - -
1987 [3]	16,819	1,724	90,693	28,026	54,330	8,337	42,452	4,494	1,210	7,081	- - -
1988 [3]	16,713	1,692	94,269	28,505	57,375	8,389	43,774	4,316	1,234	7,309	- - -
1989 [3]	16,868	1,780	103,025	29,042	63,973	10,010	47,602	4,148	1,271	8,067	- - -
1990	16,756	1,844	108,580	29,858	68,634	10,088	52,969	3,938	1,258	8,009	- - -
1991	16,876	1,950	113,526	33,437	69,869	10,220	56,176	3,961	1,207	- - -	- - -
Graduates [1]											
1950 [4]	5,553	373	25,790	- - -	- - -	- - -	2,828	2,565	961	- - -	- - -
1960	7,081	427	30,113	4,136	789	25,188	16,491	3,253	364	3,497	660
1970	8,367	432	43,103	9,069	11,483	22,551	36,456	3,749	445	4,758	642
1975	12,714	702	73,915	20,170	32,183	21,562	45,375	4,969	806	6,712	1,093
1980	15,135	1,059	75,523	24,994	36,034	14,495	41,892	5,256	1,073	7,432	2,049
1981	15,667	1,151	73,985	24,370	36,712	12,903	41,002	5,550	1,092	7,323	2,526
1982	15,985	1,017	74,052	24,081	38,289	11,682	43,299	5,371	1,106	6,859	2,631
1983	15,824	1,317	77,408	23,855	41,849	11,704	45,174	5,756	1,166	6,374	2,948
1984	16,327	1,287	80,312	23,718	44,394	12,200	44,654	5,337	1,188	5,963	- - -
1985	16,319	1,474	82,075	24,975	45,208	11,892	36,955	5,353	1,114	5,724	- - -
1986	16,125	1,560	77,027	25,170	41,333	10,524	29,599	4,957	1,085	5,800	- - -
1987	15,836	1,587	70,561	23,761	38,528	8,272	27,285	4,717	1,081	5,854	- - -
1988	15,887	1,572	64,839	21,504	37,397	5,938	26,912	4,581	1,106	6,171	2,797
1989 [5]	15,620	1,609	61,660	18,997	37,837	4,826	30,368	4,312	1,143	6,557	2,400
1990	15,336	1,529	66,088	18,571	42,318	5,199	35,417	4,233	1,115	- - -	- - -
1991 [6]	15,499	1,533	72,230	19,264	46,794	6,172	38,100	3,995	1,136	- - -	- - -
2000 [7]	16,536	1,758	61,800	15,822	41,834	4,100	- - -	3,242	1,200	7,120	2,950
Schools [1,8]											
1950 [4]	79	6	1,170	- - -	- - -	- - -	85	42	10	- - -	20
1960	86	6	1,137	172	57	908	661	47	10	76	12
1970	103	7	1,340	267	437	636	1,233	53	11	74	11
1975	114	9	1,362	326	608	428	1,315	59	12	73	12
1980	126	14	1,385	377	697	311	1,299	60	15	72	14
1981	126	15	1,401	383	715	303	1,309	60	16	72	16
1982	127	15	1,432	402	742	288	1,295	60	16	72	16
1983	127	15	1,466	421	764	281	1,297	60	16	72	17
1984	127	15	1,477	427	777	273	1,254	60	16	72	17
1985	127	15	1,473	441	776	256	1,165	60	16	72	17
1986	127	15	1,469	455	776	238	1,087	59	16	73	17
1987	127	15	1,465	467	789	209	1,068	58	16	74	17
1988	127	15	1,442	479	792	171	1,095	58	16	74	17
1989	127	15	1,457	488	812	157	1,171	58	16	74	17
1990	126	15	1,470	489	829	152	1,154	58	16	74	17
1991	126	15	1,484	501	838	145	1,125	58	16	74	17

[1]Data on the number of schools are collected at the beginning of the academic year while data on first-year enrollment and number of graduates are collected at the end of the academic year.
[2]First-year enrollment data for optometry exclude Ohio State University.
[3]First-year enrollment data for pharmacy include the University of Puerto Rico.
[4]Data for total registered nursing are for 1951.
[5]Data for chiropractic medicine are estimated.
[6]Data for medicine are estimated.
[7]Projected.
[8]Some nursing schools offer more than one type of program. Numbers shown for nursing are number of nursing programs.

NOTE: Some numbers in this table have been revised and differ from previous editions of Health, United States.

SOURCES: Association of American Medical Colleges: AAMC Data Book Statistical Information Related to Medical Education. Washington, D.C., 1991; Bureau of Health Professions: Eighth Report to the President and Congress on the Status of Health Personnel in the United States. Health Resources and Services Administration. DHHS Pub. No. HRS-P-OD-92-1. Health Resources and Services Administration: Unpublished data; National League for Nursing: Nursing Datasource, 1992; National League for Nursing: Nursing Data Review, 1989; American Nurses Association: Facts About Nursing, 1951 and 1961; American Dental Association Council on Dental Education: Annual Report on Dental Education 1990–91. Chicago, 1991; American Medical Association: Medical education in the United States. JAMA. Vol. 266, No. 7. August 21, 1991; American Association of Colleges of Osteopathic Medicine: Annual Statistical Report 1991. Rockville, Md., 1991; American Chiropractic Association: Unpublished data.

Table 105 (page 1 of 2). First-year and total enrollment of minorities in schools for selected health occupations, according to detailed race and Hispanic origin: United States, academic years 1980–81 and 1990–91

[Data are based on reporting by health professions associations]

Occupation, detailed race, and Hispanic origin	First-year enrollment [1]				Total enrollment [1]			
	1980–81	1990–91 [2]	1980–81	1990–91 [2]	1980–81	1990–91 [2]	1980–81	1990–91 [2]
Allopathic medicine	Number of students		Percent of students		Number of students		Percent of students	
All races [3]	17,186	16,876	100.0	100.0	65,189	65,163	100.0	100.0
Non-Hispanic white	14,262	11,830	83.0	70.1	55,434	47,893	85.0	73.5
Non-Hispanic black	1,128	1,263	6.6	7.5	3,708	4,241	5.7	6.5
Hispanic	818	933	4.8	5.5	2,761	3,538	4.2	5.4
Mexican American	258	285	1.5	1.7	951	1,109	1.5	1.7
Mainland Puerto Rican	95	120	0.6	0.7	329	457	0.5	0.7
Other Hispanic [4]	465	528	2.7	3.1	1,481	1,972	2.3	3.0
American Indian	67	76	0.4	0.5	221	277	0.3	0.4
Asian	572	2,527	3.3	15.0	1,924	8,436	3.0	12.9
Osteopathic medicine								
All races	1,496	1,950	100.0	100.0	4,940	6,792	100.0	100.0
Non-Hispanic white [3]	1,397	1,565	93.4	80.3	4,688	5,680	94.9	83.6
Non-Hispanic black	40	79	2.7	4.1	94	217	1.9	3.2
Hispanic	18	78	1.2	4.0	52	277	1.1	4.1
American Indian	8	14	0.5	0.7	19	36	0.4	0.5
Asian	33	214	2.2	11.0	87	582	1.8	8.6
Podiatry								
All races	695	622	100.0	100.0	2,577	2,226	100.0	100.0
Non-Hispanic white [3]	629	433	90.5	69.6	2,353	1,671	91.3	75.1
Non-Hispanic black	40	77	5.8	12.4	110	237	4.3	10.6
Hispanic	8	54	1.2	8.7	39	148	1.5	6.6
American Indian	2	2	0.3	0.3	6	7	0.2	0.3
Asian	16	56	2.3	9.0	69	163	2.7	7.3
Dentistry [5]								
All races	5,964	3,961	100.0	100.0	22,842	15,770	100.0	100.0
Non-Hispanic white [3]	5,192	2,805	87.1	70.8	20,208	11,185	88.5	70.9
Non-Hispanic black	283	265	4.7	6.7	1,022	940	4.5	6.0
Hispanic	160	240	2.7	6.1	519	1,073	2.3	6.8
American Indian	12	10	0.2	0.3	53	53	0.2	0.3
Asian	317	641	5.3	16.2	1,040	2,519	4.6	16.0
Optometry [5]								
All races	1,174	1,207	100.0	100.0	4,540	4,650	100.0	100.0
Non-Hispanic white [3]	- - -	930	- - -	77.1	4,148	3,706	91.4	79.7
Non-Hispanic black	- - -	47	- - -	3.9	57	134	1.3	2.9
Hispanic	- - -	50	- - -	4.1	80	186	1.8	4.0
American Indian	- - -	7	- - -	0.6	12	21	0.3	0.5
Asian	- - -	173	- - -	14.3	243	603	5.4	13.0
Pharmacy [6]								
All races	7,442	8,009	100.0	100.0	21,628	22,764	100.0	100.0
Non-Hispanic white [3]	6,470	- - -	86.9	- - -	19,153	18,325	88.6	80.5
Non-Hispanic black	376	- - -	5.1	- - -	945	1,301	4.4	5.7
Hispanic	210	- - -	2.8	- - -	459	945	2.1	4.2
American Indian	13	- - -	0.2	- - -	36	63	0.2	0.3
Asian	373	- - -	5.0	- - -	1,035	2,130	4.8	9.4
Veterinary medicine								
All races	2,131	2,197	100.0	100.0	7,777	8,420	100.0	100.0
Non-Hispanic white [3]	- - -	2,021	- - -	92.0	7,401	7,787	95.2	92.5
Non-Hispanic black	- - -	61	- - -	2.8	176	215	2.3	2.6
Hispanic	- - -	66	- - -	3.0	89	243	1.1	2.9
American Indian	- - -	13	- - -	0.6	32	45	0.4	0.5
Asian	- - -	36	- - -	1.6	79	130	1.0	1.5

See footnotes at end of table.

Table 105 (page 2 of 2). First-year and total enrollment of minorities in schools for selected health occupations, according to detailed race and Hispanic origin: United States, academic years 1980–81 and 1990–91

[Data are based on reporting by health professions associations]

Occupation, detailed race, and Hispanic origin	First-year enrollment [1]				Total enrollment [1]			
	1980–81	1990–91 [2]	1980–81	1990–91 [2]	1980–81	1990–91 [2]	1980–81	1990–91 [2]
Registered nurses [7]	Number of students		Percent of students		Number of students		Percent of students	
All races	110,201	113,526	100.0	100.0	230,966	221,170	100.0	100.0
Non-Hispanic white [3]	- - -	94,709	- - -	83.4	- - -	183,102	- - -	82.8
Non-Hispanic black	- - -	10,822	- - -	9.5	- - -	23,094	- - -	10.4
Hispanic.	- - -	3,619	- - -	3.2	- - -	6,580	- - -	3.0
American Indian	- - -	840	- - -	0.7	- - -	1,803	- - -	0.8
Asian	- - -	3,536	- - -	3.1	- - -	6,591	- - -	3.0

[1]Total enrollment data are collected in the beginning of the academic year while first-year enrollment data are collected at the end of the academic year.
[2]First-year and total enrollments for pharmacy students are for 1989–90, and include the University of Puerto Rico.
[3]Includes race/ethnicity unspecified.
[4]Includes Puerto Rican Commonwealth students.
[5]Excludes Puerto Rican schools.
[6]Pharmacy first-year enrollment data are for students in the first year of the final 3 years of pharmacy education. Pharmacy total enrollment data are for students in the final 3 years of pharmacy education.
[7]In 1990, the National League for Nursing developed a new system for analyzing minority data. In evaluating the former system, much underreporting was noted. Therefore, any data prior to 1989 would not be comparable.

NOTE: Some numbers in this table have been revised and differ from previous editions of Health, United States.

SOURCES: Association of American Medical Colleges: AAMC Data Book Statistical Information Related to Medical Education. Washington, D.C., 1991; American Association of Colleges of Osteopathic Medicine: 1991 Annual Statistical Report. Rockville, Md., 1991; Bureau of Health Professions: Minorities and Women in the Health Fields, 1990 Edition; American Dental Association in cooperation with the American Association of Dental Schools: Annual Report on Dental Education 1990/91. Chicago, 1991; Association of Schools and Colleges of Optometry: Unpublished data; American Association of Colleges of Pharmacy: Unpublished data; Association of American Veterinary Medical Colleges: Unpublished data; American Association of Colleges of Podiatric Medicine: Unpublished data; National League for Nursing: Nursing Datasource. New York, 1992; Nursing Data Book, New York, 1982.

Table 106. First-year and total enrollment of women in schools for selected health occupations, according to detailed race and Hispanic origin: United States, academic years 1971–72, 1980–81, and 1990–91

[Data are based on reporting by health professions associations]

Enrollment, occupation, detailed race, and Hispanic origin	Both sexes			Women		
	1971–72[1]	1980–81	1990–91[2]	1971–72[1]	1980–81	1990–91[2]
First-year enrollment [3]	Number of students			Percent of students		
Allopathic medicine [4]	12,361	17,186	16,876	13.7	28.9	38.8
Non-Hispanic white.	- - -	14,262	11,830	- - -	27.4	37.7
Non-Hispanic black.	881	1,128	1,263	22.7	45.5	55.3
Hispanic.	- - -	818	933	- - -	31.5	42.0
Mexican American	118	258	285	8.5	30.6	39.3
Mainland Puerto Rican	40	95	120	15.0	43.2	43.3
Other Hispanic [5]	- - -	465	528	- - -	29.7	43.3
American Indian	23	67	76	34.8	35.8	40.8
Asian	217	572	2,527	19.4	31.5	40.3
Osteopathic medicine.	670	1,496	1,950	4.3	22.0	34.2
Dentistry [6]	4,705	5,964	3,961	3.1	19.8	37.9
Optometry.	906	1,174	1,207	5.3	25.3	50.6
Pharmacy [7]	6,532	7,442	8,009	25.8	48.4	- - -
Veterinary medicine	1,453	2,131	2,197	15.3	43.5	61.6
Registered nurses	93,344	110,201	113,526	94.5	92.7	89.3
Total enrollment [3]						
Allopathic medicine [4]	43,650	65,189	65,163	10.9	26.5	37.3
Non-Hispanic white.	- - -	55,434	47,893	- - -	25.0	35.4
Non-Hispanic black.	2,055	3,708	4,241	20.4	44.3	55.8
Hispanic.	- - -	2,761	3,538	- - -	30.1	39.0
Mexican American	252	951	1,109	9.5	26.4	38.5
Mainland Puerto Rican	76	329	457	17.1	35.9	43.1
Other Hispanic [5]	- - -	1,481	1,972	- - -	31.1	38.4
American Indian	42	221	277	23.8	28.5	42.6
Asian	647	1,924	8,436	17.9	30.4	37.7
Osteopathic medicine.	2,304	4,940	6,792	3.4	19.7	32.7
Podiatry.	1,268	2,577	2,226	1.2	11.9	- - -
Optometry.	3,094	4,540	4,650	- - -	- - -	47.3
Veterinary medicine	5,149	7,777	8,420	11.5	38.8	60.1
Registered nurses	211,239	230,966	221,170	95.5	94.3	- - -

[1]Total enrollments for registered nurse students are for 1972–73.
[2]First-year enrollments for pharmacy students are for 1989–90, and include the University of Puerto Rico.
[3]Total enrollment data are collected at the beginning of the academic year while first-year enrollment data are collected at the end of the academic year.
[4]Includes race/ethnicity unspecified.
[5]Includes Puerto Rican Commonwealth students.
[6]Excludes Puerto Rican schools.
[7]Pharmacy first-year enrollment data are for students in the first year of the final 3 years of pharmacy education.

NOTES: Data not available on first-year enrollment of women in schools of podiatry and total enrollment of women in schools of dentistry and pharmacy. Some numbers in this table have been revised and differ from previous editions of Health, United States.

SOURCES: Association of American Medical Colleges: AAMC Data Book Statistical Information Related to Medical Education. Washington, D.C., 1991; American Association of Colleges of Osteopathic Medicine: 1991 Annual Statistical Report. Rockville, Md., 1991; Bureau of Health Professions: Minorities and Women in the Health Fields, 1990 Edition; American Dental Association in cooperation with the American Association of Dental Schools: Annual Report on Dental Education 1990/91. Chicago, 1991; Association of Schools and Colleges of Optometry: Unpublished data; American Association of Colleges of Pharmacy: Unpublished data; Association of American Veterinary Medical Colleges: Unpublished data; American Association of Colleges of Podiatric Medicine: Unpublished data; National League for Nursing: Nursing Datasource. New York, 1992; Nursing Data Book, New York, 1982; State-Approved Schools of Nursing-RN. New York, 1973.

Table 107. Short-stay hospitals, beds, and occupancy rates, according to type of ownership and size of hospital: United States, selected years 1960–91

[Data are based on reporting by a census of hospitals]

Type of ownership and size of hospital	1960	1970	1975	1980	1985	1986	1987	1988	1989	1990	1991
Hospitals					Number						
All ownerships.........	5,768	6,193	6,310	6,229	6,091	6,035	5,967	5,892	5,808	5,728	5,675
Federal..............	361	334	331	325	307	307	308	313	311	308	305
Nonfederal	5,407	5,859	5,979	5,904	5,784	5,728	5,659	5,579	5,497	5,420	5,370
Nonprofit	3,291	3,386	3,364	3,339	3,364	3,338	3,289	3,256	3,233	3,202	3,184
Proprietary..........	856	769	775	730	805	834	828	790	769	749	738
State-local government	1,260	1,704	1,840	1,835	1,615	1,556	1,542	1,533	1,495	1,469	1,448
Size of hospital:											
6–99 beds...........	- - -	- - -	3,196	2,953	2,751	2,732	2,736	2,694	2,646	2,584	2,541
100–199 beds	- - -	- - -	1,413	1,436	1,458	1,445	1,408	1,391	1,388	1,369	1,366
200–299 beds	- - -	- - -	701	742	765	781	776	779	766	773	763
300–499 beds	- - -	- - -	651	724	736	706	686	671	664	661	671
500 beds or more.....	- - -	- - -	349	374	381	371	361	357	344	341	334
Beds											
All ownerships.........	735,451	935,724	1,036,025	1,080,164	1,087,750	1,066,611	1,046,013	1,033,881	1,014,965	1,007,201	1,002,600
Federal..............	96,394	87,492	89,049	88,144	84,612	85,071	84,523	84,419	79,202	77,827	76,725
Nonfederal	639,057	848,232	946,976	992,020	1,003,138	981,540	961,490	949,462	935,763	929,374	925,875
Nonprofit	445,753	591,937	658,948	692,929	707,806	689,685	673,308	668,101	660,947	657,016	656,713
Proprietary..........	37,029	52,739	73,495	87,033	103,921	106,716	105,746	103,623	102,416	101,377	99,657
State-local government	156,275	203,556	214,533	212,058	191,411	185,139	182,436	177,738	172,400	170,981	169,505
Size of hospital:											
6–99 beds...........	- - -	- - -	165,148	155,259	147,703	146,202	145,541	143,006	139,478	136,034	134,073
100–199 beds	- - -	- - -	201,587	203,023	206,029	204,139	198,777	196,555	196,322	193,388	193,735
200–299 beds	- - -	- - -	171,057	180,047	185,033	189,017	188,294	189,236	186,675	188,833	185,944
300–499 beds	- - -	- - -	247,410	276,201	279,700	266,477	258,841	253,110	251,987	250,646	254,120
500 beds or more.....	- - -	- - -	250,823	265,634	269,285	260,776	254,560	251,974	240,503	238,300	234,728
Occupancy rate					Percent of beds occupied						
All ownerships.........	75.7	77.9	75.0	75.6	65.5	64.9	65.5	65.9	66.5	67.1	66.4
Federal..............	82.5	77.5	77.6	77.8	74.3	72.6	71.8	71.2	71.0	71.2	70.1
Nonfederal	74.7	78.0	74.8	75.4	64.8	64.2	64.9	65.5	66.2	66.8	66.1
Nonprofit	76.6	80.1	77.4	78.2	67.2	66.8	67.6	68.2	68.8	69.3	68.6
Proprietary..........	65.4	72.2	65.9	65.2	52.1	50.7	51.1	50.9	51.7	52.8	52.6
State-local government	71.6	73.2	69.7	70.7	62.8	62.6	63.1	63.8	64.8	65.3	64.4
Size of hospital:											
6–99 beds...........	- - -	- - -	61.1	60.6	48.4	47.3	47.8	48.3	49.0	49.7	49.9
100–199 beds	- - -	- - -	71.3	71.6	60.0	58.8	59.2	59.7	60.8	61.8	60.5
200–299 beds	- - -	- - -	77.1	77.3	65.9	65.5	65.6	66.0	66.9	67.3	66.8
300–499 beds	- - -	- - -	80.0	80.0	69.4	69.0	70.1	70.9	70.9	71.5	70.4
500 beds or more.....	- - -	- - -	80.9	81.9	74.9	74.9	75.6	75.8	76.5	76.6	76.2

NOTE: Excludes psychiatric and tuberculosis and other respiratory disease hospitals.

SOURCES: American Hospital Association: Hospitals. JAHA 35(15):396–401 and 45(15):463–467, Aug. 1961 and Aug. 1971; Hospital Statistics, 1976, 1981, 1985–92 Editions. Chicago, 1976, 1981, 1985–92. (Copyrights 1961, 1971, 1976, 1981, 1985–92: Used with the permission of the American Hospital Association.)

Table 108. Long-term hospitals, beds, and occupancy rates, according to type of hospital and ownership: United States, selected years 1970–91

[Data are based on reporting by a census of hospitals]

Type of hospital and ownership	1970	1975	1980	1985	1986	1987	1988	1989	1990	1991
Hospitals					Number					
General	75	44	17	23	21	21	20	25	31	30
Federal	38	23	9	14	13	13	10	10	11	9
Nonfederal	37	21	8	9	8	8	10	15	20	21
Psychiatric	459	419	381	383	390	391	393	382	362	354
Federal	33	26	23	19	18	18	17	17	16	15
Nonprofit.	56	45	47	57	55	51	53	50	45	39
Proprietary	39	51	57	81	91	96	103	96	80	76
State-local government	331	297	254	226	226	226	220	219	221	224
Tuberculosis and other respiratory diseases. .	103	34	10	5	2	3	3	3	3	3
All other	200	196	150	122	129	126	121	125	112	109
Federal	1	2	1	3	4	3	2	2	1	4
Nonprofit.	110	94	66	59	61	58	55	58	49	45
Proprietary	2	9	11	13	15	17	15	19	17	19
State-local government	87	91	72	47	49	48	49	46	45	41
Beds										
General	42,569	17,329	8,253	12,985	11,112	11,508	9,807	11,275	11,599	10,466
Federal	31,403	14,406	7,205	10,073	9,079	9,232	7,449	8,373	8,040	6,481
Nonfederal	11,166	2,923	1,048	2,912	2,033	2,276	2,358	2,902	3,559	3,985
Psychiatric	551,847	344,257	218,400	162,968	157,378	150,727	143,853	135,968	131,356	121,100
Federal	41,500	27,523	20,871	15,739	15,167	14,585	12,285	12,046	11,315	10,044
Nonprofit.	8,892	5,366	6,645	6,708	6,668	5,994	5,950	5,486	5,218	3,715
Proprietary	3,399	4,821	5,877	8,832	9,270	9,786	10,014	9,200	7,923	7,222
State-local government	498,056	306,547	185,007	131,689	126,273	120,362	115,604	109,236	106,900	100,119
Tuberculosis and other respiratory diseases. .	19,937	5,699	1,500	574	183	339	312	348	355	355
All other	49,152	49,268	37,911	29,519	29,614	27,541	26,013	25,612	22,166	24,016
Federal	357	968	357	1,599	1,812	1,451	1,043	1,010	734	3,043
Nonprofit.	12,638	12,733	10,038	9,391	9,829	8,785	8,107	8,878	7,324	7,086
Proprietary	101	879	1,356	1,364	1,844	1,681	1,472	1,606	1,197	1,226
State-local government	36,056	34,688	26,160	17,165	16,129	15,624	15,391	14,118	12,911	12,661
Occupancy rate					Percent of beds occupied					
General	79.2	84.4	83.9	80.2	79.1	76.5	78.3	81.3	78.4	81.7
Federal	80.4	85.2	84.6	80.7	77.8	74.7	76.9	81.1	76.7	80.3
Nonfederal	75.8	80.4	79.0	78.6	85.0	83.8	82.6	81.7	82.3	84.1
Psychiatric	84.9	81.3	85.9	87.2	87.0	87.9	87.5	87.7	86.1	86.7
Federal	83.4	88.3	87.9	83.5	79.6	83.1	84.5	83.0	81.0	78.7
Nonprofit.	85.2	84.8	87.2	86.5	85.5	81.7	78.9	77.1	76.5	80.0
Proprietary	78.4	74.1	76.3	77.6	75.8	75.8	77.8	77.3	72.7	69.6
State-local government	85.0	80.8	86.0	88.3	88.8	89.8	89.1	89.7	88.1	89.0
Tuberculosis and other respiratory diseases. .	61.9	57.6	66.4	64.3	59.6	70.5	76.6	73.0	65.4	79.2
All other	83.3	82.3	85.9	88.7	87.5	87.2	87.6	86.0	86.3	84.2
Federal	73.4	86.3	65.3	81.9	80.1	82.2	83.9	87.1	92.9	78.8
Nonprofit.	82.8	83.3	87.3	89.9	88.4	87.9	89.2	86.2	85.9	85.2
Proprietary	87.1	86.0	86.5	85.6	82.6	76.3	80.6	79.5	75.9	64.1
State-local government	83.6	81.7	85.6	88.9	88.4	88.5	87.6	86.5	87.2	86.9

SOURCES: American Hospital Association: Hospitals. JAHA 45(15):463–467, Aug. 1971; Hospital Statistics, 1976, 1981, 1985–92 Editions. Chicago, 1976, 1981, 1985–92. (Copyrights 1971, 1976, 1981, 1985–92: Used with the permission of the American Hospital Association.)

Table 109. Inpatient and residential treatment beds in mental health organizations and rate per 100,000 civilian population, according to type of organization: United States, selected years 1970–88

[Data are based on inventories of mental health organizations]

Organization	1970	1980 [1]	1982 [2]	1984	1986	1988
	Number					
All organizations.	524,878	274,713	247,312	262,673	267,613	271,923
State and county mental hospitals	413,066	156,482	140,140	130,411	119,033	107,109
Private psychiatric hospitals	14,295	17,157	19,011	21,474	30,201	42,255
Nonfederal general hospital psychiatric services	22,394	29,384	36,525	46,045	45,808	48,421
Veterans Administration psychiatric services [3]	50,688	33,796	24,646	23,546	26,874	25,742
Federally funded community mental health centers. .	8,108	16,264	. . .	. . .	. . .	. . .
Residential treatment centers for emotionally						
disturbed children.	15,129	20,197	18,475	16,745	24,547	25,173
All other [4,5]	1,198	1,433	8,515	24,452	21,150	23,223
	Number per 100,000 civilian population					
All organizations.	263.6	124.3	108.1	112.9	111.7	111.4
State and county mental hospitals	207.4	70.2	61.2	56.1	49.7	44.0
Private psychiatric hospitals	7.2	7.7	8.3	9.2	12.6	17.3
Nonfederal general hospital psychiatric services	11.2	13.7	16.0	19.8	19.1	19.8
Veterans Administration psychiatric services [3]	25.5	15.7	10.8	10.1	11.2	10.5
Federally funded community mental health centers. .	4.1	7.3	. . .	. . .	. . .	. . .
Residential treatment centers for emotionally						
disturbed children.	7.6	9.1	8.1	7.2	10.3	10.3
All other [4,5]	0.6	0.6	3.7	10.5	8.8	9.5

[1] During 1979–80, comparable data were not available for certain organization types, and data for either an earlier or later period were substituted.

[2] During 1981–82, some organizations were reclassified and data for some organization types were not available, resulting in a particularly large increase for the "all other" category in 1982.

[3] Includes Veterans Administration neuropsychiatric hospitals and Veterans Administration general hospitals with separate psychiatric services.

[4] Includes other multiservice mental health organizations with inpatient and residential treatment services that are not elsewhere classified.

[5] Beginning in 1983 a definitional change sharply increased the number of multiservice mental health organizations. See Appendix I.

NOTE: Changes in reporting procedures in 1979–80 and 1981–82 affect the comparability of data with those from previous years.

SOURCES: Statistical Research Branch, Division of Applied and Services Research, National Institute of Mental Health: R. W. Manderscheid and S. A. Barrett: Mental Health, United States, 1987. DHHS Pub. No. (ADM) 87-1518. U.S. Government Printing Office, 1987; R. W. Manderscheid and M. A. Sonnenschein: Mental Health, United States, 1990. DHHS Pub. No. (ADM) 90-1708. U.S. Government Printing Office, 1990; Unpublished data.

Table 110. Community hospital beds per 1,000 population and average annual percent change, according to geographic division and State: United States, selected years 1940–90

[Data are based on reporting by facilities]

Geographic division and State	Beds per 1,000 civilian population									Average annual percent change			
	1940[1]	1950[1]	1960[2]	1970	1980	1985	1988	1989	1990	1940–60[1,2]	1960–70[2]	1970–80	1980–90
United States	3.2	3.3	3.6	4.3	4.5	4.2	3.9	3.8	3.8	0.6	1.8	0.5	−1.7
New England	4.4	4.2	3.9	4.1	4.1	4.0	3.6	3.5	3.4	−0.6	0.5	0.0	−1.9
Maine	3.0	3.2	3.4	4.7	4.7	4.2	3.9	3.8	3.8	0.6	3.3	0.0	−2.1
New Hampshire	4.2	4.2	4.4	4.0	3.9	3.4	3.2	3.1	3.1	0.2	−0.9	−0.3	−2.3
Vermont	3.3	4.0	4.5	4.5	4.4	3.8	3.1	3.1	3.1	1.6	0.0	−0.2	−3.4
Massachusetts	5.1	4.8	4.2	4.4	4.4	4.4	4.0	3.8	3.6	−1.0	0.5	0.0	−2.0
Rhode Island	3.9	3.8	3.7	4.0	3.8	3.6	3.3	3.2	3.2	−0.3	0.8	−0.5	−1.7
Connecticut	3.7	3.6	3.4	3.4	3.5	3.3	3.0	3.0	2.9	−0.4	0.0	0.3	−1.9
Middle Atlantic	3.9	3.8	4.0	4.4	4.6	4.4	4.1	4.1	4.2	0.1	1.0	0.4	−0.9
New York	4.3	4.1	4.3	4.6	4.5	4.4	4.2	4.2	4.2	0.0	0.7	−0.2	−0.7
New Jersey	3.5	3.2	3.1	3.6	4.2	3.9	3.7	3.7	3.7	−0.6	1.5	1.6	−1.3
Pennsylvania	3.5	3.8	4.1	4.7	4.8	4.7	4.4	4.3	4.4	0.8	1.4	0.2	−0.9
East North Central	3.2	3.2	3.6	4.4	4.7	4.5	4.1	4.0	3.9	0.6	2.0	0.7	−1.8
Ohio	2.7	2.9	3.4	4.2	4.7	4.6	4.2	4.0	4.0	1.2	2.1	1.1	−1.6
Indiana	2.3	2.6	3.1	4.0	4.5	4.2	4.1	3.9	3.9	1.5	2.6	1.2	−1.4
Illinois	3.4	3.6	4.0	4.7	5.1	4.7	4.3	4.1	4.0	0.8	1.6	0.8	−2.4
Michigan	4.0	3.3	3.3	4.3	4.4	4.1	3.8	3.7	3.7	−1.0	2.7	0.2	−1.7
Wisconsin	3.4	3.7	4.3	5.2	4.9	4.6	4.0	3.9	3.8	1.2	1.9	−0.6	−2.5
West North Central	3.1	3.7	4.3	5.7	5.8	5.4	5.1	4.9	4.9	1.6	2.9	0.2	−1.7
Minnesota	3.9	4.4	4.8	6.1	5.7	5.2	4.8	4.5	4.4	1.0	2.4	−0.7	−2.6
Iowa	2.7	3.2	3.9	5.6	5.7	5.2	5.2	5.0	5.1	1.9	3.7	0.2	−1.1
Missouri	2.9	3.3	3.9	5.1	5.7	5.2	4.9	4.8	4.8	1.5	2.7	1.1	−1.7
North Dakota	3.5	4.3	5.2	6.8	7.4	7.4	7.0	7.0	7.0	2.0	2.7	0.8	−0.6
South Dakota	2.8	4.4	4.5	5.6	5.5	6.6	5.6	5.8	6.1	2.4	2.2	−0.2	1.0
Nebraska	3.4	4.2	4.4	6.2	6.0	6.0	5.8	5.5	5.4	1.3	3.5	−0.3	−1.0
Kansas	2.8	3.4	4.2	5.4	5.8	5.2	4.7	4.8	4.8	2.0	2.5	0.7	−1.9
South Atlantic	2.5	2.8	3.3	4.0	4.5	4.1	3.8	3.7	3.7	1.4	1.9	1.2	−1.9
Delaware	4.4	3.9	3.7	3.7	3.6	3.5	3.1	3.0	3.0	−0.9	0.0	−0.3	−1.8
Maryland	3.9	3.6	3.3	3.1	3.6	3.4	2.9	2.9	2.9	−0.8	−0.6	1.5	−2.1
District of Columbia	5.5	5.5	5.9	7.4	7.3	7.8	7.8	7.9	7.5	0.4	2.3	−0.1	0.3
Virginia	2.2	2.5	3.0	3.7	4.1	3.8	3.5	3.4	3.3	1.6	2.1	1.0	−2.1
West Virginia	2.7	3.1	4.1	5.4	5.5	5.1	4.7	4.7	4.7	2.1	2.8	0.2	−1.6
North Carolina	2.2	2.6	3.4	3.8	4.2	3.7	3.4	3.4	3.4	2.2	1.1	1.0	−2.1
South Carolina	1.8	2.4	2.9	3.7	3.9	3.6	3.3	3.2	3.3	2.4	2.5	0.5	−1.7
Georgia	1.7	2.0	2.8	3.8	4.6	4.3	4.1	4.1	4.0	2.5	3.1	1.9	−1.4
Florida	2.8	2.9	3.1	4.4	5.1	4.6	4.2	4.0	4.0	0.5	3.6	1.5	−2.4
East South Central	1.7	2.1	3.0	4.4	5.1	5.0	4.7	4.7	4.8	2.9	3.9	1.5	−0.6
Kentucky	1.8	2.2	3.0	4.0	4.5	4.4	4.3	4.3	4.4	2.6	2.9	1.2	−0.2
Tennessee	1.9	2.3	3.4	4.7	5.5	5.3	4.8	4.8	4.9	3.0	3.3	1.6	−1.1
Alabama	1.5	2.0	2.8	4.3	5.1	5.0	4.6	4.6	4.6	3.2	4.4	1.7	−1.0
Mississippi	1.4	1.7	2.9	4.4	5.3	5.2	5.4	5.2	5.3	3.7	4.3	1.9	0.0
West South Central	2.1	2.7	3.3	4.3	4.7	4.2	3.9	3.8	3.9	2.3	2.7	0.9	−1.8
Arkansas	1.4	1.6	2.9	4.2	5.0	4.8	4.5	4.5	4.7	3.7	3.8	1.8	−0.6
Louisiana	3.1	3.8	3.9	4.2	4.8	4.6	4.4	4.4	4.6	1.2	0.7	1.3	−0.4
Oklahoma	1.9	2.5	3.2	4.5	4.6	4.1	4.0	3.9	4.0	2.6	3.5	0.2	−1.4
Texas	2.0	2.7	3.3	4.3	4.7	4.1	3.7	3.6	3.5	2.5	2.7	0.9	−2.9
Mountain	3.6	3.8	3.5	4.3	3.8	3.5	3.3	3.1	3.1	−0.1	2.1	−1.2	−2.0
Montana	4.9	5.3	5.1	5.8	5.9	5.5	5.6	5.7	5.8	0.2	1.3	0.2	−0.2
Idaho	2.6	3.4	3.2	4.0	3.7	3.5	3.2	3.2	3.2	1.0	2.3	−0.8	−1.4
Wyoming	3.5	3.9	4.6	5.5	3.6	4.3	4.8	4.7	4.9	1.4	1.8	−4.1	3.1
Colorado	3.9	4.2	3.8	4.6	4.2	3.6	3.3	3.0	3.2	−0.1	1.9	−0.9	−2.7
New Mexico	2.7	2.2	2.9	3.5	3.1	2.9	2.8	2.9	2.9	0.4	1.9	−1.2	−0.7
Arizona	3.4	4.0	3.0	4.1	3.6	3.2	2.9	2.8	2.7	−0.6	3.2	−1.3	−2.8
Utah	3.2	2.9	2.8	3.6	3.1	2.7	2.7	2.6	2.6	−0.7	2.5	−1.5	−1.7
Nevada	5.0	4.4	3.9	4.2	4.2	3.7	3.2	3.0	2.9	−1.2	0.7	0.0	−3.6
Pacific	4.1	3.2	3.1	3.7	3.5	3.2	2.9	2.8	2.7	−1.4	1.8	−0.6	−2.6
Washington	3.4	3.6	3.3	3.5	3.1	3.0	2.7	2.6	2.5	−0.1	0.6	−1.2	−2.1
Oregon	3.5	3.1	3.5	4.0	3.5	3.2	2.9	2.9	2.9	0.0	1.3	−1.3	−1.9
California	4.4	3.3	3.0	3.8	3.6	3.2	2.9	2.9	2.7	−1.9	2.4	−0.5	−2.8
Alaska	. . .	. . .	2.4	2.3	2.7	2.2	2.4	2.5	2.3	. . .	−0.4	1.6	−1.6
Hawaii	. . .	. . .	3.7	3.4	3.1	2.8	2.7	2.7	2.8	. . .	−0.8	−0.9	−1.0

[1] 1940 and 1950 data are estimated based on published figures.
[2] 1960 includes hospital units of institutions.

SOURCES: American Medical Association: Hospital service in the United States. JAMA 116(11):1055–1144, 1941, and 146(2):109–184, 1951. (Copyright 1941 and 1951: Used with the permission of the American Medical Association.); American Hospital Association: Hospitals. JAHA 35(15):383–430, Aug. 1, 1961. (Copyright 1961: Used with the permission of the American Hospital Association.); Data computed by the Centers for Disease Control and Prevention, National Center for Health Statistics, Division of Analysis from data compiled by the Division of Health Care Statistics, National Master Facility Inventory and the American Hospital Association 1990 annual survey; U.S. Bureau of the Census: Current Population Reports. Series P-25, Nos. 72, 304, 460, 640, 970, 1010, 1044, and 1058. Washington. U.S. Government Printing Office, 1953, 1965, 1971, 1976, 1980, 1985, 1989, and 1990.

Table 111. Occupancy rates in community hospitals and average annual percent change, according to geographic division and State: United States, selected years 1940–90

[Data are based on reporting by facilities]

Geographic division and State	Percent of beds occupied								Average annual percent change			
	1940[1]	1960[2]	1970	1980	1985	1988	1989	1990	1940–60[1,2]	1960–70[2]	1970–80	1980–90
United States	69.9	74.7	77.3	75.2	65.1	65.7	66.1	66.7	0.3	0.3	−0.3	−1.2
New England	72.5	75.2	79.7	80.1	72.8	73.6	74.9	74.3	0.2	0.6	0.1	−0.7
Maine	72.4	73.2	73.0	74.5	66.8	70.8	71.4	71.6	0.1	−0.0	0.2	−0.4
New Hampshire	65.3	66.5	73.4	73.2	63.4	65.7	66.8	67.0	0.1	1.0	−0.0	−0.9
Vermont	68.8	68.5	76.3	73.7	68.0	66.8	65.9	66.9	−0.0	1.1	−0.3	−1.0
Massachusetts	71.8	75.8	80.3	81.7	74.1	73.4	75.7	74.6	0.3	0.6	0.2	−0.9
Rhode Island	77.7	75.7	82.9	85.9	76.2	83.2	79.9	79.5	−0.1	0.9	0.4	−0.8
Connecticut	75.9	78.2	82.6	80.4	75.4	76.4	77.7	77.0	0.1	0.5	−0.3	−0.4
Middle Atlantic	75.5	78.1	82.4	83.2	77.1	79.4	79.8	80.2	0.2	0.5	0.1	−0.4
New York	78.9	79.4	82.9	85.9	83.9	85.4	85.6	85.7	0.0	0.4	0.4	−0.0
New Jersey	72.4	78.4	82.5	82.8	74.8	78.2	79.3	80.0	0.4	0.5	0.0	−0.3
Pennsylvania	71.3	76.0	81.5	79.5	68.7	71.3	71.8	72.6	0.3	0.7	−0.2	−0.9
East North Central	71.0	78.4	79.5	76.9	64.2	63.8	63.9	64.8	0.5	0.1	−0.3	−1.7
Ohio	72.1	81.3	81.8	79.2	63.9	65.5	65.0	64.8	0.6	0.1	−0.3	−2.0
Indiana	68.5	79.6	80.3	77.6	61.6	58.3	59.8	60.6	0.8	0.1	−0.3	−2.4
Illinois	73.1	76.0	79.3	74.9	64.4	63.1	63.8	66.1	0.2	0.4	−0.6	−1.2
Michigan	71.5	80.5	80.6	78.2	67.4	66.2	65.7	65.5	0.6	0.0	−0.3	−1.8
Wisconsin	65.2	73.9	73.2	73.6	61.8	63.5	63.2	64.9	0.6	−0.1	0.1	−1.3
West North Central	65.7	71.8	73.6	71.2	60.3	60.9	61.5	61.9	0.4	0.2	−0.3	−1.4
Minnesota	71.0	72.3	73.9	73.7	63.8	64.1	65.9	66.9	0.1	0.2	−0.0	−1.0
Iowa	63.6	72.6	71.9	68.7	57.3	60.8	61.9	61.6	0.7	−0.1	−0.5	−1.1
Missouri	68.6	75.8	79.3	75.1	63.0	61.9	62.5	61.7	0.5	0.5	−0.5	−1.9
North Dakota	61.9	71.3	67.1	68.6	61.1	64.1	63.1	64.5	0.7	−0.6	0.2	−0.6
South Dakota	59.1	66.0	66.3	60.6	57.5	59.4	60.8	62.1	0.6	0.0	−0.9	0.2
Nebraska	59.0	65.6	69.9	67.4	58.4	56.1	55.9	58.6	0.5	0.6	−0.4	−1.4
Kansas	60.4	69.1	71.4	68.8	54.3	56.5	55.5	55.8	0.7	0.3	−0.4	−2.1
South Atlantic	66.7	74.8	77.9	75.5	65.5	66.6	66.6	67.2	0.6	0.4	−0.3	−1.2
Delaware	59.2	70.2	78.8	81.8	68.0	77.2	75.7	76.5	0.9	1.2	0.4	−0.7
Maryland	74.6	73.9	79.3	84.0	73.5	77.8	78.3	78.1	−0.0	0.7	0.6	−0.7
District of Columbia	76.2	80.8	77.7	83.0	75.9	75.9	79.7	76.1	0.3	−0.4	0.7	−0.9
Virginia	70.0	78.0	81.1	77.8	67.2	67.3	66.4	67.2	0.5	0.4	−0.4	−1.5
West Virginia	62.1	74.5	79.3	75.6	60.7	60.8	60.3	62.7	0.9	0.6	−0.5	−1.9
North Carolina	64.6	73.9	78.5	77.8	64.9	71.3	72.2	73.0	0.7	0.6	−0.1	−0.6
South Carolina	69.1	76.9	76.4	77.0	67.7	67.0	69.1	70.5	0.5	−0.1	0.1	−0.9
Georgia	62.7	71.7	76.5	70.4	64.4	65.7	65.0	65.1	0.7	0.7	−0.8	−0.8
Florida	57.5	73.9	76.2	71.7	62.5	61.5	61.0	61.6	1.3	0.3	−0.6	−1.5
East South Central	62.6	71.8	78.2	74.6	62.7	61.2	61.4	62.2	0.7	0.9	−0.5	−1.8
Kentucky	61.6	73.4	79.6	77.4	64.0	60.8	61.1	61.7	0.9	0.8	−0.3	−2.2
Tennessee	65.5	75.9	78.2	75.9	64.6	64.8	64.4	63.9	0.7	0.3	−0.3	−1.7
Alabama	59.0	70.8	80.0	73.3	62.3	60.1	60.7	62.6	0.9	1.2	−0.9	−1.6
Mississippi	63.8	62.8	73.6	70.5	58.1	57.1	57.5	59.2	−0.1	1.6	−0.4	−1.7
West South Central	62.5	68.7	73.2	69.7	56.9	55.9	56.9	57.8	0.5	0.6	−0.5	−1.9
Arkansas	55.6	70.0	74.4	69.6	56.0	56.8	59.2	61.7	1.2	0.6	−0.7	−1.2
Louisiana	75.0	67.9	73.6	69.7	58.6	55.8	56.4	57.4	−0.5	0.8	−0.5	−1.9
Oklahoma	54.5	71.0	72.5	68.1	56.2	57.2	58.0	57.9	1.3	0.2	−0.6	−1.6
Texas	59.6	68.2	73.0	70.1	56.6	55.5	56.4	57.3	0.7	0.7	−0.4	−2.0
Mountain	60.9	69.9	71.2	69.6	58.6	59.7	60.6	60.5	0.7	0.2	−0.2	−1.4
Montana	62.8	60.3	65.9	66.1	59.1	62.6	61.5	61.8	−0.2	0.9	0.0	−0.7
Idaho	65.4	55.9	66.1	65.2	56.6	56.7	55.2	55.9	−0.8	1.7	−0.1	−1.5
Wyoming	47.5	61.1	63.1	57.2	52.0	50.5	53.0	53.7	1.3	0.3	−1.0	−0.6
Colorado	62.1	80.6	74.0	71.6	59.0	60.7	63.8	63.3	1.3	−0.9	−0.3	−1.2
New Mexico	47.8	65.1	69.8	66.2	60.0	57.9	59.0	57.4	1.6	0.7	−0.5	−1.4
Arizona	61.2	74.2	73.3	74.2	61.5	63.6	62.8	62.4	1.0	−0.1	0.1	−1.7
Utah	65.8	70.0	73.7	70.0	58.7	56.6	58.1	58.8	0.3	0.5	−0.5	−1.7
Nevada	67.9	70.7	72.7	68.8	52.6	55.9	58.3	59.5	0.2	0.3	−0.5	−1.4
Pacific	69.7	71.4	71.0	69.0	61.6	63.6	63.4	63.5	0.1	−0.1	−0.3	−0.8
Washington	67.5	63.4	69.7	71.7	58.5	59.9	61.2	62.4	−0.3	1.0	0.3	−1.4
Oregon	71.2	65.8	69.3	69.3	55.6	56.4	58.2	56.4	−0.4	0.5	0.0	−2.0
California	69.9	74.3	71.3	68.5	62.3	64.4	63.8	63.8	0.3	−0.4	−0.4	−0.7
Alaska	. . .	53.8	59.1	58.3	62.6	49.7	48.8	49.9	. . .	0.9	−0.1	−1.5
Hawaii	. . .	61.5	75.7	74.7	76.4	83.5	83.2	84.4	. . .	2.1	−0.1	1.2

[1]1940 data are estimated based on published figures.
[2]1960 includes hospital units of institutions.

SOURCES: American Medical Association: Hospital service in the United States. JAMA 116(11):1055–1144, 1941. (Copyright 1941: Used with the permission of the American Medical Association.); American Hospital Association: Hospitals. JAHA 35(15):383–430, Aug. 1, 1961. (Copyright 1961: Used with the permission of the American Hospital Association.); Data computed by the Centers for Disease Control and Prevention, National Center for Health Statistics, Division of Analysis from data compiled by the Division of Health Care Statistics, National Master Facility Inventory and the American Hospital Association 1990 annual survey.

Table 112. Full-time equivalent employees per 100 average daily patients in community hospitals and average annual percent change, according to geographic division and State: United States, selected years 1960–90

[Data are based on reporting by facilities]

Geographic division and State	Employees per 100 average daily patients							Average annual percent change		
	1960[1]	1970	1980	1985	1988	1989	1990	1960–70[1]	1970–80	1980–90
United States	226	302	394	472	526	546	563	2.9	2.7	3.6
New England	249	351	456	532	599	617	619	3.5	2.7	3.1
Maine	227	289	409	494	534	550	551	2.4	3.5	3.0
New Hampshire	240	310	400	517	558	581	595	2.6	2.6	4.1
Vermont	227	318	348	434	528	553	574	3.4	0.9	5.1
Massachusetts	252	365	488	547	632	651	643	3.8	2.9	2.8
Rhode Island	270	383	454	547	549	579	601	3.6	1.7	2.8
Connecticut	247	347	440	529	594	605	618	3.5	2.4	3.5
Middle Atlantic	225	311	383	450	494	507	518	3.3	2.1	3.1
New York	233	336	396	436	480	492	505	3.7	1.7	2.5
New Jersey	225	278	332	423	453	465	474	2.1	1.8	3.6
Pennsylvania	214	287	390	491	544	559	567	3.0	3.1	3.8
East North Central	226	299	396	494	559	582	607	2.8	2.8	4.4
Ohio	232	302	392	526	579	605	635	2.7	2.6	4.9
Indiana	216	280	374	482	575	590	640	2.6	2.9	5.5
Illinois	226	301	407	492	553	569	586	2.9	3.1	3.7
Michigan	239	313	417	513	579	612	627	2.7	2.9	4.2
Wisconsin	199	277	367	405	471	497	521	3.4	2.9	3.6
West North Central	212	273	357	422	477	493	506	2.6	2.7	3.5
Minnesota	220	273	347	384	428	433	431	2.2	2.4	2.2
Iowa	208	258	349	427	468	478	504	2.2	3.1	3.7
Missouri	217	289	385	471	557	579	602	2.9	2.9	4.6
North Dakota	177	254	295	326	354	376	385	3.7	1.5	2.7
South Dakota	188	247	352	323	399	404	415	2.8	3.6	1.7
Nebraska	220	276	326	397	445	476	490	2.3	1.7	4.2
Kansas	210	270	368	478	508	525	538	2.5	3.1	3.9
South Atlantic	217	295	379	458	516	536	553	3.1	2.5	3.9
Delaware	243	328	405	526	601	608	665	3.0	2.1	5.1
Maryland	237	354	403	473	535	553	566	4.1	1.3	3.5
District of Columbia	240	363	483	599	619	614	623	4.2	2.9	2.6
Virginia	193	289	369	435	504	525	537	4.1	2.5	3.8
West Virginia	198	255	351	452	504	511	534	2.6	3.2	4.3
North Carolina	196	277	363	464	521	531	558	3.5	2.7	4.4
South Carolina	185	257	356	426	483	501	528	3.3	3.3	4.0
Georgia	233	294	396	458	499	524	542	2.4	3.0	3.2
Florida	245	295	375	450	514	546	555	1.9	2.4	4.0
East South Central	227	275	348	409	468	490	509	1.9	2.4	3.9
Kentucky	229	276	332	403	464	480	516	1.9	1.9	4.5
Tennessee	231	284	359	420	488	522	534	2.1	2.4	4.1
Alabama	233	266	357	410	477	494	514	1.3	3.0	3.7
Mississippi	207	270	334	392	422	435	444	2.7	2.1	2.9
West South Central	225	297	384	471	537	560	588	2.8	2.6	4.4
Arkansas	209	274	355	429	476	494	501	2.7	2.6	3.5
Louisiana	218	292	392	483	547	567	586	3.0	3.0	4.1
Oklahoma	218	296	404	480	529	548	585	3.1	3.2	3.8
Texas	232	304	383	473	547	574	607	2.7	2.3	4.7
Mountain	226	299	413	486	535	551	571	2.8	3.3	3.3
Montana	216	247	302	351	370	386	397	1.4	2.0	2.8
Idaho	255	281	374	427	491	524	543	1.0	2.9	3.8
Wyoming	217	251	445	417	437	447	467	1.5	5.9	0.5
Colorado	221	306	398	481	555	586	598	3.3	2.7	4.2
New Mexico	228	314	430	536	546	543	595	3.3	3.2	3.3
Arizona	222	327	455	523	564	571	590	3.9	3.4	2.6
Utah	243	304	460	579	661	669	702	2.3	4.2	4.3
Nevada	224	284	427	490	534	558	562	2.4	4.2	2.8
Pacific	243	327	467	545	578	602	625	3.0	3.6	3.0
Washington	263	313	428	544	613	617	666	1.8	3.2	4.5
Oregon	232	303	417	548	669	674	729	2.7	3.2	5.7
California	241	334	481	550	570	594	615	3.3	3.7	2.5
Alaska	220	301	454	515	584	599	639	3.2	4.2	3.5
Hawaii	226	278	401	435	457	580	508	2.1	3.7	2.4

[1]1960 includes hospital units of institutions, but excludes students, interns, and residents.

SOURCES: American Hospital Association: Hospitals. JAHA 35(15):383–430, Aug. 1, 1961. (Copyright 1961: Used with the permission of the American Hospital Association.); Data computed by the Centers for Disease Control and Prevention, National Center for Health Statistics, Division of Analysis from data compiled by the Division of Health Care Statistics, National Master Facility Inventory and the American Hospital Association 1990 annual survey.

Table 113. Nursing homes with 25 or more beds, beds, and bed rates, according to geographic division and State: United States, 1976, 1982, and 1986

[Data are based on reporting by facilities]

Geographic division and State	Nursing homes			Beds			Bed rate [1]		
	1976	1982	1986	1976	1982	1986	1976	1982	1986
United States	14,133	14,565	16,033	1,291,632	1,469,357	1,615,771	681.4	603.0	582.2
New England	1,211	1,246	1,235	91,885	105,293	108,474	719.7	643.4	597.2
Maine	121	155	144	7,027	9,717	9,685	602.9	630.1	561.3
New Hampshire	68	70	75	5,633	6,729	6,987	702.1	636.4	557.4
Vermont	53	51	47	3,477	3,196	3,083	678.0	501.5	434.1
Massachusetts	645	620	612	47,169	50,366	51,126	744.0	634.2	585.4
Rhode Island	85	95	101	6,766	8,885	9,927	682.6	679.6	681.2
Connecticut	239	255	256	21,813	26,400	27,666	738.0	680.7	645.8
Middle Atlantic	1,567	1,587	1,921	187,435	210,010	243,962	554.3	491.9	517.0
New York	708	732	777	97,489	108,898	114,192	587.7	524.7	501.7
New Jersey	313	332	356	31,147	36,638	39,071	511.7	465.5	439.6
Pennsylvania	546	523	788	58,799	64,474	90,699	527.9	458.2	583.6
East North Central	2,904	2,966	2,999	281,144	326,171	330,342	786.4	730.3	666.5
Ohio	750	830	886	60,680	74,276	82,522	646.4	636.2	641.8
Indiana	420	449	449	35,799	47,196	47,257	747.5	807.3	724.0
Illinois	805	809	775	84,085	99,777	96,684	844.8	813.8	713.3
Michigan	508	471	480	53,966	55,349	53,651	782.5	628.4	542.7
Wisconsin	421	407	409	46,614	49,573	50,228	986.5	816.6	745.3
West North Central	1,965	2,171	2,142	157,057	185,774	187,781	772.8	734.6	683.6
Minnesota	385	390	399	38,177	42,500	44,357	862.1	735.5	697.3
Iowa	440	475	440	31,785	38,150	34,942	812.5	790.9	686.1
Missouri	408	530	552	32,539	46,403	50,204	602.4	705.7	692.0
North Dakota	82	80	81	6,413	6,402	6,789	901.8	730.2	718.9
South Dakota	117	116	114	8,047	7,938	7,918	897.6	706.0	652.9
Nebraska	210	225	214	18,408	18,516	18,132	898.7	726.7	665.4
Kansas	323	355	342	21,688	25,865	25,439	741.6	725.7	655.9
South Atlantic	1,475	1,745	2,152	142,245	177,495	212,382	539.2	485.5	484.1
Delaware	22	27	36	2,123	2,194	3,345	490.5	376.3	485.5
Maryland	165	179	200	18,559	21,164	24,402	685.9	584.4	575.2
District of Columbia	17	16	19	2,604	2,556	3,029	440.2	377.0	383.7
Virginia	208	267	288	23,816	29,251	29,653	696.8	652.7	561.8
West Virginia	73	95	103	4,858	7,505	8,692	281.0	356.2	374.6
North Carolina	276	346	402	20,903	28,156	34,049	569.1	560.5	562.5
South Carolina	102	130	157	8,311	11,560	14,071	507.1	515.9	518.1
Georgia	304	306	298	28,732	32,194	31,738	862.4	742.0	607.5
Florida	308	379	649	32,339	42,915	63,403	365.0	318.2	382.9
East South Central	856	865	887	66,994	85,565	90,180	579.0	589.1	541.4
Kentucky	267	276	277	19,929	25,837	26,426	646.5	681.5	621.3
Tennessee	258	251	267	19,448	26,111	28,599	556.9	576.2	544.7
Alabama	209	190	203	19,207	20,490	21,736	646.7	555.6	506.5
Mississippi	122	148	140	8,410	13,127	13,419	415.2	522.2	469.0
West South Central	1,740	1,789	1,922	157,173	177,237	189,920	912.1	802.5	736.3
Arkansas	208	200	237	19,322	19,327	21,910	861.1	689.7	703.2
Louisiana	200	224	276	18,969	24,836	32,747	713.9	748.7	836.4
Oklahoma	341	359	382	25,990	28,902	30,359	877.6	788.6	751.0
Texas	991	1,006	1,027	92,892	104,172	104,904	991.4	846.9	712.7
Mountain	495	529	631	41,881	47,857	57,414	597.9	503.5	506.1
Montana	69	59	57	4,725	5,120	4,804	584.3	553.3	491.5
Idaho	54	47	60	4,263	4,102	5,240	598.1	448.6	517.0
Wyoming	22	25	27	1,753	2,060	2,301	595.2	556.8	550.0
Colorado	174	157	183	17,792	16,848	18,402	873.1	644.3	610.2
New Mexico	30	31	56	2,489	2,351	4,915	360.0	241.5	416.5
Arizona	67	109	134	5,832	9,888	12,740	402.6	428.9	424.3
Utah	63	76	84	3,707	5,025	5,995	503.3	518.8	511.2
Nevada	16	25	30	1,320	2,463	3,017	481.6	570.5	534.5
Pacific	1,920	1,667	2,144	165,818	153,955	195,316	670.9	481.0	520.8
Washington	318	309	328	29,415	30,017	32,021	835.1	670.0	623.9
Oregon	202	177	214	15,758	15,711	17,404	660.1	503.9	495.1
California	1,369	1,148	1,569	118,144	105,325	143,179	646.1	445.5	512.7
Alaska	8	10	10	738	1,031	1,082	1,232.1	1,458.3	950.0
Hawaii	23	23	23	1,763	1,871	1,630	384.0	269.4	200.5

[1]Number of beds per 1,000 resident population 85 years of age and over.

NOTE: The 1982 inventory excluded certain types of nursing homes that the 1976 and 1986 inventories included (nursing home units of hospitals, nursing homes for the blind, etc.). To make the data comparable, these types of homes and their beds were subtracted from the 1976 and 1986 figures.

SOURCES: Centers for Disease Control and Prevention, National Center for Health Statistics, Division of Health Care Statistics: Trends in nursing and related care homes and hospitals, United States, selected years 1969–80, by G. W. Strahan. Vital and Health Statistics. Series 14, No. 30. DHHS Pub. No. (PHS) 84-1825. Public Health Service. Washington. U.S. Government Printing Office, Mar. 1984; nursing and related care homes as reported from the 1982 National Master Facility Inventory Survey, by D. A. Roper. Vital and Health Statistics. Series 14, No. 32. DHHS Pub. No. (PHS) 86-1827. Public Health Service. Washington. U.S. Government Printing Office, Sept. 1986; data from the National Master Facility Inventory; final data from the 1986 Inventory of Long-term Care Places; resident population computed by the Division of Analysis, National Center for Health Statistics from the Compressed Mortality File, a county-level national mortality and population data base.

Table 114. Gross domestic product, national health expenditures, and Federal and State and local government expenditures: United States, selected years 1960–91

[Data are compiled by the Health Care Financing Administration]

Year	Gross domestic product in billions	National health expenditures			Federal government expenditures			State and local government expenditures		
		Amount in billions	Percent of gross domestic product	Amount per capita	Total in billions	Health in billions	Health as a percent of total	Total in billions	Health in billions	Health as a percent of total
1960.	$513.4	$27.1	5.3	$143	$93.4	$2.9	3.1	$48.3	$3.7	7.8
1965.	702.7	41.6	5.9	204	124.6	4.8	3.9	72.3	5.5	7.6
1966.	769.8	45.9	6.0	222	144.9	7.5	5.2	81.1	6.1	7.5
1967.	814.3	51.7	6.3	248	165.2	12.2	7.4	90.9	6.9	7.6
1968.	889.3	58.5	6.6	278	181.5	14.1	7.8	102.6	7.7	7.5
1969.	959.5	65.7	6.9	309	191.0	16.1	8.4	113.3	8.5	7.5
1970.	1,010.7	74.4	7.4	346	208.5	17.7	8.5	127.2	9.9	7.8
1971.	1,097.2	82.3	7.5	379	224.3	20.4	9.1	142.8	10.8	7.6
1972.	1,207.0	92.3	7.6	421	249.3	22.9	9.2	156.3	12.2	7.8
1973.	1,349.6	102.5	7.6	464	270.3	25.2	9.3	171.9	14.1	8.2
1974.	1,458.6	116.1	8.0	521	305.6	30.5	10.0	193.5	16.1	8.3
1975.	1,585.9	132.9	8.4	592	364.2	36.4	10.0	221.0	18.7	8.5
1976.	1,768.4	152.2	8.6	672	392.7	42.9	10.9	239.3	19.5	8.1
1977.	1,974.1	172.0	8.7	753	426.4	47.6	11.2	256.3	22.5	8.8
1978.	2,232.7	193.7	8.7	840	469.3	54.3	11.6	278.2	25.5	9.1
1979.	2,488.6	217.2	8.7	933	520.3	61.4	11.8	305.4	28.9	9.5
1980.	2,708.0	250.1	9.2	1,064	613.1	72.0	11.7	336.6	33.2	9.9
1981.	3,030.6	290.2	9.6	1,222	697.8	84.0	12.0	362.3	37.8	10.4
1982.	3,149.6	326.1	10.4	1,359	770.9	93.3	12.1	382.1	41.5	10.9
1983.	3,405.0	358.6	10.5	1,480	840.0	103.2	12.3	403.2	44.4	11.0
1984.	3,777.2	389.6	10.3	1,592	892.7	112.6	12.6	434.1	47.0	10.8
1985.	4,038.7	422.6	10.5	1,711	969.9	123.5	12.7	472.6	51.2	10.8
1986.	4,268.6	454.9	10.7	1,824	1,028.2	132.5	12.9	517.0	57.2	11.1
1987.	4,539.9	494.2	10.9	1,962	1,065.6	143.6	13.5	554.2	64.4	11.6
1988.	4,900.4	546.1	11.1	2,146	1,109.0	156.6	14.1	593.0	70.5	11.9
1989.	5,250.8	604.3	11.5	2,352	1,181.6	175.0	14.8	636.7	78.3	12.3
1990.	5,522.2	675.0	12.2	2,601	1,273.6	194.5	15.3	699.2	90.5	12.9
1991.	5,677.5	751.8	13.2	2,868	1,332.7	222.9	16.7	760.7	107.1	14.1

NOTES: These data include revisions in health expeditures back to 1985 and in population back to 1960 and differ from previous editions of Health, United States. These data reflect Bureau of Economic Analysis, Department of Commerce revisions to the gross domestic product and Federal and State and local government expenditures as of July 1992 and Social Security Administration population revisions as of July 1992.

SOURCE: Office of National Health Statistics, Office of the Actuary: National health expenditures, 1991. Health Care Financing Review. Vol. 14, Number 2. HCFA Pub. No. 03335. Health Care Financing Administration. Washington. U.S. Government Printing Office, Winter 1992.

Table 115. Total health expenditures as a percent of gross domestic product and per capita expenditures in dollars: Selected countries and years 1960–91

[Data compiled by the Organization for Economic Cooperation and Development]

Country	1960	1965	1970	1975	1980	1985	1988	1989	1990	1991[1]
	Health expenditures as a percent of gross domestic product									
Australia	4.9	5.1	5.7	7.5	7.3	7.7	7.7	7.8	8.2	8.6
Austria	4.4	4.7	5.4	7.3	7.9	8.1	8.4	8.4	8.3	8.4
Belgium	3.4	3.9	4.1	5.9	6.6	7.4	7.7	7.6	7.6	7.9
Canada	5.5	6.0	7.1	7.2	7.4	8.5	8.8	9.0	9.5	10.0
Denmark	3.6	4.8	6.1	6.5	6.8	6.3	6.5	6.5	6.3	6.5
Finland	3.9	4.9	5.7	6.3	6.5	7.2	7.2	7.2	7.8	8.9
France	4.2	5.2	5.8	7.0	7.6	8.5	8.6	8.7	8.8	9.1
Germany	4.8	5.1	5.9	8.1	8.4	8.7	8.8	8.3	8.3	8.5
Greece	2.9	3.1	4.0	4.1	4.3	4.9	5.0	5.4	5.4	5.2
Iceland	3.5	4.2	5.2	6.2	6.4	7.1	8.6	8.6	8.3	8.4
Ireland	4.0	4.4	5.6	8.0	9.2	8.2	7.3	6.9	7.0	7.3
Italy	3.6	4.3	5.2	6.1	6.9	7.0	7.6	7.6	8.1	8.3
Japan	3.0	4.5	4.6	5.6	6.6	6.5	6.6	6.6	6.5	6.6
Luxembourg	- - -	- - -	4.1	5.6	6.8	6.8	7.2	6.9	7.2	7.2
Netherlands	3.9	4.4	6.0	7.6	8.0	8.0	8.2	8.1	8.2	8.3
New Zealand	4.3	- - -	5.2	6.7	7.2	6.5	7.1	7.2	7.3	7.6
Norway	3.3	3.9	5.0	6.7	6.6	6.4	7.7	7.4	7.4	7.6
Portugal	- - -	- - -	3.1	6.4	5.9	7.0	7.1	7.2	6.7	6.8
Spain	1.5	2.5	3.7	4.8	5.6	5.7	6.0	6.3	6.6	6.7
Sweden	4.7	5.6	7.2	7.9	9.4	8.8	8.6	8.6	8.6	8.6
Switzerland	3.3	3.8	5.2	7.0	7.3	7.6	7.8	7.5	7.8	7.9
Turkey	- - -	- - -	- - -	3.5	4.0	2.8	3.8	3.9	4.0	4.0
United Kingdom	3.9	4.1	4.5	5.5	5.8	6.0	6.1	6.1	6.2	6.6
United States	5.3	5.9	7.4	8.4	9.2	10.5	11.1	11.5	12.2	13.2
	Per capita health expenditures [2]									
Australia	$99	$127	$207	$438	$663	$998	$1,171	$1,225	$1,310	$1,407
Austria	69	94	163	369	683	984	1,191	1,298	1,383	1,448
Belgium	55	84	128	303	571	879	1,081	1,153	1,242	1,377
Canada	109	154	253	435	743	1,244	1,558	1,666	1,811	1,915
Denmark	70	125	212	340	582	807	972	1,013	1,051	1,151
Finland	57	95	164	305	517	855	1,044	1,147	1,291	1,426
France	75	124	203	386	698	1,083	1,295	1,415	1,528	1,650
Germany	98	135	216	458	811	1,175	1,409	1,412	1,522	1,659
Greece	16	27	58	102	184	282	334	384	400	404
Iceland	53	88	137	290	581	889	1,331	1,373	1,379	1,447
Ireland	38	53	97	231	449	572	620	651	748	845
Italy	51	83	153	280	571	814	1,058	1,150	1,296	1,408
Japan	27	64	127	256	517	792	992	1,092	1,175	1,267
Luxembourg	- - -	- - -	154	326	632	930	1,219	1,267	1,392	1,494
Netherlands	74	106	207	410	696	931	1,101	1,176	1,286	1,360
New Zealand	94	- - -	180	364	562	747	900	954	995	1,047
Norway	49	77	134	306	549	846	1,112	1,128	1,193	1,305
Portugal	- - -	- - -	46	157	238	398	493	548	554	624
Spain	14	38	82	187	325	452	598	682	774	848
Sweden	94	151	271	470	855	1,150	1,303	1,390	1,455	1,443
Switzerland	96	141	268	512	839	1,224	1,435	1,498	1,640	1,713
Turkey	- - -	- - -	- - -	36	64	66	110	118	133	142
United Kingdom	79	102	147	273	458	685	858	912	985	1,043
United States	143	204	346	592	1,063	1,711	2,146	2,351	2,600	2,868

[1]Preliminary figures.

[2]Per capita health expenditures for each country have been adjusted to U.S. dollars using gross domestic product purchasing power parities for each year.

NOTE: Some numbers in this table have been revised and differ from previous editions of Health, United States.

SOURCES: Schieber, G. J., Poullier, J. P., Greenwald, L. G.: U.S. health expenditure performance: An international comparison and data update. Health Care Financing Review. Vol. 13, Number 4. HCFA Pub. No. 03331. Health Care Financing Administration. Washington. U.S. Government Printing Office, September 1992; Office of National Health Statistics, Office of the Actuary: National health expenditures, 1991. Health Care Financing Review. Vol. 14, Number 2. HCFA Pub. No. 03335. Health Care Financing Administration. Washington. U.S. Government Printing Office, Winter 1992; Unpublished data.

Table 116. National health expenditures, percent distribution, and average annual percent change, according to type of expenditure: United States, selected years 1960–91

[Data are compiled by the Health Care Financing Administration]

Type of expenditure	1960	1965	1970	1975	1980	1985	1987	1988	1989	1990	1991
					Amount in billions						
Total.........................	$27.1	$41.6	$74.4	$132.9	$250.1	$422.6	$494.2	$546.1	$604.3	$675.0	$751.8
					Percent distribution						
All expenditures................	100.0	100.0	100.0	100.0	100.0	100.0	100.0	100.0	100.0	100.0	100.0
Health services and supplies	93.7	91.7	92.8	93.8	95.5	96.4	96.5	96.4	96.6	96.6	96.9
Personal health care...............	88.1	85.6	87.3	87.7	87.7	87.5	88.9	88.4	87.9	87.6	87.8
Hospital care..................	34.2	33.7	37.6	39.4	40.9	39.8	39.3	38.8	38.5	38.2	38.4
Physician services..............	19.5	19.7	18.3	17.5	16.7	17.5	18.8	19.3	19.2	19.1	18.9
Dentist services................	7.2	6.7	6.3	6.2	5.7	5.5	5.5	5.4	5.2	5.0	4.9
Nursing home care	3.6	4.1	6.5	7.5	8.0	8.1	8.0	7.8	7.9	7.9	8.0
Other professional services	2.2	2.1	2.0	2.6	3.5	3.9	4.3	4.4	4.5	4.5	4.8
Home health care	0.1	0.1	0.2	0.3	0.5	0.9	0.8	0.8	0.9	1.1	1.3
Drugs and other medical nondurables	15.7	14.2	11.8	9.8	8.6	8.6	8.7	8.5	8.4	8.2	8.1
Vision products and other medical durables..................	3.0	3.0	2.7	2.3	1.8	1.7	1.8	1.9	1.7	1.7	1.6
Other personal health care..........	2.6	2.0	1.8	2.0	1.8	1.5	1.6	1.6	1.6	1.7	1.9
Program administration and net cost of health insurance	4.3	4.6	3.7	3.8	4.9	6.0	4.7	4.9	5.6	5.8	5.8
Government public health activities......	1.4	1.5	1.9	2.3	2.9	2.9	3.0	3.0	3.1	3.3	3.3
Research and construction.............	6.3	8.3	7.2	6.2	4.5	3.6	3.5	3.6	3.4	3.4	3.1
Noncommercial research.............	2.6	3.7	2.6	2.5	2.2	1.8	1.8	1.9	1.8	1.8	1.7
Construction....................	3.7	4.6	4.5	3.7	2.3	1.8	1.7	1.7	1.6	1.6	1.4

Type of expenditure	1960–65	1965–70	1970–75	1975–80	1980–85	1985–87	1987–88	1988–89	1989–90	1990–91
				Average annual percent change						
All expenditures....................	8.9	12.3	12.3	13.5	11.1	8.1	10.5	10.7	11.7	11.4
Health services and supplies	8.5	12.6	12.5	13.9	11.3	8.2	10.3	10.9	11.8	11.7
Personal health care...............	8.3	12.8	12.4	13.5	11.0	9.0	9.9	10.0	11.4	11.6
Hospital care....................	8.6	14.7	13.4	14.3	10.4	7.4	9.2	9.6	11.1	11.8
Physician services................	9.2	10.6	11.4	12.5	12.1	12.1	13.1	10.4	11.0	10.2
Dentist services.................	7.3	10.8	12.1	11.7	10.1	8.0	8.5	7.5	7.7	8.8
Nursing home care	11.6	23.4	15.4	15.0	11.3	7.8	7.8	11.1	12.3	12.4
Other professional services	7.4	11.8	18.3	19.9	13.8	12.8	12.4	13.8	13.5	16.7
Home health care	9.6	19.7	23.2	27.2	23.3	3.6	9.9	24.4	34.4	29.0
Drugs and other medical nondurables	6.8	8.4	8.1	10.7	10.8	9.3	7.2	9.1	10.3	9.0
Vision products and other medical durables..................	9.0	10.1	8.8	8.2	9.4	12.7	11.8	2.8	12.6	5.4
Other personal health care..........	3.5	10.7	14.6	11.0	6.9	10.6	12.1	11.8	17.4	21.9
Program administration and net cost of health insurance	10.5	7.5	12.8	19.3	15.5	-4.4	16.8	25.7	15.3	12.7
Government public health activities......	10.8	17.1	17.0	18.9	11.3	8.9	13.5	14.3	16.0	11.6
Research and construction.............	15.2	9.0	9.2	6.4	6.4	5.9	14.9	4.2	9.6	2.1
Noncommercial research.............	17.1	5.1	11.2	10.4	7.4	7.6	14.5	6.2	8.0	6.1
Construction....................	13.9	11.8	8.0	3.3	5.4	4.2	15.3	1.9	11.5	-2.2

NOTE: These data include revisions in health expenditures back to 1985 and differ from previous editions of Health, United States.

SOURCE: Office of National Health Statistics, Office of the Actuary: National health expenditures, 1991. Health Care Financing Review. Vol. 14, No. 2. HCFA Pub. No. 03335. Health Care Financing Administration. Washington. U.S. Government Printing Office, Winter 1992.

Table 117. Personal health care expenditures average annual percent change and percent distribution of factors affecting growth: United States, 1960–91

[Data are compiled by the Health Care Financing Administration]

Period	Average annual percent change	Factors affecting growth			
		All factors	Prices	Population	Intensity [1]
		Percent distribution			
1960–91	11.3	100	57	10	33
1960–61	6.1	100	31	27	42
1961–62	7.6	100	32	20	48
1962–63	9.3	100	22	16	62
1963–64	9.9	100	29	14	57
1964–65	8.6	100	37	15	48
1965–66	10.5	100	45	11	44
1966–67	13.6	100	43	8	49
1967–68	13.1	100	45	8	47
1968–69	13.0	100	51	8	41
1969–70	13.7	100	50	8	42
1970–71	9.9	100	65	11	24
1971–72	11.3	100	39	9	52
1972–73	11.7	100	38	7	55
1973–74	14.6	100	63	6	31
1974–75	14.7	100	75	6	19
1975–76	14.0	100	62	6	32
1976–77	12.3	100	63	7	30
1977–78	12.2	100	66	8	26
1978–79	13.0	100	70	8	22
1979–80	15.9	100	73	6	21
1980–81	16.2	100	70	6	24
1981–82	12.4	100	77	8	15
1982–83	10.0	100	72	10	18
1983–84	8.4	100	75	12	13
1984–85	8.3	100	66	12	22
1985–86	8.4	100	60	12	28
1986–87	9.6	100	61	11	28
1987–88	9.9	100	68	10	22
1988–89	10.0	100	70	10	20
1989–90	11.4	100	58	9	33
1990–91	11.6	100	54	9	37

[1]Represents changes in use or kinds of services and supplies.

NOTE: These data include revisions back to 1960 and differ from previous editions of Health, United States.

SOURCE: Office of National Health Statistics, Office of the Actuary: National health expenditures, 1991. Health Care Financing Review. Vol. 14, Number 2. HCFA Pub. No. 03335. Health Care Financing Administration. Washington. U.S. Government Printing Office, Winter 1992.

Table 118. Consumer Price Index and average annual percent change for all items and selected items: United States, selected years 1950–92

[Data are based on reporting by samples of providers and other retail outlets]

Year	All items	Medical care	Food	Apparel and upkeep	Housing	Energy	Personal care
			Consumer Price Index				
1950.	24.1	15.1	25.4	40.3	- - -	- - -	26.2
1955.	26.8	18.2	27.8	42.9	- - -	- - -	29.9
1960.	29.6	22.3	30.0	45.7	- - -	22.4	34.6
1965.	31.5	25.2	32.2	47.8	- - -	22.9	36.6
1970.	38.8	34.0	39.2	59.2	36.4	25.5	43.5
1975.	53.8	47.5	59.8	72.5	50.7	42.1	57.9
1976.	56.9	52.0	61.6	75.2	53.8	45.1	61.7
1977.	60.6	57.0	65.5	78.6	57.4	49.4	65.7
1978.	65.2	61.8	72.0	81.4	62.4	52.5	69.9
1979.	72.6	67.5	79.9	84.9	70.1	65.7	75.2
1980.	82.4	74.9	86.8	90.9	81.1	86.0	81.9
1981.	90.9	82.9	93.6	95.3	90.4	97.7	89.1
1982.	96.5	92.5	97.4	97.8	96.9	99.2	95.4
1983.	99.6	100.6	99.4	100.2	99.5	99.9	100.3
1984.	103.9	106.8	103.2	102.1	103.6	100.9	104.3
1985.	107.6	113.5	105.6	105.0	107.7	101.6	108.3
1986.	109.6	122.0	109.0	105.9	110.9	88.2	111.9
1987.	113.6	130.1	113.5	110.6	114.2	88.6	115.1
1988.	118.3	138.6	118.2	115.4	118.5	89.3	119.4
1989.	124.0	149.3	125.1	118.6	123.0	94.3	125.0
1990.	130.7	162.8	132.4	124.1	128.5	102.1	130.4
1991.	136.2	177.0	136.3	128.7	133.6	102.5	134.9
1992.	140.3	190.1	137.9	131.9	137.5	103.0	138.3
			Average annual percent change				
1950–92.	4.3	6.2	4.1	2.9	[1]6.2	[2]4.9	4.0
1950–55.	2.1	3.8	1.8	1.3	- - -	- - -	2.7
1955–60.	2.0	4.1	1.5	1.3	- - -	- - -	3.0
1960–65.	1.3	2.5	1.4	0.9	- - -	0.4	1.1
1965–70.	4.3	6.2	4.0	4.4	- - -	2.2	3.5
1970–75.	6.8	6.9	8.8	4.1	6.9	10.5	5.9
1975–80.	8.9	9.5	7.7	4.6	9.9	15.4	7.2
1975–76	5.8	9.5	3.0	3.7	6.1	7.1	6.6
1976–77	6.5	9.6	6.3	4.5	6.7	9.5	6.5
1977–78	7.6	8.4	9.9	3.6	8.7	6.3	6.4
1978–79	11.3	9.2	11.0	4.3	12.3	25.1	7.6
1979–80	13.5	11.0	8.6	7.1	15.7	30.9	8.9
1980–85.	5.5	8.7	4.0	2.9	5.8	3.4	5.7
1980–81	10.3	10.7	7.8	4.8	11.5	13.6	8.8
1981–82	6.2	11.6	4.1	2.6	7.2	1.5	7.1
1982–83	3.2	8.8	2.1	2.5	2.7	0.7	5.1
1983–84	4.3	6.2	3.8	1.9	4.1	1.0	4.0
1984–85	3.6	6.3	2.3	2.8	4.0	0.7	3.8
1985–90.	4.0	7.5	4.6	3.4	3.6	0.1	3.8
1985–86	1.9	7.5	3.2	0.9	3.0	−13.2	3.3
1986–87	3.6	6.6	4.1	4.4	3.0	0.5	2.9
1987–88	4.1	6.5	4.1	4.3	3.8	0.8	3.7
1988–89	4.8	7.7	5.8	2.8	3.8	5.6	4.7
1989–90	5.4	9.0	5.8	4.6	4.5	8.3	4.3
1990–91.	4.2	8.7	2.9	3.7	4.0	0.4	3.5
1991–92.	3.0	7.4	1.2	2.5	2.9	0.5	2.5

[1]Data are for 1970–92.
[2]Data are for 1960–92.

NOTE: 1982–84 = 100.

SOURCE: Bureau of Labor Statistics, U.S. Department of Labor: Consumer Price Index. Various releases.

Table 119. Consumer Price Index and average annual percent change for all items and medical care components: United States, selected years 1950–92

[Data are based on reporting by samples of providers and other retail outlets]

Consumer Price Index

Item and medical care component	1950	1960	1965	1970	1975	1980	1985	1989	1990	1991	1992
CPI, all items	24.1	29.6	31.5	38.8	53.8	82.4	107.6	124.0	130.7	136.2	140.3
Less medical care	---	30.2	32.0	39.2	54.3	82.8	107.2	122.4	128.8	133.8	137.5
CPI, all services	16.9	24.1	26.6	35.0	48.0	77.9	109.9	131.9	139.2	146.3	152.0
All medical care	15.1	22.3	25.2	34.0	47.5	74.9	113.5	149.3	162.8	177.0	190.1
Medical care services	12.8	19.5	22.7	32.3	46.6	74.8	113.2	148.9	162.7	177.1	190.5
Professional medical services	---	---	---	37.0	50.8	77.9	113.5	146.4	156.1	165.7	175.8
Physicians' services	15.7	21.9	25.1	34.5	48.1	76.5	113.3	150.1	160.8	170.5	181.2
Dental services	21.0	27.0	30.3	39.2	53.2	78.9	114.2	146.1	155.8	167.4	178.7
Eye care [1]	---	---	---	---	---	---	---	112.4	117.3	121.9	127.0
Services by other medical professionals [1]	---	---	---	---	---	---	---	114.2	120.2	126.6	131.7
Hospital and related services	---	---	---	---	---	69.2	116.1	160.5	178.0	196.1	214.0
Hospital rooms	4.9	9.3	12.3	23.6	38.3	68.0	115.4	158.1	175.4	191.9	208.7
Other inpatient services [1]	---	---	---	---	---	---	---	128.9	142.7	158.0	172.3
Outpatient services [1]	---	---	---	---	---	---	---	124.7	138.7	153.4	168.7
Medical care commodities	39.7	46.9	45.0	46.5	53.3	75.4	115.2	150.8	163.4	176.8	188.1
Prescription drugs	43.4	54.0	47.8	47.4	51.2	72.5	120.1	165.2	181.7	199.7	214.7
Nonprescription drugs and medical supplies [1]	---	---	---	---	---	---	---	114.6	120.6	126.3	131.2
Internal and respiratory over-the-counter drugs	---	---	39.0	42.3	51.8	74.9	112.2	138.8	145.9	152.4	158.2
Nonprescription medical equipment and supplies	---	---	---	---	---	79.2	109.6	131.1	138.0	145.0	150.9

Average annual percent change

Item and medical care component	1950–60	1960–65	1965–70	1970–75	1975–80	1980–85	1985–89	1989–90	1990–91	1991–92
CPI, all items	2.1	1.3	4.3	6.8	8.9	5.5	3.6	5.4	4.2	3.0
Less medical care	---	1.2	4.1	6.7	8.8	5.3	3.4	5.2	3.9	2.8
CPI, all services	3.6	2.0	5.6	6.5	10.2	7.1	4.7	5.5	5.1	3.9
All medical care	4.0	2.5	6.2	6.9	9.5	8.7	7.1	9.0	8.7	7.4
Medical care services	4.3	3.1	7.3	7.6	9.9	8.6	7.1	9.3	8.9	7.6
Professional medical services	---	---	---	6.5	8.9	7.8	6.6	6.6	6.1	6.1
Physicians' services	3.4	2.8	6.6	6.9	9.7	8.2	7.3	7.1	6.0	6.3
Dental services	2.5	2.3	5.3	6.3	8.2	7.7	6.4	6.6	7.4	6.8
Eye care [1]	---	---	---	---	---	---	---	4.4	3.9	4.2
Services by other medical professionals [1]	---	---	---	---	---	---	---	5.3	5.3	4.0
Hospital and related services	---	---	---	---	---	10.9	8.4	10.9	10.2	9.1
Hospital rooms	6.6	5.8	13.9	10.2	12.2	11.2	8.2	10.9	9.4	8.8
Other inpatient services [1]	---	---	---	---	---	---	---	10.7	10.7	9.1
Outpatient services [1]	---	---	---	---	---	---	---	11.2	10.6	10.0
Medical care commodities	1.7	−0.8	0.7	2.8	7.2	8.8	7.0	8.4	8.2	6.4
Prescription drugs	2.2	−2.4	−0.2	1.6	7.2	10.6	8.3	10.0	9.9	7.5
Nonprescription drugs and medical supplies [1]	---	---	---	---	---	---	---	5.2	4.7	3.9
Internal and respiratory over-the-counter drugs	---	---	1.6	4.1	7.7	8.4	5.5	5.1	4.5	3.8
Nonprescription medical equipment and supplies	---	---	---	---	---	6.7	4.6	5.3	5.1	4.1

[1]Dec. 1986 = 100.

NOTE: 1982–84 = 100, except where noted.

SOURCE: Bureau of Labor Statistics, U.S. Department of Labor: Consumer Price Index. Various releases.

Table 120. Hospital expenses and personnel and average annual percent change in nonfederal short-stay hospitals: United States, 1971–91

[Data are based on reporting by a census of hospitals]

Year and period	Expenses for inpatient care				Personnel[2]	
	Total in billions	Per inpatient day	Per inpatient stay	Employee costs as percent of total[1]	Number in thousands	Number per 100 patients
1971.	$22.4	$83	$667	63.9	1,999	272
1972.	25.5	95	747	62.6	2,056	278
1973.	28.5	102	794	61.8	2,149	280
1974.	32.8	113	883	60.7	2,289	289
1975.	39.1	133	1,025	59.4	2,399	298
1976.	45.4	152	1,172	57.9	2,483	304
1977.	51.8	173	1,317	57.5	2,581	315
1978.	58.3	194	1,470	57.2	2,662	323
1979.	66.2	216	1,631	57.0	2,762	328
1980.	77.0	244	1,844	56.4	2,879	334
1981.	90.7	284	2,168	56.7	3,039	347
1982.	105.1	327	2,493	56.7	3,110	353
1983.	116.6	368	2,776	56.5	3,102	357
1984.	123.6	410	2,984	56.1	3,023	367
1985.	130.7	460	3,239	55.2	3,003	385
1986.	140.9	499	3,530	53.9	3,032	392
1987.	152.9	537	3,849	53.1	3,120	400
1988.	168.9	581	4,194	52.9	3,209	404
1989.	185.2	631	4,572	53.0	3,307	411
1990.	203.9	682	4,930	53.6	3,423	417
1991.	225.2	745	5,346	53.8	3,539	427
	Average annual percent change					
1971–91.	12.2	11.6	11.0	. . .	2.9	2.3
1971–72.	14.1	14.5	12.0	. . .	2.9	2.2
1972–73.	11.5	7.4	6.3	. . .	4.5	0.7
1973–74.	14.9	10.8	11.2	. . .	6.5	3.2
1974–75.	19.4	17.7	16.1	. . .	4.8	3.1
1975–76.	16.1	14.3	14.3	. . .	3.5	2.0
1976–77.	14.2	13.8	12.4	. . .	3.9	3.6
1977–78.	12.6	12.1	11.6	. . .	3.1	2.5
1978–79.	13.4	11.3	11.0	. . .	3.8	1.5
1979–80.	16.3	13.0	13.1	. . .	4.2	1.8
1980–81.	17.9	16.4	17.6	. . .	5.6	3.9
1981–82.	15.8	15.1	15.0	. . .	2.3	1.7
1982–83.	11.0	12.5	11.4	. . .	−0.3	1.1
1983–84.	5.9	11.4	7.5	. . .	−2.5	2.8
1984–85.	5.8	12.2	8.5	. . .	−0.7	4.9
1985–86.	7.8	8.5	9.0	. . .	1.0	1.8
1986–87.	8.5	7.6	9.0	. . .	2.9	2.0
1987–88.	10.5	8.2	9.0	. . .	2.9	1.0
1988–89.	9.7	8.6	9.0	. . .	3.1	1.7
1989–90.	10.1	8.1	7.8	. . .	3.5	1.5
1990–91.	10.4	9.2	8.4	. . .	3.4	2.4

[1]Includes employee payroll and benefit costs. Does not include contracted labor services.
[2]Full-time equivalent personnel.

NOTE: Data refer to nonfederal short-term general and other specialty hospitals.

SOURCE: American Hospital Association: Hospital Statistics, 1992 Edition. Chicago, 1992. (Copyright 1992: Used with the permission of the American Hospital Association.)

Table 121. Hospital expenses in short-stay hospitals, according to type of ownership and size of hospital: United States, selected years 1970–91

[Data are based on reporting by a census of hospitals]

Type of ownership and size of hospital	1970	1975	1980	1985	1987	1988	1989	1990	1991
Total expenses	Amount in billions								
All ownership	$19.7	$42.7	$83.8	$141.3	$164.9	$182.0	$198.6	$217.4	$240.2
Federal [1]	1.1	3.6	6.8	10.6	12.0	13.1	13.4	13.5	15.0
Department of Defense	0.2	1.1	1.9	3.5	4.0	4.5	4.3	3.9	4.6
Department of Veterans Affairs	0.9	2.3	4.5	6.6	7.5	8.0	8.5	8.9	9.6
Indian Health Service	0.0	0.1	0.2	0.3	0.3	0.4	0.4	0.4	0.5
Nonfederal short-stay [2]	18.6	39.1	77.0	130.7	152.9	168.9	185.2	203.9	225.2
Nonprofit	13.6	28.0	55.8	96.2	112.4	124.8	136.9	150.7	166.8
Proprietary	0.7	2.6	5.8	11.5	14.1	15.5	17.2	18.8	20.5
State-local government	4.1	8.6	15.3	23.0	26.4	28.6	31.0	34.4	37.9
Size of hospital:									
6–99 beds	2.2	4.4	8.0	12.5	14.6	16.1	17.5	18.6	20.8
100–199 beds	3.4	7.1	13.4	22.5	26.5	29.4	32.7	35.4	39.2
200–299 beds	3.4	7.0	13.8	23.9	29.4	33.0	36.5	40.7	43.9
300–499 beds	5.6	11.3	23.7	40.3	45.5	50.0	55.0	60.4	67.4
500 beds or more	5.1	12.9	24.9	42.2	48.9	53.5	56.9	62.4	68.9
Expenses per inpatient day	Amount								
Nonfederal short-stay [2]	$68	$133	$244	$460	$537	$581	$631	$682	$745
Nonprofit	72	133	246	463	544	591	642	692	757
Proprietary	50	133	257	500	585	649	708	752	820
State-local government	67	132	236	429	490	514	554	610	668
Size of hospital:									
6–99 beds	45	102	198	381	426	456	483	506	551
100–199 beds	58	119	218	409	481	520	561	595	654
200–299 beds	68	128	235	447	523	572	614	664	719
300–499 beds	74	138	257	482	569	615	679	733	803
500 beds or more	72	155	275	503	600	654	717	783	872
Expenses per inpatient stay	Amount								
Nonfederal short-stay [2]	$579	$1,025	$1,844	$3,239	$3,849	$4,194	$4,572	$4,930	$5,346
Nonprofit	597	1,045	1,900	3,308	3,912	4,267	4,638	4,995	5,388
Proprietary	348	886	1,676	3,033	3,617	4,023	4,406	4,727	5,134
State-local government	585	1,016	1,724	3,073	3,720	3,990	4,389	4,769	5,281
Size of hospital:									
6–99 beds	339	665	1,234	2,276	2,700	2,971	3,173	3,348	3,742
100–199 beds	470	865	1,554	2,739	3,301	3,603	3,913	4,204	4,558
200–299 beds	585	990	1,773	3,070	3,684	4,023	4,376	4,683	5,054
300–499 beds	665	1,147	2,047	3,535	4,161	4,569	5,007	5,352	5,748
500 beds or more	870	1,637	2,627	4,387	5,216	5,756	6,310	6,873	7,567

[1] Includes other Federal hospitals not listed separately.
[2] Includes nonfederal short-stay general and other specialty hospitals.

SOURCES: American Hospital Association: Hospitals. JAHA 45(15):463–467, Aug. 1971; Hospital Statistics, 1976, 1981, 1985–92 Editions. Chicago, 1976, 1981, 1985–92. (Copyrights 1971, 1976, 1981, 1985–92: Used with the permission of the American Hospital Association.); Unpublished data.

Table 122. National health expenditures and average annual percent change, according to source of funds: United States, selected years 1929-91

[Data are compiled by the Health Care Financing Administration]

Year	All health expenditures in billions	Private funds			Public funds		
		Amount in billions	Amount per capita	Percent of total	Amount in billions	Amount per capita	Percent of total
1929	$3.6	$3.2	$25	86.4	$0.5	$4	13.6
1935	2.9	2.4	18	80.8	0.6	4	19.2
1940	4.0	3.2	23	79.7	0.8	6	20.3
1950	12.7	9.2	58	72.8	3.4	22	27.2
1955	17.7	13.2	75	74.3	4.6	27	25.7
1960	27.1	20.5	108	75.5	6.7	35	24.5
1965	41.6	31.3	154	75.3	10.3	50	24.7
1966	45.9	32.3	157	70.4	13.6	66	29.6
1967	51.7	32.5	156	62.9	19.2	92	37.1
1968	58.5	36.7	174	62.8	21.8	103	37.2
1969	65.7	41.1	193	62.5	24.6	116	37.5
1970	74.4	46.7	217	62.8	27.7	129	37.2
1971	82.3	51.1	235	62.1	31.2	144	37.9
1972	92.3	57.2	261	62.0	35.1	160	38.0
1973	102.5	63.2	286	61.6	39.3	178	38.4
1974	116.1	69.4	312	59.8	46.6	209	40.2
1975	132.9	77.8	346	58.5	55.1	246	41.5
1976	152.2	89.8	396	59.0	62.4	276	41.0
1977	172.0	102.0	446	59.3	70.1	307	40.7
1978	193.7	113.9	494	58.8	79.8	346	41.2
1979	217.2	126.9	545	58.4	90.4	388	41.6
1980	250.1	145.0	617	58.0	105.2	447	42.0
1981	290.2	168.5	709	58.0	121.8	513	42.0
1982	326.1	191.3	797	58.7	134.8	562	41.3
1983	358.6	211.0	871	58.8	147.6	609	41.2
1984	389.6	230.0	940	59.0	159.6	652	41.0
1985	422.6	248.0	1,004	58.7	174.6	707	41.3
1986	454.9	265.2	1,063	58.3	189.6	760	41.7
1987	494.2	286.2	1,136	57.9	208.0	826	42.1
1988	546.1	319.0	1,254	58.4	227.1	893	41.6
1989	604.3	351.0	1,366	58.1	253.3	986	41.9
1990	675.0	390.0	1,502	57.8	285.1	1,098	42.2
1991	751.8	421.8	1,609	56.1	330.0	1,259	43.9
Average annual percent change							
1929-65	7.0	6.6	5.2	...	8.8	7.3	...
1965-91	11.8	10.5	9.5	...	14.3	13.2	...
1929-35	-3.6	-4.6	-5.1	...	2.2	1.4	...
1935-40	6.3	6.0	4.7	...	7.6	6.8	...
1940-50	12.2	11.2	9.7	...	15.5	13.8	...
1950-55	7.0	7.4	5.3	...	5.8	4.2	...
1955-60	8.9	9.2	7.5	...	7.9	5.3	...
1960-65	8.9	8.9	7.3	...	9.1	7.6	...
1965-70	12.3	8.3	7.2	...	21.9	20.6	...
1970-75	12.3	10.7	9.8	...	14.8	13.8	...
1975-80	13.5	13.3	12.2	...	13.8	12.7	...
1980-85	11.1	11.3	10.2	...	10.7	9.6	...
1980-81	16.0	16.2	15.1	...	15.8	14.6	...
1981-82	12.4	13.6	12.4	...	10.7	9.6	...
1982-83	10.0	10.3	9.2	...	9.5	8.5	...
1983-84	8.7	9.0	8.0	...	8.1	7.1	...
1984-85	8.5	7.8	6.8	...	9.4	8.3	...
1985-90	9.8	9.5	8.4	...	10.3	9.2	...
1985-86	7.6	7.0	5.9	...	8.6	7.6	...
1986-87	8.6	7.9	6.9	...	9.7	8.6	...
1987-88	10.5	11.5	10.4	...	9.2	8.1	...
1988-89	10.7	10.0	8.9	...	11.5	10.4	...
1989-90	11.7	11.1	10.0	...	12.5	11.4	...
1990-91	11.4	8.2	7.1	...	15.7	14.6	...

NOTES: These data include revisions in health expenditures back to 1985 and in population back to 1960 and differ from previous editions of Health, United States. They reflect Social Security Administration population revisions as of July 1992.

SOURCE: Office of National Health Statistics, Office of the Actuary: National health expenditures, 1991. Health Care Financing Review. Vol. 14, No. 2. HCFA Pub. No. 03335. Health Care Financing Administration. Washington. U.S. Government Printing Office, Winter 1992.

Table 123. Personal health care expenditures and percent distribution, according to source of funds: United States, selected years 1929–91

[Data are compiled by the Health Care Financing Administration]

Year	Total in billions [1]	Per capita	All sources	Out-of-pocket payments	Private health insurance	Other private funds	Government Total	Government Federal	Government State and local
				Percent distribution					
1929	$3.2	$26	100.0	[2]88.4	([2])	2.6	9.0	2.7	6.3
1935	2.7	21	100.0	[2]82.4	([2])	2.8	14.7	3.4	11.3
1940	3.5	26	100.0	[2]81.3	([2])	2.6	16.1	4.1	12.0
1950	10.9	70	100.0	65.5	9.1	2.9	22.4	10.4	12.0
1955	15.7	93	100.0	58.1	16.1	2.8	23.0	10.5	12.5
1960	23.9	126	100.0	55.9	21.0	1.7	21.4	8.9	12.5
1965	35.6	175	100.0	53.4	24.3	1.9	20.4	8.3	12.0
1970	64.9	302	100.0	39.5	23.4	2.6	34.6	22.6	12.0
1971	71.3	329	100.0	38.0	23.8	2.6	35.6	23.7	11.9
1972	79.4	362	100.0	37.5	23.6	2.7	36.1	24.0	12.2
1973	88.6	401	100.0	37.1	23.9	2.6	36.4	23.8	12.6
1974	101.6	456	100.0	35.0	24.6	2.5	37.8	25.6	12.2
1975	116.6	519	100.0	33.1	25.6	2.5	38.9	26.6	12.3
1976	132.8	587	100.0	32.0	26.4	3.0	38.6	27.6	11.0
1977	149.2	653	100.0	31.0	27.3	2.9	38.8	27.6	11.2
1978	167.5	726	100.0	30.0	27.9	3.0	39.1	28.0	11.1
1979	189.3	813	100.0	28.6	28.9	3.0	39.5	28.4	11.1
1980	219.4	933	100.0	27.1	29.7	3.5	39.7	28.9	10.8
1981	254.8	1,073	100.0	26.4	30.3	3.5	39.9	29.4	10.5
1982	286.4	1,194	100.0	25.9	30.9	3.6	39.6	29.3	10.3
1983	314.9	1,300	100.0	25.8	30.9	3.5	39.8	29.7	10.1
1984	341.2	1,395	100.0	25.7	31.2	3.4	39.8	29.8	9.9
1985	369.7	1,497	100.0	25.5	30.9	3.5	40.1	30.2	9.9
1986	400.8	1,607	100.0	25.2	31.0	3.5	40.3	30.0	10.3
1987	439.3	1,744	100.0	24.8	31.4	3.4	40.4	29.7	10.7
1988	482.8	1,898	100.0	24.5	32.1	3.5	39.9	29.3	10.5
1989	530.9	2,066	100.0	23.8	32.1	3.6	40.5	29.9	10.6
1990	591.5	2,279	100.0	23.1	32.3	3.6	41.0	29.9	11.0
1991	660.2	2,518	100.0	21.9	31.7	3.6	42.9	30.9	12.0

[1]Includes all expenditures for health services and supplies other than expenses for program administration and net cost of private health insurance and government public health activities.
[2]Out-of-pocket payments and private health insurance are combined for these years.

NOTES: These data include revisions in health expenditures back to 1985 and in population back to 1960 and differ from previous editions of Health, United States. They reflect Social Security Administration population revisions as of July 1992.

SOURCE: Office of National Health Statistics, Office of the Actuary: National health expenditures, 1991. Health Care Financing Review. Vol. 14, No. 2. HCFA Pub. No. 03335. Health Care Financing Administration. Washington. U.S. Government Printing Office, Winter 1992.

Table 124 (page 1 of 2). Expenditures for health services and supplies and percent distribution, by type of payer: United States, selected calendar years 1965–91

[Data are compiled by the Health Care Financing Administration]

Type of payer	1965	1967	1970	1975	1980	1985	1987	1988	1989	1990	1991
	Amount in billions [1]										
Total [1]	$38.2	$47.9	$69.1	$124.7	$238.9	$407.2	$476.9	$526.2	$583.6	$652.4	$728.6
Private	30.3	35.0	50.1	86.2	162.0	279.0	327.5	362.5	398.3	436.6	474.1
Private business	6.0	8.3	13.7	27.8	64.3	113.5	131.8	151.0	167.0	187.9	205.4
Private employer share of private health insurance premiums	4.9	5.6	9.8	19.9	47.9	83.9	95.0	110.9	122.8	140.2	152.7
Private employer contribution to Medicare hospital insurance trust fund [2]	0.0	1.4	2.1	5.0	10.5	20.3	24.6	26.2	28.1	29.5	32.8
Workers' compensation and temporary disability insurance medical benefits and administration	0.8	1.0	1.4	2.4	5.1	7.8	10.5	12.0	14.1	16.0	17.5
Industrial inplant health services	0.2	0.2	0.3	0.5	0.9	1.4	1.7	1.9	2.1	2.2	2.4
Household (individuals)	23.7	26.0	35.0	55.9	90.8	153.6	181.9	196.1	213.8	228.9	247.0
Employee share of private health insurance premiums and individual policy premiums	4.6	4.9	6.0	9.9	16.6	30.0	37.5	37.7	42.7	46.6	52.2
Employee and self-employment contributions and voluntary premiums paid to Medicare hospital insurance trust fund [2]	0.0	1.6	2.4	5.7	12.0	24.0	29.4	31.2	33.7	35.6	39.9
Premiums paid by individuals to Medicare supplementary medical insurance trust fund	0.0	0.6	1.0	1.7	2.7	5.2	6.1	8.7	11.2	10.2	10.7
Out-of-pocket health spending by individuals	19.0	18.9	25.6	38.5	59.5	94.4	108.8	118.5	126.2	136.5	144.3
Non-patient revenue	0.6	0.8	1.5	2.5	7.0	12.0	13.8	15.4	17.5	19.8	21.7
Public	7.9	12.8	18.9	38.5	76.8	128.2	149.4	163.7	185.4	215.8	254.5
Federal Government	3.4	7.0	10.4	21.3	42.6	68.9	77.0	84.3	96.5	113.7	133.8
Employer contributions to private health insurance	0.2	0.2	0.3	1.2	2.2	4.3	4.8	6.4	8.0	9.1	9.8
Other [3]	3.3	6.8	10.1	20.1	40.3	64.5	72.2	77.9	88.5	104.6	124.0
State and local government	4.5	5.8	8.5	17.2	34.2	59.3	72.4	79.4	88.8	102.1	120.7
Employer contributions to private health insurance	0.3	0.4	0.6	1.9	6.7	16.0	17.9	20.4	23.6	26.3	29.7
Other [4]	4.2	5.5	7.9	15.2	27.5	43.3	54.5	59.1	65.2	75.8	91.0
	Percent distribution										
Total	100.0	100.0	100.0	100.0	100.0	100.0	100.0	100.0	100.0	100.0	100.0
Private	79.3	73.2	72.6	69.2	67.8	68.5	68.7	68.9	68.2	66.9	65.1
Private business	15.6	17.3	19.8	22.3	26.9	27.9	27.6	28.7	28.6	28.8	28.2
Private employer share of private health insurance premiums	12.9	11.7	14.2	16.0	20.0	20.6	19.9	21.1	21.0	21.5	21.0
Private employer contribution to Medicare hospital insurance trust fund [2]	0.0	2.9	3.0	4.0	4.4	5.0	5.2	5.0	4.8	4.5	4.5
Workers' compensation and temporary disability insurance medical benefits and administration	2.2	2.2	2.1	2.0	2.1	1.9	2.2	2.3	2.4	2.4	2.4
Industrial inplant health services	0.6	0.5	0.5	0.4	0.4	0.4	0.4	0.4	0.4	0.3	0.3
Household (individuals)	62.0	54.2	50.7	44.8	38.0	37.7	38.1	37.3	36.6	35.1	33.9
Employee share of private health insurance premiums and individual policy premiums	12.2	10.2	8.7	7.9	6.9	7.4	7.9	7.2	7.3	7.1	7.2
Employee and self-employment contributions and voluntary premiums paid to Medicare hospital insurance trust fund [2]	0.0	3.3	3.4	4.6	5.0	5.9	6.2	5.9	5.8	5.5	5.5
Premiums paid by individuals to Medicare supplementary medical insurance trust fund	0.0	1.3	1.4	1.4	1.1	1.3	1.3	1.7	1.9	1.6	1.5
Out-of-pocket health spending by individuals	49.8	39.5	37.1	30.9	24.9	23.2	22.8	22.5	21.6	20.9	19.8
Non-patient revenue	1.7	1.7	2.2	2.0	2.9	2.9	2.9	2.9	3.0	3.0	3.0

See footnotes at end of table.

Table 124 (page 2 of 2). Expenditures for health services and supplies and percent distribution, by type of payer: United States, selected calendar years 1965–91

[Data are compiled by the Health Care Financing Administration]

Type of payer	1965	1967	1970	1975	1980	1985	1987	1988	1989	1990	1991
					Percent distribution						
Public . . . . : . . .	20.7	26.8	27.4	30.8	32.2	31.5	31.3	31.1	31.8	33.1	34.9
Federal Government	9.0	14.6	15.0	17.1	17.8	16.9	16.2	16.0	16.5	17.4	18.4
Employer contributions to private health insurance.	0.4	0.5	0.4	0.9	0.9	1.1	1.0	1.2	1.4	1.4	1.3
Other [3]	8.6	14.1	14.7	16.1	16.9	15.9	15.1	14.8	15.2	16.0	17.0
State and local government	11.7	12.2	12.3	13.8	14.3	14.6	15.2	15.1	15.2	15.6	16.6
Employer contributions to private health insurance.	0.7	0.8	0.9	1.5	2.8	3.9	3.7	3.9	4.0	4.0	4.1
Other [4]	11.0	11.4	11.4	12.2	11.5	10.6	11.4	11.2	11.2	11.6	12.5

[1]Excludes research and construction.

[2]Includes one-half of self-employment contribution to Medicare hospital insurance trust fund.

[3]Includes expenditures for Federal programs such as Medicaid and Medicare with adjustments for contributions by employers and individuals and premiums paid to the Medicare insurance trust fund.

[4]Includes expenditures for State and local programs such as Medicaid and maternal and child health, and employer contributions to Medicare hospital insurance trust fund.

NOTES: This table disaggregates health expenditures according to four classes of payers: businesses, households (individuals), Federal Government, and State and local governments. Where businesses or households pay dedicated funds into government health programs (e.g., Medicare) or employers and employees share in the cost of health premiums, these costs are assigned to businesses or households accordingly. This results in a lower share of expenditures being assigned to the Federal Government than for tabulations of expenditures by source of funds. Estimates of national health expenditure by source of funds aim to track government sponsored health programs over time, and do not delineate the role of business employers in paying for health care. These data include revisions and differ from previous editions of Health, United States.

SOURCE: Office of National Health Statistics, Office of the Actuary: Business, households, and governments - Health Spending 1991. Health Care Financing Review. Vol. 14, No. 3. Health Care Financing Administration. Washington. U.S. Government Printing Office, Winter 1993.

Table 125. Expenditures on hospital care, nursing home care, physician services, and all other personal health care expenditures and percent distribution, according to source of funds: United States, selected years, 1960–91

[Data are compiled by the Health Care Financing Administration]

Service and year	Total in billions	Out-of-pocket payments	Private health insurance	Other private funds	Government Total [1]	Medicaid	Medicare
Hospital care		Percent distribution					
1960	$9.3	20.7	35.6	1.2	42.5	. . .	. . .
1965	14.0	19.6	40.9	1.9	37.6	. . .	. . .
1970	27.9	9.0	34.4	3.2	53.4	8.1	18.8
1975	52.4	8.4	34.4	2.8	54.5	8.8	21.9
1980	102.4	5.2	36.6	4.9	53.3	9.4	25.8
1984	157.5	5.1	36.1	4.6	54.1	9.1	28.8
1985	168.3	5.2	35.4	4.9	54.4	9.2	28.9
1986	179.8	4.8	35.5	5.0	54.7	9.2	28.2
1987	194.2	4.5	35.7	5.0	54.8	9.5	27.7
1988	212.0	4.9	36.0	5.3	53.9	9.4	27.1
1989	232.4	4.7	36.3	5.4	53.7	9.8	26.9
1990	258.1	4.0	36.6	5.4	54.0	11.2	26.1
1991	288.6	3.4	35.2	5.1	56.3	15.0	25.4
Nursing home care							
1960	1.0	80.0	0.0	6.4	13.6	. . .	. . .
1965	1.7	64.5	0.1	5.8	29.5	. . .	. . .
1970	4.9	48.2	0.3	4.9	46.6	28.0	5.0
1975	9.9	42.1	0.7	4.8	52.3	47.5	2.9
1980	20.0	43.3	0.9	3.1	52.7	48.6	2.1
1984	31.2	47.8	1.1	2.1	48.9	44.9	1.8
1985	34.1	48.6	1.0	1.9	48.5	44.6	1.7
1986	36.7	49.1	1.0	1.9	48.0	44.1	1.6
1987	39.7	47.9	1.0	1.9	49.2	45.2	1.6
1988	42.8	48.1	1.1	1.9	48.9	44.4	2.2
1989	47.5	44.2	1.1	1.9	52.7	43.4	7.2
1990	53.3	45.3	1.1	1.9	51.7	45.1	4.5
1991	59.9	43.1	1.1	1.9	53.9	47.4	4.4
Physician services							
1960	5.3	62.7	30.2	0.1	7.1	. . .	. . .
1965	8.2	60.6	32.5	0.1	6.8	. . .	. . .
1970	13.6	42.8	35.2	0.1	21.9	4.6	11.8
1975	23.3	32.8	39.3	0.1	27.9	7.1	14.6
1980	41.9	26.9	42.9	0.1	30.2	5.1	19.0
1984	67.1	23.4	45.2	0.0	31.4	3.8	21.6
1985	74.0	21.8	45.6	0.0	32.6	3.9	22.5
1986	82.1	20.8	45.7	0.0	33.5	3.9	23.1
1987	93.0	20.4	45.8	0.0	33.8	3.8	23.3
1988	105.1	19.9	46.7	0.0	33.4	3.6	23.0
1989	116.1	19.4	46.4	0.0	34.1	3.7	23.6
1990	128.8	18.7	47.1	0.0	34.2	4.1	23.1
1991	142.0	18.1	47.0	0.0	34.8	4.9	23.1
All other personal health care [2]							
1960	8.4	87.8	1.4	2.7	8.0	. . .	. . .
1965	11.7	87.4	2.2	2.6	7.8	. . .	. . .
1970	18.5	80.6	4.3	2.7	12.4	4.4	0.7
1975	31.0	72.2	8.5	3.0	16.4	6.2	1.7
1980	55.1	62.1	17.5	3.5	16.9	6.0	3.1
1984	85.5	57.4	21.9	4.0	16.7	6.1	4.7
1985	93.4	56.6	21.9	4.3	17.2	6.5	4.8
1986	102.2	56.1	22.2	4.1	17.7	6.9	4.8
1987	112.4	55.3	22.9	3.9	17.9	7.3	4.7
1988	122.9	54.3	23.7	3.9	18.1	7.6	4.7
1989	135.0	53.2	23.6	4.0	19.1	8.4	5.2
1990	151.2	51.5	23.6	4.3	20.7	9.0	5.9
1991	169.7	48.8	23.8	4.5	22.9	10.5	6.8

[1]Includes other government expenditures for these health care services, for example, care funded by the Department of Veterans Affairs and state and locally financed subsidies to hospitals.

[2]Includes expenditures for dental services, other professional services, home health care, drugs and other medical nondurables, vision products and other medical durables, and other personal health care.

SOURCE: Office of National Health Statistics, Office of the Actuary: National health expenditures, 1991. Health Care Financing Review. Vol. 14, No. 2. HCFA Pub. No. 03335. Health Care Financing Administration. Washington. U.S. Government Printing Office, Winter 1992.

Table 126. Nursing home average monthly charges per resident and percent of residents, according to primary source of payments and selected facility characteristics: United States, 1977 and 1985

[Data are based on reporting by a sample of nursing homes]

Facility characteristic	Own income or family support 1977	Own income or family support 1985	Medicare 1977	Medicare 1985	Medicaid 1977	Medicaid 1985	Public assistance welfare 1977	Public assistance welfare 1985	All other sources 1977	All other sources 1985
	Average monthly charge [1]									
All facilities	$690	$1,450	$1,167	$2,141	$720	$1,504	$508	$863	$440	$1,099
Ownership										
Proprietary	686	1,444	1,048	2,058	677	1,363	501	763	562	1,174
Nonprofit and government	698	1,462	1,325	*2,456	825	1,851	534	1,237	324	1,029
Certification										
Skilled nursing facility	866	1,797	1,136	2,315	955	2,000	575	*1,338	606	1,589
Skilled nursing and intermediate facility.	800	1,643	1,195	2,156	739	1,509	623	1,215	630	1,702
Intermediate facility	567	1,222	. . .	. . .	563	1,150	479	900	*456	1,460
Not certified	447	999	. . .	. . .	. . .	. . .	401	664	*155	464
Bed size										
Less than 50 beds	516	886	*869	*1,348	663	1,335	394	*835	*295	*749
50–99 beds	686	1,388	*1,141	1,760	634	1,323	493	774	468	1,116
100–199 beds.	721	1,567	1,242	2,192	691	1,413	573	855	551	1,504
200 beds or more.	823	1,701	*1,179	2,767	925	1,919	602	1,071	370	*866
Geographic region										
Northeast.	909	1,645	1,369	2,109	975	2,035	*511	738	395	1,244
Midwest.	652	1,398	*1,160	2,745	639	1,382	537	1,241	524	1,416
South.	585	1,359	*1,096	2,033	619	1,200	452	727	342	1,057
West	663	1,498	*868	1,838	663	1,501	564	837	*499	*843
	Percent of residents									
All facilities	38.4	41.6	2.0	1.4	47.8	50.4	6.4	3.4	5.3	3.2
Ownership										
Proprietary	37.5	40.1	1.7	1.6	49.6	52.1	7.3	3.9	3.8	2.3
Nonprofit and government	40.4	44.9	2.7	*0.9	43.8	46.6	4.4	2.3	8.6	5.3
Certification										
Skilled nursing facility	41.5	39.1	4.6	2.6	41.4	53.7	7.7	2.1	4.8	2.4
Skilled nursing and intermediate facility.	31.6	36.8	2.6	1.9	58.3	57.8	3.2	1.3	4.1	2.2
Intermediate facility	36.3	41.4	. . .	. . .	55.3	55.9	5.3	*1.5	3.1	*1.1
Not certified	64.2	65.5	. . .	. . .	. . .	. . .	19.0	18.0	16.7	12.9
Bed size										
Less than 50 beds	49.6	53.1	*1.8	*1.2	32.7	33.8	10.5	11.2	5.4	*0.6
50–99 beds	39.5	49.5	*1.2	*1.3	46.5	42.9	8.1	3.9	4.7	2.5
100–199 beds.	38.4	39.6	2.6	1.5	50.4	55.2	4.6	1.6	4.0	2.1
200 beds or more.	28.6	30.1	2.3	*1.5	55.5	57.7	4.6	3.0	9.1	7.7
Geographic region										
Northeast.	34.6	34.8	3.3	1.7	53.3	52.9	3.8	7.1	5.1	3.5
Midwest.	44.5	49.1	1.5	*0.8	42.1	45.9	6.5	2.5	5.4	1.6
South.	32.2	39.4	*1.4	*1.2	52.5	53.8	8.2	2.5	5.7	3.1
West	41.3	40.4	2.5	*2.7	44.7	49.2	6.7	*1.2	4.8	6.6

[1]Includes life-care residents and no-charge residents.

*Relative standard error greater than 30 percent.

SOURCES: Centers for Disease Control and Prevention, National Center for Health Statistics: The National Nursing Home Survey, 1977 summary for the United States, by J. F. Van Nostrand, A. Zappolo, E. Hing, et al. Vital and Health Statistics. Series 13, No. 43. DHEW Pub. No. (PHS) 79-1794. Public Health Service. Washington. U.S. Government Printing Office, July 1979; and The National Nursing Home Survey: 1985 summary for the United States, by E. Hing, E. Sekscenski, and G. Strahan. Vital and Health Statistics. Series 13, No. 97. DHHS Pub. No. (PHS) 89-1758. Public Health Service. Washington. U.S. Government Printing Office, Jan. 1989.

Table 127. Nursing home average monthly charges per resident and percent of residents, according to selected facility and resident characteristics: United States, 1964, 1973–74, 1977, and 1985

[Data are based on reporting by a sample of nursing homes]

Facility and resident characteristic	Average monthly charge [1]				Percent of residents			
	1964	1973–74 [2]	1977	1985	1964	1973–74 [2]	1977	1985
Facility characteristic								
All facilities	$186	$479	$689	$1,456	100.0	100.0	100.0	100.0
Ownership:								
Proprietary	205	489	670	1,379	60.2	69.8	68.2	68.7
Nonprofit and government	145	456	732	1,624	39.8	30.2	31.8	31.3
Certification [3]:								
Skilled nursing facility	. . .	566	880	1,905	. . .	39.8	20.7	18.5
Skilled nursing and intermediate facility	. . .	514	762	1,571	. . .	24.5	40.5	45.2
Intermediate facility	. . .	376	556	1,179	. . .	22.4	28.3	24.9
Not certified	. . .	329	390	875	. . .	13.3	10.6	11.4
Bed size:								
Less than 50 beds.	- - -	397	546	1,036	- - -	15.2	12.9	8.9
50–90 beds	- - -	448	643	1,335	- - -	34.1	30.5	27.6
100–199 beds.	- - -	502	706	1,478	- - -	35.6	38.8	43.2
200 beds or more	- - -	576	837	1,759	- - -	15.1	17.9	20.2
Geographic region:								
Northeast	213	651	918	1,781	28.6	22.0	22.4	23.6
Midwest	171	433	640	1,399	36.6	34.6	34.5	32.5
South.	161	410	585	1,256	18.1	26.0	27.2	29.4
West	204	454	653	1,458	16.7	17.4	15.9	14.5
Resident characteristic								
All residents	186	479	689	1,456	100.0	100.0	100.0	100.0
Age:								
Under 65 years	155	434	585	1,379	12.0	10.6	13.6	11.6
65–74 years	184	473	669	1,372	18.9	15.0	16.2	14.2
75–84 years	191	488	710	1,468	41.7	35.5	35.7	34.1
85 years and over	194	485	719	1,497	27.5	38.8	34.5	40.0
Sex:								
Male.	171	466	652	1,438	35.0	29.1	28.8	28.4
Female.	194	484	705	1,463	65.0	70.9	71.2	71.6

[1]Includes life-care residents and no-charge residents.
[2]Data exclude residents of personal care homes.
[3]Medicare extended care facilities and Medicaid skilled nursing homes from the 1973–74 survey were considered to be equivalent to Medicare or Medicaid skilled nursing facilities in 1977 and 1985 for the purposes of this comparison.

SOURCES: Centers for Disease Control and Prevention, National Center for Health Statistics: Charges for care and sources of payment for residents in nursing homes, United States, June–August 1969, by J. F. Van Nostrand and J. F. Sutton. Vital and Health Statistics. Series 12, No. 21. DHEW Pub. No. (HRA) 74-1706. Public Health Service. Washington. U.S. Government Printing Office, July 1973; Charges for care and sources of payment for residents in nursing homes, United States, National Nursing Home Survey, Aug. 1973–Apr. 1974, by E. Hing. Vital and Health Statistics. Series 13, No. 32. DHEW Pub. No. (PHS) 78-1783. Public Health Service. Washington. U.S. Government Printing Office. Nov. 1977; The National Nursing Home Survey: 1977 summary for the United States, by J. F. Van Nostrand, A. Zappolo, E. Hing, et al. Vital and Health Statistics. Series 13, No. 43. DHEW Pub. No. (PHS) 79-1794. Public Health Service. Washington. U.S. Government Printing Office, July 1979; and The National Nursing Home Survey: 1985 summary for the United States, by E. Hing, E. Sekscenski, and G. Strahan. Vital and Health Statistics. Series 13, No. 97. DHHS Pub. No. (PHS) 89-1758. Public Health Service. Washington. U.S. Government Printing Office, Jan. 1989.

Table 128. National funding for health research and development and average annual percent change, according to source of funds: United States, selected years 1960–91

[Data are compiled by the National Institutes of Health from multiple sources]

Year and period	All funding	Federal	State and local	Industry [1]	Private nonprofit organizations
			Amount in millions		
1960	$886	$448	$46	$253	$139
1965	1,890	1,174	90	450	176
1970	2,847	1,667	170	795	215
1971	3,168	1,877	198	860	233
1972	3,536	2,147	228	934	227
1973	3,750	2,225	245	1,048	232
1974	4,443	2,754	254	1,183	252
1975	4,701	2,832	286	1,319	264
1976	5,107	3,059	312	1,469	267
1977	5,568	3,396	338	1,614	220
1978	6,273	3,811	416	1,800	246
1979	7,162	4,321	465	2,093	284
1980	7,967	4,723	480	2,459	305
1981	8,738	4,848	564	2,998	328
1982	9,595	4,970	642	3,593	390
1983	10,778	5,399	718	4,205	456
1984	12,159	6,087	800	4,765	507
1985	13,565	6,791	884	5,352	538
1986	14,900	6,895	1,034	6,188	782
1987	16,940	7,847	1,191	7,103	800
1988	19,011	8,425	1,300	8,432	854
1989	20,977	9,163	1,471	9,404	939
1990 [2]	23,076	9,791	1,632	10,634	1,020
1991 [2]	25,560	10,711	1,702	12,020	1,128
			Average annual percent change		
1960–91	11.5	10.8	12.4	13.3	7.0
1960–65	16.4	21.2	14.4	12.2	4.8
1965–70	8.5	7.3	13.6	12.1	4.1
1970–75	10.6	11.2	11.0	10.7	4.2
1970–71	11.3	12.6	16.5	8.2	8.4
1971–72	11.6	14.4	15.2	8.6	−2.6
1972–73	6.1	3.6	7.5	12.2	2.2
1973–74	18.5	23.8	3.7	12.9	8.6
1974–75	5.8	2.8	12.6	11.5	4.8
1975–80	11.1	10.8	10.9	13.3	2.9
1975–76	8.6	8.0	9.1	11.4	1.1
1976–77	9.0	11.0	8.3	9.9	−17.6
1977–78	12.7	12.2	23.1	11.5	11.8
1978–79	14.2	13.4	11.8	16.3	15.4
1979–80	11.2	9.3	3.2	17.5	7.4
1980–85	11.2	7.5	13.0	16.8	12.0
1980–81	9.7	2.6	17.5	21.9	7.5
1981–82	9.8	2.5	13.8	19.8	18.9
1982–83	12.3	8.6	11.8	17.0	16.9
1983–84	12.8	12.7	11.4	13.3	11.2
1984–85	11.6	11.6	10.5	12.3	6.1
1985–90	11.2	7.6	13.0	14.7	13.6
1985–86	9.8	1.5	17.0	15.6	45.4
1986–87	13.7	13.8	15.2	14.8	2.3
1987–88	12.2	7.4	9.2	18.7	6.8
1988–89	10.3	8.8	13.2	11.5	10.0
1989–90	10.0	6.9	10.9	13.1	8.6
1990–91	10.8	9.4	4.3	13.0	10.6

[1]Includes expenditures for drug research. These expenditures are included in the "drugs and sundries" component of the Health Care Financing Administration's National Health Expenditure Series, not under "research."
[2]Preliminary figures.

NOTE: These data include revisions and may differ from previous editions of Health, United States.

SOURCES: National Institutes of Health: NIH Data Book, 1992. Public Health Service, U.S. Department of Health and Human Services, NIH Pub. No. 92-1261, Sept. 1992; National Institutes of Health, Office of Science Policy and Legislation: Selected data.

Table 129. Federal funding for health research and development and percent distribution, according to agency: United States, selected fiscal years 1970–91

[Data are compiled by the National Institutes of Health from Federal Government sources]

Agency	1970 [1]	1975 [1]	1980	1984	1985	1986	1987	1988	1989	1990	1991 [2]
					Amount in millions						
Total	$1,667	$2,832	$4,723	$6,087	$6,791	$6,895	$7,847	$8,425	$9,163	$9,791	$10,711
					Percent distribution						
All Federal agencies	100.0	100.0	100.0	100.0	100.0	100.0	100.0	100.0	100.0	100.0	100.0
Department of Health and Human Services	70.6	77.6	78.2	78.9	79.7	81.1	83.3	84.1	84.9	85.2	86.0
National Institutes of Health	52.4	66.4	67.4	69.9	71.1	72.6	74.6	74.7	74.0	72.9	72.0
Centers for Disease Control and Prevention	- - -	1.5	1.8	0.7	0.7	0.8	0.8	1.1	1.3	1.0	1.1
Other Public Health Service	16.2	8.3	7.9	7.5	7.3	7.3	7.7	8.0	9.1	10.8	12.3
Other Department of Health and Human Services	2.0	1.3	1.1	0.7	0.6	0.5	0.4	0.4	0.6	0.5	0.7
Other agencies	29.4	22.4	21.8	21.1	20.3	18.9	16.7	15.9	15.1	14.8	14.0
Department of Agriculture	3.0	2.2	3.1	2.4	2.1	1.1	1.3	1.3	1.3	1.1	1.1
Department of Defense	7.5	4.1	4.5	6.8	6.5	7.2	5.2	5.1	4.2	4.4	3.2
Department of Education [3]	. . .	. . .	0.7	0.7	0.6	0.6	0.6	0.7	0.6	0.6	0.4
Department of Energy [4]	6.3	5.8	4.5	3.0	2.6	2.4	2.3	2.4	2.4	2.8	3.4
Department of the Interior	0.7	0.3	0.5	0.4	0.4	0.4	0.4	0.4	0.4	0.4	0.4
Environmental Protection Agency	. . .	1.3	1.7	0.7	0.8	0.5	0.6	0.3	0.6	0.3	0.3
International Development Cooperation Agency [5]	0.6	0.2	0.3	0.3	0.6	0.4	0.4	0.3	0.3	0.2	0.2
National Aeronautics and Space Administration	5.2	2.6	1.5	1.8	1.7	1.9	1.7	1.6	1.5	1.5	1.5
National Science Foundation	1.7	1.6	1.6	1.4	1.3	1.2	1.1	1.0	1.0	0.8	0.7
Department of Veterans Affairs	3.5	3.3	2.8	3.1	3.3	2.7	2.7	2.6	2.6	2.4	2.4
All other departments and agencies	0.9	1.0	0.4	0.3	0.4	0.4	0.4	0.3	0.3	0.2	0.3

[1] Data for fiscal year ending June 30; all other data for fiscal year ending September 30.
[2] Preliminary figures.
[3] Office of Handicapped Research, formerly included in other Department of Health and Human Services.
[4] Includes Atomic Energy Commission and Energy Research and Development Administration.
[5] Includes Department of State and Agency for International Development.

SOURCES: National Institutes of Health: NIH Data Book, 1992. Public Health Service, U.S. Department of Health and Human Services, NIH Pub. No. 92-1261, Sept. 1992; Office of Science Policy and Legislation, National Institutes of Health, Public Health Service: Unpublished data.

Table 130. Federal spending for human immunodeficiency virus (HIV)–related activities, according to agency and type of activity: United States, fiscal years 1982–91

[Data are compiled from Federal Government appropriations]

Agency and type of activity	1982	1983	1984	1985	1986	1987	1988	1989	1990	1991
Agency					Amount in millions					
All Federal spending............................	$8	$44	$104	$208	$507	$926	$1,591	$2,275	$2,978	$3,648
Department of Health and Human Services, total..........................	6	39	97	197	402	777	1,420	2,002	2,597	3,246
Public Health Service, total	6	29	61	109	234	502	962	1,301	1,590	1,888
National Institutes of Health	4	22	44	64	135	261	474	602	744	807
Alcohol, Drug Abuse, and Mental Health Administration....................	–	1	3	3	12	48	112	173	215	237
Centers for Disease Control and Prevention....	2	6	14	33	62	136	305	378	443	497
Food and Drug Administration	–	–	1	9	10	16	30	74	57	63
Health Resources and Services Administration	–	–	–	–	15	12	37	60	113	266
Agency for Health Care Policy and Research....	–	–	–	–	–	–	1	7	8	10
Office of the Assistant Secretary for Health.....	–	–	–	–	–	30	3	6	8	6
Indian Health Service	–	–	–	–	–	–	–	1	3	2
Health Care Financing Administration	–	10	30	75	135	215	360	545	780	1,050
Social Security Administration	–	–	6	13	33	60	98	153	224	305
Other Department of Health and Human Services Agencies	–	–	–	–	–	–	–	3	3	3
Department of Veterans Affairs	2	5	7	11	23	55	84	142	208	217
Department of Defense........................	–	–	–	–	79	74	53	86	125	127
Agency for International Development	–	–	–	–	2	17	30	40	41	50
Other departments............................	–	–	–	–	1	3	4	5	7	8
Activity										
Research.........................	4	24	47	85	193	344	659	981	1,164	1,282
Public Health Service	4	23	47	84	166	316	635	943	1,116	1,230
Department of Veterans Affairs...............	–	1	–	1	2	4	7	11	14	8
Department of Defense	–	–	–	–	25	24	17	27	34	44
Education and prevention	3	7	15	27	84	197	367	403	470	504
Public Health Service	2	6	14	25	52	145	300	303	366	400
Department of Veterans Affairs...............	1	1	1	2	5	11	17	28	29	29
Department of Defense	–	–	–	–	24	22	16	26	28	19
Agency for International Development..........	–	–	–	–	2	17	30	40	41	50
Other....................................	–	–	–	–	1	2	4	6	6	6
Medical care	1	13	36	83	197	325	467	738	1,120	1,557
Health Care Financing Administration:										
Medicaid (Federal share)...................	–	10	30	70	130	200	330	490	670	870
Medicare	–	–	–	5	5	15	30	55	110	180
Public Health Service	–	–	–	–	16	41	27	55	108	258
Department of Veterans Affairs...............	1	3	6	8	16	40	60	103	165	180
Department of Defense	–	–	–	–	30	28	20	33	63	64
Other....................................	–	–	–	–	–	1	–	2	4	5
Cash assistance.............................	–	–	6	13	33	60	98	153	224	305
Social Security Administration:										
Disability Insurance........................	–	–	5	10	25	45	80	125	185	240
Supplemental Security Income...............	–	–	1	3	8	15	18	28	39	65

NOTES: These data include revisions and differ from previous editions of Health, United States. Federal expenditures on HIV-related activities are estimated at about 35 to 40 percent of total HIV-related expenditures which include, for example, expenditures covered by private health insurance, out-of-pocket costs to patients, and the States' share of Medicaid, public hospital, and other local expenditures.

SOURCE: Budget Office, Public Health Service: Unpublished data.

Table 131. Public health expenditures by State and territorial health agencies, according to source of funds and program area: United States, selected fiscal years 1976–89

[Data are based on reporting by State and territorial health agencies]

Funds and program area	1976	1978	1980	1982	1984	1985	1986	1987	1988	1989
	Amount in millions									
Total	$2,540	$3,256	$4,451	$5,145	$6,242	$6,950	$7,491	$8,128	$8,540	$9,669
Source of funds										
Federal grants and contracts.	797	1,133	1,573	1,778	2,344	2,556	2,700	2,822	3,072	3,503
Department of Agriculture	154	351	678	916	1,307	1,455	1,551	1,652	1,690	1,988
Other.	643	782	895	861	1,037	1,101	1,148	1,170	1,381	1,515
State.	1,486	1,802	2,513	2,923	3,352	3,810	4,124	4,562	4,696	5,184
Local.	96	87	114	123	151	149	148	140	144	154
Fees, reimbursements, and other . .	161	234	250	321	395	435	520	604	628	829
Program area										
WIC [1]	138	337	661	890	1,269	1,431	1,534	1,622	1,660	1,938
Noninstitutional personal health other than WIC [2].	1,079	1,356	1,698	1,905	2,380	2,521	2,777	3,130	3,483	3,972
State health agency-operated institutions.	531	641	819	950	979	1,153	1,236	1,227	1,342	1,459
Environmental health	199	237	298	355	415	467	480	528	464	520
Health resources	208	297	357	360	563	627	651	709	720	824
Laboratory.	104	131	161	182	214	229	238	265	279	308
Other [3]	281	256	457	504	423	521	576	647	592	649
	Percent distribution									
Total	100.0	100.0	100.0	100.0	100.0	100.0	100.0	100.0	100.0	100.0
Source of funds										
Federal grants and contracts.	31.4	34.8	35.3	34.6	37.6	36.8	36.0	34.7	36.0	36.2
Department of Agriculture	6.1	10.8	15.2	17.8	20.9	20.9	20.7	20.3	19.8	20.6
Other.	25.3	24.0	20.1	16.7	16.6	15.8	15.3	14.4	16.2	15.7
State.	58.5	55.3	56.5	56.8	53.7	54.8	55.0	56.1	55.0	53.6
Local.	3.8	2.7	2.6	2.4	2.4	2.1	2.0	1.7	1.7	1.6
Fees, reimbursements, and other . .	6.3	7.2	5.6	6.2	6.3	6.3	6.9	7.4	7.3	8.6
Program area										
WIC [1]	5.4	10.4	14.8	17.3	20.3	20.6	20.5	20.0	19.4	20.0
Noninstitutional personal health other than WIC [2].	42.5	41.6	38.2	37.0	38.1	36.3	37.1	38.5	40.8	41.1
State health agency-operated institutions.	20.9	19.7	18.4	18.5	15.7	16.6	16.5	15.1	15.7	15.1
Environmental health	7.8	7.3	6.7	6.9	6.6	6.7	6.4	6.5	5.4	5.4
Health resources	8.2	9.1	8.0	7.0	9.0	9.0	8.7	8.7	8.4	8.5
Laboratory.	4.1	4.0	3.6	3.5	3.4	3.3	3.2	3.3	3.3	3.2
Other [3]	11.0	7.9	10.3	9.8	6.8	7.5	7.7	8.0	6.9	6.7

[1]Supplemental Food Program for Women, Infants, and Children.
[2]Includes funds for maternal and child health services other than WIC, handicapped children's services, communicable disease control, dental health, chronic disease control, mental health, alcohol and drug abuse, and supporting personal health programs.
[3]Funds for general administration and funds to local health departments not allocated to program areas.

NOTE: Data are reported for 55 health agencies in 50 States, the District of Columbia, and 4 territories (Puerto Rico, American Samoa, Guam, and the Virgin Islands).

SOURCES: Public Health Foundation: Public Health Agencies 1987: Expenditures and Sources of Funds. Washington. 1987; Unpublished data.

Table 132. Personal health care per capita expenditures and average annual percent change, according to geographic division and State: United States, selected years 1966–82

[Data are compiled by the Health Care Financing Administration]

Geographic division and State	Amount per capita						Average annual percent change	
	1966	1969	1972	1976	1980	1982	1966–80	1980–82
United States	$201	$280	$381	$605	$958	$1,220	11.8	12.8
New England	234	328	441	686	1,058	1,356	11.4	13.2
Maine	173	242	328	542	870	1,091	12.2	12.0
New Hampshire	188	245	330	507	759	986	10.5	14.0
Vermont	197	274	352	531	778	978	10.3	12.1
Massachusetts	253	360	489	760	1,175	1,508	11.6	13.3
Rhode Island	231	315	413	672	1,062	1,351	11.5	12.8
Connecticut	236	330	438	675	1,046	1,348	11.2	13.5
Middle Atlantic	227	319	425	662	1,017	1,310	11.3	13.5
New York	258	366	488	745	1,107	1,417	11.0	13.1
New Jersey	192	264	355	578	877	1,115	11.5	12.8
Pennsylvania	201	279	372	590	972	1,273	11.9	14.4
East North Central	203	278	378	610	978	1,249	11.9	13.0
Ohio	195	264	361	597	958	1,247	12.0	14.1
Indiana	182	252	337	542	861	1,101	11.7	13.1
Illinois	220	300	407	634	1,033	1,308	11.7	12.5
Michigan	211	286	388	635	1,014	1,281	11.9	12.4
Wisconsin	192	269	373	610	952	1,219	12.1	13.2
West North Central	200	273	369	597	973	1,241	12.0	12.9
Minnesota	216	287	389	602	976	1,229	11.4	12.2
Iowa	197	265	351	563	935	1,176	11.8	12.1
Missouri	198	273	365	627	997	1,285	12.2	13.5
North Dakota	197	273	367	676	1,034	1,325	12.6	13.2
South Dakota	181	241	327	522	887	1,154	12.0	14.1
Nebraska	195	268	371	598	948	1,216	12.0	13.3
Kansas	195	270	379	568	988	1,271	12.3	13.4
South Atlantic	169	242	342	551	879	1,115	12.5	12.6
Delaware	209	286	381	599	912	1,153	11.1	12.4
Maryland	190	273	390	609	957	1,232	12.2	13.5
District of Columbia	430	667	958	1,349	2,198	2,838	12.4	13.6
Virginia	151	213	301	493	811	1,054	12.8	14.0
West Virginia	161	227	313	508	808	1,057	12.2	14.4
North Carolina	143	204	282	461	737	931	12.4	12.4
South Carolina	125	182	251	423	686	857	12.9	11.8
Georgia	150	217	319	515	843	1,048	13.1	11.5
Florida	184	264	377	623	975	1,228	12.6	12.2
East South Central	148	211	294	483	798	1,025	12.8	13.3
Kentucky	155	218	286	444	739	957	11.8	13.8
Tennessee	166	232	324	531	874	1,144	12.6	14.4
Alabama	145	210	300	501	809	1,033	13.1	13.0
Mississippi	115	163	242	425	730	897	14.1	10.8
West South Central	170	242	331	533	859	1,096	12.3	13.0
Arkansas	142	198	284	470	766	994	12.8	13.9
Louisiana	156	226	322	511	857	1,106	12.9	13.6
Oklahoma	183	263	351	539	852	1,086	11.6	12.9
Texas	177	249	338	549	876	1,110	12.1	12.6
Mountain	189	259	346	541	849	1,070	11.3	12.3
Montana	175	236	325	510	801	1,036	11.5	13.7
Idaho	153	210	292	455	695	868	11.4	11.8
Wyoming	200	268	327	451	710	873	9.5	10.9
Colorado	233	311	396	605	942	1,209	10.5	13.3
New Mexico	157	214	282	458	722	904	11.5	11.9
Arizona	190	271	376	582	882	1,112	11.6	12.3
Utah	158	211	286	458	714	896	11.4	12.0
Nevada	196	282	389	658	1,163	1,380	13.6	8.9
Pacific	234	328	440	691	1,093	1,380	11.6	12.4
Washington	219	297	390	584	915	1,165	10.8	12.8
Oregon	197	274	364	587	912	1,165	11.6	13.0
California	242	340	460	727	1,152	1,451	11.8	12.2
Alaska	227	289	340	560	961	1,187	10.9	11.1
Hawaii	208	300	401	598	932	1,228	11.3	14.8

NOTES: Per capita spending estimates are the expenditure level of services rendered in a geographic area per resident population. Per capita figures cannot be interpreted directly as spending per resident unless substantially all of the services provided in a State are consumed by residents of that State. U.S. estimates do not include services provided in U.S. territories or possessions, services rendered by U.S. taxpayers while living abroad, and services furnished to U.S. personnel living abroad or on military vessels.

SOURCE: Office of the Actuary: Personal health care expenditures by State, selected years 1966–1982, by K. R. Levit. Health Care Financing Review. HCFA Pub. No. 03199. Health Care Financing Administration. Washington. U.S. Government Printing Office, Summer 1985.

Table 133. Hospital care per capita expenditures and average annual percent change, according to geographic division and State: United States, selected years 1966–82

[Data are compiled by the Health Care Financing Administration]

Geographic division and State	Amount per capita						Average annual percent change	
	1966	1969	1972	1976	1980	1982	1966–80	1980–82
United States	$80	$119	$166	$276	$441	$577	13.0	14.4
New England	101	151	207	335	515	669	12.3	14.0
Maine	74	107	138	246	411	517	13.0	12.2
New Hampshire	73	98	134	213	334	458	11.5	17.1
Vermont	86	126	162	242	338	443	10.3	14.5
Massachusetts.	116	178	247	400	624	810	12.8	13.9
Rhode Island	101	148	196	328	492	623	12.0	12.5
Connecticut.	91	133	185	296	444	578	12.0	14.1
Middle Atlantic	94	144	200	328	495	641	12.6	13.8
New York	110	171	236	377	540	679	12.0	12.1
New Jersey	71	103	145	254	371	498	12.5	15.9
Pennsylvania	82	127	178	300	505	675	13.9	15.6
East North Central.	81	117	167	286	465	615	13.3	15.0
Ohio	74	107	154	273	446	599	13.7	15.9
Indiana	63	95	134	235	383	512	13.8	15.6
Illinois	90	132	195	323	539	700	13.6	14.0
Michigan	90	123	170	295	477	628	12.7	14.7
Wisconsin	76	117	163	268	401	539	12.6	15.9
West North Central	79	117	158	270	451	592	13.3	14.6
Minnesota	89	122	168	272	425	540	11.8	12.7
Iowa	69	103	139	238	404	536	13.5	15.2
Missouri	81	123	164	295	510	679	14.0	15.4
North Dakota	83	121	156	283	479	624	13.3	14.1
South Dakota.	75	101	133	234	398	530	12.7	15.4
Nebraska.	75	115	157	259	429	568	13.3	15.1
Kansas	76	116	160	269	451	593	13.6	14.7
South Atlantic	68	103	151	252	411	539	13.7	14.5
Delaware.	91	131	174	291	437	552	11.9	12.4
Maryland	84	122	185	287	464	606	13.0	14.3
District of Columbia	192	334	564	903	1,516	2,021	15.9	15.5
Virginia	63	92	132	218	372	506	13.5	16.6
West Virginia	70	107	152	264	424	564	13.7	15.3
North Carolina	57	85	121	201	324	428	13.2	14.9
South Carolina.	51	79	107	188	303	397	13.6	14.5
Georgia.	56	86	135	228	386	492	14.8	12.9
Florida.	66	103	151	268	434	569	14.4	14.5
East South Central	60	91	131	226	383	507	14.2	15.1
Kentucky.	60	91	121	202	326	433	12.9	15.2
Tennessee.	67	102	149	252	430	578	14.2	15.9
Alabama.	61	92	134	238	408	541	14.5	15.2
Mississippi.	48	73	111	198	343	431	15.1	12.1
West South Central	66	97	135	229	380	500	13.3	14.7
Arkansas.	56	77	114	197	324	443	13.4	16.9
Louisiana.	63	94	145	239	412	549	14.4	15.4
Oklahoma	63	102	132	224	378	498	13.7	14.8
Texas	69	101	137	233	379	495	12.9	14.3
Mountain	76	109	145	234	377	483	12.1	13.2
Montana	67	95	122	193	336	445	12.2	15.1
Idaho	50	75	104	162	254	335	12.3	14.8
Wyoming.	85	116	123	188	313	398	9.8	12.8
Colorado.	100	136	171	274	422	557	10.8	14.9
New Mexico.	69	96	122	222	348	449	12.3	13.6
Arizona.	78	119	169	256	396	498	12.3	12.1
Utah	58	81	114	188	307	399	12.6	14.0
Nevada	68	108	151	273	540	630	16.0	8.0
Pacific	85	123	169	280	445	583	12.6	14.5
Washington.	72	102	133	223	337	434	11.7	13.5
Oregon	66	96	127	219	347	468	12.6	16.1
California.	88	129	180	298	479	626	12.9	14.3
Alaska.	149	173	164	255	446	552	8.1	11.3
Hawaii.	79	115	146	222	352	479	11.3	16.7

NOTES: Per capita spending estimates are the expenditure level of services rendered in a geographic area per resident population. Per capita figures cannot be interpreted directly as spending per resident unless substantially all of the services provided in a State are consumed by residents of that State.

SOURCE: Office of the Actuary: Personal health care expenditures by State, selected years 1966–1982, by K. R. Levit. Health Care Financing Review. HCFA Pub. No. 03199. Health Care Financing Administration. Washington. U.S. Government Printing Office, Summer 1985.

Table 134. Nursing home care per capita expenditures and average annual percent change, according to geographic division and State: United States, selected years 1966–82

[Data are compiled by the Health Care Financing Administration]

Geographic division and State	Amount per capita						Average annual percent change	
	1966	1969	1972	1976	1980	1982	1966–80	1980–82
United States	$12	$19	$31	$52	$90	$114	15.5	12.5
New England	20	28	47	85	145	186	15.2	13.3
Maine	15	23	40	70	134	176	16.9	14.6
New Hampshire	16	20	35	43	71	90	11.2	12.6
Vermont	19	27	39	75	121	149	14.1	11.0
Massachusetts	22	32	52	94	152	192	14.8	12.4
Rhode Island	15	21	34	78	169	214	18.9	12.5
Connecticut	19	29	49	90	156	206	16.2	14.9
Middle Atlantic	14	21	36	66	108	145	15.7	15.9
New York	16	26	46	85	135	184	16.5	16.7
New Jersey	10	15	24	45	77	97	15.7	12.2
Pennsylvania	12	18	28	48	88	116	15.3	14.8
East North Central	12	19	31	54	97	125	16.1	13.5
Ohio	12	18	27	53	99	143	16.3	20.2
Indiana	12	20	33	57	102	129	16.5	12.5
Illinois	13	20	33	52	90	109	14.8	10.1
Michigan	10	17	27	48	86	106	16.6	11.0
Wisconsin	14	22	39	71	120	150	16.6	11.8
West North Central	18	28	44	69	131	172	15.2	14.6
Minnesota	22	33	57	91	175	235	16.0	15.9
Iowa	22	36	51	81	143	168	14.3	8.4
Missouri	12	19	29	47	95	139	15.9	21.0
North Dakota	19	33	47	60	112	154	13.5	17.3
South Dakota	18	30	49	69	132	165	15.3	11.8
Nebraska	17	27	42	68	112	140	14.4	11.8
Kansas	18	26	42	65	130	163	15.2	12.0
South Atlantic	8	12	20	33	59	77	15.3	14.2
Delaware	8	12	20	42	67	86	16.4	13.3
Maryland	9	17	24	46	75	102	16.4	16.6
District of Columbia	6	10	18	22	43	55	15.1	13.1
Virginia	6	9	16	30	63	85	18.3	16.2
West Virginia	3	5	12	20	41	62	20.5	23.0
North Carolina	6	11	16	30	58	75	17.6	13.7
South Carolina	6	9	16	28	62	76	18.2	10.7
Georgia	8	13	23	37	67	79	16.4	8.6
Florida	11	15	25	31	48	65	11.1	16.4
East South Central	7	11	20	35	67	86	17.5	13.3
Kentucky	9	14	23	40	81	104	17.0	13.3
Tennessee	6	10	17	28	56	76	17.3	16.5
Alabama	8	14	22	40	62	79	15.8	12.9
Mississippi	4	7	15	30	71	90	22.8	12.6
West South Central	12	19	31	48	79	94	14.4	9.1
Arkansas	13	21	34	50	95	112	15.3	8.6
Louisiana	8	13	22	38	68	89	16.5	14.4
Oklahoma	19	31	47	58	91	111	11.8	10.4
Texas	11	18	30	48	78	88	15.0	6.2
Mountain	10	15	23	35	59	74	13.5	12.0
Montana	12	17	33	43	66	92	12.9	18.1
Idaho	12	17	26	45	69	84	13.3	10.3
Wyoming	6	12	23	24	38	49	14.1	13.6
Colorado	15	21	33	54	86	104	13.3	10.0
New Mexico	5	9	15	16	34	49	14.7	20.0
Arizona	8	13	17	22	41	53	12.4	13.7
Utah	9	12	17	30	55	63	13.8	7.0
Nevada	7	10	20	29	60	82	16.6	16.9
Pacific	12	18	31	48	82	97	14.7	8.8
Washington	16	21	43	61	109	137	14.7	12.1
Oregon	17	24	37	57	94	113	13.0	9.6
California	11	18	30	47	78	91	15.0	8.0
Alaska	1	2	9	17	14	26	20.7	36.3
Hawaii	6	10	18	28	36	63	13.7	32.3

NOTES: Per capita spending estimates are the expenditure level of services rendered in a geographic area per resident population. Per capita figures cannot be interpreted directly as spending per resident unless substantially all of the services provided in a State are consumed by residents of that State.

SOURCE: Office of the Actuary: Personal health care expenditures by State, selected years 1966–1982, by K. R. Levit. Health Care Financing Review. HCFA Pub. No. 03199. Health Care Financing Administration. Washington. U.S. Government Printing Office, Summer 1985.

Table 135. Health care coverage for persons under 65 years of age, according to type of coverage and selected characteristics: United States, 1980, 1984, and 1989

[Data are based on household interviews of a sample of the civilian noninstitutionalized population]

Characteristic	Private insurance			Medicaid [1]			Not covered [2]		
	1980	1984	1989	1980	1984	1989	1980	1984	1989
	Percent of population								
Total [3,4]	78.8	76.9	76.6	5.9	6.0	6.4	12.5	15.4	15.7
Age									
Under 15 years	74.7	71.9	71.7	10.2	10.8	11.4	12.8	16.1	15.9
Under 5 years	70.3	67.6	68.1	12.0	13.4	13.3	15.2	18.0	17.0
5–14 years .·.	76.7	74.2	73.6	9.4	9.4	10.4	11.7	15.0	15.3
15–44 years	79.3	77.0	76.6	4.2	4.4	4.4	14.2	17.6	18.1
45–64 years	83.6	83.6	83.3	3.1	2.7	3.4	8.6	10.2	10.6
Sex [3]									
Male.	79.5	77.5	76.9	4.7	5.0	5.2	12.7	15.8	16.4
Female.	78.2	76.3	76.2	7.1	7.1	7.6	12.2	15.1	14.9
Race [3]									
White	81.9	80.0	79.7	3.9	4.1	4.5	11.4	14.2	14.5
Black	60.1	58.9	59.2	17.9	17.5	17.1	19.0	22.3	22.0
Family income [3,5]									
Less than $14,000.	38.6	34.1	34.6	27.6	26.5	26.6	31.0	37.8	37.3
$14,000–$24,999.	61.1	71.3	71.4	9.2	4.2	4.8	25.9	22.1	21.4
$25,000–$34,999.	79.0	88.3	87.9	3.0	1.2	1.2	15.0	8.7	9.3
$35,000–$49,999.	90.2	93.1	92.4	1.1	0.4	0.8	6.2	4.8	5.6
$50,000 or more	93.7	95.2	95.7	0.6	0.4	0.4	3.9	3.1	3.2
Geographic region [3]									
Northeast	81.7	80.4	83.4	7.0	7.4	5.8	10.3	11.8	10.3
Midwest	83.8	80.6	81.9	5.8	7.0	7.1	9.0	11.8	10.7
South.	75.6	74.4	71.8	4.8	4.4	5.7	15.0	18.4	20.0
West	74.3	72.3	72.1	6.5	6.2	7.2	15.3	19.0	19.1
Location of residence [3]									
Within MSA.	79.7	77.6	77.2	6.2	6.5	6.4	11.3	14.4	15.1
Outside MSA.	77.0	75.4	74.3	5.2	5.2	6.5	14.8	17.5	17.8

[1] Includes persons receiving Aid to Families with Dependent Children or Supplemental Security Income or those with current Medicaid cards.

[2] Includes persons not covered by private insurance, Medicaid, Medicare, and military plans.

[3] Age adjusted.

[4] Includes all other races not shown separately and unknown family income.

[5] Family income categories for 1989. Income categories for 1980 are: less than $7,000; $7,000–$9,999; $10,000–$14,999; $15,000–$24,999; $25,000 or more; and, in 1984 are: less than $10,000; $10,000–$18,999; $19,000–$29,999; $30,000–$39,999; and $40,000 or more.

NOTES: Percents do not add to 100 because the percent with other types of health insurance (e.g., Medicare, military) is not shown, and because persons with both private insurance and Medicaid appear in both columns. 1980 denominators include persons with unknown health insurance (1.0 percent).

SOURCE: Centers for Disease Control and Prevention, National Center for Health Statistics, Division of Health Interview Statistics and Division of Analysis: Data from the National Health Interview Survey.

Table 136. Health care coverage for persons 65 years of age and over, according to type of coverage and selected characteristics: United States, 1980, 1984, and 1989

[Data are based on household interviews of a sample of the civilian noninstitutionalized population]

Characteristic	Medicare and private insurance			Medicare and Medicaid [1]			Medicare only [2]		
	1980	1984	1989	1980	1984	1989	1980	1984	1989
	Percent of population								
Total [3,4]	64.4	70.9	73.5	8.1	5.4	5.7	22.7	20.0	16.8
Age									
65–74 years	67.0	73.3	74.2	6.8	4.5	5.0	20.6	17.7	15.5
75 years and over	59.9	66.8	72.3	10.3	7.0	6.8	26.4	24.1	19.0
75–84 years	61.9	69.2	74.1	9.7	6.5	6.4	24.8	22.0	17.4
85 years and over	51.2	56.2	64.8	12.7	9.3	8.5	33.0	33.4	26.1
Sex [3]									
Male	65.6	71.6	73.9	5.7	3.3	4.0	23.1	20.8	17.2
Female	63.6	70.5	73.4	9.6	6.9	6.8	22.4	19.4	16.4
Race [3]									
White	68.3	74.4	77.3	6.6	4.0	4.5	21.0	18.5	14.7
Black	26.5	38.1	39.3	23.3	19.9	16.5	40.6	35.4	37.9
Family income [3,5]									
Less than $14,000	53.4	57.5	64.8	15.7	12.3	11.4	28.2	27.3	21.5
$14,000–$24,999	72.9	79.8	81.2	4.8	1.8	2.6	19.1	15.1	13.4
$25,000–$34,999	74.1	80.3	80.0	3.9	2.2	2.4	18.3	13.7	12.5
$35,000–$49,999	74.4	81.0	80.3	2.5	*2.3	*1.9	16.8	11.9	10.2
$50,000 or more	71.9	78.5	76.5	2.2	*1.8	*1.1	18.3	14.4	12.6
Geographic region [3]									
Northeast	67.4	74.3	73.1	5.6	3.5	4.0	22.3	18.4	18.0
Midwest	71.2	77.6	79.6	4.9	3.2	2.9	19.9	16.8	14.1
South	58.9	65.1	70.6	10.8	7.9	7.7	25.6	23.0	18.3
West	60.7	68.2	71.4	10.9	6.5	7.6	21.7	21.0	16.0
Location of residence [3]									
Within MSA	64.2	71.6	73.6	7.5	4.7	5.1	23.0	19.6	16.8
Outside MSA	64.9	69.8	73.4	9.2	6.6	7.2	22.2	20.7	16.8

[1]Includes persons receiving Aid to Families with Dependent Children or Supplemental Security Income or those with current Medicaid cards.

[2]Includes persons not covered by private insurance or Medicaid and a small proportion of persons with other types of coverage, such as CHAMPUS or public assistance.

[3]Age adjusted.

[4]Includes all other races not shown separately and unknown family income.

[5]Family income categories for 1989. Income categories for 1980 are: less than $7,000; $7,000–$9,999; $10,000–$14,999; $15,000–$24,999; $25,000 or more; and, in 1984 are: less than $10,000; $10,000–$18,999; $19,000–$29,999; $30,000–$39,999; and $40,000 or more.

*Relative standard error greater than 30 percent.

NOTES: Percents do not add to 100 because the percent without Medicare is not shown and persons with Medicare, private insurance, and Medicaid appear in both columns. 1980 denominators include persons with unknown health insurance (less than 1 percent). In 1989, 5.2 percent of all persons 65 years of age and over had no Medicare, but only 0.9 percent were without health insurance.

SOURCE: Centers for Disease Control and Prevention, National Center for Health Statistics, Division of Health Interview Statistics and Division of Analysis: Data from the National Health Interview Survey.

Table 137. Health maintenance organizations and enrollment, according to model type, geographic region, and Federal program: United States, selected years 1976–92

[Data are based on a census of health maintenance organizations]

Plans and enrollment	1976	1980	1984	1985 [1]	1986	1987	1989	1990	1991	1992
Plans					Number					
All plans	174	235	304	478	623	647	604	572	553	555
Model type [2]:										
Individual practice association [3]	41	97	125	244	384	409	385	360	346	340
Group [4]	122	138	179	234	239	238	219	212	168	166
Mixed	- - -	- - -	- - -	- - -	- - -	- - -	- - -	- - -	39	49
Geographic region:										
Northeast	29	55	67	81	105	114	118	115	116	111
Midwest	52	72	106	157	202	203	183	160	157	165
South	23	45	66	141	188	194	172	176	163	161
West	70	63	65	99	128	136	131	121	117	118
Enrollment [5]					Number of persons in thousands					
Total	5,987	9,078	15,101	21,005	25,725	29,232	31,883	33,028	34,004	36,076
Model type [2]:										
Individual practice association [3]	390	1,694	2,929	6,379	9,932	12,014	13,542	13,741	13,619	14,665
Group [4]	5,562	7,384	12,172	14,625	15,793	17,217	18,342	19,287	17,063	16,543
Mixed	- - -	- - -	- - -	- - -	- - -	- - -	- - -	- - -	3,322	4,868
Federal program [6]:										
Medicaid [7]	- - -	265	349	561	802	811	1,043	1,187	1,446	1,728
Medicare	- - -	391	671	1,064	1,490	1,674	1,761	1,842	2,029	2,161
					Number enrolled per 1,000 population					
Geographic region:										
Northeast	19.9	31.4	57.8	79.4	100.5	117.0	137.7	145.6	153.7	161.1
Midwest	15.2	28.1	61.6	96.8	116.4	130.5	129.2	126.2	126.5	128.3
South	4.3	8.3	20.4	37.5	54.4	64.2	70.5	70.5	71.4	78.1
West	96.9	121.8	148.0	172.5	190.4	205.6	225.5	232.1	237.7	247.0

[1]Increases partly due to changes in reporting methods (see Appendix I).

[2]Eleven HMO's with 35,000 enrollment did not report model type in 1976.

[3]An HMO operating under an individual practice association model contracts with an association of physicians from various settings (a mixture of solo and group practices) to provide health services.

[4]Group includes staff, group, and network model types.

[5]Open-ended enrollment in HMO plans, amounting to 1.2 million on Jan. 1, 1991, is not included in this table.

[6]Federal program enrollment in HMO's refers to enrollment by Medicaid or Medicare beneficiaries, where the Medicaid or Medicare program contracts directly with the HMO to pay the appropriate annual premium.

[7]Data for 1989 and later include enrollment in managed care health insuring organizations.

NOTES: Data as of June 30 in 1976–84, December 31 in 1985–87, and January 1 in 1989–92. Medicaid enrollment in 1989–90 are as of June 30. HMO's in Guam are not included.

SOURCES: Office of Health Maintenance Organizations: Summary of the National HMO census of prepaid plans—June 1976 and National HMO Census 1980. Public Health Service. Washington. U.S. Government Printing Office. DHHS Pub. No. (PHS) 80-50159; InterStudy: National HMO Census: Annual Report on the Growth of HMO's in the U.S., 1984–1985 Editions; The InterStudy Edge, 1989, 1990, vol. 2; Competitive Edge, vols. 1 and 2, issues 1, 1991 and 1992; 1986 December Update of Medicare Enrollment in HMO's. 1988 January Update of Medicare Enrollment in HMO's. Excelsior, Minnesota (Copyrights 1983, 1984, 1985, 1986, 1987, 1988, 1989: Used with the permission of InterStudy); U.S. Bureau of the Census: Current Population Reports. Series P-25, Nos. 998 and 1058. Washington. U.S. Government Printing Office, Dec. 1986 and Mar. 1990. U.S. Dept. of Commerce: Press release CB 91-100. Mar. 11, 1991. Health Care Financing Administration: Unpublished data; Centers for Disease Control and Prevention, National Center for Health Statistics: Data computed by the Division of Analysis.

Table 138. Medicare enrollees and expenditures and percent distribution, according to type of service: United States and other areas, selected years 1967–91

[Data are compiled by the Health Care Financing Administration]

Type of service	1967	1970	1975	1980	1985	1988	1989	1990	1991 [1]
Enrollees					Number in millions				
Total [2]	19.5	20.5	25.0	28.5	31.1	33.0	33.6	34.2	34.9
Hospital insurance	19.5	20.4	24.6	28.1	30.6	32.4	33.0	33.7	34.4
Supplementary medical insurance	17.9	19.6	23.9	27.4	30.0	31.6	32.1	32.6	33.2
Expenditures					Amount in millions				
Total	$4,737	$7,493	$16,316	$36,822	$72,294	$88,561	$100,586	$110,984	$121,340
Total hospital insurance [3]	3,430	5,281	11,581	25,577	48,414	53,331	60,803	66,997	72,570
Inpatient hospital	3,034	4,827	10,877	24,082	44,680	49,062	53,822	59,301	63,167
Skilled nursing facility	282	246	278	401	577	816	2,978	2,876	2,520
Home health agency	29	51	160	568	2,144	2,313	2,765	3,517	5,130
Hospice	...	...	...	...	43	156	238	356	500
Administrative expenses [4]	77	157	266	512	834	815	792	758	1,021
Peer Review activity	...	...	...	14	136	169	208	189	232
Total supplementary medical insurance	1,307	2,212	4,735	11,245	23,880	35,230	39,783	43,987	48,770
Physician	1,128	1,790	3,415	8,188	17,311	24,372	27,057	29,628	32,231
Outpatient hospital	33	114	652	1,935	4,304	6,534	7,662	8,475	9,756
Home health agency	10	34	87	195	54	62	73	81	70
Group practice prepayment	19	26	80	203	720	2,019	2,308	2,827	3,524
Independent laboratory	7	11	39	114	558	983	1,194	1,457	1,648
Administrative expenses	110	237	462	610	933	1,260	1,489	1,519	1,541
					Percent distribution of expenditures				
Total hospital insurance [3]	100.0	100.0	100.0	100.0	100.0	100.0	100.0	100.0	100.0
Inpatient hospital	88.5	91.4	93.9	94.2	92.3	92.0	88.5	88.5	87.0
Skilled nursing facility	8.2	4.7	2.4	1.6	1.2	1.5	4.9	4.3	3.5
Home health agency	0.8	1.0	1.4	2.2	4.4	4.3	4.5	5.2	7.1
Hospice	...	...	...	...	0.1	0.3	0.4	0.5	0.7
Administrative expenses [4]	2.2	3.0	2.3	2.0	1.7	1.5	1.3	1.1	1.4
Peer Review activity	...	...	...	0.1	0.3	0.3	0.3	0.3	0.3
Total supplementary medical insurance	100.0	100.0	100.0	100.0	100.0	100.0	100.0	100.0	100.0
Physician	86.3	80.9	72.1	72.8	72.5	69.2	68.0	67.4	66.1
Outpatient hospital	2.5	5.2	13.8	17.2	18.0	18.5	19.3	19.3	20.0
Home health agency	0.8	1.5	1.8	1.7	0.2	0.2	0.2	0.2	0.1
Group practice prepayment	1.5	1.2	1.7	1.8	3.0	5.7	5.8	6.4	7.2
Independent laboratory	0.5	0.5	0.8	1.0	2.3	2.8	3.0	3.3	3.4
Administrative expenses	8.4	10.7	9.8	5.4	3.9	3.6	3.7	3.5	3.2

[1]Preliminary figures.
[2]Number enrolled in the hospital insurance and/or supplementary medical insurance programs on July 1.
[3]In 1967 includes coverage for outpatient hospital diagnostic services.
[4]Includes costs of experiments and demonstration projects.

NOTE: Table includes Medicare data for residents of the United States, Puerto Rico, Virgin Islands, Guam, other outlying areas, foreign countries, and unknown residence.

SOURCE: Office of Medicare Cost Estimates, Office of the Actuary and Bureau of Data Management and Strategy. Health Care Financing Administration. Washington.

Table 139. Medicare enrollment, persons served, and payments for Medicare enrollees 65 years of age and over, according to selected characteristics: United States and other areas, selected years 1967–90

[Data are compiled by the Health Care Financing Administration]

Characteristic	Enrollment in millions [1]				Persons served per 1,000 enrollees [2]				Payments per person served [3]				Payments per enrollee			
	1967	1977	1987	1990	1967	1977	1987	1990	1967	1977	1987	1990	1967	1977	1987	1990
Total	19.5	23.8	29.4	30.9	367	570	754	802	$592	$1,332	$3,025	$3,578	$217	$759	$2,281	$2,869
Age																
65–66 years	2.8	3.3	4.0	4.0	300	533	700	753	496	1,075	2,214	2,463	149	573	1,550	1,854
67–68 years	2.6	3.2	3.7	3.9	326	511	667	721	521	1,173	2,536	2,995	170	599	1,691	2,160
69–70 years	2.4	2.9	3.4	3.7	339	531	705	741	530	1,211	2,700	3,131	180	643	1,902	2,322
71–72 years	2.3	2.6	3.1	3.2	351	555	740	788	560	1,228	2,904	3,393	197	681	2,150	2,673
73–74 years	2.1	2.3	2.9	2.9	369	576	762	808	574	1,319	3,048	3,595	212	759	2,322	2,906
75–79 years	3.9	4.5	5.7	6.1	398	597	787	838	624	1,430	3,312	3,924	248	853	2,608	3,287
80–84 years	2.2	3.0	3.7	4.0	430	623	828	869	693	1,549	3,496	4,222	298	965	2,894	3,668
85 years and over	1.3	2.1	3.0	3.3	465	652	841	883	740	1,636	3,708	4,486	345	1,068	3,119	3,962
Sex																
Male	8.3	9.6	11.8	12.4	357	546	712	759	647	1,505	3,432	4,018	231	821	2,443	3,049
Female.	11.3	14.2	17.6	18.5	373	586	782	830	554	1,223	2,778	3,309	207	717	2,173	2,747
Race [4]																
White.	17.4	21.1	25.7	26.9	375	576	760	810	593	1,328	2,993	3,530	222	765	2,275	2,857
Other.	1.5	2.1	2.8	3.1	260	514	699	738	557	1,404	3,403	4,090	145	722	2,379	3,019
Geographic region [5]																
Northeast.	5.1	5.7	6.6	6.8	385	613	793	833	604	1,426	3,171	3,842	233	874	2,513	3,201
Midwest.	5.6	6.3	7.4	7.6	352	541	756	823	599	1,401	2,969	3,445	211	757	2,246	2,834
South.	5.6	7.5	9.6	10.3	351	556	768	831	528	1,198	2,893	3,485	186	666	2,221	2,894
West	2.9	3.8	5.2	5.6	455	632	726	730	620	1,341	3,222	3,694	282	848	2,339	2,695

[1]Includes fee-for-service and Health Maintenance Organization (HMO) enrollees and is as of July 1 each year.
[2]Excludes HMO enrollees.
[3]Excludes amounts for HMO services.
[4]Excludes persons of unknown race.
[5]Includes the resident population of the United States but not residence unknown.

NOTE: Table includes Medicare data for residents of the United States, Puerto Rico, Virgin Islands, Guam, other outlying areas, foreign countries, and unknown residence.

SOURCE: Bureau of Data Management and Strategy, Health Care Financing Administration: Unpublished data.

Table 140. Hospital utilization and benefit payments for aged and disabled Medicare enrollees in nonfederal short-stay hospitals, according to geographic division: United States, 1980, 1985, and 1990

[Data are compiled by the Health Care Financing Administration]

Geographic division	Discharges 1980	Discharges 1985	Discharges 1990	Days of care 1980	Days of care 1985	Days of care 1990	Average length of stay 1980	Average length of stay 1985	Average length of stay 1990
	Number per 1,000 hospital insurance enrollees						Number of days per hospital discharge		
United States [1]	372	347	313	4,016	2,835	2,783	10.8	8.2	8.9
New England	333	312	296	4,130	3,125	3,037	12.4	10.0	10.3
Middle Atlantic	329	421	322	4,528	3,569	3,721	13.8	8.5	11.6
East North Central	373	325	324	4,243	2,791	2,804	11.4	8.6	8.7
West North Central	426	355	319	4,371	2,745	2,505	10.3	7.7	7.8
South Atlantic	372	314	300	3,880	2,655	2,669	10.4	8.5	8.9
East South Central	436	415	385	4,260	3,311	3,170	9.8	8.0	8.2
West South Central	433	374	351	4,025	2,792	2,840	9.3	7.5	8.1
Mountain	360	312	277	3,243	2,195	1,943	9.0	7.0	7.0
Pacific	338	293	259	2,988	2,111	1,881	8.8	7.2	7.3

Geographic division	Average total charges [3] 1980	Average total charges [3] 1985	Average total charges [3] 1990	Benefit payments [2] Hospital insurance 1980	Benefit payments [2] Hospital insurance 1985	Benefit payments [2] Hospital insurance 1990	Benefit payments [2] Supplementary medical insurance 1980	Benefit payments [2] Supplementary medical insurance 1985	Benefit payments [2] Supplementary medical insurance 1990
	Amount per inpatient day			Amount per enrollee					
United States [1]	$296	$623	$1,072	$909	$1,585	$1,989	$390	$770	$1,276
New England	295	559	931	978	1,661	2,085	402	769	1,224
Middle Atlantic	304	559	902	965	1,792	2,275	428	893	1,475
East North Central	298	623	1,060	1,008	1,603	1,999	370	706	1,220
West North Central	246	580	1,019	888	1,476	1,715	304	643	953
South Atlantic	277	613	1,065	818	1,486	1,845	384	771	1,326
East South Central	249	561	991	754	1,413	2,046	281	544	1,096
West South Central	259	599	1,106	798	1,488	2,011	352	653	1,302
Mountain	310	706	1,295	782	1,309	1,710	368	667	1,145
Pacific	424	907	1,623	1,003	1,713	2,002	509	1,008	1,365

[1]Includes residence unknown.
[2]Benefit payments represent cash-flow disbursements from the Medicare Hospital Insurance and Supplementary Medical Insurance Trust Funds for all types of covered services and include retroactive adjustments for nonbilling reimbursement such as capital, direct medical education, kidney acquisitions, and bad debts by Medicare patients; indirect medical education; lump sum interim payments; and audited fiscal year cost adjustments. Approximately 90 percent of total benefit payments are for short-stay hospital services.
[3]Includes charges for Medicare covered and noncovered services and days.

SOURCE: Bureau of Data Management and Strategy, Health Care Financing Administration: Unpublished data.

Table 141. Medicaid recipients and medical vendor payments, according to basis of eligibility: United States, selected fiscal years 1972–91

[Data are compiled by the Health Care Financing Administration]

Basis of eligibility	1972	1975	1980	1985	1986	1987	1988	1989	1990	1991
Recipients					Number in millions					
All recipients	17.6	22.0	21.6	21.8	22.5	23.1	22.9	23.5	25.3	28.3
					Percent of recipients [1]					
Aged (65 years and over)	18.8	16.4	15.9	14.0	13.9	14.1	13.8	13.3	12.7	11.9
Blind and disabled	9.8	11.2	13.5	13.8	14.2	14.6	15.2	15.3	14.7	14.4
Adults in AFDC [2] families	17.8	20.6	22.6	25.3	25.1	24.2	24.0	24.3	23.8	24.0
Children in AFDC [2] families	44.5	43.6	43.2	44.7	44.4	44.0	43.8	43.9	44.4	46.1
Other Title XIX [3]	9.0	8.2	6.9	5.6	6.0	6.1	5.9	5.0	3.9	3.3
Vendor payments					Amount in billions					
All payments	$6.3	$12.2	$23.3	$37.5	$41.0	$45.0	$48.7	$54.5	$64.9	$77.0
					Percent distribution					
Total	100.0	100.0	100.0	100.0	100.0	100.0	100.0	100.0	100.0	100.0
Aged (65 years and over)	30.6	35.6	37.5	37.6	36.8	35.6	35.2	34.1	33.2	33.1
Blind and disabled	22.2	25.7	32.7	35.9	36.4	37.3	38.2	38.3	37.6	36.7
Adults in AFDC [2] families	15.3	16.8	13.9	12.7	11.9	12.4	12.1	12.7	13.2	13.5
Children in AFDC [2] families	18.1	17.9	13.4	11.8	12.5	12.2	12.0	12.6	14.0	15.1
Other Title XIX [3]	13.9	4.0	2.6	2.1	2.4	2.4	2.5	2.1	1.6	1.3
Vendor payments per recipient					Amount					
All recipients	$358	$556	$1,079	$1,719	$1,821	$1,949	$2,126	$2,318	$2,568	$2,725
Aged (65 years and over)	580	1,206	2,540	4,605	4,808	4,974	5,426	5,926	6,717	7,577
Blind and disabled	807	1,276	2,618	4,459	4,686	4,974	5,332	5,817	6,564	6,979
Adults in AFDC [2] families	307	455	662	860	864	999	1,069	1,206	1,429	1,540
Children in AFDC [2] families	145	228	335	452	512	542	583	668	811	892
Other Title XIX [3]	555	273	398	657	720	763	892	967	1,062	1,096

[1]Recipients included in more than one category for 1980–89. From 1988 to 1991 between 0.2 and 0.5 percent of recipients have unknown basis of eligibility.
[2]Aid to Families with Dependent Children.
[3]Includes some participants in Supplemental Security Income program and other people deemed medically needy in participating States.

NOTES: 1972 and 1975 data are for fiscal year ending June 30. All other years are for fiscal year ending September 30.

SOURCE: Bureau of Data Management and Strategy, Health Care Financing Administration: Unpublished data.

Table 142 (page 1 of 2). Medicaid recipients and medical vendor payments, according to type of service: United States, selected fiscal years 1972–91

[Data are compiled by the Health Care Financing Administration]

Type of service	1972	1975	1980	1985	1986	1987	1988	1989	1990	1991
Recipients					Number in millions					
All recipients	17.6	22.0	21.6	21.8	22.5	23.1	22.9	23.5	25.3	28.3
					Percent of recipients					
Inpatient:										
General hospitals	16.1	15.6	17.0	15.7	15.7	16.3	16.7	17.7	18.2	17.9
Mental hospitals	0.2	0.3	0.3	0.3	0.2	0.2	0.3	0.4	0.4	0.2
Mentally retarded intermediate care facilities	- - -	0.3	0.6	0.7	0.6	0.6	0.6	0.6	0.6	0.5
Nursing facilities	- - -	- - -	- - -	- - -	- - -	- - -	- - -	- - -	- - -	5.3
Skilled	3.1	2.9	2.8	2.5	2.5	2.5	2.5	2.4	2.4	- - -
Intermediate care	- - -	3.1	3.7	3.8	3.7	3.7	3.8	3.8	3.4	- - -
Physician	69.8	69.1	63.7	66.0	66.2	66.5	66.6	66.7	67.6	68.3
Dental	13.6	17.9	21.5	21.4	22.9	22.2	22.1	17.9	18.0	18.4
Other practitioner	9.1	12.1	15.0	15.4	15.3	15.3	15.2	15.1	15.3	15.1
Outpatient hospital	29.6	33.8	44.9	46.2	47.5	47.5	46.0	48.3	49.0	50.0
Clinic	2.8	4.9	7.1	9.7	9.0	9.4	9.8	10.2	11.1	12.4
Laboratory and radiological	20.0	21.5	14.9	29.1	31.6	32.9	33.1	33.0	35.5	37.1
Home health	0.6	1.6	1.8	2.5	2.6	2.6	2.5	2.6	2.8	2.9
Prescribed drugs	63.3	64.3	63.4	63.8	65.3	65.3	66.9	67.7	68.5	69.3
Family planning	. . .	5.5	5.2	7.5	7.7	7.1	6.7	6.7	6.9	7.7
Early and periodic screening	. . .	. . .	. . .	8.7	9.5	9.7	10.0	10.7	11.7	14.0
Rural health clinic	. . .	. . .	. . .	0.4	0.5	0.6	0.6	0.7	0.9	1.4
Other care	14.4	13.2	11.9	15.5	14.7	15.6	18.2	19.5	20.3	21.1
Vendor payments					Amount in billions					
All payments	$6.3	$12.2	$23.3	$37.5	$41.0	$45.0	$48.7	$54.5	$64.9	$77.0
					Percent distribution					
Total	100.0	100.0	100.0	100.0	100.0	100.0	100.0	100.0	100.0	100.0
Inpatient:										
General hospitals	40.6	27.6	27.5	25.2	25.3	25.1	24.8	24.5	25.7	25.8
Mental hospitals	1.8	3.3	3.3	3.2	2.7	3.1	2.8	2.7	2.6	2.6
Mentally retarded intermediate care facilities	- - -	3.1	8.5	12.6	12.4	12.4	12.4	12.2	11.3	10.0
Nursing facilities	- - -	- - -	- - -	- - -	- - -	- - -	- - -	- - -	- - -	26.9
Skilled	23.3	19.9	15.8	13.5	13.8	13.2	13.0	12.2	12.4	- - -
Intermediate care	- - -	15.4	18.0	17.4	16.5	16.2	16.3	16.3	14.9	- - -
Physician	12.6	10.0	8.0	6.3	6.2	6.2	6.1	6.3	6.2	6.4
Dental	2.7	2.8	2.0	1.2	1.3	1.2	1.2	0.9	0.9	0.9
Other practitioner	0.9	1.0	0.8	0.7	0.6	0.6	0.6	0.6	0.6	0.6
Outpatient hospital	5.8	3.0	4.7	4.8	4.8	4.9	5.0	5.2	5.1	5.6
Clinic	0.7	3.2	1.4	1.9	2.0	2.1	2.3	2.3	2.6	2.9
Laboratory and radiological	1.3	1.0	0.5	0.9	1.0	1.1	1.1	1.1	1.1	1.2
Home health	0.4	0.6	1.4	3.0	3.3	3.8	4.1	4.7	5.2	5.3
Prescribed drugs	8.1	6.7	5.7	6.2	6.6	6.6	6.8	6.8	6.8	7.0
Family planning	. . .	0.5	0.3	0.5	0.6	0.5	0.4	0.4	0.4	0.5
Early and periodic screening	. . .	. . .	. . .	0.2	0.2	0.3	0.3	0.3	0.3	0.4
Rural health clinic	. . .	. . .	. . .	0.0	0.0	0.0	0.0	0.0	0.1	0.1
Other care	1.8	1.9	1.9	2.5	2.7	2.7	2.9	3.5	3.7	3.9

See footnotes at end of table.

Table 142 (page 2 of 2). Medicaid recipients and medical vendor payments, according to type of service: United States, selected fiscal years 1972–91

[Data are compiled by the Health Care Financing Administration]

Type of service	1972	1975	1980	1985	1986	1987	1988	1989	1990	1991
Vendor payments per recipient						Amount				
Total payment per recipient	$358	$556	$1,079	$1,719	$1,821	$1,949	$2,126	$2,318	$2,568	$2,725
Inpatient:										
General hospitals	903	983	1,742	2,753	2,924	3,000	3,151	3,208	3,630	3,922
Mental hospitals	2,825	6,045	11,742	19,867	21,000	24,719	22,917	16,397	18,548	30,948
Mentally retarded intermediate										
care facilities	- - -	5,507	16,438	32,102	34,979	37,523	41,531	44,999	50,048	52,750
Nursing facilities	- - -	- - -	- - -	- - -	- - -	- - -	- - -	- - -	- - -	13,811
Skilled	2,665	3,863	6,081	9,274	9,912	10,432	10,974	11,809	13,356	- - -
Intermediate care	- - -	2,764	5,326	7,882	8,180	8,575	9,149	9,994	11,236	- - -
Physician	65	81	136	163	171	181	193	217	235	256
Dental	71	86	99	98	103	105	114	118	130	136
Other practitioner	37	48	61	75	73	74	82	89	96	102
Outpatient hospital	70	50	113	178	185	203	229	250	269	303
Clinic	82	358	209	337	398	441	490	523	602	629
Laboratory and radiological	23	27	38	53	60	63	72	76	80	85
Home health	229	204	847	2,093	2,280	2,775	3,541	4,225	4,733	5,048
Prescribed drugs	46	58	96	166	183	198	215	232	256	277
Family planning	. . .	55	72	119	130	138	135	145	151	164
Early and periodic screening	. . .	. . .	. . .	45	48	51	54	58	67	81
Rural health clinic	. . .	. . .	. . .	81	93	101	107	133	154	154
Other care	44	80	172	274	331	340	343	418	465	503

NOTES: 1972 and 1975 data are for fiscal year ending June 30. All other years are for fiscal year ending September 30.

SOURCE: Bureau of Data Management and Strategy, Health Care Financing Administration: Unpublished data.

Table 143. Department of Veterans Affairs health care expenditures and use, and persons treated according to selected characteristics: United States, selected fiscal years 1965–91

[Data are compiled by Department of Veterans Affairs]

	1965 [1]	1970 [1]	1975 [1]	1980	1985	1988	1989	1990	1991
Health care expenditures	Amount in millions								
All expenditures [2]	$1,150	$1,689	$3,328	$5,981	$8,936	$10,230	$10,949	$11,500	$12,400
	Percent distribution								
All services.	100.0	100.0	100.0	100.0	100.0	100.0	100.0	100.0	100.0
Inpatient hospital	81.9	71.3	66.4	64.3	60.3	53.9	54.1	57.5	56.9
Outpatient care.	12.0	14.0	17.8	19.1	18.9	22.6	23.3	25.3	25.8
Department of Veterans Affairs nursing homes and domiciliaries	2.9	4.3	4.8	5.1	5.4	6.5	6.7	7.1	7.7
Community nursing homes	0.0	1.2	1.4	2.0	3.0	3.5	2.6	2.4	2.3
All other [3].	3.2	9.1	9.6	9.6	12.4	13.4	13.3	7.7	7.3
Health care use	Number in thousands								
Inpatient hospital stays [4]	731	787	1,114	1,248	1,306	1,086	1,028	1,029	984
Outpatient visits	5,987	7,312	14,630	17,971	19,601	23,232	22,643	22,602	23,035
Department of Veterans Affairs nursing homes and domiciliary stays	32	32	29	28	34	44	44	46	48
Community nursing home stays.	0	15	22	29	39	42	32	29	29
Inpatients [5]	Number in thousands								
Total	- - -	- - -	- - -	- - -	- - -	650	617	598	574
	Percent distribution								
Total	- - -	- - -	- - -	- - -	- - -	100.0	100.0	100.0	100.0
Veterans with service connected disability . . .	- - -	- - -	- - -	- - -	- - -	36.9	38.2	38.9	39.1
Veterans without service connected disability.	- - -	- - -	- - -	- - -	- - -	62.2	61.1	60.3	60.0
Low income	- - -	- - -	- - -	- - -	- - -	51.9	53.9	54.8	55.4
Exempt [6].	- - -	- - -	- - -	- - -	- - -	2.8	2.5	2.5	2.7
Other [7]	- - -	- - -	- - -	- - -	- - -	5.6	4.2	2.8	1.8
Unknown	- - -	- - -	- - -	- - -	- - -	1.9	0.5	0.2	0.1
Non-veterans	- - -	- - -	- - -	- - -	- - -	0.8	0.8	0.8	0.9
Outpatients [5]	Number in thousands								
Total	- - -	- - -	- - -	- - -	- - -	2,763	2,597	2,564	2,557
	Percent distribution								
Total	- - -	- - -	- - -	- - -	- - -	100.0	100.0	100.0	100.0
Veterans with service connected disability . . .	- - -	- - -	- - -	- - -	- - -	34.5	37.6	38.3	38.5
Veterans without service connected disability.	- - -	- - -	- - -	- - -	- - -	48.4	50.3	49.8	50.1
Low income	- - -	- - -	- - -	- - -	- - -	34.5	39.9	41.1	42.1
Exempt [6].	- - -	- - -	- - -	- - -	- - -	2.7	2.8	2.9	2.9
Other [7]	- - -	- - -	- - -	- - -	- - -	5.7	5.2	3.6	2.6
Unknown	- - -	- - -	- - -	- - -	- - -	5.5	2.4	2.2	2.4
Non-veterans	- - -	- - -	- - -	- - -	- - -	17.0	12.0	11.8	11.4

[1]Data for fiscal year ending June 30; all other data for fiscal year ending September 30.
[2]Health care expenditures exclude construction, medical administration, and miscellaneous operating expenses.
[3]Includes miscellaneous benefits and services, contract hospitals, education and training, subsidies to State veterans hospitals, nursing homes, and domiciliaries, and the Civilian Health and Medical Program of the Department of Veterans Affairs.
[4]One-day dialysis patients were included in fiscal years 1975, 1980, and 1985. Interfacility transfers were included beginning in fiscal year 1990.
[5]Individuals.
[6]Prisoner of war, exposed to agent orange, etc.
[7]Financial means tested veterans who receive medical care subject to copayments according to income level.

NOTES: The veteran population was estimated at 26.6 million in 1991 with 29 percent age 65 or over compared with 11 percent in 1980. Thirty-two percent had served prior to and during World War II, 15 percent during the Korean conflict, 29 percent during the Vietnam era, 1 percent during the Persian Gulf War, and 23 percent during peacetime.

SOURCE: Office of Policy and Planning and the Office of Finance and Information Resources Management, Department of Veterans Affairs: Unpublished data.

Table 144. Mental health expenditures, percent distribution, and per capita expenditures, according to type of mental health organization: United States, selected years 1969–88

[Data are based on inventories of mental health organizations]

Type of organization	1969	1975	1979	1983	1986	1988
	Amount in millions					
All organizations	$3,293	$6,564	$8,764	$14,432	$18,458	$23,028
State and county mental hospitals	1,814	3,185	3,757	5,491	6,326	6,978
Private psychiatric hospitals	220	467	743	1,712	2,629	4,588
Nonfederal general hospitals with separate psychiatric services	298	621	723	2,176	2,878	3,610
Veterans Administration medical centers[1]	450	699	848	1,316	1,338	1,290
Federally funded community mental health centers	143	776	1,481	–	–	–
Residential treatment centers for emotionally disturbed children	123	279	436	573	978	1,305
Freestanding psychiatric outpatient clinics	186	422	589	430	518	657
All other organizations[2]	59	116	187	2,734	3,792	4,600
	Percent distribution					
All organizations	100.0	100.0	100.0	100.0	100.0	100.0
State and county mental hospitals	55.1	48.5	42.9	38.0	34.4	30.3
Private psychiatric hospitals	6.7	7.1	8.5	11.9	14.2	19.9
Nonfederal general hospitals with separate psychiatric services	9.0	9.5	8.2	15.1	15.6	15.7
Veterans Administration medical centers[1]	13.7	10.6	9.7	9.1	7.2	5.6
Federally funded community mental health centers	4.4	11.8	16.9	–	–	–
Residential treatment centers for emotionally disturbed children	3.7	4.3	5.0	4.0	5.3	5.7
Freestanding psychiatric outpatient clinics	5.6	6.4	6.7	3.0	2.8	2.8
All other organizations[2]	1.8	1.8	2.1	18.9	20.5	20.0
	Amount per capita[3]					
All organizations	$17	$31	$40	$62	$77	$95
State and county mental hospitals	9	15	17	24	26	29
Private psychiatric hospitals	1	2	3	7	11	19
Nonfederal general hospitals with separate psychiatric services	2	3	3	9	12	15
Veterans Administration medical centers[1]	2	3	4	6	6	5
Federally funded community mental health centers	1	4	7	–	–	–
Residential treatment centers for emotionally disturbed children	1	1	2	2	4	5
Freestanding psychiatric outpatient clinics	1	2	3	2	2	3
All other organizations[2]	0	1	1	12	16	19

[1]Includes Veterans Administration neuropsychiatric hospitals, general hospital psychiatric services, and psychiatric outpatient clinics.
[2]Includes freestanding psychiatric partial care organizations and multiservice mental health organizations. Multiservice mental health organizations were redefined in 1983; see Appendix I.
[3]Civilian population.

NOTES: Changes in reporting procedures in 1983 affect the comparability of data with those from previous years. Mental health expenditures include salaries, other operating expenditures, and capital expenditures.

SOURCES: Survey and Reports Branch, Division of Applied and Services Research, National Institute of Mental Health: R. W. Manderscheid and S. A. Barrett: Mental Health, United States, 1987. DHHS Pub. No. (ADM) 87-1518. U.S. Government Printing Office, 1987; Unpublished data.

Table 145. State mental health agency per capita expenditures for mental health services, and average annual percent change, according to State: United States, selected fiscal years 1981–90

[Data are based on reporting by State mental health agencies]

State	1981	1983	1985	1987	1990	Average annual percent change 1981–90
	Amount per capita					
United States.	$27	$31	$35	$38	[1]$48	6.7
Alabama.	20	24	28	29	38	7.4
Alaska.	38	41	45	50	72	7.4
Arizona.	10	10	12	16	27	11.7
Arkansas.	17	20	24	23	26	5.0
California.	28	29	34	30	42	4.4
Colorado.	24	25	28	30	34	4.0
Connecticut.	32	39	44	56	73	9.7
Delaware.	44	51	46	41	55	2.4
District of Columbia [2]	- - -	23	28	130	268	- - -
Florida	20	23	26	25	37	7.1
Georgia.	25	26	23	32	51	8.2
Hawaii.	19	22	23	26	38	8.1
Idaho.	13	15	15	17	20	4.6
Illinois.	18	21	24	25	34	7.4
Indiana	19	23	27	31	47	10.7
Iowa	8	10	11	12	17	8.9
Kansas	17	22	27	28	35	8.0
Kentucky.	15	17	19	23	23	5.0
Louisiana	19	23	26	25	28	4.5
Maine	25	32	36	42	67	11.5
Maryland.	33	37	40	49	61	7.1
Massachusetts.	32	36	46	62	84	11.4
Michigan.	32	39	49	61	74	9.6
Minnesota [3].	17	30	32	42	54	- - -
Mississippi	14	16	24	22	34	10.6
Missouri	24	25	28	31	35	4.5
Montana	24	28	29	28	28	1.5
Nebraska	16	19	21	21	29	6.5
Nevada.	22	25	26	28	33	4.7
New Hampshire.	35	39	42	36	63	6.9
New Jersey.	26	31	36	43	57	9.0
New Mexico	24	25	25	24	23	-0.3
New York	67	74	90	99	118	6.5
North Carolina.	24	29	38	41	46	7.6
North Dakota.	38	42	36	42	40	0.4
Ohio.	25	28	30	33	41	5.8
Oklahoma.	22	33	31	30	36	5.6
Oregon.	20	21	25	28	41	8.0
Pennsylvania.	41	47	52	50	57	3.9
Rhode Island.	36	32	35	41	50	3.7
South Carolina.	31	33	33	45	51	5.8
South Dakota	17	21	22	27	25	4.3
Tennessee	18	20	23	24	29	5.6
Texas	13	16	17	18	23	6.5
Utah	13	16	17	19	21	5.2
Vermont	32	40	44	44	54	5.9
Virginia.	23	29	32	35	45	7.9
Washington.	18	24	30	37	43	10.3
West Virginia.	20	20	22	23	24	2.3
Wisconsin	22	27	28	31	37	5.7
Wyoming.	23	28	31	30	35	4.7

[1]Puerto Rico is included in U.S. total.
[2]Between 1985 and 1990, St. Elizabeth's Hospital was transferred from the National Institute of Mental Health to the District of Columbia Office of Mental Health.
[3]Data for 1981 not comparable with 1983–90 data for Minnesota.

NOTE: Expenditures for mental illness, excluding mental retardation and substance abuse.

SOURCE: National Association of State Mental Health Program Directors and the National Association of State Mental Health Program Directors Research Institute, Inc.: Final Report: Funding Sources and Expenditures of State Mental Health Agencies: Revenue/Expenditure Study Results, Fiscal Year 1990. Nov. 1992.

Appendixes

Appendix Contents

I. Sources and Limitations of Data

Introduction_____ 196
Department of Health and Human Services
  Public Health Service
    Centers for Disease Control and Prevention
      National Center for Health Statistics
        National Vital Statistics System_____ 196
        National Linked File of Live Births and
          Infant Deaths_____ 198
        Compressed Mortality File_____ 198
        National Survey of Family Growth_____ 198
        National Health Interview Survey_____ 199
        National Health and Nutrition
          Examination Survey_____ 200
        National Master Facility Inventory_____ 201
        National Hospital Discharge Survey_____ 202
        National Nursing Home Survey_____ 202
        National Ambulatory Medical Care
          Survey_____ 203
      National Center for Infectious Diseases
        AIDS Surveillance_____ 204
      Epidemiology Program Office
        National Notifiable Diseases Surveillance
          System_____ 204
      National Center for Chronic Disease
        Prevention and Health Promotion
        Abortion Surveillance_____ 204
      National Center for Prevention Services
        U.S. Immunization Survey_____ 205
      National Institute for Occupational Safety
        and Health
        National Traumatic Occupational
          Fatalities Data Base_____ 205
        National Occupational Hazard Survey____ 205
        National Occupational Exposure Survey__ 205
    Health Resources and Services Administration
      Bureau of Health Professions
        Physician Supply Projections_____ 206
        Nurse Supply Estimates_____ 206
    Substance Abuse and Mental Health Services
      Administration
      Office of Applied Studies
        National Household Surveys on Drug
          Abuse_____ 206
        The Drug Abuse Warning Network_____ 206
      Center for Mental Health Services
        Surveys of Mental Health Organizations__ 207
    National Institutes of Health
      National Cancer Institute
        Surveillance, Epidemiology, and End
          Results Program_____ 207
      National Institute on Drug Abuse
        High School Senior Survey (Monitoring
          the Future Survey)_____ 208

Health Care Financing Administration
  Office of the Actuary
    Estimates of National Health
      Expenditures_____ 208
    Medicare Statistical System_____ 209
    Medicaid Data System_____ 209
Department of Commerce
  Bureau of the Census
    Census of Population_____ 209
    Current Population Survey_____ 209
    Population Estimates_____ 210
Department of Labor
  Bureau of Labor Statistics
    Annual Survey of Occupational Injuries
      and Illnesses_____ 210
    Consumer Price Index_____ 211
    Employment and Earnings_____ 211
Department of Veterans Affairs
    The Patient Treatment File_____ 211
    The Patient Census File_____ 211
    The Outpatient Clinic File_____ 211
Environmental Protection Agency
  National Aerometric Surveillance
    Network_____ 211
United Nations
    Demographic Yearbook_____ 211
    World Health Statistics Annual_____ 212
Alan Guttmacher Institute
    Abortion Survey_____ 212
American Association of Colleges of Osteopathic
  Medicine_____ 212
American Dental Assocation_____ 212
American Hospital Association
    Annual Survey of Hospitals_____ 212
American Medical Association
    Physician Masterfile_____ 213
    Annual Census of Hospitals_____ 213
Association of American Medical Colleges_____ 213
InterStudy
    National Health Maintenance
      Organization Census_____ 213
National League for Nursing_____ 214
Public Health Foundation
    Association of State and Territorial
      Health Officials Reporting System_____ 214

II. Glossary

Alphabetical Listing of Terms_____ 215

List of Glossary Tables

I.   Standard million age distribution used to
      adjust death rates to the U.S. population in
      1940_____ 215
II.   Numbers of live births and mother's age
      groups used to adjust maternal mortality rates
      to live births in the United States in 1970____ 215
III. Population and age groups used to adjust
      data to the U.S. civilian noninstitutionalized
      population in 1970: Selected surveys_____ 216

IV. Revision of the *International Classification of Diseases*, according to year of conference by which adopted and years in use in the United States_____ 217

V. Cause-of-death codes, according to applicable revision of *International Classification of Diseases*_____ 217

VI. Codes for industries, according to the *Standard Industrial Classification (SIC) Manual*_____ 221

VII. Codes for diagnostic categories from the *International Classification of Diseases, Ninth Revision, Clinical Modification*_____ 222

VIII. Codes for surgical categories from the *International Classification of Diseases, Ninth Revision, Clinical Modification*_____ 222

IX. Codes for diagnostic and other nonsurgical procedure categories from the *International Classification of Diseases, Ninth Revision, Clinical Modification*_____ 223

X. Mental illness codes, according to applicable revision of the *Diagnostic and Statistical Manual of Mental Disorders* and *International Classification of Diseases*_____ 224

Appendix I
Sources and Limitations of Data

Introduction

This report consolidates the most current data on the health of the population of the United States, the availability and use of health resources, and health care expenditures. The information was obtained from the data files and/or published reports of many governmental and nongovernmental agencies and organizations. In each case, the sponsoring agency or organization collected data using its own methods and procedures. Therefore, the data in this report vary considerably with respect to source, method of collection, definitions, and reference period.

Much of the data presented in the detailed tables are from the ongoing data collection systems of the National Center for Health Statistics. For an overview of these systems, see National Center for Health Statistics, M.G. Kovar: Data systems of the National Center for Health Statistics. *Vital and Health Statistics.* Series 1, No. 23. DHHS Pub. No. (PHS) 89–1325. Public Health Service. Hyattsville, Md. 1989. However, health care personnel data come primarily from the Bureau of Health Professions, Health Resources and Services Administration, and the American Medical Association. National health expenditures data were compiled by the Office of the Actuary, Health Care Financing Administration.

Although a detailed description and comprehensive evaluation of each data source is beyond the scope of this appendix, users should be aware of the general strengths and weaknesses of the different data collection systems. For example, population-based surveys obtain socioeconomic data, data on family characteristics, and information on the impact of an illness, such as days lost from work or limitation of activity. They are limited by the amount of information a respondent remembers or is willing to report. Detailed medical information, such as precise diagnoses or the types of operations performed, may not be known and so will not be reported. Conversely, health care providers, such as physicians and hospitals, usually have good diagnostic information but little or no information about the socioeconomic characteristics of individuals or the impact of illnesses on individuals.

The population covered by different data collection systems may not be the same, and understanding the differences is critical to interpreting the data. Data on vital statistics and national expenditures cover the entire population. Most data on morbidity and utilization of health resources cover only the civilian noninstitutionalized population. Thus, statistics are not included for military personnel, who are usually young; for institutionalized people, who may be any age; or for nursing home residents, who are usually old.

All data collection systems are subject to error, and records may be incomplete or contain inaccurate information. People may not remember essential information, a question may not mean the same thing to different respondents, and some institutions or individuals may not respond at all. It is not always possible to measure the magnitude of these errors or their impact on the data. Where possible, the tables have notes describing the universe and the method of data collection to enable the user to place his or her own evaluation on the data. In many instances data do not add to totals because of rounding.

Overall estimates generally have relatively small sampling errors, but estimates for certain population subgroups may be based on small numbers and have relatively large sampling errors. Numbers of births and deaths from the vital statistics system represent complete counts (except for births in those States where data are based on a 50-percent sample for certain years). Therefore, they are not subject to sampling error. However, when the figures are used for analytical purposes, such as the comparison of rates over a time period, the number of events that actually occurred may be considered as one of a large series of possible results that could have arisen under the same circumstances. When the number of events is small and the probability of such an event is small, considerable caution must be observed in interpreting the conditions described by the figures. Estimates that are unreliable because of large sampling errors or small numbers of events have been noted with asterisks in selected tables. The criteria used to designate unreliable estimates are indicated as notes to the applicable tables.

The descriptive summaries that follow provide a general overview of study design, methods of data collection, and reliability and validity of the data. More complete and detailed discussions are found in the publications referenced at the end of each summary. The data set or source is listed under the agency or organization that sponsored the data collection.

Department of Health and Human Services

Public Health Service

Centers for Disease Control and Prevention

National Center for Health Statistics

National Vital Statistics System

Through the National Vital Statistics System, the National Center for Health Statistics (NCHS) collects and publishes data on births, deaths, marriages, and divorces in the United States. Fetal deaths are classified and tabulated separately from other deaths. The Division of Vital Statistics obtains information on births and deaths from the registration offices of all States, New York City, the District of Columbia, Puerto Rico, the U.S. Virgin Islands, and Guam. Geographic coverage for births and deaths has been complete since 1933.

Until 1972, microfilm copies of all death certificates and a 50-percent sample of birth certificates were received from all registration areas and processed by NCHS. Beginning in 1972, some States began sending their data to NCHS through the Cooperative Health Statistics System (CHSS). States that participated in the CHSS program processed 100 percent of their death and birth records and sent the entire data file to NCHS on computer tapes. Currently, the data are sent to NCHS through the Vital Statistics Cooperative Program (VSCP), following the same procedures as the CHSS. The number of participating States grew from 6 in 1972 to 46 in 1984. All 50 States and the District of Columbia participated in the VSCP starting in 1985.

In most areas, practically all births and deaths are registered. The most recent test of the completeness of birth registration, conducted on a sample of births from 1964 to 1968, showed that 99.3 percent of all births in the United States during that period were registered. No comparable information is available for deaths, but it is generally believed that death registration in the United States is at least as complete as birth registration.

Demographic information on the birth certificate such as race and ethnicity is provided by the mother at the time of birth. Medical and health information is based on hospital records. Demographic information on the death certificate is provided by the funeral director based on information supplied by an informant. Medical certification of cause of death is provided by a physician, medical examiner, or coroner.

U.S. Standard Live Birth and Death Certificates and Fetal Death Reports are revised periodically, allowing careful evaluation of each item and addition, modification, and deletion of items. Beginning with 1989, revised standard certificates replaced the 1978 versions. The 1989 revision of the birth certificate includes items to identify the Hispanic parentage of newborns and to expand information about maternal and infant health characteristics. The 1989 revision of the death certificate includes items on educational attainment and Hispanic origin of decedents as well as changes to improve the medical certification of cause of death. Standard certificates recommended by NCHS are modified in each registration area to serve the area's needs. However, most certificates conform closely in content and arrangement to the standard certificate, and all certificates contain a minimum data set specified by NCHS. For selected items, reporting areas expanded during the years spanned by this report. For items on the birth certificate, the number of reporting States increased for mother's education, prenatal care, marital status, and Hispanic parentage; and on the death certificate, for educational attainment and Hispanic origin of the decedent.

Mother's education was reported on the birth certificate by 38 States in 1970. Data were not available from Alabama, Arkansas, California, Connecticut, Delaware, District of Columbia, Georgia, Idaho, Maryland, New Mexico, Pennsylvania, Texas, and Washington. In 1975 these data were available from four additional States, Connecticut, Delaware, Georgia, Maryland, and the District of Columbia, increasing the number of States reporting mother's education to 42 and the District of Columbia. Between 1980 and 1988 only three States, California, Texas, and Washington did not

report mother's education. In 1988 mother's education was also missing from New York State outside of New York City. In 1989 and 1990 mother's education was missing only from Washington and New York State outside of New York City.

Prenatal care was reported on the birth certificate by 38 States and the District of Columbia in 1970. Data were not available from Alabama, Alaska, Arkansas, Colorado, Connecticut, Delaware, Georgia, Idaho, Massachusetts, New Mexico, Pennsylvania, and Virginia. In 1975 these data were available from four additional States, Colorado, Connecticut, Delaware, and Georgia, increasing the number of States reporting prenatal care to 42 and the District of Columbia. Between 1980 and 1990 prenatal care information was available for the entire United States.

In 1970 **mother's marital status** was reported on the birth certificate by 39 States and the District of Columbia, and in 1975, by 38 States and the District of Columbia. In 1970 and 1975 data were not available from California, Connecticut, Georgia, Idaho, Maryland, Massachusetts, Montana, New Mexico, New York, Ohio, and Vermont; and in 1975 also from Nevada. Between 1980 and 1990 information about mother's marital status was available for the entire United States. During this period, marital status of mother was reported on the birth certificates of 41–42 States. For the remaining eight–nine States that lacked the item, marital status was inferred from a comparison of the child's and parents' surnames.

In 1980 and 1981 information on **births of Hispanic parentage** was reported on the birth certificate by the following 22 States: Arizona, Arkansas, California, Colorado, Florida, Georgia, Hawaii, Illinois, Indiana, Kansas, Maine, Mississippi, Nebraska, Nevada, New Jersey, New Mexico, New York, North Dakota, Ohio, Texas, Utah, and Wyoming. In 1982, Tennessee, and in 1983 the District of Columbia began reporting this information. Between 1983 and 1987 information on births of Hispanic parentage was available for 23 States and the District of Columbia. In 1988 this information became available for Alabama, Connecticut, Kentucky, Massachusetts, Montana, North Carolina, and Washington, increasing the number of States reporting information on births of Hispanic parentage to 30 States and the District of Columbia. In 1989 this information became available from an additional 17 States, increasing the number of Hispanic-reporting States to 47 and the District of Columbia. In 1989 only Louisiana, New Hampshire, and Oklahoma did not report Hispanic parentage on the birth certificate. In 1990 Louisiana began reporting Hispanic parentage. In 1990 about 99 percent of the total U.S. Hispanic population resided in the Hispanic-reporting area comprised of 48 States and the District of Columbia.

Information on **educational attainment of decedents** became available for the first time in 1989 due to the revision of the U.S. Standard Certificate of Death. Mortality data by educational attainment for 1989 are based on deaths to residents of the following 21 States whose data were at least 90 percent complete: Arizona, California, Colorado, Delaware, Florida, Hawaii, Idaho, Illinois, Iowa, Kansas, Michigan, Minnesota, Missouri,

Montana, New Hampshire, Oregon, South Carolina, Utah, Vermont, Wisconsin, and Wyoming. In 1990 the reporting area encompassed 28 States and the District of Columbia with the addition of the following States: Alabama, Massachusetts, Nebraska, North Dakota, Ohio, Pennsylvania, and Texas. The reporting areas in 1989 and 1990 represent 40 and 62 percent of U.S. deaths in those years.

In 1980–84 mortality data by **Hispanic origin of decedent** were based on deaths to residents of the following 15 States whose data on the death certificate were at least 90 percent complete and of comparable format: Arizona, Colorado, Georgia, Hawaii, Illinois, Indiana, Kansas, Mississippi, Nebraska, New York, North Dakota, Ohio, Texas, Utah, and Wyoming. In 1985 Arkansas, California, and the District of Columbia, and in 1986 New Jersey, were added to the Hispanic reporting area, increasing the number of reporting States in 1985 to 17 and the District of Columbia and in 1986–87 to 18 and the District of Columbia. In 1988 Alabama, Kentucky, Maine, Montana, North Carolina, Oregon, Rhode Island, and Washington were added to the reporting area, increasing the number of States to 26 and the District of Columbia. In 1989 an additional 18 States were added, increasing the Hispanic reporting area to 44 States and the District of Columbia. In 1989 only Connecticut, Louisiana, Maryland, New Hampshire, Oklahoma, and Virginia were not included in the reporting area. In 1990 Maryland and Virginia were added to the reporting area; however, New York was excluded due to the high proportion of not stated or unknown origin from New York City. The 1990 reporting area for Hispanic origin of decedent included 45 States and the District of Columbia. Based on data from the Bureau of the Census, the 1990 reporting area encompassed an estimated 88 percent of the U.S. Hispanic population.

Provisional death rates by cause, age, race, and sex are estimated from the Current Mortality Sample. The Current Mortality Sample is a 10-percent systematic sample of death certificates received each month in the vital statistics offices in the 50 States, the District of Columbia, and the independent registration area of New York City. All death certificates received during the 1-month period are sampled regardless of the month or year in which the death occurred.

For more information, see: National Center for Health Statistics, Technical Appendix, *Vital Statistics of the United States, 1988*, Vol. I, Natality, DHHS Pub. No. (PHS) 90–1100 and Vol. II, Mortality, Part A, DHHS Pub. No. (PHS) 91–1101, Public Health Service. Washington. U.S. Government Printing Office, 1991.

National Linked File of Live Births and Infant Deaths

The national linked file of live births and infant deaths is a data file for research on infant mortality. It is comprised of linked vital records for infants born in a given year who died in that year or the next year before their first birthday. It includes all of the variables on the national natality file, as well as the medical information reported for the same infant on the death record and the age of the infant at death. The use of linked files avoids discrepancies in the reporting of race between the birth and infant death certificates. Although discrepancies are relatively rare for white and black infants, they can be substantial for other races. The match completeness for the 1983–87 files is 98 percent. The linked files are available after the regular vital statistics files because construction of the linked file requires 2 years of mortality data to be linked to each birth cohort. For more information, see: National Center for Health Statistics, K. Prager: Infant mortality by birthweight, age of mother, and other characteristics: United States, 1985 birth cohort. *Vital and Health Statistics.* Forthcoming.

Compressed Mortality File

The Compressed Mortality File (CMF) used to compute death rates by urbanization level is a county level national mortality and population data base spanning the years 1968–90. The mortality data base of the CMF is derived from the detailed mortality files of the National Vital Statistics System comprised of approximately 2 million micro-data death records for each of the years. The population data base of the CMF is derived from intercensal estimates and census counts of the resident population of each U.S. county by 5-year age groups, race, and sex. These estimates reflect adjustments based on the 1970, 1980, and 1990 censuses. Counties are categorized according to level of urbanization based on the rural-urban continuum codes for metropolitan and nonmetropolitan counties developed by the Economic Research Service, U.S. Department of Agriculture. See Appendix II, Urbanization. For more information about the CMF, contact: Chief, Analytical Coordination Branch, Division of Analysis, National Center for Health Statistics, 6525 Belcrest Road, Hyattsville, MD 20782.

National Survey of Family Growth

Data from the National Survey of Family Growth (NSFG) are based on samples of women ages 15–44 years in the civilian noninstitutionalized population living in the coterminous United States. The first and second cycles excluded women who had never been married, except those with offspring in the household. The third and fourth cycles include all women ages 15–44 years, regardless of whether they have ever been married.

The purpose of the survey is to provide national data on the demographic and social factors associated with childbearing, adoption, and maternal and child health. These factors include sexual activity, marriage, unmarried cohabitation, divorce and remarriage, contraception and sterilization, infertility, breastfeeding, pregnancy loss, low birth weight, use of medical care for family planning, infertility, and prenatal care. Interviews are conducted in person by professional female interviewers using a standardized, printed questionnaire. The average interview length is about 1 hour.

Cycle I of the NSFG was conducted from June 1973–February 1974. The counties and independent cities of the United States were combined to form a frame of primary sampling units (PSU's), and 101 PSU's were selected as the first-stage sample. The next three stages produced a clustered sample of 28,998 households within the 101 PSU's. At 26,028 of these households (89.8 percent), household screener interviews were completed. These screeners produced a fifth-stage sample of 10,879 women of whom 9,797 were interviewed. Never-married women (except those with offspring in the household) were excluded from Cycle I.

Cycle II of NSFG was conducted from January–September 1976. The sample consisted of 27,162 households in 79 PSU's. Household screener interviews were completed at 25,479 of these households (93.8 percent). Of the 10,202 women in the sample, 8,611 were interviewed. Again, never-married women (except those with offspring in the household) were excluded from the sample for Cycle II.

Interviewing for Cycle III of the NSFG was conducted from August 1982–February 1983. The sample design was similar to that in Cycle II: 31,027 households were selected in 79 PSU's. Household screener interviews were completed in 29,511 households (95.1 percent). Of the 9,964 eligible women identified, 7,969 were interviewed. The sample for Cycle III included black women and women 15–19 years of age at higher rates than other women. Women of all marital statuses were interviewed in Cycle III.

Cycle IV was conducted between January and August 1988. The sample was obtained from households that had been interviewed in the 1985, 1986, or 1987 National Health Interview Surveys. Women living in Alaska and Hawaii were included, so that the survey covered women from the noninstitutionalized population of the entire United States. Interviews were completed with 8,450 women. As in previous cycles, black women were oversampled.

In order to produce estimates for the entire population of eligible women in the United States, data for the interviewed sample women were inflated by the reciprocal of the probability of selection at each stage of sampling and adjusted for screener and interview nonresponse. Cycles I and II estimates for ever-married women were poststratified to benchmark population values for 12 age-race categories based on data from the Current Population Survey of the U.S. Bureau of the Census. Cycle III estimates were poststratified within 24 categories of age, race, and marital status. In Cycle IV the poststratification was done within categories of age, race, marital status, and parity.

Quality control procedures for interviewer selection, interviewer training, field listing, and data processing were built into the NSFG to minimize nonsampling error and bias. In addition, the nonresponse adjustments in the estimator were designed to minimize the effect of nonresponse bias by assigning to nonrespondents the characteristics of similar respondents. Sampling errors for NSFG were estimated by balanced half-sample replication.

Detailed information on the NSFG sample design is available in the following reports: National Center for Health Statistics, D. K. French: National Survey of Family Growth, Cycle I, sample design, estimation procedures, and variance estimation. *Vital and Health Statistics.* Series 2, No. 76. DHEW Pub. No. (PHS) 78–1350. Public Health Service. Washington. U.S. Government Printing Office, Jan. 1979; National Center for Health Statistics, W. R. Grady: National Survey of Family Growth, Cycle II: Sample design, estimation procedures, and variance estimation. *Vital and Health Statistics.* Series 2, No. 87. DHHS Pub. No. (PHS) 81–1361. Public Health Service. Washington. U.S. Government Printing Office, Feb. 1981; National Center for Health Statistics, C. Bachrach, M. Horn, W. Mosher, and I. Shimizu: National Survey of Family Growth, Cycle III: Estimation procedures, weighting, and variance estimation. *Vital and Health Statistics.* Series 2, No. 98. DHHS Pub. No. (PHS) 85–1372. Public Health Service. Washington. U.S. Government Printing Office, Sept. 1985; and National Center for Health Statistics, D. Judkins, S. Botman, and W. Mosher: National Survey of Family Growth: Design, Estimation, and Inference. *Vital and Health Statistics.* Series 2, No. 109. DHHS Pub. No. (PHS) 91–1386. Public Health Service. Washington. U.S. Government Printing Office, Sept. 1991.

National Health Interview Survey

The National Health Interview Survey (NHIS) is a continuing nationwide sample survey in which data are collected through personal household interviews. Information is obtained on personal and demographic characteristics including race and ethnicity by self-reporting or as reported by an informant; illnesses, injuries, impairments, chronic conditions, utilization of health resources, and other health topics. The household questionnaire is reviewed each year, with special health topics being added or deleted. For most health topics, data are collected over an entire calendar year.

The sample design plan of the NHIS follows a multistage probability design that permits a continuous sampling of the civilian noninstitutionalized population residing in the United States. The survey is designed in such a way that the sample scheduled for each week is representative of the target population and the weekly samples are additive over time. The response rate for the survey has been between 95 and 98 percent over the years.

In 1985 the NHIS adopted several new sample design features although, conceptually, the sampling plan remained the same as the previous design. Two major changes included reducing the number of primary sampling locations from 376 to 198 for sampling efficiency and oversampling the black population to improve the precision of the statistics.

The sample was designed so that a typical NHIS sample for the data collection years 1985–94 will consist of approximately 7,500 segments containing about 59,000 assigned households. Of these households, an expected 10,000 will be vacant, demolished, or occupied by persons not in the target population of the survey. The expected sample of 49,000 occupied households will yield a probability sample of about 127,000 persons. In 1990 there was a sample of 119,631 persons and in 1991 a sample of 120,032 persons.

A description of the survey design, the methods used in estimation, and general qualifications of the data obtained from the survey are presented in: National Center for Health Statistics, P. F. Adams and V. Benson: Current estimates from the National Health Interview Survey, United States, 1991. *Vital and Health*

Statistics. Series 10, No. 184. DHHS Pub. No. (PHS) 93–1512. Public Health Service. Washington. U.S. Government Printing Office, Dec. 1992.

National Health and Nutrition Examination Survey

For the first program or cycle of the National Health Examination Survey (NHES I), 1960–62, data were collected on the total prevalence of certain chronic diseases as well as the distributions of various physical and physiological measures, including blood pressure and serum cholesterol levels. For that program, a highly stratified, multistage probability sample of 7,710 adults, of whom 86.5 percent were examined, was selected to represent the 111 million civilian noninstitutionalized adults 18–79 years of age in the United States at that time. The sample areas consisted of 42 primary sampling units from the 1,900 geographic units. In 1971 a nutrition surveillance component was added and the survey name was changed to the National Health and Nutrition Examination Survey.

For more information on NHES I, see: National Center for Health Statistics: Cycle I of the National Health Examination Survey, sample and response, United States, 1960–62. T. Gordon and H. W. Miller. *Vital and Health Statistics.* Series 11, No. 1. PHS Pub. No. 1000. Public Health Service. Washington. U.S. Government Printing Office, May 1964.

In the first National Health and Nutrition Examination Survey (NHANES I), conducted from 1971 through 1974, a major purpose was to measure and monitor indicators of the nutrition and health status of the American people through dietary intake data, biochemical tests, physical measurements, and clinical assessments for evidence of nutritional deficiency. Detailed examinations were given by dentists, ophthalmologists, and dermatologists with an assessment of need for treatment. In addition, data were obtained for a subsample of adults on overall health care needs and behavior, and more detailed examination data were collected on cardiovascular, respiratory, arthritic, and hearing conditions.

The NHANES I target population was the civilian noninstitutionalized population 1–74 years of age residing in the coterminous United States, except for people residing on any of the reservation lands set aside for the use of American Indians. The sample design was a multistage, stratified probability sample of clusters of persons in land-based segments. The sample areas consisted of 65 primary sampling units (PSU's) selected from the 1,900 PSU's in the coterminous United States. A subsample of persons 25–74 years of age was selected to receive the more detailed health examination. Groups at high risk of malnutrition were oversampled at known rates throughout the process.

Household interviews were completed for more than 96 percent of the 28,043 persons selected for the NHANES I sample, and about 75 percent (20,749) were examined.

For NHANES II, conducted from 1976–80, the nutrition component was expanded from the one fielded for NHANES I. In the medical area primary emphasis was placed on diabetes, kidney and liver functions, allergy, and speech pathology.

The NHANES II target population was the civilian noninstitutionalized population 6 months–74 years of age residing in the United States, including Alaska and Hawaii. NHANES II utilized a multistage probability design that involved selection of PSU's, segments (clusters of households) within PSU's, households, eligible persons, and finally, sample persons. The sample design provided for oversampling among those persons 6 months–5 years of age, those 60–74 years of age, and those living in poverty areas.

A sample of 27,801 persons was selected for NHANES II. Of this sample 20,322 (73.1 percent) were examined.

Race information for NHANES I and NHANES II was determined primarily by interviewer observation. The estimation procedure used to produce national statistics for NHANES I and NHANES II involved inflation by the reciprocal of the probability of selection, adjustment for nonresponse, and poststratified ratio adjustment to population totals. Sampling errors also were estimated to measure the reliability of the statistics.

For more information on NHANES I, see: National Center for Health Statistics, H. W. Miller: Plan and operation of the National Health and Nutrition Examination Survey, United States, 1971–73. *Vital and Health Statistics.* Series 1, Nos. 10a and 10b. DHEW Pub. No. (HSM) 73–1310. Health Services and Mental Health Administration. Washington. U.S. Government Printing Office, Feb. 1973; and National Center for Health Statistics, A. Engel, R. S. Murphy, K. Maurer, and E. Collins: Plan and operation of the NHANES I Augmentation Survey of Adults 25–74 Years, United States, 1974–75. *Vital and Health Statistics.* Series 1, No. 14. DHEW Pub. No. (PHS) 78–1314. Public Health Service. Washington. U.S. Government Printing Office, June 1978.

For more information on NHANES II, see: National Center for Health Statistics, A. McDowell, A. Engel, J. T. Massey, and K. Maurer: Plan and operation of the Second National Health and Nutrition Examination Survey, 1976–80. *Vital and Health Statistics.* Series 1, No. 15. DHHS Pub. No. (PHS) 81–1317. Public Health Service. Washington. U.S. Government Printing Office, July 1981. For information on nutritional applications of these surveys, see: Yetley, E., and C. Johnson, 1987. Nutritional applications of the Health and Nutrition Examination Surveys (HANES). *Ann Rev Nutr* 7:441–63.

The Hispanic Health and Nutrition Examination Survey (HHANES), conducted during 1982–84, was similar in content and design to the previous National Health and Nutrition Examination Surveys. The major difference between HHANES and the previous national surveys is that HHANES employed a probability sample of three special subgroups of the population living in selected areas of the United States rather than a national probability sample. The three HHANES universes included approximately 84, 57, and 59 percent of the respective 1980 Mexican, Cuban, and Puerto Rican-origin populations in the continental United States. The Hispanic ethnicity of these populations was determined by self-report.

In the HHANES three geographically and ethnically distinct populations were studied: Mexican Americans in

Texas, New Mexico, Arizona, Colorado, and California; Cuban Americans living in Dade County, Florida; and Puerto Ricans living in parts of New York, New Jersey, and Connecticut. In the Southwest 9,894 persons were selected (75 percent or 7,462 were examined), in Dade County 2,244 persons were selected (60 percent or 1,357 were examined), and in the Northeast 3,786 persons were selected (75 percent or 2,834 were examined).

For more information on HHANES, see: National Center for Health Statistics: Plan and operation of the Hispanic Health and Nutrition Examination Survey, 1982–84. *Vital and Health Statistics.* Series 1, No. 19. DHHS Pub. No. (PHS) 85–1321. Public Health Service. Washington. U.S. Government Printing Office, Sept. 1985.

The third National Health and Nutrition Examination Survey (NHANES III) is a 6-year survey covering the years 1988–94 and consists of two phases. The first phase, 1988–91, and the second phase, 1991–94, both separately constitute national samples of the U.S. population as does the complete 6-year survey. For the first phase of NHANES III (1988–91), a sample of 20,277 persons was selected. Of this sample, 15,630 (77 percent) were examined in the mobile examination center. Over the 6-year period, approximately 40,000 persons will be selected for the survey and approximately 30,000 are expected to be examined.

The NHANES III target population is the civilian noninstitutionalized population aged 2 months and over. The sample design provides for oversampling among children 2–35 months of age, persons aged 70 years and over, Black Americans, and Mexican Americans. Race is reported for the household by the respondent.

Although some of the specific health areas have changed from earlier NHANES surveys, the goals of the NHANES III are similar to those of earlier NHANES surveys:

■ To estimate the national prevalence of selected diseases and risk factors;
■ To estimate national population reference distributions of selected health parameters; and
■ To document and investigate reasons for secular trends in selected diseases and risk factors.

Two additional goals are new for the NHANES III Survey:

■ To contribute to an understanding of disease etiology; and
■ To investigate the natural history of selected diseases.

For more information on NHANES III, see: National Center for Health Statistics: Sample Design: Third National Health and Nutrition Examination Survey. *Vital and Health Statistics.* Series 2, No. 113. DHHS Pub. No. (PHS) 92–1387. Public Health Service. Washington. U.S. Government Printing Office, Sept. 1992.

National Master Facility Inventory

The National Master Facility Inventory (NMFI) is a comprehensive file of inpatient health facilities in the United States. The three broad categories of facilities in NMFI are hospitals, nursing and related care homes, and other custodial or remedial care facilities. To be included in NMFI, hospitals must have at least six inpatient beds; nursing and related care homes and other facilities must have at least three inpatient beds.

NMFI is kept current by the periodic addition of names and addresses obtained from State licensing and other agencies for all newly established inpatient facilities. In addition, annual surveys of hospitals and periodic surveys of nursing homes and other facilities are conducted to update name and location, type of business, number of beds, and number of residents or patients in the facilities, and to identify those facilities that have gone out of business.

From 1968–75 the hospital survey was conducted in conjunction with the American Hospital Association (AHA) Annual Survey of Hospitals. AHA performed the data collection for its member hospitals, while the National Center for Health Statistics (NCHS) collected the data for the approximately 400 non-AHA registered hospitals. Since 1976, however, all of the data collection has been performed by AHA.

Hospitals are requested to report data for the full year ending September 30. More than half of the responding hospitals used this reporting period for the 1982 survey. The remaining hospitals used various other reporting periods. The response rate for the 1982 hospital survey was about 90 percent and was 96 percent for the 1986 survey.

The nursing home and other facilities surveys were conducted by NCHS in 1963, 1967, 1969, 1971, 1973, 1976, 1978, 1980, 1982, and 1986. In the 1980 and 1982 NMFI surveys, only nursing and related care homes were covered. In 1986 nursing and related care homes and facilities for the mentally retarded were covered and called the Inventory of Long-Term Care Places. In 1982 arrangements were made with 35 States for obtaining their data on nursing and related care homes. NCHS surveyed certain types of homes that were excluded from the State surveys.

Statistics derived from the hospital and nursing home and other facilities surveys were adjusted for facility and item nonresponse. Missing items on the questionnaire were imputed, when possible, by using information reported by the same facility in a previous survey. When data were not available from a previous census for a responding facility, the data were imputed by using data from similar responding facilities. Similar facilities are defined as those with the same types of business, ownership, service, and approximately the same bed size.

For more detailed information on NMFI, see: National Center for Health Statistics, D. A. Roper: Nursing and related care homes as reported from the 1982 NMFI survey. *Vital and Health Statistics.* Series 14, No. 32. DHHS Pub. No. (PHS) 86–1827. Public Health Service. Washington. U.S. Government Printing Office, Sept. 1986; and National Center for Health Statistics, A. Sirrocco. The 1986 Inventory of Long-Term Care Places: An overview of facilities for the mentally retarded. *Advance Data From Vital and Health Statistics.* No. 143.

DHHS Pub. No. (PHS) 87–1250. Public Health Service. Hyattsville, Md., 1987.

National Hospital Discharge Survey

The National Hospital Discharge Survey (NHDS) is a continuing nationwide sample survey of short-stay hospitals in the United States. Before 1988 the scope of NHDS encompassed patients discharged from noninstitutional hospitals, exclusive of military and Veterans Administration hospitals, located in the 50 States and the District of Columbia. Only hospitals having six or more beds for patient use and those in which the average length of stay for all patients is less than 30 days are included in the survey. Beginning in 1988 the scope was altered slightly to include all general and children's general hospitals regardless of the length of stay. Although all discharges of patients from these hospitals are within the scope of the survey, discharges of newborn infants from all hospitals are excluded from this report as well as discharges of all patients from Federal hospitals.

The original sample was selected in 1964 from a frame of short-stay hospitals listed in the National Master Facility Inventory. A two-stage stratified sample design was used, and hospitals were stratified according to bed size and geographic region. Sample hospitals were selected with probabilities ranging from certainty for the largest hospitals to 1 in 40 for the smallest hospitals. Within each sample hospital, a systematic random sample of discharges was selected from the daily listing sheet. Initially, the within-hospital sampling rates for selecting discharges varied inversely with the probability of hospital selection so that the overall probability of selecting a discharge was approximately the same across the sample. Those rates were adjusted for individual hospitals in subsequent years to control the reporting burden of those hospitals.

In 1985, for the first time, two data collection procedures were used for the survey. The first was the traditional manual system of sample selection and data abstraction. In the manual system, sample selection and transcription of information from the hospital records to abstract forms were performed by either the hospital staff or representatives of the National Center for Health Statistics (NCHS) or both. The second was an automated method, used in approximately 17 percent of the sample hospitals in 1985, involving the purchase of data tapes from commercial abstracting services. Upon receipt of these tapes they were subject to NCHS sampling, editing, and weighting procedures.

In 1988 the NHDS was redesigned. The hospitals with the most beds and/or discharges annually were selected with certainty, but the remaining sample was selected using a three-stage stratified design. The first stage is a sample of the primary sampling units (PSU's) used by the National Health Interview Survey. Within PSU's, hospitals were stratified or arrayed by abstracting status (whether subscribing to a commercial abstracting service) and within abstracting status arrayed by type of service and bed size. Within these strata and arrays, a systematic sampling scheme with probability proportional to the number of discharges annually was used to select hospitals. The rates for systematic sampling of discharges within hospitals vary inversely with probability of hospital selection within PSU. Discharge records from hospitals submitting data via commercial abstracting services (approximately 30 percent of sample hospitals in 1991) were arrayed by primary diagnoses, patient sex and age group, and date of discharge before sampling. Otherwise, the procedures for sampling discharges within hospitals is the same as that used in the prior design.

In 1991 the hospital sample was updated by continuing the sampling process among hospitals which were NHDS-eligible for the sampling frame in 1991, but not 1987. That is, the additional hospitals were added at the end of the list for the strata where they belonged, and the systematic sampling was continued as if the additional hospitals had been present during the initial sample selection. Hospitals which were no longer NHDS-eligible were deleted. The updating process will be repeated every third year.

The basic unit of estimation for NHDS is the sample patient abstract. The estimation procedure involves inflation by the reciprocal of the probability of selection, adjustment for nonresponding hospitals and missing abstracts, and ratio adjustments to fixed totals. Of the 529 hospitals selected for the survey, 521 were within the scope of the survey, and 484 participated in the survey in 1991. Data were abstracted from about 275,000 medical records.

For more detailed information on the design of NHDS and the magnitude of sampling errors associated with NHDS estimates, see: National Center for Health Statistics, E. J. Graves: National Hospital Discharge Survey: Annual Summary, 1990. *Vital and Health Statistics.* Series 13, No. 112. DHHS Pub. No. (PHS) 92–1773. Public Health Service. Washington. U.S. Government Printing Office, June 1992; and Haupt, B. J., Kozak, L. J.: National Hospital Discharge Survey: Estimates from two survey designs. *Vital and Health Statistics.* Series 13, No. 111. DHHS Pub. No. (PHS) 92–1772. Public Health Service. Washington. U.S. Government Printing Office, May 1992.

National Nursing Home Survey

The National Center for Health Statistics (NCHS) has conducted three National Nursing Home Surveys. The first survey was conducted from August 1973–April 1974; the second survey from May–December 1977; and the third from August 1985–January 1986.

Much of the background information and experience used to develop the first National Nursing Home Survey was obtained from a series of three ad hoc sample surveys of nursing and personal care homes called the Resident Places Surveys (RPS–1, –2, –3). The three surveys were conducted by the National Center for Health Statistics during April–June 1963, May–June 1964, and June–August 1969. During the first survey, RPS–1, data were collected on nursing homes, chronic disease and geriatric hospitals, nursing home units, and chronic disease wards of general and mental hospitals. RPS–2 concentrated mainly on nursing homes and geriatric hospitals. During the third survey, RPS–3, nursing and personal care homes in the coterminous United States were sampled.

For the initial National Nursing Home Survey (NNHS) conducted in 1973–74, the universe included only those nursing homes that provided some level of nursing care. Thus, homes providing only personal or domiciliary care were excluded. The sample of 2,118 homes was selected from the 17,685 homes that provided some level of nursing care and were listed in the 1971 National Master Facility Inventory (NMFI) or those that opened for business in 1972. Data were obtained from about 20,600 staff and 19,000 residents. Response rates were 97 percent for facilities, 88 percent for expenditures, 98 percent for residents, and 82 percent for staff.

The scope of the 1977 NNHS encompassed all types of nursing homes, including personal care and domiciliary care homes. The sample of about 1,700 facilities was selected from 23,105 nursing homes in the sampling frame, which consisted of all homes listed in the 1973 NMFI and those opening for business between 1973 and December 1976. Data were obtained from about 13,600 staff, 7,000 residents, and 5,100 discharged residents. Response rates were 95 percent for facilities, 85 percent for expenses, 81 percent for staff, 99 percent for residents, and 97 percent for discharges.

The scope of the 1985 NNHS was similar to the 1977 survey in that it included all types of nursing homes. The sample of 1,220 homes was selected from a sampling frame of 20,479 nursing and related care homes. The frame consisted of all homes in the 1982 NMFI; homes identified in the 1982 Complement Survey of the NMFI as "missing" from the 1982 NMFI; facilities that opened for business between 1982 and June 1984; and hospital-based nursing homes obtained from the Health Care Financing Administration. Information on the facility was collected through a personal interview with the administrator. Accountants were asked to complete a questionnaire on expenditures or provide a financial statement. Resident data were provided by a nurse familiar with the care provided to the resident. The nurse relied on the medical record and personal knowledge of the resident. In addition to employee data that were collected during the interview with the administrator, a sample of registered nurses completed a self-administered questionnaire. Discharge data were based on information recorded in the medical record. Additional data about the current and discharged residents were obtained in telephone interviews with next of kin. Data were obtained from 1,079 facilities, 2,763 registered nurses, 5,243 current residents, and 6,023 discharges. Response rates were 93 percent for facilities, 68 percent for expenses, 80 percent for registered nurses, 97 percent for residents, 95 percent for discharges, and 90 percent for next of kin.

Statistics for all three surveys were derived by a ratio-estimation procedure. Statistics were adjusted for failure of a home to respond, failure to fill out one of the questionnaires, and failure to complete an item on a questionnaire.

For more information on the 1973–74 NNHS, see: National Center for Health Statistics, M. R. Meiners: Selected operating and financial characteristics of nursing homes, United States, 1973–74 National Nursing Home Survey. *Vital and Health Statistics.* Series 13, No.

22. DHEW Pub. No. (HRA) 76–1773. Health Resources Administration. Washington. U.S. Government Printing Office, Dec. 1975. For more information on the 1977 NNHS, see: National Center for Health Statistics, J. F. Van Nostrand, A. Zappolo, E. Hing, et al.: The National Nursing Home Survey, 1977 Summary for the United States. *Vital and Health Statistics.* Series 13, No. 43. DHHS Pub. No. (PHS) 79–1794. Public Health Service. Washington. U.S. Government Printing Office, July 1979. For more information on the 1985 NNHS, see: National Center for Health Statistics, E. Hing, E. Sekscenski, G. Strahan: The National Nursing Home Survey, 1985 Summary for the United States. *Vital and Health Statistics.* Series 13, No. 97. DHHS Pub. No. (PHS) 89–1758. Public Health Service. Washington. U.S. Government Printing Office, Jan. 1989.

National Ambulatory Medical Care Survey

The National Ambulatory Medical Care Survey (NAMCS) is a continuing national probability sample of ambulatory medical encounters. The scope of the survey covers physician-patient encounters in the offices of nonfederally employed physicians classified by the American Medical Association or American Osteopathic Association as "office-based, patient care" physicians. Excluded are visits to hospital-based physicians, visits to specialists in anesthesiology, pathology, and radiology and visits to physicians who are principally engaged in teaching, research, or administration. Telephone contacts and nonoffice visits are also excluded.

A multistage probability design is employed. The first-stage sample consists of 84 primary sampling units (PSU's) in 1985 and 112 PSU's in 1989 selected from about 1,900 such units into which the United States has been divided. In each sample PSU a sample of practicing nonfederal office-based physicians is selected from masterfiles maintained by the American Medical Association and the American Osteopathic Association. The final stage involves systematic random samples of office visits during randomly assigned 7-day reporting periods. In 1985 the survey excluded Alaska and Hawaii. In 1989 the survey included all 50 States.

For the 1985 survey a sample of 5,032 physicians was selected. The physician response rate for 1985 was 70 percent providing data on 71,594 patient records. For the 1990 survey a sample of 3,063 physicians was selected. The physician response rate for 1990 was 74 percent providing data on 43,469 patient records. Race and ethnicity in patient records are based on observation by physician or staff.

The estimation procedure used in NAMCS basically has three components: inflation by the reciprocal of the probability of selection, adjustment for nonresponse, and ratio adjustment to fixed totals.

For more detailed information on the design of NAMCS and the magnitude of sampling errors associated with NAMCS estimates, see: National Center for Health Statistics, S. Schappert. 1990 Summary: National Ambulatory Medical Care Survey. *Advance Data From Vital and Health Statistics.* No. 213. DHHS Pub. No. (PHS) 92–1250. Public Health Service. Hyattsville, Md., 1992.

National Center for Infectious Diseases

AIDS Surveillance

Acquired immunodeficiency syndrome (AIDS) surveillance is conducted by health departments in each State, territory, and the District of Columbia. Although surveillance activities range from passive to active, most areas employ multifaceted active surveillance programs, which include four major reporting sources of AIDS information: hospitals and hospital-based physicians, physicians in nonhospital practice, public and private clinics, and medical record systems (death certificates, tumor registries, hospital discharge abstracts, and communicable disease reports). Using a standard confidential case report form, the health departments collect information without personal identifiers, which is coded and computerized either at the Centers for Disease Control and Prevention (CDC) or at health departments from which it is then transmitted electronically to CDC.

AIDS surveillance data are used to detect epidemiologic trends, to identify unusual cases requiring follow up, and for publication in the *HIV/AIDS Surveillance Report.* Studies to determine the completeness of reporting of AIDS cases meeting the national surveillance definition suggest reporting at greater than or equal to 90 percent. The number of deaths among AIDS cases reported to the CDC AIDS Surveillance System differs from the number of HIV infection deaths based on the National Vital Statistics System. The major reasons for these differences are that not all persons diagnosed with AIDS are reported to the AIDS Surveillance System, not all deaths among persons with AIDS are due to AIDS, and not all deaths due to HIV infection are reported as such on the death certificate.

For more information on AIDS surveillance, contact: Chief, Surveillance Section, Surveillance and Evaluation Branch, AIDS Program, National Center for Infectious Diseases, Centers for Disease Control and Prevention, Atlanta, Ga. 30333.

Epidemiology Program Office

National Notifiable Diseases Surveillance System

The Epidemiology Program Office (EPO) of the Centers for Disease Control and Prevention (CDC), in partnership with the Council of State and Territorial Epidemiologists (CSTE), operates the National Notifiable Diseases Surveillance System. The purpose of this system is primarily to provide weekly provisional information on the occurrence of diseases defined as notifiable by CSTE. In addition, the system also provides summary data on an annual basis. State epidemiologists report cases of notifiable diseases to EPO, and EPO tabulates and publishes these data in the *Morbidity and Mortality Weekly Report (MMWR)* and the *Summary of Notifiable Diseases, United States* (entitled *Annual Summary* before 1985). Notifiable disease surveillance is used by public health practitioners at local, State, and national levels as part of disease prevention and control activities.

Notifiable disease reports are received from 52 areas in the United States and 5 territories. To calculate U.S. rates, data reported by 50 States, New York City, and the District of Columbia, are used (New York State is reported as Upstate New York, which excludes New York City).

Completeness of reporting varies because not all cases receive medical care and not all treated conditions are reported. Although State laws and regulations mandate disease reporting, reporting to CDC by States and territories is voluntary. Reporting of varicella (chickenpox) and mumps to CDC is not done by some States in which these diseases are not notifiable to local or State authorities. The number of areas reporting varicella was 31 in 1985, 33 in 1988, 30 in 1989, and 31 in 1990 and 1991. The number of areas reporting mumps was 48 in 1985 and 1988, and 50 in 1989, 1990, and 1991.

Estimates of underreporting of some diseases have been made. For example, it is estimated that only 10 percent of cases of congenital rubella syndrome are reported. Only 10–15 percent of all measles cases were reported prior to the institution of the Measles Elimination Program in 1978. A recent investigation following an outbreak in an inner city suggests that fewer than 50 percent of measles cases are reported. Data from a study of pertussis suggest that only one-third of severe cases causing hospitalization or death are reported. Data from a study of tetanus deaths suggest that only 40 percent of tetanus cases are reported to CDC.

For more information, see: Centers for Disease Control and Prevention, Final 1991 reports of notifiable diseases, *Morbidity and Mortality Weekly Report*, 40(53), Public Health Service, DHHS, Atlanta, Ga., Oct. 1992, or write to Centers for Disease Control and Prevention, Director, Division of Surveillance and Epidemiology, Atlanta, Ga. 30333.

National Center for Chronic Disease Prevention and Health Promotion

Abortion Surveillance

The Centers for Disease Control and Prevention (CDC) acquires abortion service statistics by State of occurrence from three sources—central health agencies, hospitals and other medical facilities, and the National Center for Health Statistics. Most of the central health agencies have established direct reporting systems, although a few collected data by surveying abortion facilities. Epidemiologic surveillance of abortion was initiated in eight States in 1969, and now statewide abortion data are also reported by the remaining States.

The total number of abortions reported to CDC is about 16 percent less than the total estimated independently by the Alan Guttmacher Institute, the research and development division of the Planned Parenthood Federation of America, Inc.

For more information, contact: Director, Division of Reproductive Health, Center for Health Promotion and Education, Centers for Disease Control and Prevention, Atlanta, Ga. 30333.

National Center for Prevention Services

U.S. Immunization Survey

This system is the result of a contractual agreement between the Centers for Disease Control and Prevention and the U.S. Bureau of the Census. Estimates from the U.S. Immunization Survey are based on data obtained during the third week of September in certain years for a subsample of households interviewed for the Current Population Survey, which is described separately in this appendix.

The reporting system contains demographic variables and vaccine history along with disease history when relevant to vaccine history. The system is used to estimate the immunization level of the Nation's child population against the vaccine-preventable diseases; from time to time, immunization level data on the adult population are collected.

The scope of the U.S. Immunization Survey covers the 50 States and the District of Columbia. For example, the 1981 sample included approximately 45,000 household units. Six thousand sample units were found to be vacant or otherwise not to be interviewed. Of the approximately 39,000 occupied households eligible for interview, about 1,500 were not interviewed because the occupants were not at home after repeated calls or were unavailable for some other reason.

The estimating procedure that was used involves the inflation of weighted sample results to independent estimates of the civilian noninstitutionalized population of the United States by age and race.

In 1979 the questionnaire was modified to solicit information regarding the source of immunization responses given by the interviewee. This change was made to measure the percent of responses for which a family immunization record was the source of the information.

For more information about the survey methodology, contact: Director, Division of Immunization, Center for Preventive Services, Centers for Disease Control and Prevention, Atlanta, Ga. 30333.

National Institute for Occupational Safety and Health

National Traumatic Occupational Fatalities Data Base

The National Traumatic Occupational Fatalities (NTOF) data base is compiled by the National Institute for Occupational Safety and Health (NIOSH) based on information taken from death certificates. Certificates are collected from 52 vital statistics reporting units (the 50 States, New York City, and the District of Columbia) based on the following criteria: (1) age 16 years or older; (2) an external cause of death (ICD–9, E800–E999); and (3) a positive response to the injury at work item.

There is no standardized definition of a work-related injury and no national guidelines exist regarding the completion of this item on the death certificate. Thus, numbers and rates of occupational injury deaths from NTOF should be regarded as the lower bound for the true number of these events. Denominator data for the calculation of rates by industry division were obtained from the U.S. Bureau of the Census' County Business Patterns, supplemented by employment data for agriculture derived from the U.S. Bureau of the Census' 1982 Census of Agriculture and public administration employment data taken from the Bureau of Labor Statistics' annual average employment data for 1980–86. The rates presented are for the U.S. civilian labor force.

For further information on NTOF, contact: Director, Division of Safety Research, National Institute for Occupational Safety and Health, 944 Chestnut Ridge Road, Mailstop S–133, Morgantown, W.Va. 26505.

National Occupational Hazard Survey

The National Occupational Hazard Survey (NOHS) was conducted by the National Institute for Occupational Safety and Health (NIOSH) to obtain data on employee exposure to particular chemicals and physical agents in various industries.

A random sample of 4,636 urban workplaces was selected by the U.S. Department of Labor, Bureau of Labor Statistics. Because mining and government activities are not within the coverage of the Occupational Safety and Health Act and agricultural and rural areas were beyond the logistical capacity of the survey, the sample excluded those types of facilities. Included were facilities in 66 different two-digit Standard Industrial Classifications (SICs), located in 67 standard metropolitan statistical areas. Field work was performed by 20 industrial hygiene surveyors who collected data from February 1972 through June 1974.

Information in Part I, elicited during a questionnaire interview of management, profiled the SIC and size of facility, along with its medical, safety, and industrial hygiene programs. Part II, the greatest part of the NOHS data, contained the recorded observations of the surveyor's management-escorted "walk-through" of all facility work areas. Part II listed, by job title, the number of employees who were potentially exposed to the same chemicals and physical agents. The surveyor recorded all materials and physical agents each employee group encountered, regardless of toxicity; hazardous nature; conditions of use; and the presence, absence, or effectiveness of any exposure control measures. For each potential exposure listed within an occupational group, the surveyor also recorded the duration, intensity, form, and the control utilized and whether it functioned.

For more information on NOHS, see: National Institute for Occupational Safety and Health, National Occupational Hazard Survey, Vol. I, Survey manual, DHEW Pub. No. (NIOSH) 74–127; Vol. II, Data editing and data base development, DHEW Pub. No. (NIOSH) 77–213; Vol. III, Survey analysis and supplemental tables, DHEW Pub. No. (NIOSH) 78–114.

National Occupational Exposure Survey

During 1981–83 NIOSH conducted a second national survey of worksites patterned after the NOHS. In this second survey, known as the National Occupational Exposure Survey (NOES), information was collected essentially identical to the NOHS in a sample of 4,490 facilities over a 30-month period.

For further information on NOES, see: National Institute for Occupational Safety and Health, National Occupational Exposure Survey, Vol. I, Survey Manual, DHHS Pub. No. (NIOSH) 86–106; Vol. II, Sampling Methodology, DHHS Pub. No. (NIOSH) 89–102; and Vol. III, Analysis of Management Interview Responses, DHHS Pub. No. (NIOSH) 89–103.

Health Resources and Services Administration

Bureau of Health Professions

Physician Supply Projections

Physician supply projections in this report are based on a model developed by the Bureau of Health Professions to forecast the supply of physicians by specialty, activity, and State of practice. The 1986 supply of active physicians (M.D.s) was used as the starting point for the most recent projections of active physicians. The major source of data used to obtain 1986 figures was the American Medical Association (AMA) Physician Masterfile.

In the first stage of the projections, graduates from U.S. schools of allopathic (M.D.) and osteopathic (D.O.) medicine and internationally-trained additions were estimated on a year-by-year basis. Estimates of first-year enrollments, student attrition, other medical school-related trends, and a model of net internationally-trained medical graduate immigration were used in deriving these annual additions. These year-by-year additions were then combined with the already existing active supply in a given year to produce a preliminary estimate of the active work force in each succeeding year. These estimates were then reduced to account for mortality and retirement. Gender-specific mortality and retirement losses were computed by 5-year age cohorts on an annual basis, using age distributions and mortality and retirement rates based on AMA data.

For more information, see: Bureau of Health Professions, *Eighth Report to the President and Congress on the Status of Health Personnel in the United States*, DHHS Pub. No. HRS–P–OD–92–1, Health Resources and Services Administration, Rockville, Md.

Nurse Supply Estimates

Nursing estimates in this report are based on a model developed by the Bureau of Health Professions to meet the requirements of Section 951, P.L. 94–63. The model estimates the following for each State: (1) nurse population—those with current licenses to practice; (2) nurse supply—all practicing nurses either full or part time (or all of those available to practice at that time); and (3) full-time equivalent supply—nurses practicing full time plus one-half of those practicing part time (or available on that basis).

Each of the three estimates are divided into three levels of highest educational preparation: associate degree or diploma; baccalaureate; master's and doctorate.

Among the factors considered are new graduates, changes in educational status, nursing employment rates, age, migration patterns, death rates, and licensure phenomena. Data sources include National League for Nursing for data on nursing education and National Council of State Boards of Nursing for data on licensure. Data on the number and characteristics of registered nurses are based on data from the National Sample Survey of Registered Nurses conducted by the Division of Nursing, Bureau of Health Professions in March 1988.

Substance Abuse and Mental Health Services Administration

Office of Applied Studies

National Household Surveys on Drug Abuse

Data on trends in use of marijuana, cigarettes, and alcohol among youths 12–17 years of age and young adults 18–25 years of age are from the National Household Survey on Drug Abuse. The 1991 survey is the 11th in a series that began in 1971 under the auspices of the National Commission on Marijuana and Drug Abuse. Since 1974, the survey has been sponsored by the National Institute on Drug Abuse.

The National Household Survey covers the population group 12 years of age and over living in households in the United States. The 1991 survey is based on home personal interviews of 32,594 randomly selected persons 12 years of age and over. Youths (12–17 years of age) and young adults (18–25 years of age) are oversampled as are black persons and Hispanics. The interview response rate in this survey was 85 percent for the youth and young adult sample. In 1991 the sample was broadened to include college students in dormitories, homeless people in shelters, civilians in military installations, and special expanded samples of six major metropolitan areas. Alaska and Hawaii were included for the first time in 1991.

For more information on the National Household Survey on Drug Abuse, see: Population Estimates, 1991. For further information on the National Household Survey on Drug Abuse, write: Office of Applied Studies, Substance Abuse and Mental Health Services Administration, 5600 Fishers Lane, Rockwall II, Suite 6–15, Rockville, Md. 20857.

The Drug Abuse Warning Network

The Drug Abuse Warning Network (DAWN) is a large-scale, ongoing drug abuse data collection system based on information from emergency room and medical examiner facilities. DAWN collects information about those drug abuse occurrences that have resulted in a medical crisis or death. The major objectives of the DAWN data system include: the monitoring of drug abuse patterns and trends, identification of substances associated with drug abuse episodes, and the assessment of drug-related consequences and other health hazards.

Before 1989 DAWN data were collected from a nonrandom panel of emergency rooms located primarily in 21 metropolitan areas throughout the continental United States. The same group of emergency rooms contributed DAWN data during these years, and were referred to as a consistent panel. In 1989 the DAWN was redesigned from a nonrandom sample to a national probability sample of emergency rooms located throughout the continental United States. For the 1989 sample, a sample of 685 hospitals was selected from the American Hospital Association inventory of nonfederal short-stay hospitals. A response rate of 78 percent was obtained in 1991.

Within each facility, a designated DAWN reporter is responsible for identifying drug abuse episodes by reviewing official records and transcribing and submitting data on each case.

For further information, see: The Drug Abuse Warning Network (DAWN), Annual Data, 1991, Parts A and B, or write to: Office of Applied Studies, Substance Abuse and Mental Health Services Administration, 5600 Fishers Lane, Rockwall II, Suite 6–15, Rockville, Md. 20857.

Center for Mental Health Services

Surveys of Mental Health Organizations

The Survey and Analysis Branch of the Division of State and Community Systems Development conducts a biennial inventory of mental health organizations and general hospital mental health services (IMHO/ GHMHS). One version is designed for specialty mental health organizations and another for nonfederal general hospitals with separate psychiatric services. The response rate to most of the items on these inventories is relatively high (90 percent or better) as is the rate for data presented in this report. However, for some inventory items, the response rate may be somewhat lower.

The IMHO/GHMHS is the primary source for Center for Mental Health Services data included in this report. This data system is based on questionnaires mailed every other year to mental health organizations in the United States, including psychiatric hospitals, nonfederal general hospitals with psychiatric services, Veterans Administration psychiatric services, residential treatment centers for emotionally disturbed children, freestanding outpatient psychiatric clinics, partial care organizations, and freestanding and multiservice mental health organizations, not elsewhere classified.

Federally funded community mental health centers (CMHC's) were included separately through 1980. In 1981, with the advent of block grants, the changes in definition of CMHC's, and the discontinuation of CMHC monitoring by the Center for Mental Health Services, organizations formerly classified as CMHC's have been reclassified as other organization types, primarily "multiservice mental health organizations, not elsewhere classified" and "freestanding psychiatric outpatient clinics."

Beginning in 1983 any organization that provides services in any combination of two or more services (for example, outpatient plus partial care, residential treatment plus outpatient plus partial care) and is neither a hospital nor a residential treatment center for emotionally disturbed children is classified as a multiservice mental health organization. Before 1983 an organization had to have either inpatient or residential

treatment services in combination with at least one other service to be a "multiservice mental health organization." The result of this definitional change is to increase sharply the number of multiservice mental health organizations, therefore, decreasing the number of freestanding psychiatric outpatient clinics.

Other surveys conducted by the Survey and Analysis Branch encompass samples of patients admitted to State, county, and private mental hospitals, outpatient psychiatric services, and Veterans Administration psychiatric services. The purpose of these surveys is to determine the sociodemographic, clinical, and treatment characteristics of patients served by these facilities.

For more information, write: Survey and Analysis Branch, Division of State and Community Systems Development Center for Mental Health Services, Room 18C–07, 5600 Fishers Lane, Rockville, Md. 20857. For further information on mental health, see: National Institute of Mental Health, *Mental Health, United States, 1990.* R. W. Manderscheid and M. A. Sonnenschein, eds. DHHS Pub. No. (ADM) 90–1708. U.S. Government Printing Office, 1990.

National Institutes of Health

National Cancer Institute

Surveillance, Epidemiology, and End Results Program

In the Surveillance, Epidemiology, and End Results (SEER) Program the National Cancer Institute (NCI) contracts with 11 population-based registries throughout the United States and Puerto Rico to provide data on all residents diagnosed with cancer during the year and to provide current follow-up information on all previously diagnosed patients.

All patients included in this report were residents of one of the following geographic areas at the time of their initial diagnosis of cancer: Atlanta, Georgia; Detroit, Michigan; Seattle-Puget Sound, Washington; San Francisco-Oakland, California; Connecticut; Iowa; New Mexico; Utah; and Hawaii. Data from New Jersey were excluded because those data are available only since 1979. Further, data from Puerto Rico were also excluded because this analysis focuses on trends occurring within the United States exclusive of its territories.

Population estimates used to calculate incidence rates are obtained from the U.S. Bureau of the Census. NCI uses estimation procedures as needed to obtain estimates for years and races not included in the data provided by the U.S. Bureau of the Census. Rates presented in this report may differ somewhat from previous reports due to revised population estimates and the addition and deletion of small numbers of incidence cases.

Life tables used to determine normal life expectancy when calculating relative survival rates were obtained from the National Center for Health Statistics. Separate life tables are used for each race-sex-specific group included in the SEER Program.

For further information, see: National Cancer Institute, *Cancer Statistics Review, 1973–90* by

L. Gloeckler Ries, et al., NIH Pub. No. 93–2789. Public Health Service. Bethesda, Md., 1993.

National Institute on Drug Abuse

High School Senior Survey (Monitoring the Future Survey)

The High School Senior Survey is a large-scale epidemiological survey of drug abuse initiated by the National Institute on Drug Abuse (NIDA) in 1975 and conducted annually through a NIDA grant awarded to the University of Michigan's Institute for Social Research. Each year data are collected in 125–135 public and private high schools, yielding a sample of approximately 16,000 high school seniors.

The survey design is a multistage random sample with stage one being the selection of particular geographic areas, stage two the selection of one or more high schools in each area, and stage three the selection of seniors within each high school. Data are collected through written questionnaires administered in the classroom by the Institute for Social Research representatives. High school dropouts and absentees (on the day of the survey) are excluded from the survey. Data from the Census Bureau show that between 1980 and 1990 the percent of persons 16–24 years of age who had not finished high school and were not enrolled in school declined slightly from 11 to 9 percent of white persons and dropped from 19 to 13 percent of black persons.

For further information on the High School Senior Survey, see: National Institute for Drug Abuse, Drug Use Among American High School Seniors, College Students, and Young Adults, 1975–1990, Vols. I and II. DHHS Pub. No. (ADM) 92–1940. U.S. Government Printing Office, 1992.

Health Care Financing Administration

Office of the Actuary

Estimates of National Health Expenditures

Estimates of expenditures for health (National Health Accounts) are compiled annually by type of expenditure and source of funds.

Estimates of expenditures for health services come from an array of sources. The American Hospital Association data on hospital finances are the primary source for estimates relating to hospital care. The salaries of physicians and dentists on the staffs of hospitals, hospital outpatient clinics, hospital-based home health agencies, and nursing home care provided in the hospital setting are considered to be components of hospital care. Expenditures for services of health professionals (doctors, dentists, chiropractors, private duty nurses, therapists, podiatrists, etc.) are estimated using a combination of data from the U.S. Bureau of the Census' Services Annual Survey and the quinquenniel census of Service Industries, from the Internal Revenue Service and from tabulations on the operations of health maintenance organizations. Expenditures for drugs and other medical nondurables and vision products and other medical durables purchased in retail outlets are based on estimates of personal consumption expenditures prepared by the U.S. Department of Commerce's Bureau of Economic Analysis and on industry data on prescription drug transactions. Those durable and nondurable products provided to inpatients in hospitals or nursing homes, and those provided by licensed professionals or through home health agencies are excluded here, but are included with the expenditure estimates for those in the provider service category. Nursing home expenditures cover care rendered in establishments providing inpatient nursing and health-related personal care through active treatment programs for medical and health-related conditions. These establishments cover skilled nursing and intermediate care facilities, including those for the mentally retarded. Spending estimates are based upon revenue data from the National Nursing Home Survey conducted by the National Center for Health Statistics. Expenditures for construction include the erection or renovation of hospitals, nursing homes, medical clinics, and medical research facilities, but not for private office buildings providing office space for private practitioners. Expenditures for noncommercial research (the cost of commerical research by drug companies are assumed to be imbedded in the price charged for the product; to include this item again would result in double counting) are developed from information gathered by the National Institutes of Health.

Source of funding estimates likewise come from a multiplicity of sources. Data on the Federal health programs are taken from administrative records maintained by the servicing agencies. Among the sources used to estimate State and local government spending for health are the U.S. Bureau of the Census' *Government Finances* and Social Security Administration reports on State-operated Workers' Compensation programs. Federal and State-local expenditures for education and training of medical personnel are excluded from these measures where they are separable. For the private financing of health care, data on the financial experience of health insurance organizations come from special Health Care Financing Administration analyses of private health insurers. Information on out-of-pocket spending from the U.S. Bureau of Labor Statistics' Consumer Expenditure Survey, from the 1977 National Medical Care Expenditure Survey conducted by the National Center for Health Services Research and from private surveys conducted by the American Hospital Association, American Medical Association, and the American Dental Association is used to develop estimates of direct spending by consumers.

For more specific information on definitions, sources, and methods used in the National Health Accounts, see: National Health Expenditures, 1991, by Suzanne Letsch, Helen Lazenby, Cathy Cowan and Katharine Levit, Office of the Actuary, *Health Care Financing Review*, Vol. 14, No. 2. HCFA Pub. No. 03335. Health Care Financing Administration. Washington. U.S. Government Printing Office, Winter 1992.

Medicare Statistical System

The Medicare Statistical System (MSS) provides data for examining the program's effectiveness and for tracking the eligibility of enrollees and the benefits they use, the certification status of institutional providers, and the payments made for covered services. Records are maintained on about 33 million enrollees and 24,000 participating institutional providers; and about 420 million bills for services are processed annually.

The MSS contains four major computer files: the health insurance master file, the service provider file, the Hospital Insurance (HI) claims file, and the Supplementary Medical Insurance (SMI) payment records file.

The health insurance master file contains records for each aged and disabled enrollee and includes data on type of entitlement, deductible status, benefit period status and benefits used, as well as demographic information such as age, sex, race, and residence.

The service provider file contains information on hospitals, home health agencies, skilled nursing facilities, independent clinical laboratories, and suppliers of portable x ray or outpatient physical therapy services that participate in Medicare. For hospitals, data on number of beds, type of ownership, and other characteristics are included.

The HI claims file contains information on the beneficiaries' entitlement and their use of benefits during the benefit period for hospital, skilled nursing facility, and home health agency services.

The SMI payment record file provides information on whether the enrollee has met the deductible and on amounts paid for physicians' services and other SMI-covered services and supplies.

Data from the Medicare statistical system provide information about enrollee use of benefits for a point in time or over an extended period. Statistical reports are produced on enrollment, characteristics of participating providers, reimbursements, and services used.

For further information on the Medicare statistical system, see: Health Care Financing Administration, Medicare Statistical File Manual, HCFA Pub. No. 03272, Baltimore, Md., July 1988.

Medicaid Data System

The majority of Medicaid data are compiled from forms submitted annually by State Medicaid agencies to the Health Care Financing Administration (HCFA) for federal fiscal years ending September 30 on the Form HCFA–2082, *Statistical Report on Medical Care: Eligibles, Recipients, Payments, and Services.*

When using the data keep the following caveats in mind:

■ Counts of recipients and eligibles categorized by basis of eligibility generally count each person only once—based on the person's basis of eligibility as of first appearance on the Medicaid rolls during the federal fiscal year covered by the report. Note, however, that some States report duplicated counts of recipients; that is, they report an individual in as many categories as the individual had different eligibility statuses during the

year. In such cases, the sum of all basis-of-eligibility cells will be greater than the "total recipients" number.

■ Expenditure data include payments for all claims adjudicated or paid during the fiscal year covered by the report. Note that this is not the same as summing payments for services that were rendered during the reporting period.

■ Some States fail to submit the HCFA–2082 for a particular year. When this happens, HCFA estimates the current year's HCFA–2082 data for missing States based upon prior year's submissions and information the State entered on Form HCFA–64 (the form States use to claim reimbursement for Federal matching funds for Medicaid).

■ HCFA–2082's submitted by States frequently contain obvious errors in one or more cells in the form. For cells obviously in error, HCFA estimates values that appear to be more reasonable.

For further information on Medicaid data, see: *Health Care Financing Program Statistics: Analysis of State Medicaid Program Characteristics, 1986,* by C. Howe and R. Terrell, HCFA Pub. No. 03249, Health Care Financing Administration, Baltimore, Md. U.S. Government Printing Office, Aug. 1987.

Department of Commerce

Bureau of the Census

Census of Population

The census of population has been taken in the United States every 10 years since 1790. In the 1990 census, data were collected on sex, race, age, and marital status from 100 percent of the enumerated population. More detailed information such as income, education, housing, occupation, and industry were collected from a representative sample of the population. For most of the country, one out of six households (about 17 percent) received the more detailed questionnaire. In places of residence estimated to have less than 2,500 population, 50 percent of households received the long form.

For more information on the 1990 census, see: U.S. Bureau of the Census, *1990 Census of Population, General Population Characteristics,* Series 1990, CP–1.

Current Population Survey

The Current Population Survey (CPS) is a household sample survey of the civilian noninstitutionalized population conducted monthly by the Bureau of the Census. The CPS provides estimates of employment, unemployment, and other characteristics of the general labor force, the population as a whole, and various other subgroups of the population.

A list of housing units from the 1980 census, supplemented by newly constructed units and households known to be missed in the 1980 census, provides the sampling frame in most areas for the present CPS. In some rural locations, current household listings of selected land areas serve as the frame.

The present CPS sample is located in 729 sample areas, with coverage in every State and the District of Columbia. In an average month during 1991, the number of housing units or living quarters eligible for interview was about 60,000; of these between 4 and 5 percent were, for various reasons, unavailable for interview.

The estimation procedure used involves inflation by the reciprocal of the probability of selection, adjustment for nonresponse, and ratio adjustment.

For more information, see: U.S. Bureau of the Census, *The Current Population Survey, Design and Methodology*, Technical Paper 40, Washington, U.S. Government Printing Office, Jan. 1978.

Population Estimates

National population estimates are derived by using decennial census data as benchmarks and data available from various agencies as follows: Births and deaths (National Center for Health Statistics); immigrants (Immigration and Naturalization Service); Armed Forces (Department of Defense); net movement between Puerto Rico and the U.S. mainland (Puerto Rico Planning Board); and federal employees abroad (Office of Personnel Management and Department of Defense). State estimates are based on similar data and also on a variety of data series, including school statistics from State departments of education and parochial school systems. Current estimates are consistent with official decennial census figures and do not reflect estimated decennial census underenumeration.

After decennial population censuses, intercensal population estimates for the preceding decade are prepared to replace postcensal estimates. Intercensal population estimates are more accurate than postcensal estimates because they take into account the census of population at the beginning and end of the decade. Intercensal estimates have been prepared for the 1960's, 1970's, and 1980's to correct the "error of closure" or difference between the estimated population at the end of the decade and the census count for that date. The error of closure at the national level was quite small during the 1960's (379,000). However, for the 1970's it amounted to almost 5 million.

For more information, see: U.S. Bureau of the Census, Estimates of the population of the United States, by age, sex, and race: 1980–1989, *Current Population Reports*, Series P–25, No. 1057, Washington, U.S. Government Printing Office, 1990.

Department of Labor

Bureau of Labor Statistics

Annual Survey of Occupational Injuries and Illnesses

Since 1971 the Bureau of Labor Statistics (BLS) has conducted an annual survey of establishments in the private sector to collect statistics on occupational injuries and illnesses. The Annual Survey of Occupational Injuries and Illnesses is based on records that employers maintain under the Occupational Safety and Health Act. Excluded from the survey are self-employed individuals;

farmers with fewer than 11 employees; employers regulated by other Federal safety and health laws; and Federal, State, and local government agencies.

Data are obtained from a sample of approximately 280,000 establishments, that is, single physical locations where business is conducted or where services of industrial operations are performed. An independent sample is selected for each State and the District of Columbia that represents industries in that jurisdiction. The BLS then subsamples the State samples to select the establishments to be included in the national sample.

Establishments included in the survey are instructed in a mailed questionnaire to provide summary totals of all entries for the previous calendar year to its Log and Summary of Occupational Injuries and Illnesses (OSHA No. 200 form). Occupational injuries include any injury—such as a cut, fracture, sprain, or amputation, which results from a work accident or from exposure involving a single incident in the work environment. Occupational illnesses are any abnormal condition or disorder, other than one resulting from an occupational injury, caused by exposure to environmental factors associated with employment. Lost workday cases are cases that involve days away from work, or days of restricted work activity, or both. The response rate is about 94 percent.

For more information, see: Bureau of Labor Statistics, *Occupational Injuries and Illnesses in the United States by Industry, 1988.* BLS Bulletin 2366, U.S. Department of Labor, Washington, August 1990.

Consumer Price Index

The Consumer Price Index is a monthly measure of the average change in the prices paid by urban consumers for a fixed market basket of goods and services. The all-urban index (CPI–U) introduced in 1978 is representative of the buying habits of about 80 percent of the noninstitutionalized population of the United States.

In calculating the index, price changes for the various items in each location were averaged together with weights that represent their importance in the spending of all urban consumers. Local data were then combined to obtain a U.S. city average.

The index measures price changes from a designated reference date, 1982 to 1984, which equals 100. An increase of 22 percent, for example, is shown as 122. This change can also be expressed in dollars as follows: The price of a base period "market basket" of goods and services bought by all urban consumers has risen from $10 in 1982 to 1984 and to $11.83 in 1988.

The most recent revision of the CPI, completed in 1987, reflected spending patterns based on the Survey of Consumer Expenditures from 1982 to 1984, the 1980 Census of Population, and the ongoing Point-of-Purchase Survey. Using this improved sample design, prices for the goods and services required to calculate the index are collected in 85 urban areas throughout the country and from about 21,000 retail and service establishments. In addition, data on rents are collected from about 40,000 tenants and 20,000 owner-occupied housing units. Food, fuels, and a few other items are priced monthly in all 85 locations. Prices of most other goods and services are collected bimonthly in the remaining areas. All price information is obtained through visits or calls by trained Bureau of Labor Statistics field representatives.

The 1987 revision changed the treatment of health insurance in the cost-weight definitions for medical care items. This change has no effect on the final index result but provides a clearer picture of the role of health insurance in the CPI. As part of the revision, three new indexes have been created by separating previously combined items, for example, eye care from other professional services, and inpatient and outpatient treatment from other hospital and medical care services.

For more information, see: Bureau of Labor Statistics, *Handbook of Methods,* BLS Bulletin 2285, U.S. Department of Labor, Washington, April 1988; I. K. Ford and P. Sturm. CPI revision provides more accuracy in the medical care services component, *Monthly Labor Review,* U.S. Department of Labor, Bureau of Labor Statistics, Washington, April 1988.

Employment and Earnings

The Division of Monthly Industry Employment Statistics and the Division of Employment and Unemployment Analysis of the Bureau of Labor Statistics publish data on employment and earnings. The data are collected by the U.S. Bureau of the Census, State Employment Security Agencies, and State Departments of Labor in cooperation with BLS.

The major data source is the Current Population Survey (CPS), a household interview survey conducted monthly by the U.S. Bureau of the Census to collect labor force data for BLS. CPS is described separately in this appendix. Data based on establishment records are also compiled each month from mail questionnaires by BLS, in cooperation with State agencies.

For more information, see: U.S. Department of Labor, Bureau of Labor Statistics, *Employment and Earnings, January 1992,* Vol. 39, No. 1, Washington, U.S. Government Printing Office, Jan. 1992.

Department of Veterans Affairs

Data are obtained from the Department of Veterans Affairs (VA) administrative data systems. These include budget information, patient treatment file, patient census file, and outpatient clinic file. Data from the three patient files are stored locally at each VA medical facility. At established intervals, data are transmitted to the national databank at the Austin Automated Center where they are compiled for nationwide statistics, reports, and comparisons.

The Patient Treatment File

The patient treatment file (PTF) collects data on each episode of inpatient care provided to patients including patients admitted to VA hospitals, VA nursing homes, and VA domiciliaries. In addition, when the Department of Veterans Affairs provides payments to non-VA hospitals and nursing homes, these episodes of care are entered into the PTF system. The PTF record includes the patient's name, dates of inpatient treatment, social security number, date of birth, State and county of residence, as well as the ICD–9–CM diagnostic and procedure or operative codes for each episode of treatment.

The Patient Census File

The patient census file (census) collects data on each episode of inpatient care provided to patients who remain in the medical facility at midnight on a selected date of each year, normally September 30. This file includes patients admitted to VA hospitals, VA nursing homes, and VA domiciliaries. The census record includes the same information as reported on the patient treatment file record at the time of the patient's discharge.

The Outpatient Clinic File

The outpatient clinic file (OPC) collects data on each instance of medical treatment provided to a veteran in an outpatient setting. The OPC record includes the patient's name, date of birth, social security number, and VA eligibility. The purpose and type of treatment provided to the veteran during each episode of outpatient treatment is also recorded. This encompasses the medical treating specialty (for example, orthopedics, general surgery, or hypertension); diagnostic procedures and/or testing; date of visit and disposition after treatment.

For more information, write: Department of Veterans Affairs, Biometrics Division 008B22, 810 Vermont Ave., NW., Washington, DC 20420.

Environmental Protection Agency

National Aerometric Surveillance Network

The Environmental Protection Agency (EPA), through extensive monitoring of activities conducted by Federal, State, and local air pollution control agencies, collects data on the six pollutants for which National Ambient Air Quality Standards have been set. These pollution control agencies submit data quarterly to EPA's National Aerometric Data Bank (NADB). There are about 3,400 total stations reporting. Data from some short-term or sporadic monitoring for such purposes as special studies and complaint investigations are usually not included in NADB because the data are not extensive enough to provide equitable comparisons with routine data from permanent monitoring sites.

For more information, see: Environmental Protection Agency, *National Air Pollutant Emission Estimates, 1940–91,* EPA–450/R–92–013, Research Triangle Park, N.C., Oct. 1992, or write to Office of Air Quality Planning and Standards, Environmental Protection Agency, Research Triangle Park, N.C. 27711.

United Nations

Demographic Yearbook

The Statistical Office of the United Nations prepares the *Demographic Yearbook,* a comprehensive collection of international demographic statistics.

Questionnaires are sent annually and monthly to more than 220 national statistical services and other appropriate government offices. Data forwarded on these questionnaires are supplemented, to the extent possible, by data taken from official national publications and by correspondence with the national statistical services. To insure comparability, rates, ratios, and percentages have been calculated in the Statistical Office of the United Nations.

Lack of international comparability between estimates arises from differences in concepts, definitions, and time of data collection. The comparability of population data is affected by several factors, including (1) the definitions of the total population, (2) the definitions used to classify the population into its urban and rural components, (3) difficulties relating to age reporting, (4) the extent of over- or underenumeration, and (5) the quality of population estimates. The completeness and accuracy of vital statistics data also vary from one country to another. Differences in statistical definitions of vital events may also influence comparability.

For more information, see: United Nations, *Demographic Yearbook 1990,* Pub. No. ST/ESA/STAT/SER.R/18, United Nations, New York, NY, 1990.

World Health Statistics Annual

The World Health Organization (WHO) prepares the *World Health Statistics Annual,* an annual volume of information on vital statistics and causes of death designed for use by the medical and public health professions. Each volume is the result of a joint effort by the national health and statistical administrations of many countries, the United Nations, and WHO.

United Nations estimates of vital rates and population size and composition, where available, are reprinted directly in the *Statistics Annual.* For those countries for which the United Nations does not prepare demographic estimates, primarily smaller populations, the latest available data reported to the United Nations and based on reasonably complete coverage of events are used.

Information published on late fetal and infant mortality is based entirely on official national data either reported directly or made available to the World Health Organization.

Selected life table functions are calculated from the application of a uniform methodology to national mortality data provided to WHO, in order to enhance their value for international comparisons. The life table procedure used by WHO may often lead to discrepancies with national figures published by countries, due to differences in methodology or degree of age detail maintained in calculations.

The international comparability of estimates published in the *World Health Statistics Annual* is affected by the same problems discussed above for the *Demographic Yearbook.* Cross-national differences in statistical definitions of vital events, in the completeness and accuracy of vital statistics data, and in the comparability of population data are the primary factors affecting comparability.

For more information, see: World Health Organization, *World Health Statistics Annual 1991,* World Health Organization, Geneva, Switzerland, 1991.

Alan Guttmacher Institute

Abortion Survey

The Alan Guttmacher Institute (AGI) conducts an annual survey of abortion providers. Data are collected from hospitals, nonhospital clinics, and physicians identified as providers of abortion services. A universal survey of 3,092 hospitals, nonhospital clinics, and individual physicians was compiled. To assess the completeness of the provider and abortion counts, supplemental surveys were conducted of a sample of obstetrician-gynecologists and a sample of hospitals (not in original universe) that were identified as providing abortion services through the AHA survey.

The number of abortions estimated by AGI is about 20 percent more than the number reported to the Centers for Disease Control and Prevention.

For more information, write to: The Alan Guttmacher Institute, 111 5th Avenue, 11th Floor, New York, NY 10003–1089.

American Association of Colleges of Osteopathic Medicine

The American Association of Colleges of Osteopathic Medicine compiles data on various aspects of osteopathic medical education for distribution to the profession, the government, and the public. Questionnaires are sent annually to all schools of osteopathic medicine requesting information on characteristics of applicants and students, curricula, faculty, grants, contracts, revenues, and expenditures. The response rate is 100 percent.

For more information, see: *Annual Statistical Report, 1991,* American Association of Colleges of Osteopathic Medicine, Rockville, Md., 1991.

American Dental Association

The Division of Educational Measurement of the American Dental Association conducts annual surveys of predoctoral dental educational institutions. The questionnaire, mailed to all dental schools, collects information on student characteristics, financial management, and curricula.

For more information, see: American Dental Association, *Annual Report on Dental Education 1990/91.* Chicago, Ill.

American Hospital Association

Annual Survey of Hospitals

Data from the American Hospital Association (AHA) annual survey are based on questionnaires that were sent to all hospitals, both AHA-registered and nonregistered, in the United States and its associated areas. U.S. government hospitals located outside the United States were excluded. Questionnaires were mailed to all hospitals on AHA files. Overall, in 1991, 6,044 hospitals reported data, a response rate of 91 percent. For nonreporting hospitals and for the survey questionnaires of reporting hospitals on which some information was missing, estimates were made for all data except those on beds, bassinets, and facilities. Data for beds and bassinets of nonreporting hospitals were based on the most recent information available from those hospitals. Facilities and services and inpatient service area data include only reporting hospitals and, therefore, do not include estimates.

Estimates of other types of missing data were based on data reported the previous year, if available. When unavailable, the estimates were based on data furnished by reporting hospitals similar in size, control, major service provided, length of stay, and geographic and demographic characteristics.

Hospitals are requested to report data for the full year ending September 30. In the 1991 survey 36 percent of the responding hospitals used this reporting period; the remaining hospitals used various reporting periods.

For more information on the AHA Annual Survey of Hospitals, see: American Hospital Association, *Hospital Statistics, 1991–92 Edition, Data from the American Hospital Association 1991 Annual Survey,* Chicago, 1992.

American Medical Association

Physician Masterfile

A masterfile of physicians has been maintained by the American Medical Association (AMA) since 1906. Today, the Physician Masterfile contains data on almost every physician in the United States, members and nonmembers of AMA, and on those graduates of American medical schools temporarily practicing overseas. The file also includes graduates of international medical schools who are in the United States and meet education standards for primary recognition as physicians.

A file is initiated on each individual upon entry into medical school or, in the case of international graduates, upon entry into the United States. Between 1969–85 a mail questionnaire survey was conducted every 4 years to update the file information on professional activities, self-designated area of specialization, and present employment status. Since 1985 approximately one-third of all physicians are surveyed each year.

For more information on the AMA Physician Masterfile, see: Division of Survey and Data Resources, American Medical Association, *Physician Characteristics and Distribution in the U.S.,* 1992 edition, Chicago, 1992.

Annual Census of Hospitals

From 1920 to 1953 the Council on Medical Education and Hospitals of the American Medical Association (AMA) conducted annual censuses of all hospitals registered by AMA.

In each annual census, questionnaires were sent to hospitals asking for the number of beds, bassinets, births, patients admitted, average census of patients, lists of staff doctors and interns, and other information of importance at the particular time. Response rates were always nearly 100 percent.

The community hospital data from 1940 and 1950 presented in this report were calculated using published figures from the AMA Annual Census of Hospitals. Although the hospital classification scheme used by AMA in published reports is not strictly comparable with the definition of community hospitals, methods were employed to achieve the greatest comparability possible.

For more information on the AMA Annual Census of Hospitals, see: American Medical Association, Hospital service in the United States, *Journal of the American Medical Association,* 116(11):1055–1144, 1941.

Association of American Medical Colleges

The AAMC collects information on student enrollment in medical schools through the annual Liaison Committee on Medical Education questionnaire, the fall enrollment questionnaire, and the American Medical College Application Service (AMCAS) data system. Other data sources are the institutional profile system, the premedical students questionnaire, the graduation questionnaire, the minority student opportunities in medicine questionnaire, the faculty roster system, data from the Medical College Admission Test, and one-time surveys developed for special projects.

For more information, see: Association of American Medical Colleges' Data Book: Statistical Information Related to Medical Education. Washington, DC, 1991.

InterStudy

National Health Maintenance Organization Census

From 1976 to 1980 the Office of Health Maintenance Organizations conducted a census of health maintenance organizations (HMO). Since 1981 InterStudy has conducted the census. A questionnaire is sent to all HMO's in the United States asking for updated enrollment, profit status, and Federal qualification status. New HMO's are also asked to provide information on model type. When necessary, information is obtained, supplemented, or clarified by telephone. For nonresponding HMO's, State-supplied information or the most current available data are used.

In 1985 a large increase in the number of HMO's and enrollment was partly attributable to a change in the categories of HMO's included in the census: Medicaid-only and Medicare-only HMO's have been added. Also component HMO's, which have their own discrete management, can be listed separately; whereas, previously the oldest HMO reported for all of its component or expansion sites, even when the components had different operational dates or were different model types.

For further information, see: InterStudy, *National HMO Census: Annual Report on the Growth of HMO's in the U.S., 1982–1986 Editions*; *The InterStudy Edge*, Spring 1987 and 1988 editions and 1989, 1990, volume 2. Excelsior, Minn., 1983–90.

National League for Nursing

The division of research of the National League for Nursing, conducts The Annual Survey of Schools of Nursing in October of each year. Questionnaires are sent to all graduate nursing programs (master's and doctoral), baccalaureate programs designed exclusively for registered nurses, basic registered nursing programs (baccalaureate, associate degree, and diploma), and licensed practical nursing programs. A 100-percent response rate has been achieved for many years on questionnaire items on enrollments, first-time admissions, and graduates. Response rates of approximately 80 percent are achieved for other areas of inquiry.

For more information, see: National League for Nursing, Nursing Data Source 1991, New York, N.Y.

Public Health Foundation

Association of State and Territorial Health Officials Reporting System

The Association of State and Territorial Health Officials (ASTHO) Reporting System, operated by the Public Health Foundation (PHF), is a statistical system that provides comprehensive information about the public health programs of State and local health departments. The Reporting System was established in 1970 by ASTHO in response to congressional requests for information about State health agency uses of block grant funds (that is, PHS Act, Section 314(d) grant monies). Data collected through the Reporting System are maintained in a comprehensive data base and are published in annual reports, chartbooks, and newsletters.

PHF, through the ASTHO Reporting System conducts an annual survey of the official State health agency (SHA) in each of the 50 States, the District of Columbia, and 4 U.S. territories. The survey includes extensive detail on the agencies' expenditures, funding sources, staffing, services, and activities.

Recently, PHF revised the ASTHO Reporting System's core data base to be outcome-oriented and focused on national health priorities. The new data base will provide the necessary data on States' efforts to meet the national objectives outlined by the Department of Health and Human Services in *Healthy People 2000: National Health Promotion and Disease Prevention Objectives.*

For more information, contact: Public Health Foundation, 1220 L Street, NW., Suite 350, Washington, DC 20005.

Appendix II
Glossary

Alphabetical Listing of Terms

The glossary is an alphabetical listing of terms used in *Health, United States*. It includes cross references to related terms and synonyms. It also contains the standard populations used for age adjustment and *International Classification of Diseases* (ICD) codes for cause of death and diagnostic and procedure categories.

Abortion — The Centers for Disease Control and Prevention's surveillance program counts legal abortions only. For surveillance purposes, legal abortion is defined as a procedure performed by a licensed physician or someone acting under the supervision of a licensed physician to induce the termination of a pregnancy.

Acquired immunodeficiency syndrome (AIDS) — All 50 States and the District of Columbia report AIDS cases to CDC using a uniform case definition and case report form. The case reporting definitions were expanded in 1985 (*MMWR* 1985; 34:373–5); 1987 (*MMWR* 1987; 36 (supp. no. 1S): 1S-15S); and 1993 (*MMWR* 1993; 41 (supp. no. RR-17)). These data are published quarterly by CDC in *HIV/AIDS Surveillance Report*. See related *Human immunodeficiency virus infection*.

Active physician — See *Physician*.

Acute condition — See *Condition*.

Addition — An addition to a psychiatric organization is defined by the National Institute of Mental Health as a new admission, a readmission, a return from leave, or a transfer from another service of the same organization or another organization. See related *Inpatient care episodes; Mental disorder; Mental health organization; Mental health service type*.

Admission — The American Hospital Association defines admissions as patients, excluding newborns, accepted for inpatient services during the survey reporting period. See related *Discharge; Patient*.

Age — Age is reported as age at last birthday, that is, age in completed years, often calculated by subtracting date of birth from the reference date, with the reference date being the date of the examination, interview, or other contact with an individual.

Age adjustment — Age adjustment, using the direct method, is the application of the age-specific rates in a population of interest to a standardized age distribution in order to eliminate the differences in observed rates that result from age differences in population composition. This adjustment is usually done when comparing two or more populations at one point in time or one population at two or more points in time.

In this report the death rates are age adjusted to the U.S. population enumerated in 1940. Computations may be simplified by expressing the 1940 U.S. population on a per million basis (table I). Adjustment is based on 11

Table I. Standard million age distribution used to adjust death rates to the U.S. population in 1940

Age	Standard million
All ages	1,000,000
Under 1 year	15,343
1–4 years	64,718
5–14 years	170,355
15–24 years	181,677
25–34 years	162,066
35–44 years	139,237
45–54 years	117,811
55–64 years	80,294
65–74 years	48,426
75–84 years	17,303
85 years and over	2,770

age groups with two exceptions. First, age-adjusted death rates for black males and black females in 1950 are based on nine age groups, with under 1 year and 1–4 years of age combined as one group and 75–84 years and 85 years of age and over combined as one group. Second, cause-specific provisional death rates are based on 10 age groups, with 1–4 years and 5–14 years of age combined as one group. Maternal mortality rates for Complications of pregnancy, childbirth, and the puerperium are calculated as the number of deaths per 100,000 live births. These rates are age adjusted to the 1970 distribution of live births by mother's age in the United States as shown in table II.

The data from the National Health Interview Survey (NHIS), National Health Examination Survey (NHES), National Health and Nutrition Examination Survey (NHANES), and the National Hospital Discharge Survey (NHDS) are age adjusted to the 1970 civilian noninstitutionalized population. Most of the data from the NHIS and NHDS are age adjusted using the following four age groups: under 15 years, 15–44 years, 45–64 years, and 65 years and over. The NHES and NHANES data are age adjusted using the following six age groups: 20–24 years, 25–34 years, 35–44 years, 45–54 years, 55–64 years, and 65–74 years. The 1970 civilian noninstitutionalized population used to age adjust data from each survey are shown in table III and derived as follows: Institutionalized population = (1 – proportion of total population not institutionalized on April 1, 1970) × total population on July 1, 1970. Civilian noninstitutionalized population = civilian population on July 1, 1970 – institutionalized population.

Table II. Numbers of live births and mother's age groups used to adjust maternal mortality rates to live births in the United States in 1970

Mother's age	Number
All ages	3,731,386
Under 20 years	656,460
20–24 years	1,418,874
25–29 years	994,904
30–34 years	427,806
35 years and over	233,342

SOURCE: U.S. Bureau of the Census: Population estimates and projections. *Current Population Reports*. Series P-25, No. 499. Washington. U.S. Government Printing Office, May 1973.

Table III. Population and age groups used to adjust data to the U.S. civilian noninstitutionalized population in 1970: Selected surveys

Survey and age	Number in thousands
NHIS and NHDS	
All ages.	199,584
Under 15 years	57,745
15–44 years	81,189
45–64 years	41,537
65 years and over	19,113
NHIS health care coverage	
65 years and over	19,113
65–74 years	12,224
75 years and over	6,889
NHIS smoking data	
18 years and over	130,158
18–24 years	22,464
25–34 years	24,430
35–44 years	22,614
45–64 years	41,537
65 years and over	19,113
NHES and NHANES	
20–74 years	116,182
20–24 years	15,378
25–34 years	24,430
35–44 years	22,614
45–54 years	23,070
55–64 years	18,467
65–74 years	12,223

SOURCE: Calculated from U.S. Bureau of Census: Estimates of the Population of the United States by Age, Sex, and Race: 1970 to 1977. Population Estimates and Projections. *Current Population Reports.* Series P-25, No. 721, Washington. U.S. Government Printing Office, April 1978.

AIDS — See *Acquired immunodeficiency syndrome.*

Air pollution — See *Pollutant.*

Average annual rate of change (percent change) — In this report average annual rates of change or growth rates are calculated as follows:

$$((P_n / P_o)^{1/N} - 1) \times 100$$

where P_n = later time period
P_o = earlier time period
N = number of years in interval.

This geometric rate of change assumes that a variable increases or decreases at the same rate during each year between the two time periods.

Average length of stay — In the National Health Interview Survey, the average length of stay per discharged patient is computed by dividing the total number of hospital days for a specified group by the total number of discharges for that group. Similarly, in the National Hospital Discharge Survey, the average length of stay is computed by dividing the total number of days of care, counting the date of admission but not the date of discharge, by the number of patients discharged. The American Hospital Association computes the average length of stay by dividing the number of inpatient days by the number of admissions.

As measured in the National Nursing Home Survey, length of stay for residents is the time from their admission until the reporting time, and the length of stay for discharges is the time between the date of admission and the date of discharge. See related *Days of care; Discharge; Patient; Resident.*

Bed — Any bed that is set up and staffed for use by inpatients is counted as a bed in a facility. In the National Master Facility Inventory, the count is of beds at the end of the reporting period; for the American Hospital Association, it is of the average number of beds, cribs, and pediatric bassinets during the entire period. The World Health Organization defines a hospital bed as one regularly maintained and staffed for the accommodation and full-time care of a succession of inpatients and situated in a part of the hospital where continuous medical care for inpatients is provided. The National Institute of Mental Health counts the number of beds set up and staffed for use in inpatient and residential treatment services on the last day of the survey reporting period. See related *Hospital; Inpatient care episodes; Mental health organization; Mental health service type; Occupancy rate.*

Bed-disability day — See *Disability day.*

Birth cohort — A birth cohort consists of all persons born within a given period of time, such as a year.

Birth rate — See *Rate: Birth and related rates.*

Birth weight — The first weight of the newborn obtained after birth. Low birth weight is defined as less than 2,500 grams or 5 pounds 8 ounces. Before 1979 low birth weight was defined as 2,500 grams or less. Very low birth weight is defined as less than 1,500 grams or 3 pounds 4 ounces.

Cause of death — For the purpose of national mortality statistics, every death is attributed to one underlying condition, based on information reported on the death certificate and utilizing the international rules for selecting the underlying cause of death from the reported conditions. Beginning with 1979, the *International Classification of Diseases, Ninth Revision* (ICD-9) has been used for coding cause of death. Data from earlier time periods were coded using the appropriate revision of the ICD for that time period. (See tables IV and V.) Changes in classification of causes of death in successive revisions of the ICD may introduce discontinuities in cause-of-death statistics over time. For further discussion, see Technical Appendix in National Center for Health Statistics: *Vital Statistics of the United States, 1988, Volume II, Mortality, Part A.* DHHS Pub. No. (PHS) 91–1101, Public Health Service, Washington, U.S. Government Printing Office, 1991. See related *International Classification of Diseases, Ninth Revision; Human immunodeficiency virus infection.*

Cause-of-death ranking — Cause-of-death ranking is based on the List of 72 Selected Causes of Death and the category Human immunodeficiency virus infection (ICD-9 Nos. *042–*044). The List of 72 Selected Causes of Death was adapted from one of the special lists for mortality tabulations recommended by the World Health Organization for use with the Ninth Revision of the *International Classification of Diseases.* Two group

Table IV. Revision of the *International Classification of Diseases,* according to year of conference by which adopted and years in use in the United States

Revision of the International Classification of Diseases	Year of conference by which adopted	Years in use in United States
First.	1900	1900–1909
Second	1909	1910–1920
Third	1920	1921–1929
Fourth	1929	1930–1938
Fifth.	1938	1939–1948
Sixth	1948	1949–1957
Seventh	1955	1958–1967
Eighth	1965	1968–1978
Ninth	1975	1979–present

titles—Major cardiovascular diseases and Symptoms, signs, and ill-defined conditions—are not ranked. In addition, category titles that begin with the words "Other" and "All other" are not ranked. The remaining category titles are ranked according to number of deaths to determine the leading causes of death. When one of the titles that represents a subtotal is ranked (for example, unintentional injuries), its component parts are not ranked (in this case, motor vehicle crashes and all other unintentional injuries). See related *International Classification of Diseases, Ninth Revision.*

Civilian noninstitutionalized population; Civilian population — See *Population.*

Cocaine-related emergency room episodes — The Drug Abuse Warning Network monitors selected adverse medical consequences of cocaine and other drug abuse episodes by measuring contacts with hospital emergency rooms. Contacts may be for drug overdose, unexpected drug reactions, chronic abuse, detoxification, or other reasons in which drug use is known to have occurred.

Community hospitals — See *Hospital.*

Completed fertility rate — See *Rate: Birth and related rates.*

Condition — A health condition is a departure from a state of physical or mental well-being. An impairment is a health condition that includes chronic or permanent health defects resulting from disease, injury, or congenital malformations. All health conditions, except impairments, are coded according to the *International Classification of Diseases, Ninth Revision, Clinical Modification* (ICD-9-CM).

Based on duration, there are two categories of conditions, acute and chronic. In the National Health Interview Survey, an *acute condition* is a condition that has lasted less than 3 months and has involved either a physician visit (medical attention) or restricted activity. A *chronic condition* refers to any condition lasting 3 months or more or is a condition classified as chronic regardless of its time of onset (for example, diabetes,

Table V. Cause-of-death codes, according to applicable revision of *International Classification of Diseases*

Cause of death	Code numbers			
	Sixth Revision	Seventh Revision	Eighth Revision	Ninth Revision
Diseases of heart	400–402, 410–443	400–402, 410–443	390–398, 402, 404, 410–429	390–398, 402, 404–429
Ischemic heart disease	. . .	. . .	. . .	410–414
Cerebrovascular diseases.	330–334	330–334	430–438	430–438
Malignant neoplasms	140–205	140–205	140–209	140–208
Respiratory system	160–164	160–164	160–163	160–165
Colorectal	153–154	153–154	153–154	153,154
Breast	170	170	174	174,175
Prostate	177	177	185	185
Chronic obstructive pulmonary diseases. . . .	241, 501, 502, 527.1	241, 501, 502, 527.1	490–493, 519.3	490–496
Pneumonia and influenza	480–483, 490–493	480–483, 490–493	470–474, 480–486	480–487
Chronic liver disease and cirrhosis	581	581	571	571
Diabetes mellitus	260	260	250	250
Nephritis, nephrotic syndrome, and nephrosis.	. . .	. . .	. . .	580–589
Septicemia	. . .	. . .	. . .	038
Atherosclerosis	. . .	. . .	. . .	440
Unintentional injuries[1]	E800–E962	E800–E962	E800–E949	E800–E949
Motor vehicle crashes[1]	E810–E835	E810–E835	E810–E823	E810–E825
Suicide	E963, E970–E979	E963, E970–E979	E950–E959	E950–E959
Homicide and legal intervention	E964, E980–E985	E964, E980–E985	E960–E978	E960–E978
Complications of pregnancy, childbirth, and the puerperium	640–689	640–689	630–678	630–676
Human immunodeficiency virus infection . . .	. . .	. . .	. . .	*042–*044
Drug-induced causes			. . .	292, 304, 305.2–305.9, E850–E858, E950.0–E950.5, E962.0, E980.0–E980.5
Alcohol-induced causes	. . .	. . .	. . .	291, 303, 305.0, 357.5, 425.5, 535.3, 571.0–571.3, 790.3, E860
Firearm injuries	. . .	. . .	E922, E955, E965, E970, E985	E922, E955.0–E955.4, E965.0–E965.4, E970, E985.0–E985.4
Malignant neoplasm of peritoneum and pleura	. . .	. . .	158, 163.0	158, 163
Coalworkers' pneumoconiosis	. . .	. . .	515.1	500
Asbestosis	. . .	. . .	515.2	501
Silicosis	. . .	. . .	515.0	502

[1]In the public health community, the term "unintentional injuries" is preferred to "accidents and adverse effects" and "motor vehicle crashes" to "motor vehicle accidents."

heart conditions, emphysema, and arthritis). The National Nursing Home Survey uses a specific list of chronic conditions, also disregarding time of onset. See related *Disability; Limitation of activity; International Classification of Diseases, Ninth Revision, Clinical Modification.*

Consumer Price Index (CPI) — The CPI is prepared by the U.S. Bureau of Labor Statistics. It is a monthly measure of the average change in the prices paid by urban consumers for a fixed market basket of goods and services. The medical care component of the CPI shows trends in medical care prices based on specific indicators of hospital, medical, dental, and drug prices. A revision of the definition of CPI has been in use since January 1988. See related *Health expenditures, national; Gross National Product.*

Crude birth rate; Crude death rate — See *Rate: Birth and related rates; Death and related rates.*

Days of care — According to the American Hospital Association and National Master Facility Inventory, days, hospital days, or inpatient days are the number of adult and pediatric days of care rendered during the entire reporting period. Days of care for newborns are excluded.

In the National Health Interview Survey, hospital days during the year refer to the total number of hospital days occurring in the 12-month period before the interview week. A hospital day is a night spent in the hospital for persons admitted as inpatients.

In the National Hospital Discharge Survey, days of care refers to the total number of patient days accumulated by patients at the time of discharge from nonfederal short-stay hospitals during a reporting period. All days from and including the date of admission but not including the date of discharge are counted. See related *Admission; Average length of stay; Discharge; Hospital; Patient.*

Death rate — See *Rate: Death and related rates.*

Dental visit — The National Health Interview Survey considers dental visits to be visits to a dentist's office for treatment or advice, including services by a technician or hygienist acting under the dentist's supervision. Services provided to hospital inpatients are not included. Dental visits are based on a 2-week recall period and are weighted to produce average annual number of visits.

Diagnosis — See *First-listed diagnosis.*

Diagnostic and other nonsurgical procedures — See *Procedure.*

Disability — In the National Health Interview Survey, a disability is any short- or long-term reduction of a person's activity as a result of an acute or chronic condition. It is often measured in terms of the number of days that a person's activity has been reduced. See related *Condition; Limitation of activity.*

Disability day — The National Health Interview Survey identifies several types of days on which a person's usual activity is reduced due to illness or injury (reported for the 2-week period preceding the week of the interview). The following types of short-term disability days are not mutually exclusive categories:

A *restricted-activity day* is any day on which a person reduces his or her usual activities by more than one half day due to an illness or an injury. Restricted-activity days are unduplicated counts of bed-disability, work-loss, and school-loss days, as well as other days during which a person reduces his or her usual activities.

A *bed-disability day* is a day on which a person stays in bed for more than half of the daylight hours (or normal waking hours) due to a specific illness or injury. All hospital days are bed-disability days. Bed-disability days may also be work-loss or school-loss days.

A *work-loss day* is a day on which a person did not work at his or her job or business for at least half of his or her normal workday due to a specific illness or injury. The number of work-loss days is determined only for currently employed persons.

A *school-loss day* is a day on which a child did not attend school for at least half of his or her normal school day due to a specific illness or injury. Beginning in 1982 school-loss days are determined only for children 5–17 years of age.

Discharge — The National Health Interview Survey defines a hospital discharge as the completion of any continuous period of stay of 1 night or more in a hospital as an inpatient, not including the period of stay of a well newborn infant. According to the National Hospital Discharge Survey, American Hospital Association, and National Master Facility Inventory, discharge is the formal release of an inpatient by a hospital (excluding newborn infants), that is, the termination of a period of hospitalization (including stays of 0 nights) by death or by disposition to a place of residence, nursing home, or another hospital. In the National Nursing Home Survey, discharge is the formal release of a resident by a nursing home. See related *Admission; Average length of stay; Days of care; Patient; Resident.*

Domiciliary care homes — See *Nursing home.*

Expenditures — See *Health expenditures, national.*

Family income — For purposes of the National Health Interview Survey and National Health and Nutrition Examination Survey, all people within a household related to each other by blood, marriage, or adoption constitute a family. Each member of a family is classified according to the total income of the family. Unrelated individuals are classified according to their own income. Family income is the total income received by the members of a family (or by an unrelated individual) in the 12 months before the interview. Family income includes wages, salaries, rents from property, interest, dividends, profits and fees from their own businesses, pensions, and help from relatives. Family income has generally been categorized into approximate quintiles in the tables.

Federal physicians — See *Physician.*

Federal hospitals — See *Hospital.*

Fertility rate — See *Rate: Birth and related rates.*

Fetal death — In the World Health Organization's definition, also adopted by the United Nations and the National Center for Health Statistics, a fetal death is death prior to the complete expulsion or extraction from its mother of a product of conception, irrespective of the duration of pregnancy; the death is indicated by the fact that after such separation, the fetus does not breathe or show any other evidence of life, such as beating of the heart, pulsation of the umbilical cord, or definite movement of voluntary muscles. For statistical purposes, fetal deaths are classified according to gestational age. In this report tabulations are shown for fetal deaths with stated or presumed gestation of 20 weeks or more and of 28 weeks or more, the latter gestational age group also known as late fetal deaths. See related *Live birth; Gestation; Rate: Death and related rates.*

First-listed diagnosis — In the National Hospital Discharge Survey this is the first recorded final diagnosis on the medical record face sheet (summary sheet).

Freestanding psychiatric outpatient clinics — See *Mental health organization.*

Full-time equivalent employee — The American Hospital Association and National Master Facility Inventory use an estimate of full-time equivalent employees in which two part-time employees are counted as one full-time employee. A full-time employee is defined as someone working 35 hours or more per week. The National Nursing Home Survey uses an estimate of full-time employees in which 35 hours of part-time employees' work per week is equivalent to one full-time employee. The National Institute of Mental Health calculates person-weeks of full-time equivalent employees by dividing the sum of hours worked by all full-time employees, part-time employees, and trainees in each staff discipline in 1 week by 40 hours per week.

General hospitals — See *Hospital.*

General hospitals providing separate psychiatric services — See *Mental health organization.*

Geographic division and region — The 50 States and the District of Columbia are grouped for statistical purposes by the U.S. Bureau of the Census into 9 geographic divisions within 4 regions. The groupings are as follows:

- Northeast
  New England
      Maine, New Hampshire, Vermont, Massachusetts, Rhode Island, and Connecticut
  Middle Atlantic
      New York, New Jersey, and Pennsylvania

- Midwest
  East North Central
      Ohio, Indiana, Illinois, Michigan, and Wisconsin

  West North Central
      Minnesota, Iowa, Missouri, North Dakota, South Dakota, Nebraska, and Kansas

- South
  South Atlantic
      Delaware, Maryland, District of Columbia, Virginia, West Virginia, North Carolina, South Carolina, Georgia, and Florida
  East South Central
      Kentucky, Tennessee, Alabama, and Mississippi
  West South Central
      Arkansas, Louisiana, Oklahoma, and Texas

- West
  Mountain
      Montana, Idaho, Wyoming, Colorado, New Mexico, Arizona, Utah, and Nevada
  Pacific
      Washington, Oregon, California, Alaska, and Hawaii

Gestation — For the National Vital Statistics System and the Centers for Disease Control and Prevention's Abortion Surveillance, the period of gestation is defined as beginning with the first day of the last normal menstrual period and ending with the day of birth. See related *Abortion; Fetal death; Live birth.*

Gross National Product (GNP) and **Gross Domestic Product (GDP)** — These are two broadly comparable measures of a nation's total output of goods and services. GNP represents the value of all goods and services produced for sale by the nation plus the estimated value of certain imputed outputs (that is, goods and services that are neither bought nor sold). The GNP is the sum of: (1) consumption expenditures by individuals and nonprofit organizations plus certain imputed values; (2) business investment in equipment, inventories, and new construction; (3) federal, State, and local government purchases of goods and services; and (4) the sale of goods and services abroad minus purchases from abroad. GDP equals GNP plus an adjustment (typically small) for the value of productive services performed domestically by foreign-born workers minus the value of productive services performed abroad by U.S. nationals. See related *Health expenditures, national.*

Health expenditures, national — See related *Consumer Price Index; Gross National Product.*

Health services and supplies expenditures — These are outlays for goods and services relating directly to patient care plus expenses for administering health insurance programs and government public health activities. This category is equivalent to total national health expenditures minus expenditures for research and construction.

National health expenditures — This measure estimates the amount spent for all health services and supplies and health-related research and construction activities consumed in the United States during the calendar year. Detailed estimates are available by source of expenditures (for example, out-of-pocket payments, private health insurance, and government programs), type of expenditures (for example, hospital care, physician services, and drugs), and are in current dollars for the year of report. Data are compiled from a variety of sources.

Nursing home expenditures — These cover care rendered in skilled nursing and intermediate care facilities, including those for the mentally retarded. The costs of long-term care provided by hospitals are excluded.

Personal health care expenditures — These are outlays for goods and services relating directly to patient care. The expenditures in this category are total national health expenditures minus expenditures for research and construction, expenses for administering health insurance programs, and government public health activities.

Private expenditures — These are outlays for services provided or paid for by nongovernmental sources—consumers, insurance companies, private industry, and philanthropic and other nonpatient care sources.

Public expenditures — These are outlays for services provided or paid for by federal, State, and local government agencies or expenditures required by governmental mandate (such as workmen's compensation insurance payments).

Health, self-assessment of — Health status was measured in the National Health Interview Survey by asking the respondent, "Would you say _____'s health is excellent, very good, good, fair, or poor?"

Health maintenance organization (HMO) — An HMO is a prepaid health plan delivering comprehensive care to members through designated providers, having a fixed monthly payment for health care services, and requiring members to be in plan for a specified period of time (usually 1 year). HMO model types are:

Group — An HMO that delivers health services through a physician group that is controlled by the HMO unit or an HMO that contracts with one or more independent group practices to provide health services.

Individual Practice Association (IPA) — An HMO that contracts directly with physicians in independent practice, and/or contracts with one or more associations of physicians in independent practice, and/or contracts with one or more multi-specialty group practices. The plan is predominantly organized around solo-single-specialty practices.

Mixed — An HMO that combines features of group and IPA.

Health services and supplies expenditures — See *Health expenditures, national.*

Hispanic origin — Hispanic ethnicity includes persons of Mexican, Puerto Rican, Cuban, Central and South American, and other or unknown Spanish origins. Persons of Hispanic origin may be of any race. See related *Race.*

HIV — See *Human immunodeficiency virus infection.*

Hospital — According to the American Hospital Association and National Master Facility Inventory, hospitals are licensed institutions with at least six beds whose primary function is to provide diagnostic and therapeutic patient services for medical conditions by an organized physician staff, and have continuous nursing services under the supervision of registered nurses. The World Health Organization considers an establishment to be a hospital if it is permanently staffed by at least one physician, can offer inpatient accommodation, and can provide active medical and nursing care. Hospitals may be classified by type of service, ownership, size in terms of number of beds, and length of stay. See related *Average length of stay; Bed; Days of care; Patient.*

Community hospitals include all nonfederal short-stay hospitals classified by the American Hospital Association according to one of the following services: general medical and surgical; obstetrics and gynecology; eye, ear, nose, and throat; rehabilitation; orthopedic; other specialty; children's general; children's eye, ear, nose, and throat; children's rehabilitation; children's orthopedic; and children's other specialty.

Federal hospitals are operated by the Federal Government.

General hospitals provide diagnostic, treatment, and surgical services for patients with a variety of medical conditions. According to the World Health Organization, these hospitals provide medical and nursing care for more than one category of medical discipline (for example, general medicine, specialized medicine, general surgery, specialized surgery, and obstetrics). Excluded are hospitals, usually in rural areas, that provide a more limited range of care.

Long-term hospitals are defined by the American Hospital Association and the National Master Facility Inventory as hospitals in which more than half the patients are admitted to units with an average length of stay of 30 days or more.

Nonprofit hospitals are operated by a church or other nonprofit organization.

Proprietary hospitals are operated for profit by individuals, partnerships, or corporations.

Psychiatric hospitals are ones whose major type of service is psychiatric care. See *Mental health organization.*

Registered hospitals are hospitals registered with the American Hospital Association. About 98 percent of hospitals are registered.

Short-stay hospitals in the National Hospital Discharge Survey are those in which the average length of stay is less than 30 days. The American

Hospital Association and National Master Facility Inventory define short-term hospitals as hospitals in which more than half the patients are admitted to units with an average length of stay of less than 30 days. The National Health Interview Survey defines short-stay hospitals as any hospital or hospital department in which the type of service provided is general; maternity; eye, ear, nose, and throat; children's; or osteopathic.

Specialty hospitals, such as psychiatric, tuberculosis, chronic disease, rehabilitation, maternity, and alcoholic or narcotic, provide a particular type of service to the majority of their patients.

Hospital-based physician — See *Physician*.

Hospital days — See *Days of care*.

Human immunodeficiency virus (HIV) infection — Mortality coding: Beginning with data for 1987, NCHS introduced category numbers *042–*044 for classifying and coding human immunodeficiency virus (HIV) infection as a cause of death. HIV infection was formerly referred to as human T-cell lymphotropic virus-III/lymphadenopathy-associated virus (HTLV-III/LAV) infection. The asterisk before the category numbers indicates that these codes are not part of the Ninth Revision of the *International Classification of Diseases* (ICD-9). Before 1987 deaths involving HIV infection were classified to Deficiency of cell-mediated immunity (ICD-9 No. 279.1) contained in the title All other diseases; to Pneumocystosis (ICD-9 No. 136.3) contained in the title All other infectious and parasitic diseases; to Malignant neoplasms, including neoplasms of lymphatic and hematopoietic tissues; and to a number of other causes. Therefore, beginning with 1987, death statistics for HIV infection are not strictly comparable with data for earlier years.

Morbidity coding: The National Hospital Discharge Survey codes diagnosis data using the *International Classification of Diseases, Ninth Revision, Clinical Modification* (ICD-9-CM). During 1984 and 1985 only data for AIDS (ICD-9-CM 279.19) were included. Beginning with data for 1986 discharges with the diagnosis Human immunodeficiency virus (HIV) infection (ICD-9-CM 042–044, 279.19 and 795.8) were included. See related *Acquired immunodeficiency syndrome; Cause of death; International Classification of Diseases, Ninth Revision; International Classification of Diseases, Ninth Revision, Clinical Modification*.

ICD; ICD codes — See *Cause of death; International Classification of Diseases, Ninth Revision*.

Incidence — Incidence is the number of cases of disease having their onset during a prescribed period of time. It is often expressed as a rate (for example, the incidence of measles per 1,000 children 5–15 years of age during a specified year). Incidence is a measure of morbidity or other events that occur within a specified period of time. See related *Prevalence*.

Individual Practice Association (IPA) — See *Health maintenance organization*.

Industry of employment — Industries are classified according to the *Standard Industrial Classification (SIC)*

Table VI. Codes for industries, according to the *Standard Industrial Classification (SIC) Manual*

Industry	Code numbers
Agriculture, forestry, and fishing	01–09
Mining	10–14
Construction	15–17
Manufacturing	20–39
Textile mill products	22
Apparel and other finished products made from fabrics and similar materials	23
Lumber and wood products, except furniture	24
Printing, publishing, and allied industries	27
Chemicals and allied products	28
Rubber and miscellaneous plastics products	30
Stone, clay, glass, and concrete products	32
Primary metal industries	33
Fabricated metal products, except machinery and transportation equipment	34
Industrial and commercial machinery and computer equipment	35
Electronic and other electrical equipment and components, except computer equipment	36
Transportation equipment	37
Measuring, analyzing, and controlling instruments; photographic, medical, and optical goods; watches and clocks	38
Miscellaneous manufacturing industries	39
Transportation, communication, and public utilities	40–49
Wholesale trade	50–51
Retail trade	52–59
Finance, insurance, and real estate	60–67
Services	70–89
Public administration	91–97

Manual of the Office of Management and Budget. Three editions of the SIC are used for coding industry data in Health, United States: the 1972 edition; the 1977 supplement to the 1972 edition; and the 1987 edition. The changes between versions include a few detailed titles created to correct or clarify industries or to recognize changes within the industry. Codes for major industrial divisions (table VI) were not changed between versions.

The category "Private sector" includes all industrial divisions except public administration and military. The category "Civilian sector" includes "Private sector" and the public administration division. The category "Not classified" is comprised of the following entries from the death certificate: housewife, student, or self-employed; information inadequate to code industry; establishments not elsewhere classified.

Infant death — An infant death is the death of a live-born child before his or her first birthday. Deaths in the first year of life may be further classified according to age as neonatal and postneonatal. *Neonatal deaths* are those that occur during the first 27 days of life; *postneonatal deaths* are those that occur between 28 days and 1 year of age. See *Live birth; Rate: Death and related rates*.

Inpatient care — See *Mental health service type*.

Inpatient care episodes — The National Institute of Mental Health defines episodes as the number of residents in inpatient organizations at the beginning of the year plus the total number of additions to these organizations during the year. Total additions during the year include new admissions and readmissions. In counting additions rather than persons, the same individual may be counted more than once. For example, if the same person is admitted more than once to a particular organization during the year, that person is counted as many times as admitted. In addition, if the same person is admitted to two or more different organizations during the year, that person is counted as an addition for each organization. See related *Addition; Patient; Mental health service type.*

Inpatient days — See *Days of care.*

Intermediate care facilities — See *Nursing homes, certification of.*

International Classification of Diseases, Ninth Revision (ICD-9) — The *International Classification of Diseases* (ICD) classifies mortality information for statistical purposes. The ICD was first used in 1900 and has been revised about every 10 years since then. The ICD-9, published in 1977, is used to code U.S. mortality data beginning with data year 1979. (See tables IV and V.) See related *Cause of death; International Classification of Diseases, Ninth Revision, Clinical Modification.*

International Classification of Diseases, Ninth Revision, Clinical Modification (ICD-9-CM) — The ICD-9-CM is based on and is completely compatible with the *International Classification of Diseases, Ninth Revision.* The ICD-9-CM is used to code morbidity data and the ICD-9 is used to code mortality data. Diagnostic groupings and code number inclusions for ICD-9-CM are shown in table VII; surgical groupings and code number inclusions are shown in table VIII; and diagnostic and other nonsurgical procedure groupings and code number inclusions are shown in table IX. See related *Condition; International Classification of Diseases, Ninth Revision; Mental disorder.*

Table VII. Codes for diagnostic categories from the *International Classification of Diseases, Ninth Revision, Clinical Modification*

Diagnostic category	Code numbers
Females with delivery	V27
Human immunodeficiency virus (HIV)	042–044, 279.19, 795.8
Malignant neoplasms	140–208, 230–234
Benign neoplasms	210–229, 235–239
Diabetes	250
Psychoses	290–299
Alcohol dependence syndrome	303
Eye diseases and conditions	360–379
Otitis media and eustachian tube disorders	381–382
Diseases of heart	391–392.0, 393–398, 402, 404, 410–416, 420–429
Cerebrovascular diseases	430–438
Acute respiratory infection	460–466
Chronic disease of tonsils and adenoids	474
Pneumonia, all forms	480–486
Bronchitis, emphysema, and asthma	490–493
Inguinal hernia	550
Noninfectious enteritis and colitis	555–556, 558
Cholelithiasis	574
Hyperplasia of prostate	600
Inflammatory disease of female pelvic organs	614–616
Disorders of menstruation	626
Pregnancy with abortive outcome	630–639
Intervertebral disc disorders	722
Congenital anomalies	740–759
Fracture, all sites	800–829
Lacerations and open wounds	870–904

Table VIII. Codes for surgical categories from the *International Classification of Diseases, Ninth Revision, Clinical Modification*

Surgical category	Code numbers
Extraction of lens	13.1–13.6
Insertion of prosthetic lens (pseudophakos)	13.7
Myringotomy	20.0
Tonsillectomy, with or without adenoidectomy	28.2–28.3
Adenoidectomy without tonsillectomy	28.6
Direct heart revascularization (coronary bypass)	36.1
Cardiac catheterization	37.21–37.23
Pacemaker insertion or replacement	37.7–37.8
Biopsies on the digestive system (Beginning in 1989)	42.24, 44.14, 44.15, 45.14, 45.15, 45.25, 45.27, 48.24, 48.26, 49.22, 49.23, 50.11, 50.12, 51.12, 51.14, 52.11, 52.12, 52.14, 54.22, 54.24
Appendectomy, excluding incidental	47.0
Cholecystectomy	51.2
Repair of inguinal hernia	53.0–53.1
Prostatectomy	60.2–60.6
Circumcision	64.0
Oophorectomy and salpingo-oophorectomy	65.3–65.6
Bilateral destruction or occlusion of fallopian tubes	66.2–66.3
Hysterectomy	68.3–68.7
Diagnostic dilation and curettage of uterus	69.09
Procedures to assist delivery (Prior to 1989)	72–73
(Beginning in 1989)	72, 73.0–73.3, 73.6–73.8, 73.93–73.99
Cesarean section	74.0–74.2, 74.4, 74.99
Repair of current obstetrical laceration	75.5–75.6
Reduction of fracture (excluding skull, nose, and jaw)	76.70, 76.78–76.79, 79.0–79.6
Excision or destruction of intervertebral disc and spinal fusion	80.5, 81.0
Excision of semilunar cartilage of knee	80.6
Arthroplasty and replacement of hip (Prior to 1989)	81.5–81.6
(Beginning in 1990)	81.40, 81.51–81.53
Operations on muscles, tendons, fascia, and bursa	82–83.1, 83.3–83.9
Biopsies on the integumentary system (breast, skin, and subcutaneous tissue)	85.11–85.12, 86.11
Debridement of wound, infection, or burn	86.22, 86.28

ICD-9 and ICD-9-CM are arranged in 17 main chapters. Most of the diseases are arranged according to their principal anatomical site, with special chapters for infective and parasitic diseases; neoplasms; endocrine, metabolic, and nutritional diseases; mental diseases; complications of pregnancy and childbirth; certain diseases peculiar to the perinatal period; and ill-defined conditions. In addition, two supplemental classifications are provided: the classification of factors influencing health status and contact with health service and the classification of external causes of injury and poisoning.

Late fetal death rate — See *Rate: Death and related rates.*

Leading causes of death — See *Cause-of-death ranking.*

Length of stay — See *Average length of stay.*

Life expectancy — Life expectancy is the average number of years of life remaining to a person at a particular age and is based on a given set of age-specific death rates, generally the mortality conditions existing in the period mentioned. Life expectancy may be determined by race, sex, or other characteristics using age-specific death rates for the population with that characteristic. See related *Rate: Death and related rates.*

Table IX. Codes for diagnostic and other nonsurgical procedure categories from the *International Classification of Diseases, Ninth Revision, Clinical Modification*

Procedure category	Code numbers
Spinal tap	03.31
Endoscopy of small intestine without biopsy. . . .	45.11–45.13
Endoscopy of large intestine without biopsy. . . .	45.21–45.24
Laparoscopy (excluding that for ligation and division of fallopian tubes)	54.21
Cystoscopy	57.31–57.32
Arthroscopy of knee.	80.26
Computerized axial tomography (CAT scan)	87.03, 87.41, 87.71, 88.01, 88.38
Contrast myelogram.	87.21
Biliary tract x ray	87.5
Arteriography using contrast material	88.4
Angiocardiography using contrast material.	88.5
Diagnostic ultrasound.	88.7
Electroencephalogram	89.14
Radioisotope scan	92.0–92.1

Limitation of activity — In the National Health Interview Survey, limitation of activity refers to a long-term reduction in a person's capacity to perform the usual kind or amount of activities associated with his or her age group. Each person identified as having a chronic condition is classified according to the extent to which his or her activities are limited, as follows:

■ Persons unable to carry on major activity;
■ Persons limited in the amount or kind of major activity performed;
■ Persons not limited in major activity but otherwise limited; and
■ Persons not limited in activity.

See related *Condition; Disability; Major activity.*

Live birth — In the World Health Organization's definition, also adopted by the United Nations and the National Center for Health Statistics, a live birth is the complete expulsion or extraction from its mother of a product of conception, irrespective of the duration of the pregnancy, which, after such separation, breathes or shows any other evidence of life such as heartbeat, umbilical cord pulsation, or definite movement of voluntary muscles, whether or not the umbilical cord has been cut or the placenta is attached. Each product of such a birth is considered live born. See related *Gestation; Rate: Birth and related rates.*

Live-birth order — In the National Vital Statistics System this item from the birth certificate refers to the total number of live births the mother has had, including the present birth as recorded on the birth certificate. Fetal deaths are excluded. See related *Live birth.*

Long-term hospital — See *Hospital.*

Low birth weight — See *Birth weight.*

Major activity (or usual activity) — This is the principal activity of a person or of his or her age-sex group. For children 1–5 years of age, it refers to ordinary play with other children; for children 5–17 years of age, it refers to school attendance; for adults 18 years of age and over, it usually refers to a job, housework, or school attendance. See related *Limitation of activity.*

Marital status — Marital status is classified through self-reporting into the categories married and unmarried. The term married encompasses all married people including those separated from their spouses. Unmarried includes those who are single (never married), divorced, or widowed. The Abortion Surveillance Reports of the Centers for Disease Control and Prevention classify separated people as unmarried for all States except Rhode Island.

Maternal mortality rate — See *Rate: Death and related rates.*

Medicaid — This program is State operated and administered but has federal financial participation. Within certain broad federally-determined guidelines, States decide who is eligible; the amount, duration, and scope of services covered; rates of payment for providers; and methods of administering the program. Medicaid provides health care services for certain low-income persons. Medicaid does not provide health services to all poor people in every State. It categorically covers participants in the Aid to Families with Dependent Children program and in the Supplemental Security Income program. In most States it also covers certain other people deemed to be medically needy. The program was authorized in 1965 by Title XIX of the Social Security Act. See related *Health expenditures, national; Health maintenance organization; and Medicare.*

Medical specialties — See *Physician specialty.*

Medical vendor payments — Under the Medicaid program, medical vendor payments are payments (expenditures) to medical vendors from the State through a fiscal agent, or to a health insurance plan. Adjustments are made for Indian Health Service payments to Medicaid, cost settlements, third party recoupments, refunds, voided checks, and other financial settlements that cannot be related to specific provided claims. Excluded are payments made for medical care under the emergency assistance provisions, payments made from State medical assistance funds that are not federally matchable, cost sharing or enrollment fees collected from recipients or a third party, and administration and training costs.

Medicare — This is a nationwide health insurance program providing health insurance protection to people 65 years of age and over, people entitled to social security disability payments for 2 years or more, and people with end-stage renal disease, regardless of income. The program was enacted July 30, 1965, as Title XVIII, *Health Insurance for the Aged* of the Social Security Act, and became effective on July 1, 1966. It consists of two separate but coordinated programs, hospital insurance (Part A) and supplementary medical insurance (Part B). See related *Health expenditures, national; Health maintenance organization; Medicaid.*

Mental disorder — The National Institute of Mental Health defines a mental disorder as any of several disorders listed in the *International Classification of Diseases, Ninth Revision, Clinical Modification* (ICD-9-CM) or *Diagnostic and Statistical Manual of Mental Disorders, Third Edition* (DSM-IIIR). Table X

Table X. Mental illness codes, according to applicable revision of the *Diagnostic and Statistical Manual of Mental Disorders* and *International Classification of Diseases*

Diagnostic category	DSM-II/ICDA-8	DSM-IIIR/ICD-9-CM
Alcohol related	291; 303; 309.13	291; 303; 305.0
Drug related	294.3; 304; 309.14	292; 304; 305.1–305.9; 327; 328
Organic disorders (other than alcoholism and drug) . .	290; 292; 293; 294 (except 294.3); 309.0; 309.2–309.9	290; 293; 294; 310
Affective disorders	296; 298.0; 300.4	296; 298.0; 300.4; 301.11; 301.13
Schizophrenia	295	295; 299

shows diagnostic categories and code numbers for ICD-9-CM/DSM-IIIR and corresponding codes for the *International Classification of Diseases, Adapted for Use in the United States, Eighth Revision* (ICDA-8) and *Diagnostic and Statistical Manual of Mental Disorders, Second Edition* (DSM-II). See related *International Classification of Diseases, Ninth Revision, Clinical Modification.*

Mental health organization — The National Institute of Mental Health defines a mental health organization as an administratively distinct public or private agency or institution whose primary concern is the provision of direct mental health services to the mentally ill or emotionally disturbed. The major types of mental health organizations are described below.

Freestanding psychiatric outpatient clinics provide only ambulatory mental health services on either a regular or emergency basis. The medical responsibility for services is generally assumed by a psychiatrist.

General hospitals providing separate psychiatric services are general hospitals that provide psychiatric services in either a separate psychiatric inpatient, outpatient, or partial hospitalization service with assigned staff and space.

Multiservice mental health organizations directly provide two or more of the program elements defined under Mental health service type and are not classifiable as a psychiatric hospital, general hospital, or a residential treatment center for emotionally disturbed children. (The classification of a psychiatric or general hospital or a residential treatment center for emotionally disturbed children takes precedence over a multiservice classification, even if two or more services are offered.)

Partial care organizations provide a program of ambulatory mental health services.

Private mental hospitals are operated by a sole proprietor, partnership, limited partnership, corporation, or nonprofit organization, primarily for the care of persons with mental disorders.

Psychiatric hospitals are hospitals primarily concerned with providing inpatient care and treatment for the mentally ill. Psychiatric inpatient units of Veterans Administration general hospitals and Veterans Administration neuropsychiatric hospitals are combined into the category Veterans Administration psychiatric hospitals because of their similarity in size, operation, and length of stay.

Residential treatment centers for emotionally disturbed children must meet all of the following criteria: (a) Not licensed as a psychiatric hospital and primary purpose is to provide individually-planned mental health treatment services in conjunction with residential care; (b) Include a clinical program that is directed by a psychiatrist, psychologist, social worker, or psychiatric nurse with a graduate degree; (c) Serve children and youth primarily under the age of 18; and (d) Primary diagnosis for the majority of admissions is mental illness, classified as other than mental retardation, developmental disability, and substance-related disorders, according to DSM-II/ICDA-8 or DSM-IIIR/ ICD-9-CM codes. See related table X and *Mental disorder.*

State and county mental hospitals are under the auspices of a State or county government or operated jointly by a State and county government.

See related *Addition; Inpatient care episode; Mental health service type.*

Mental health service type refers to the following kinds of mental health services:

Inpatient care is the provision of 24-hour mental health care in a mental health hospital setting.

Outpatient care is the provision of ambulatory mental health services for less than 3 hours at a single visit on an individual, group, or family basis, usually in a clinic or similar organization. Emergency care on a walk-in basis, as well as care provided by mobile teams who visit patients outside these organizations are included. "Hotline" services are excluded.

Partial care treatment is a planned program of mental health treatment services generally provided in visits of 3 or more hours to groups of patients. Included are treatment programs that emphasize intensive short-term therapy and rehabilitation; programs that focus on recreation, and/or occupational program activities, including sheltered workshops; and education and training programs, including special education classes, therapeutic nursery schools, and vocational training.

Residential treatment care is the provision of overnight mental health care in conjunction with an intensive treatment program in a setting other than a hospital. Facilities may offer care to emotionally disturbed children or mentally ill adults.

See related *Addition; Inpatient care episode; Mental health organization.*

Metropolitan statistical area (MSA) — The definitions and titles of MSA's are established by the U.S. Office of Management and Budget with the advice of the Federal Committee on Metropolitan Statistical Areas. Generally speaking, an MSA consists of a county or group of counties containing at least one city (or twin cities) having a population of 50,000 or more plus adjacent counties that are metropolitan in character and are economically and socially integrated with the central city. In New England, towns and cities rather than counties are the units used in defining MSA's. There is no limit to the number of adjacent counties included in the MSA as long as they are integrated with the central city. Nor is an MSA limited to a single state; boundaries may cross state lines. Metropolitan population, as used in this report, is based on MSA's as defined in the 1980 census and does not include any subsequent additions or changes.

Multiservice mental health organizations — See *Mental health organization.*

Neonatal mortality rate — See *Rate: Death and related rates.*

Nonfederal physicians — See *Physician.*

Nonprofit hospitals — See *Hospital.*

Notifiable disease — A notifiable disease is one that, when diagnosed, health providers are required, usually by law, to report to State or local public health officials. Notifiable diseases are those of public interest by reason of their contagiousness, severity, or frequency.

Nursing care — The following definition of nursing care applies to data collected in National Nursing Home Surveys through 1977. Nursing care is the provision of any of the following services: application of dressings or bandages; bowel and bladder retraining; catheterization; enema; full bed bath; hypodermic, intramuscular, or intravenous injection; irrigation; nasal feeding; oxygen therapy; and temperature-pulse-respiration or blood pressure measurement. See related *Nursing home.*

Nursing care homes — See *Nursing home.*

Nursing home — A nursing home is an establishment with three or more beds that provides nursing or personal care services to the aged, infirm, or chronically ill. The following definitions of nursing home types apply to data collected in National Nursing Home Surveys through 1977.

Nursing care homes must employ one or more full-time registered or licensed practical nurses and must provide nursing care to at least half the residents.

Personal care homes with nursing have some but fewer than half the residents receiving nursing care. In addition, such homes must employ one or more registered or licensed practical nurses or must provide administration of medications and treatments in accordance with physicians' orders, supervision of self-administered medications, or three or more personal services.

Personal care homes without nursing have no residents who are receiving nursing care. These homes provide administration of medications and treatments in accordance with physicians' orders, supervision of self-administered medications, or three or more personal services.

Domiciliary care homes primarily provide supervisory care but also provide one or two personal services.

Nursing homes are certified by the Medicare and/or Medicaid program. The following definitions of certification levels apply to data collected in National Nursing Home Surveys of 1973–74, 1977, and 1985.

Skilled nursing facilities provide the most intensive nursing care available outside of a hospital. Facilities certified by Medicare provide posthospital care to eligible Medicare enrollees. Facilities certified by Medicaid as skilled nursing facilities provide skilled nursing services on a daily basis to individuals eligible for Medicaid benefits.

Intermediate care facilities are certified by the Medicaid program to provide health-related services on a regular basis to Medicaid eligibles who do not require hospital or skilled nursing facility care but do require institutional care above the level of room and board.

Not certified facilities are not certified as providers of care by Medicare or Medicaid.

See related *Nursing care; Resident.*

Nursing home expenditures — See *Health expenditures, national.*

Occupancy rate — The National Master Facility Inventory and American Hospital Association define hospital occupancy rate as the average daily census divided by the average number of hospital beds during a reporting period. Average daily census is defined by the American Hospital Association as the average number of inpatients, excluding newborns, receiving care each day during a reporting period. The occupancy rate for facilities other than hospitals is calculated as the number of residents reported at the time of the interview divided by the number of beds reported.

Office — In the National Health Interview Survey, an office refers to the office of any physician in private practice not located in a hospital. In the National Ambulatory Medical Care Survey, an office is any location for a physician's ambulatory practice other than hospitals, nursing homes, other extended care facilities, patients' homes, industrial clinics, college clinics, and family planning clinics. However, private offices in hospitals are included. See related *Office visit; Outpatient visit; Physician; Physician contact.*

Office-based physician — See *Physician.*

Office visit — In the National Ambulatory Medical Care Survey, an office visit is any direct personal exchange between an ambulatory patient and a physician or members of his or her staff for the purposes of seeking care and rendering health services. See related *Outpatient visit; Physician contact.*

Operations — See *Procedure.*

Outpatient surgery — The American Hospital Association defines outpatient surgery as scheduled surgical services provided to patients who do not remain in the hospital overnight. The surgery may be performed in operating suites also used for inpatient surgery, specially designated surgical suites for ambulatory surgery, or procedure rooms within an ambulatory care facility. Ambulatory surgery conducted in the private office of a physician not located in a hospital is not included in the American Hospital Association's reporting system. See related *Procedure.*

Outpatient visit — The American Hospital Association defines outpatient visits as visits for receipt of medical, dental, or other services by patients who are not lodged in the hospital. Each appearance by an outpatient to each unit of the hospital is counted individually as an outpatient visit. See related *Office; Office visit; Physician contact.*

Partial care organization — See *Mental health organization.*

Partial care treatment — See *Mental health service type.*

Particulate matter — Particulate matter is defined as particles of solid or liquid matter in the air, including both nontoxic materials (soot, dust, and dirt) and toxic materials (lead, asbestos, suspended sulfates and nitrates, etc.). See related *Pollutant.*

Patient — A patient is a person who is formally admitted to the inpatient service of the hospital for observation, care, diagnosis, or treatment. See related *Admission; Average length of stay; Days of care; Discharge.*

Percent change — See *Average annual rate of change.*

Perinatal mortality rate, ratio — See *Rate: Death and related rates.*

Personal care homes with/without nursing — See *Nursing home.*

Personal health care expenditures — See *Health expenditures, national.*

Physician — Physicians, through self-reporting, are classified by the American Medical Association and others as licensed doctors of medicine or osteopathy, as follows:

Active (or professionally active) physicians are currently practicing medicine, regardless of the number of hours worked per week.

Federal physicians are employed by the Federal Government; *nonfederal* or *civilian physicians* are not.

Office-based physicians spend the plurality of their time working in practices based in private offices.

Hospital-based physicians spend the plurality of their time as salaried physicians in hospitals.

Data for physicians are presented by type of education (doctors of medicine, doctors of osteopathy); place of education (U.S. medical graduates and international medical graduates); activity status (professionally active and inactive); employment setting (federal and nonfederal); area of specialty; and geographic area. See related *Office; Physician specialty.*

Physician contact — In the National Health Interview Survey, a physician contact is defined as a consultation with a physician in person or by telephone, for examination, diagnosis, treatment, or advice. The service may be provided by the physician or by another person working under the physician's supervision. Contacts involving services provided on a mass basis (for example, blood pressure screenings) and contacts for hospital inpatients are not included.

Place of contact includes office, hospital outpatient clinics, emergency room, telephone (advice given by a physician in a telephone call), home (any place in which a person was staying at the time a physician was called there), clinics, HMO's, and other places located outside a hospital.

In the National Health Interview Survey, physician contacts are based on a 2-week recall period and are adjusted to produce average annual number of visits. The interval since the last physician contact is the length of time before the week of interview in which the physician was last consulted. See related *Office; Office visit.*

Physician specialty — A physician specialty is any specific branch of medicine in which a physician may concentrate. Data are based on physician reports of their specialty. The specialty classification system used by the Bureau of Health Professions and National Ambulatory Medical Care Survey (NAMCS) is based on the categories established by the American Medical Association.

Primary care specialties include general practice (or family practice), internal medicine, and pediatrics.

Medical specialties include, along with internal medicine and pediatrics, the areas of allergy, cardiovascular disease, dermatology, gastroenterology, pediatric allergy and cardiology, and pulmonary diseases.

Surgical specialties include general surgery, neurological surgery, obstetrics and gynecology, ophthalmology, orthopedic surgery, otolaryngology, plastic surgery, colon and rectal surgery, thoracic surgery, and urology.

Other specialties covered by NAMCS are geriatrics, neurology, preventive medicine, psychiatry, and public health. Other specialties covered by the Bureau of Health Professions are aerospace medicine, anesthesiology, child psychiatry, neurology, occupational medicine, pathology, physical medicine and rehabilitation, psychiatry, public health, and radiology.

See related *Physician.*

Pollutant — A pollutant is any substance that renders the atmosphere or water foul or noxious to health. See related *Particulate matter*.

Population — The U.S. Bureau of the Census collects and publishes data on populations in the United States according to several different definitions. Various statistical systems then use the appropriate population for calculating rates.

Total population is the population of the United States, including all members of the Armed Forces living in foreign countries, Puerto Rico, Guam, and the U.S. Virgin Islands. Other Americans abroad (for example, civilian federal employees and dependents of members of the Armed Forces or other federal employees) are not included.

Resident population is the population of U.S. residents living in the United States. It includes members of the Armed Forces stationed in the United States and their families. It excludes international military, naval, and diplomatic personnel and their families located here and residing in embassies or similar quarters. Also excluded are international workers and international students in this country and Americans living abroad. The resident population is usually the denominator when calculating birth and death rates and incidence of disease.

Civilian population is the resident population excluding members of the Armed Forces. However, families of members of the Armed Forces are included. This population is the denominator in rates calculated for the NCHS National Hospital Discharge Survey.

Civilian noninstitutionalized population is the civilian population not residing in institutions. Institutions include correctional institutions, detention homes, and training schools for juvenile delinquents; homes for the aged and dependent (for example, nursing homes and convalescent homes); homes for dependent and neglected children; homes and schools for the mentally or physically handicapped; homes for unwed mothers; psychiatric, tuberculosis, and chronic disease hospitals; and residential treatment centers. This population is the denominator in rates calculated for the NCHS National Health Interview Survey, National Health and Nutrition Examination Survey, and National Ambulatory Medical Care Survey.

Postneonatal mortality rate — See *Rate: Death and related rates*.

Poverty level — Poverty statistics are based on definitions developed by the Social Security Administration. These include a set of money income thresholds that vary by family size and composition. Families or individuals with income below their appropriate thresholds are classified as below the poverty level. These thresholds are updated annually to reflect changes in the Consumer Price Index for all urban consumers (CPI-U). For example, the average poverty

threshold for a family of four was $13,924 in 1991 and $13,359 in 1990. See related *Consumer Price Index*.

Prevalence — Prevalence is the number of cases of a disease, infected persons, or persons with some other attribute present during a particular interval of time. It is often expressed as a rate (for example, the prevalence of diabetes per 1,000 persons during a year). See related *Incidence*.

Primary care specialties — See *Physician specialty*.

Private expenditures — See *Health expenditures, national*.

Procedure — The National Hospital Discharge Survey (NHDS) defines a procedure as a surgical or nonsurgical operation, diagnostic procedure, or special treatment assigned by the physician and recorded on the medical record of patients discharged from the inpatient service of short-stay hospitals. All terms listed on the face sheet of the medical record under captions such as "operation," "operative procedures," and "operations and/or special treatments" are transcribed in the order listed. A maximum of four 4-digit ICD-9-CM codes are assigned per discharge. In accordance with ICD-9-CM coding, procedures are classified as diagnostic and other nonsurgical procedures or as surgical operations.

Diagnostic and other nonsurgical procedures are procedures generally not considered to be surgery. These include diagnostic endoscopy and radiography, radiotherapy and related therapies, physical medicine and rehabilitation, and other nonsurgical procedures. In 1989 the list of nonsurgical procedures was revised to include selected procedures previously classified as surgical. Selected diagnostic and other non-surgical procedures are listed with their ICD-9-CM code numbers in table IX. For further discussion, see National Hospital Discharge Survey: Annual Summary, 1989. National Center for Health Statistics. Vital Health Stat 13(109). 1992.

Surgical operations encompass all ICD-9-CM procedures, except those listed under "Nonsurgical procedures." Selected surgical operations are listed with their ICD-9-CM codes in table VIII. In 1989 the list of surgical operations was revised and certain procedures previously classified as surgical were reclassified as diagnostic and other nonsurgical. The American Hospital Association defines surgery as a surgical episode in the operating or procedure room. During a single episode, multiple surgical procedures may be performed.

See related *International Classification of Diseases, Ninth Revision, Clinical Modification; Outpatient surgery*.

Proprietary hospitals — See *Hospital*.

Provisional death rates — See *Rate: Death and related rates*.

Psychiatric hospitals — See *Hospital; Mental health organization*.

Public expenditures — See *Health expenditures, national*.

Race — Beginning in 1976 the Federal Government's data systems classified individuals into the following racial groups: American Indian or Alaskan Native, Asian or Pacific Islander, Black, and White. Depending on the data source, the classification by race may be based on self-classification or on observation by an interviewer or other persons filling out the questionnaire. Starting in 1989 data from the National Vital Statistics System for newborn infants was tabulated according to race of mother. Before 1989 race of newborn was based on race of both parents. If the parents were of different races and one parent was white, the child was classified according to the race of the other parent. When neither parent was white, the child was classified according to father's race, with one exception; if either parent was Hawaiian, the child was classified Hawaiian. Before 1964 the National Vital Statistics System classified all births for which race was unknown as white. Beginning in 1964 these births were classified according to information on the previous record. In the National Health Interview Survey, children whose parents are of different races are classified according to the race of the mother. See related *Hispanic origin*.

Rate — A rate is a measure of some event, disease, or condition in relation to a unit of population, along with some specification of time. See related *Age adjustment; Population*.

■ *Birth and related rates*

Birth rate is calculated by dividing the number of live births in a population in a year by the mid-year resident population. It is expressed as the number of live births per 1,000 population. The rate may be restricted to births to women of specific age, race, marital status, or geographic location (specific rate), or it may be related to the entire population (crude rate). See related *Live birth*.

Fertility rate is the number of live births per 1,000 women of reproductive age, 15–44 years.

Completed fertility rate is the sum of the central birth rates over all ages (14–49 years) of childbearing for a given birth cohort.

■ *Death and related rates*

Death rate is calculated by dividing the number of deaths in a population in a year by the mid-year resident population. It is expressed as the number of deaths per 1,000 or per 100,000 population. The rate may be restricted to deaths in specific age, race, sex, or geographic groups or from specific causes of death (specific rate) or it may be related to the entire population (crude rate).

Provisional death rate – See *National Vital Statistics System* in Appendix I.

Fetal death rate is the number of fetal deaths with stated or presumed gestation of 20 weeks or more divided by the sum of live births plus fetal deaths, stated per 1,000 live births plus fetal deaths. *Late fetal death rate* is the number of fetal deaths with stated or presumed gestation of 28 weeks or more divided by the sum of live births plus late fetal deaths, stated per 1,000 live births plus late fetal deaths. See related *Fetal death; Gestation*.

Infant mortality rate is calculated by dividing the number of infant deaths during a year by the number of live births reported in the same year. It is expressed as the number of infant deaths per 1,000 live births. *Neonatal mortality rate* is the number of deaths of children under 28 days of age, per 1,000 live births. *Postneonatal mortality rate* is the number of deaths of children that occur between 28 days and 365 days after birth, per 1,000 live births. See related *Infant death*.

Perinatal relates to the period surrounding the birth event. Rates and ratios are based on events reported in a calendar year. *Perinatal mortality rate* is the sum of late fetal deaths plus infant deaths within 7 days of birth divided by the sum of live births plus late fetal deaths, stated per 1,000 live births plus late fetal deaths. *Perinatal mortality ratio* is the sum of late fetal deaths plus infant deaths within 7 days of birth divided by the number of live births, stated per 1,000 live births. *Feto-infant mortality rate* is the sum of late fetal deaths plus all infant deaths divided by the sum of live births plus late fetal deaths, stated per 1,000 live births plus late fetal deaths. See related *Fetal death; Gestation; Infant death; Live birth*.

Maternal death is one for which the certifying physician has designated a maternal condition as the underlying cause of death. Maternal conditions are those assigned to Complications of pregnancy, childbirth, and the puerperium. (See related table V.) *Maternal mortality rate* is the number of maternal deaths per 1,000 live births. The maternal mortality rate indicates the likelihood that a pregnant woman will die from maternal causes. The number of live births used in the denominator is an approximation of the population of pregnant women who are at risk of a maternal death.

Region — See *Geographic division and region*.

Registered hospitals — See *Hospital*.

Registered nursing education — Registered nursing data are shown by level of educational preparation. Baccalaureate education requires at least 4 years of college or university; associate degree programs are based in community colleges and are usually 2 years in length; and diploma programs are based in hospitals and are usually 3 years in length.

Registration area — The United States has separate registration areas for birth, death, marriage, and divorce statistics. In general, registration areas correspond to States and include two separate registration areas for the District of Columbia and New York City. All States have adopted laws that require the registration of births and deaths and the reporting of fetal deaths. It is believed that more than 99 percent of the births and deaths occurring in this country are registered.

The *death registration area* was established in 1900 with 10 States and the District of Columbia, and the *birth registration area* was established in 1915, also with 10 States and the District of Columbia. Both areas have covered the entire United States since 1933. Currently, Puerto Rico, U.S. Virgin Islands, and Guam comprise separate registration areas, although their data are not included in statistical tabulations of U.S. resident data. See related *Reporting area*.

Relative survival rate — The relative survival rate is the ratio of the observed survival rate for the patient group to the expected survival rate for persons in the general population similar to the patient group with respect to age, sex, race, and calendar year of observation. The 5-year relative survival rate is used to estimate the proportion of cancer patients potentially curable. Because over half of all cancers occur in persons 65 years of age and over, many of these individuals die of other causes with no evidence of recurrence of their cancer. Thus, because it is obtained by adjusting observed survival for the normal life expectancy of the general population of the same age, the relative survival rate is an estimate of the chance of surviving the effects of cancer.

Reporting area — In the National Vital Statistics System, reporting requirements for selected items such as Hispanic origin, educational attainment, and marital status vary by State. Accordingly, the reporting areas for these selected items are comprised of only the States that require the item to be reported. For example, in 1989, the reporting area for educational attainment of mother on the birth certificate included 48 States, the District of Columbia, and New York City. See related *Registration area; National Vital Statistics System* in Appendix I.

Resident — In the National Nursing Home Survey, a resident is a person on the roster of the nursing home as of the night before the survey. Included are all residents for whom beds are maintained even though they may be on overnight leave or in a hospital. See related *Discharge; Nursing home*.

Resident population — See *Population*.

Residential treatment care — See *Mental health service type*.

Residential treatment centers for emotionally disturbed children — See *Mental health organization*.

Restricted-activity day — See *Disability day*.

School-loss day — See *Disability day*.

Self-assessment of health — See *Health, self-assessment of*.

Short-stay hospitals — See *Hospital*.

Skilled nursing facilities — See *Nursing homes, certification of*.

Specialty hospitals — See *Hospital*.

State health agency — The agency or department within State government headed by the State or territorial health official. Generally, the State health agency is responsible for setting State-wide public health priorities, carrying out national and State mandates, responding to public health hazards, and assuring access to health care for underserved State residents.

Surgical operations — See *Procedure*.

Surgical specialties — See *Physician specialty*.

Urbanization — In this report death rates are presented according to the level of urbanization of the decedent's county of residence. This categorization is based on the rural-urban continuum codes for metropolitan and nonmetropolitan counties developed by the Economic Research Service, U.S. Department of Agriculture. Counties are categorized as metropolitan and nonmetropolitan by using the 1983 U.S. Office of Management and Budget definition of Metropolitan Statistical Areas (MSA's). The codes classify metropolitan counties by size and nonmetropolitan counties by degree of urbanization or proximity to metropolitan areas. The original 10 categories of counties have been collapsed into five categories for this report: (1) Large core metropolitan counties contain the primary central city of an MSA with a 1980 population of 1 million or more; (2) Large fringe metropolitan counties are the noncore counties of an MSA with 1980 population of 1 million or more; (3) Medium or small metropolitan counties are in MSA's with 1980 populations under 1 million; (4) Urban nonmetropolitan counties are not in MSA's and have 2,500 or more urban residents in 1980; and (5) Rural counties are not in MSA's and have fewer than 2,500 urban residents in 1980.

Work-loss day — See *Disability day*.

Years of potential life lost — Years of potential life lost are calculated over the age range from birth to 65 years of age. The number of deaths for each age group is multiplied by the years of life lost, calculated as the difference between age 65 years and the midpoint of the age group. For example, the death of a person age 15–24 years counts as 45 years of life lost. Years of potential life lost is derived by summing years of life lost over all age groups. For more information, see Centers for Disease Control. *MMWR*. Dec. 19, 1986. Vol. 35, Supp. No. 2S.

Healthy
People
2000
Review

List of Figures

1. Years of healthy life: United States, 1990 _____ **241**

2. Infant mortality rates: United States, 1987–91, 1990 goal and year 2000 target _____ **242**

3. Death rates for children 1–14 years of age: United States, 1987–90, 1990 goal and year 2000 target _____ **242**

4. Death rates for adolescents and young adults 15–24 years of age: United States, 1987–90, 1990 goal and year 2000 target _____ **243**

5. Death rates for adults 25–64 years of age: United States, 1987–90, 1990 goal and year 2000 target _____ **243**

6. Older noninstitutionalized adults who have difficulty in performing two or more personal care activities: United States, 1984 and 1986 _____ **244**

7. Persons 18–74 years and over who engage in light to moderate physical activity for at least 30 minutes per occasion 5 or more times per week: United States, 1985, 1990, 1991, and year 2000 target for objective 1.3 _____ **245**

8. Overweight adults 20–74 years of age according to selected characteristics targeted by year 2000 objective 2.3: United States, 1991 _____ **252**

9. Current cigarette smokers among persons 20 years of age and over, according to selected characteristics targeted by year 2000 objective 3.4: United States, 1991 _____ **260**

10. Average age of first use of cigarettes, alcohol, and marijuana by adolescents 12–17 years of age: United States, 1988–91 and year 2000 targets for objective 4.5 _____ **266**

11. Persons 18 years and over with adverse health effects of stress in the past year: United States, 1985, 1990, and year 2000 target for objective 6.5 _____ **275**

12. Death rates for homicide among black males 15–34 years of age: United States, 1987–90 and year 2000 target for objective 7.1 _____ **279**

13. Percent of worksites offering health promotion activities: United States, 1985, 1992, and year 2000 target for objective 8.6 _____ **283**

14. Number of States with laws requiring safety belt and motorcycle helmet use for all ages: United States, 1989–91 and year 2000 target for objective 9.14 _____ **287**

15. Death rates for work-related injuries among full-time workers according to selected occupations: United States, 1983–90, and year 2000 targets for objective 10.1 _____ **293**

16. Outbreaks of waterborne disease: United States, 1981–88 average, 1989–90, and year 2000 target for objective 11.3 _____ **297**

17. Outbreaks due to Salmonella enteritidis: United States, 1989–91 and year 2000 target for objective 12.2 _____ **303**

18. Percent of persons 65 years and over who have lost all of their natural teeth: United States, 1986–91 and year 2000 targets for objective 13.4 _____ **306**

19. Proportion of live births that are low birth weight and are very low birth weight by race of mother: United States, 1987–90 and year 2000 targets for objective 14.5 _____ **313**

20. Age-adjusted death rates for coronary heart disease: United States, 1987–90 and year 2000 targets for objective 15.1 _____ **319**

21. Age-adjusted death rates for cancer: United States, 1987–90 and year 2000 target for objective 16.1 _____ **327**

22. Limitation of major activity caused by chronic conditions, according to selected characteristics targeted by year 2000 objective 17.2: United States, 1991 _____ **333**

23. Annual incidence of diagnosed AIDS cases according to selected characteristics targeted by year 2000 objective 18.1: United States, 1989–91 _____ **341**

24. Annual incidence of gonorrhea, according to selected characteristics: United States, 1989–91 and year 2000 targets for objective 19.1 _____ **346**

25. Annual incidence of tuberculosis, according to race and ethnicity: United States, 1988–91 and year 2000 targets for objective 20.4 _____ **350**

26. Adults with a usual source of medical care, according to selected characteristics related to year 2000 objective 21.3: United States, 1991 _____ **357**

List of Tables

1. Physical activity and fitness objective status____ 247
2. Nutrition objective status_____ 254
3. Tobacco objective status_____ 262
4. Alcohol and other drugs objective status_____ 268
5. Family planning objective status_____ 272
6. Mental health and mental disorders objective
status_____ 276
7. Violent and abusive behavior objective status___ 280
8. Educational and community based programs
objective status_____ 284
9. Unintentional injuries objective status_____ 288
10. Occupational safety and health objective
status_____ 294
11. Environmental health objective status_____ 299
12. Food and drug safety objective status_____ 304
13. Oral health objective status_____ 308
14. Maternal and infant health objective status___ 314
15. Heart disease and stroke objective status_____ 321
16. Cancer objective status_____ 328
17. Diabetes and chronic disabling conditions
objective status_____ 334
18. HIV objective status_____ 343
19. Sexually transmitted diseases objective status__ 347
20. Immunization and infectious diseases objective
status_____ 352
21. Clinical preventive services objective status___ 359
22. Surveillance and data systems objective
status_____ 364

Introduction

Background and Summary

Healthy People 2000: National Health Promotion and Disease Prevention Objectives (1) is a statement of national opportunities. This prevention initiative presents a national strategy for significantly improving the health of the American people in the decade preceding the year 2000. *Healthy People 2000* recognizes that lifestyle and environmental factors are major determinants in disease prevention and health promotion. It provides strategies to significantly reduce preventable death and disability, to enhance quality of life, and to reduce disparities in health status between various population groups within our society.

Healthy People 2000 defines three broad goals: to increase the span of healthy life for Americans; to reduce health disparities among Americans; and to achieve access to preventive services for all Americans. These goals are supported by 300 specific objectives that set priorities for public health during the 1990's. Subobjectives for minorities and other special populations were also established to meet the unique needs and health problems of these populations. *Healthy People 2000* uses the three approaches of health promotion, health protection, and preventive services as organizing categories for 22 priority areas. For each of these priority areas, a U.S. Public Health Service agency was designated to develop an implementation plan and to coordinate activities directed toward attaining the objectives (see table A).

Work on the report began in 1987 with the establishment of a consortium that has grown to include over 300 national membership organizations and all the State health departments. The *Healthy People 2000* Consortium, facilitated by the Institute of Medicine of the National Academy of Sciences, helped the U.S. Public Health Service convene eight regional hearings at which over 750 individuals and organizations presented testimony. This testimony became the primary resource material for the working groups of professionals who crafted the health objectives. After further extensive public review and comment from more than 10,000 people, the objectives were refined, revised, and published as *Healthy People 2000*.

The first national health promotion and disease prevention objectives were set in 1979, to be achieved by 1990 (2). During the 1980's, progress toward the 1990 objectives was tracked in five *Prevention Profiles* (3) and in *The 1990 Health Objectives for the Nation: A Midcourse Review* (4). The *Healthy People 2000* Review will monitor the progress of the Nation's health promotion and disease prevention objectives for the year 2000 throughout this decade.

The Reviews will be published annually. *Healthy People 2000 Review, 1992* presents an overview of the current status of progress toward all of the year 2000 objectives. The Public Health Service reviews progress toward the year 2000 objectives periodically. Summaries of these reviews are published in *Public Health Service Progress Reports on Healthy People 2000* (5). This report contains the most recent national data available and supercedes data published in *Healthy People 2000*, progress review reports, and all other earlier publications containing national data on the year 2000 objectives.

There are 300 unduplicated main objectives. Some priority areas share identical objectives; there are 332 objectives counting the duplicates. Special targets were set for higher-risk population groups. These population groups include people with low incomes, people who are members of some racial and ethnic minority groups, and people with disabilities (1). There are 223 special population targets excluding duplicates; with duplicates there are 284. Thus, without duplicates there are a total of 520 health promotion and disease prevention objectives and subobjectives for the year 2000; 616 with duplicates.

This summary of progress incorporates all priority area objectives and is therefore a duplicated count (i.e., 332 objectives). At this early point in the decade, three percent of objectives have already been met. Progress toward the targets has been made on another 28 percent of the objectives. Fifteen percent of the objectives show movement away from the targets. Data for four percent of the objectives show mixed results (these objectives have more than one data point to measure and have shown progress for some and movement away from the targets for others), and three percent have updates but show no change. Ten percent of the objectives have new baselines where baselines did not originally exist. Twenty-eight percent have no new data with which to evaluate progress. Baselines have yet to be obtained for ten percent of objectives. Data sources have been identified for all but one *Healthy People 2000* objective, which is listed in two priority areas.

Priority areas (PA's) showing the most progress are Heart Disease and Stroke (PA 15) with 9 of 17 objectives showing progress; Unintentional Injuries (PA 9) with 11 of 22 objectives showing progress including three objectives that have met or exceeded their targets; and Alcohol and Other Drugs (PA 4) with progress for 9 of 19 objectives including one objective that has exceeded its target.

Priority areas with the most objectives showing movement away from the targets are Maternal and Infant Health (PA 14) with five of 16 objectives in this category, and Diabetes and Chronic Disabling Conditions (PA 17) with six of 20 objectives in this category.

Ninety-two objectives have had no new data since the baseline published in *Healthy People 2000*. The priority areas with over half of their objectives in this category are Family Planning (PA 5) with six of 11 objectives, and Oral Health (PA 13) with 9 of 16 objectives.

Organization and Scope of This Review

This *Review* is divided into four major sections—(1) a section on the general data issues involved in the monitoring of the year 2000 objectives, (2) a section highlighting the year 2000 goals and age-related objectives, (3) a section of 22 chapters, one for each *Healthy People 2000* priority area, and (4) a four-part section of information tables.

A number of major cross-cutting data issues involved in the monitoring of the objectives and subobjectives are presented in the first section. Because these issues relate to objectives in numerous priority areas, they are discussed here rather than in each individual chapter.

The second section highlights the year 2000 goals and progress toward the year 2000 age-related objectives, continuing the tracking of the five broad 1990 goals for the five major life stages.

The third section consists of 22 chapters, one for each *Healthy People 2000* priority area. Each chapter contains a discussion of specific data issues, a figure representing one of the priority area objectives, an objective status summary table, and the full text of the objectives in that priority area.

The text for each chapter presents a brief discussion of the reasons the priority area was included in the initiative, a summary of the overall status of the objectives, and monitoring data issues that are not obvious from the summary table or the text of the objective, such as proxy measures, differing tracking systems, and operational definitions. A few caveats must be made regarding summaries of the progress (or lack of progress) on the objectives. At this early point in tracking, many summary statements are based on data from only 1 or 2 years beyond the baseline. Many data points are derived from sample surveys and are therefore subject to sampling and nonsampling errors. A small change between a baseline level and more recent information may or may not indicate progress toward achievement of the year 2000 target. A more thorough assessment of progress, taking into account trends over several years, will be made as the decade progresses.

Most figures show the progress of one of the priority area objectives toward the objective target. Some show the latest data for population groups that were targeted because of especially high risk. In some cases, choice of figures depended on the availability of data; the choice does not confer more relative importance to any of the objectives depicted.

The objective summary table presents the baselines, targets, and current progress toward the priority area objectives. Most baselines use 1987 data. The most current vital statistics data are from 1990; the most current estimates from the National Health Interview Survey are from 1991, and approximately one-quarter of the objectives are tracked with data from this survey.

There are four tables at the end of the *Review*. Table A lists the priority area lead agencies. Table B displays the cause-of-death categories used for the *Healthy People 2000* mortality objectives. Table C presents current data sources for all the *Healthy People 2000* objectives and subobjectives, and table D lists the Health Status Indicators developed for objective 22.1.

Data Issues

There are several major cross-cutting data issues involved in the monitoring of the objectives and subobjectives. These include revised baselines, issues regarding minority group subobjectives, age-adjusted versus crude mortality rates, data source comparability, cause-of-death category issues, and years of healthy life.

Revised Baselines

For a number of *Healthy People 2000* objectives, the baselines shown in this Review have been revised from the original baselines published in *Healthy People 2000*. Fifty revisions were the result of the revised Census population estimates and are discussed below. In priority area 14, 11 baselines were revised in response to a change in the method for tabulating the race of infants (see Chapter 14, Maternal and Infant Health). For 44 specific objectives (unduplicated), the baselines have been changed because of modifications in methodology, typographical errors, changes in data sources, or because the baseline data were based on preliminary analyses.

Except for objectives 6.3 and 7.6, which were revised by the lead agency responsible for achieving the objectives (table A), as of this writing, all *Healthy People 2000* targets are being shown as originally published.

Revised Death Rates

The 1986–87 baselines for population-based mortality objectives and subobjectives tracked with data from the National Vital Statistics System (NVSS), as well as subsequent data for the 1980's, have been recomputed using intercensal population estimates based on the 1990 Census enumeration (see *Health, United States, 1992*,

Appendix I). Data for the three mortality objectives (4.1, 9.3, and 10.1) tracked by sources other than the NVSS are not revised for this reason. With the exception of American Indian/Alaska Native death rates (see below), the changes are relatively small. The objectives affected by this change are shown in table B. Cases where the recomputed baseline rate was the same as the original rate are denoted in the objective status tables by "no change."

American Indian and Alaska Native Mortality Rates

The baseline rates for some American Indian/Alaska Native (AI/AN) mortality subobjectives have been revised to reflect the new intercensal populations and the inclusion of the entire U.S. AI/AN population. The objectives affected by this change are:

4.2b	Cirrhosis deaths
6.1d/7.2d	Suicide deaths
7.1f	Homicide deaths
9.1a	Unintentional injury deaths
9.3d	Motor vehicle crash deaths
17.9b	Diabetes-related deaths

The original baselines and targets for these objectives were established using data from the 33 States in which AI/AN health services are provided by the Indian Health Service Regional Service Offices. The Indian Health Service provides health care to approximately 60 percent of the AI/AN population (5); most of the population served live on or near reservations. "Reservation States" include approximately 90 percent of the AI/AN population in the United States, but exclude some urban centers with large American Indian populations.

The revised baselines are substantially lower than the original figures. These large differences are partially due to the substantially larger intercensal population estimates (death rate denominators) based on the 1990 Census compared with those based on the 1980 Census. They may also reflect the relatively greater failure to identify AI/AN deaths on death certificates in non-Reservation States compared with Reservation States (7).

Minority Group Subobjectives

The guideline for drafting the objectives required the identification of a data source to track progress before a subobjective for a minority or special population could be set. Although there are virtually no data gaps for existing subobjectives, lack of data sources prevented the establishment of subobjectives for some population groups. Many subpopulations are small and geographically clustered and cannot be measured through national surveys using standard sampling techniques. Developing techniques to assess the health of minorities and other special subpopulations will be a significant challenge during the coming decade.

Another concern is the availability of reliable denominator data. Although national surveys can provide numbers of responses for some subpopulations, intercensal population estimates may not be obtainable for these groups. County population estimates and State-specific estimates for major racial and ethnic subgroups may also be unavailable.

Age Adjustment

Most of the original baselines for mortality objectives published in *Healthy People 2000* are derived from the National Vital Statistics System and are age adjusted to the 1940 population. Exceptions are objectives 4.1, 9.3, and 10.1. Data for 4.1 and 9.3 are crude rates from the National Highway and Traffic Safety Administration's

Fatal Accident Reporting System (FARS); data for 10.1 are crude rates from the Department of Labor's Annual Survey of Occupational Injuries and Illnesses. Most of the previously published mortality subobjective baselines are age adjusted as well; the exceptions are subobjectives 4.1a (a crude rate from FARS), 9.1b, 9.1c, 9.5c, 9.6c, and 9.6d. With the publication of this Review, all mortality objectives and subobjectives, except for those tracked with FARS or Department of Labor data, will be tracked with age-adjusted rates (see *Health United States, 1992*, Appendix II).

Data Source Comparability

For some objectives the baseline data source differs from the source that will be used to monitor progress. Comparability between different data sources or even within the same data source for different years is not assured. Unless the data for an objective are obtained from the same questions of the same survey system each year, unless operational definitions remain the same, and unless analytical techniques are constant, tracking can be compromised. Comparability, if an issue, is discussed in priority area chapters. For a number of objectives that will be tracked with the third National Health and Nutrition Examination Survey (NHANES III), proxy data from various surveys are being used until the NHANES III data are available. See table C for a list of sources for each *Healthy People 2000* objective.

Cause-of-death Terminology and Codes

Twenty-four objectives (excluding duplicates) in *Healthy People 2000* are tracked using mortality data (table B). For most of these objectives, the cause-of-death terminology used in *Healthy People 2000* is different from that used in *Health, United States*; *Vital Statistics of the United States, Mortality*, and other NCHS publications; in some cases, the terminology and the identifying International Classification of Disease (ICD–9) codes are different (8).

Specifically, for five objectives, the terminology and the codes are different from those used for similar cause-of-death categories in the NCHS tabulation lists. One example, objective 7.1, concerns reduction of "homicides." Progress toward this objective is measured using ICD–9 numbers E960–E969. The NCHS tabulation lists generally use "Homicide and legal intervention" (ICD–9 numbers E960–E978), which includes police action. For 14 objectives, only the terminology differs; the defining ICD–9 identifying codes are the same. For example, objective 15.2 calls for reduction in mortality from "stroke;" NCHS tabulation lists use the term "Cerebrovascular diseases" (both use ICD–9 numbers 430–438). Only one objective, suicide, has the same title and the same code in both uses. The remaining four mortality objectives have no comparable category in NCHS publications. With the exception of heart disease, the differences between mortality rates defined by the *Healthy People 2000* ICD categories and those defined by the NCHS rubrics are relatively small, if not trivial.

Years of Healthy Life

Increasing years of healthy life is one of the three *Healthy People 2000* goals and is included as three specific objectives (8.1, 17.1, and 21.1). The 1980 baseline has been updated to 1990, using a revised methodology developed by NCHS and external consultants. This interim measure, which will be used to monitor progress until the year 2000, combines mortality data from the National Vital Statistics System with health status data from the National Health Interview Survey. The definition and measurement of years of healthy life are still being refined; research will continue

in this area. The methodology used for the interim measure will be
published elsewhere (9).

References

1. U.S. Department of Health and Human Services. Healthy people
2000: National health promotion and disease prevention objectives.
Washington: Public Health Service. 1991.

2. U.S. Department of Health and Human Services. Promoting
health/preventing disease: Objectives for the Nation. Washington:
Public Health Service. 1984.

3. National Center for Health Statistics. Prevention profile. Health,
United States, 1991. Hyattsville, Maryland: Public Health Service.
1992.

4. U.S. Department of Health and Human Services. The 1990
health objectives for the Nation: A midcourse review. Washington:
U.S. Department of Health and Human Services. 1986.

5 U.S. Department of Health and Human Services. Public Health
Service Progress Reports on Healthy People 2000. Washington:
Public Health Service. 1991–93.

6. American Indian Health Care Association. Enhancing Health
Statistics for American Indians and Alaska Native Communities:
An agenda for action. St. Paul: American Indian Health Care
Assocation. 1992.

7. Indian Health Service. Personal communication. Rockville,
Maryland: Public Health Service. November 1992.

8. World Health Organization. Manual of the International
Statistical Classification of Diseases, Injuries, and Causes of Death,
based on the recommendations of the Ninth Revision Conference,
1975. Geneva: World Health Organization. 1977.

9. National Center for Health Statistics. Years of healthy life.
Statistical notes. Hyattsville, Maryland: National Center for Health
Statistics. In press. 1993.

Year 2000 Goals and Age-Related Objectives

Healthy People 2000 has three goals: to increase the span of healthy life for all Americans, to decrease health disparities among Americans, and to achieve access to preventive services for all Americans. In addition to these goals, there are four age-related objectives that cut across the 22 priority areas and the organizing categories of health promotion, health protection, and preventive services.

The primary goal recognizes the importance of preventing disability, as well as further impairment or morbidity for those people with disabilities, so that long life will be accompanied by good health. *Healthy People 2000* emphasizes the full range of functional capacity from infancy through old age, including measures of health outcomes.

Years of healthy life can be measured by modifying life expectancy by a value representing the portion of life spent in an "unhealthy" state (for example, impaired by disabilities, disease, or injuries). As figure 1 indicates, in 1990, life expectancy in the United States was 75.4 years while years of healthy life was 64.0. On average, Americans spend 85 percent of their lifespan in a healthy state. *Healthy People 2000* is directed at increasing this percentage. The measurement of years of healthy life is discussed in the Data Issues section of the Introduction.

Specific strategies are needed to assess the unique needs of disadvantaged and high-risk populations. The second goal is to reduce disparities in death, disease, and disability rates of these groups as compared with the total population. The specific groups targeted are racial and ethnic minority populations, people with low income, and people with disabilities.

Healthy People 2000 also recognizes that many Americans lack access to an ongoing source of primary care and therefore to essential preventive services. The third goal addresses the many

Figure 1. Years of healthy life: United States, 1990

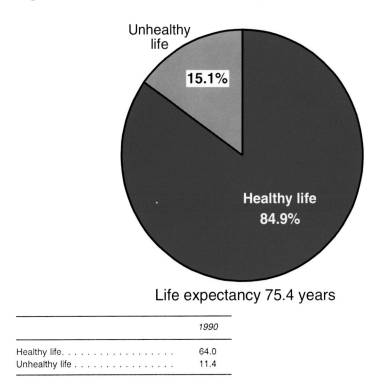

Life expectancy 75.4 years

	1990
Healthy life.	64.0
Unhealthy life	11.4

SOURCE: Centers for Disease Control and Prevention, National Center for Health Statistics, National Vital Statistics System and National Health Interview Survey.

barriers to access to health care. These barriers include inadequate health insurance, the mal-distribution of primary care providers, geographic barriers, and language and cultural barriers.

The four age-related objectives continue the emphasis of the 1990 health initiative. The 1990 Objectives for the Nation (1) identified five broad quantifiable goals to reduce preventable death and disability among Americans at major life stages: as infants, children, adolescents and young adults, adults, and older adults. Impressive progress was made toward these goals during the 1980's (2).

Continuing the tracking of the 1990 goals for infants and children, the year 2000 age-related objective is to reduce the infant mortality rate by approximately 30 percent to no more than 7 per 1,000 live births and reduce the death rate for children by 15 percent to no more than 28 per 100,000 children 1–14 years of age. The 1990 goal of 9 per 1,000 live births for infant mortality was reached and exceeded in 1991 (figure 2). For children, the 1990 goal was met by 1985 (figure 3). If the present rate of decline continues, the year 2000 target will be reached in 1993.

The year 2000 age-related objective for adolescents and young adults is to reduce the death rate by 15 percent to no more than 85 per 100,000 people 15–24 years of age. Death rates fluctuated between 1987 and 1990, showing little change and no decline (figure 4). They remain far above the 1990 goal of 93 and the year 2000 target.

For adults, the year 2000 age-related objective is to reduce the death rate by 20 percent to no more than 340 per 100,000 people 25–64 years of age. At the present average annual rate of decline of 1.6, the year 2000 objective will not be reached until 2009 (figure 5).

People who reach the age of 65 can now expect to live into their eighties (*Health, United States, 1992*, detailed table 27). The data regarding the years of healthy life indicate the likelihood that not all those years will be active and independent ones. Thus, improving the functional independence, not just the length, of later life is an important element in promoting the health of this age

Figure 2. Infant mortality rates: United States, 1987–91, 1990 goal and year 2000 target

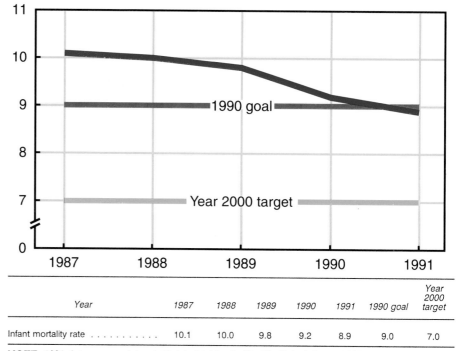

Deaths per 1,000 live births

Year	1987	1988	1989	1990	1991	1990 goal	Year 2000 target
Infant mortality rate	10.1	10.0	9.8	9.2	8.9	9.0	7.0

NOTE: 1991 data are provisional. Related tables in *Health, United States, 1992*, are 18–23 and 25.

SOURCE: Centers for Disease Control and Prevention, National Center for Health Statistics, National Vital Statistics System.

Figure 3. Death rates for children 1–14 years of age: United States, 1987–90, 1990 goal and year 2000 target

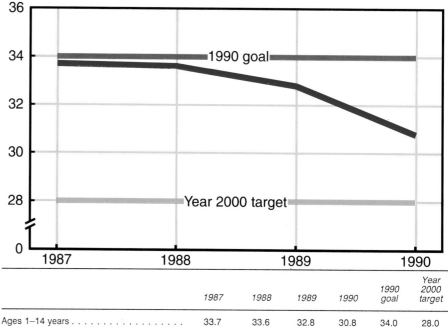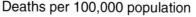

Deaths per 100,000 population

	1987	1988	1989	1990	1990 goal	Year 2000 target
Ages 1–14 years	33.7	33.6	32.8	30.8	34.0	28.0

NOTE: Related tables in *Health, United States, 1992*, are 31, 34–37, 40, 42–45, 48 and 50.

SOURCE: Centers for Disease Control and Prevention, National Center for Health Statistics, National Vital Statistics System.

group. The 1990 goal for older adults was to reduce the average annual number of days of restricted activity due to acute and chronic conditions to fewer than 30 days per year. Because of the difficulties in interpreting the meaning of restricted activity days, the year 2000 age-related objective for older adults is to reduce to no more than 90 per 1,000 people the proportion of all people 65 years of age and over who have difficulty in performing two or more personal care activities, thereby preserving independence. Data beyond the baseline were available for noninstitutionalized people only (figure 6). For people 65 years of age and over the proportion who have difficulty remained the same between 1984 and 1986. For people 85 years of age and over, the proportion who have difficulty declined by about 9 percent between 1984 and 1986.

References

1. U.S. Department of Health and Human Services. Promoting health/preventing disease: Objectives for the Nation. Washington: Public Health Service. 1984.

2. McGinnis JM, Richmond JB, Brandt EN, et al. Health progress in the United States: Results of the 1990 objectives for the Nation. Am J Med 268(18): 2545–52.

Figure 4. Death rates for adolescents and young adults 15–24 years of age: United States, 1987–90, 1990 goal and year 2000 target

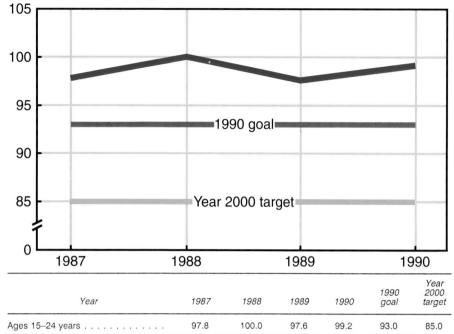

Deaths per 100,000 population

Year	1987	1988	1989	1990	1990 goal	Year 2000 target
Ages 15–24 years	97.8	100.0	97.6	99.2	93.0	85.0

NOTE: Related tables in *Health, United States, 1992* are 31, 34–37, 40, 42–45, 48, and 50.

SOURCE: Centers for Disease Control and Prevention, National Center for Health Statistics, National Vital Statistics System.

Figure 5. Death rates for adults 25–64 years of age: United States, 1987–90, 1990 goal and year 2000 target

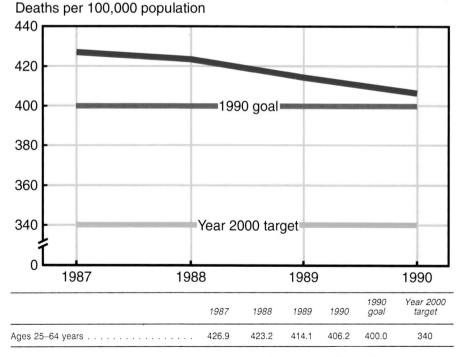

Deaths per 100,000 population

	1987	1988	1989	1990	1990 goal	Year 2000 target
Ages 25–64 years	426.9	423.2	414.1	406.2	400.0	340

NOTE: Related tables in *Health, United States, 1992*, are 31–40, 42–45, 48, and 50.

SOURCE: Centers for Disease Control and Prevention, National Center for Health Statistics, National Vital Statistics System.

Figure 6. Older noninstitutionalized adults who have difficulty in performing two or more personal care activities: United States, 1984 and 1986

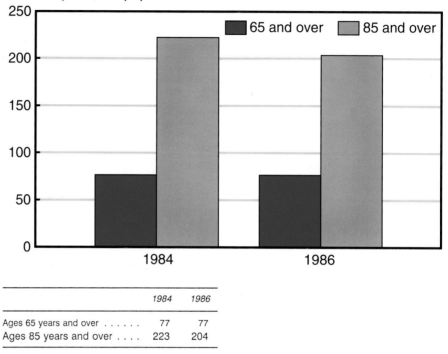

Number per 1,000 population

	1984	1986
Ages 65 years and over	77	77
Ages 85 years and over	223	204

NOTE: This objective is a duplicate of objective 17.3. A related table in *Health, United States, 1992*, is 61.

SOURCE: Centers for Disease Control and Prevention, National Center for Health Statistics, National Health Interview Survey.

Priority Area 1
Physical Activity and Fitness

Background and Data Summary

Regular physical activity can help to prevent and manage coronary heart disease, hypertension, noninsulin-dependent diabetes mellitus, osteoporosis, obesity, and mental health problems such as depression and anxiety (1). Regular physical activity has also been associated with lower rates of colon cancer (2) and stroke (3), and may be linked to reduced back injury (4). On average, physically active people outlive those who are inactive (5). Regular physical activity can also help to maintain the functional independence of older adults and enhance the quality of life for people of all ages (6).

Of the 12 Physical Activity and Fitness objectives, one has been met (objective 1.10), four show progress toward the year 2000 targets (1.1, 1.3, 1.4, and 1.6) while two are moving away from the targets (1.2 and 1.7). Data for one objective (1.5), show no change, and data to update progress for the remaining four objectives (1.8, 1.9, 1.11, and 1.12) are not yet available. Trends for special population subgroups are mixed. The decline in coronary heart disease mortality has been slower in the black population than in the total population. For objective 1.4 (vigorous physical activity), 1991 data indicate that the target for adults with annual incomes of less than $20,000 has been surpassed. The proportion of adults with a sedentary lifestyle may be increasing among the total population, although it has declined among people 65 years of age and over and people with disabilities.

Data Issues

Definitions

Physical activity and fitness as a recognized risk factor for health outcomes is a relatively new concept, contributing to present difficulties in

tracking some objectives. Calculations vary from simple counts (for example, weight-training 3 or more times a week) to complex formulas (for example, calculating average kilocalories expended per kilogram per day) (7). The intent of objective 1.3 (light to moderate physical activity) is to generate calorie-burning activity from a health standpoint by emphasizing the importance of regular physical activity that can be sustained throughout the lifespan. The sum of all physical activities performed at least 30 minutes per occasion 5 or more or 7 or more times a week regardless of the intensity has been defined as measuring this objective.

To measure the proportion of adults performing vigorous physical activity (1.4), the predicted maximum

cardiorespiratory capacity was estimated using age-sex based regression equations and then multiplying by 50 percent (see Note with the text of objective 1.4). Then all the activities that were performed for at least 20 minutes that had a kilocalorie value that was equal to or greater than that 50 percent level were counted (8,9). The estimated number of people who exercise vigorously were respondents who performed these activities 3 or more times per week.

Comparability of Data Sources

The baseline data source for objective 1.3 was the Behavioral Risk Factor Surveillance System; because this objective will be tracked with the National Health Interview Survey

Figure 7. Persons 18–74 years of age who engage in light to moderate physical activity for at least 30 minutes per occasion 5 or more times per week: United States, 1985, 1990, 1991, and year 2000 target for objective 1.3

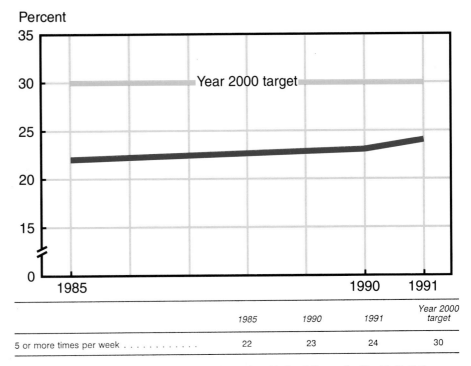

	1985	1990	1991	Year 2000 target
5 or more times per week	22	23	24	30

SOURCE: Centers for Disease Control and Prevention, National Center for Health Statistics, National Health Interview Survey.

(NHIS), and 1985 data were available from this survey, the baseline has been revised to reflect the estimates from the NHIS. The method of measuring the objective has also been modified from that used in the baseline measure, although the revised estimate did not differ for people exercising 5 or more times per week. Although data from the NHIS were used for all 3 years (1985, 90 and 91), the questionnaire changed in 1991. Databases were made as similar as possible before estimates were made.

Objectives 1.3, 1.4, 1.6, 1.8, and 1.9 for children and adolescents will be tracked with the Youth Risk Behavior Survey (YRBS) for students in grades 9–12. Although baseline and tracking data are available for objectives 1.4, 1.8, and 1.9, trends for these objectives cannot currently be ascertained for this age group because the baseline data were for other age groups and from other sources.

Proxy Measures

In late 1993 data comparable to the baseline on measured overweight will be available from the National Health and Nutrition Examination Survey III to measure progress. As an interim measure, self-reported overweight from the National Health Interview Survey (NHIS) is being used for objective 1.2. In comparisons of measured and self-reported heights and weights, women underestimate overweight and overestimate underweight, while men underestimate overweight and underweight (10,11).

Regular performance of physical activities that enhance and maintain muscular strength, muscular endurance, and flexibility (1.6) most likely requires participation in a variety of physical activities as not all activities will satisfy all three factors. However, scoring parameters for strength, endurance, and flexibility are not yet available. Until research into these areas can provide such measures, for adults this objective will be tracked using data on an activity that increases muscular strength only—weight-lifting. The 1991 data shown for students in grades 9–12 are based on self-reported participation in stretching exercises or

strengthening exercises that were done 4 or more days per week.

Objective 1.7 is to increase to at least 50 percent the proportion of overweight people who use sound dietary practices combined with regular physical activity to attain appropriate body weight. Respondents who reported they were overweight and were currently trying to lose weight or control their weight by eating fewer calories or exercising more were counted for this objective. However, an assessment of the quality of dietary practices has not yet been coupled with a measure of regular physical activity. The design of the questions used to track this objective changed between 1990 and 1991, and may have effected the estimates.

Objective 1.9 targets time spent in school physical education classes devoted to activities that may be readily carried into adulthood because their performance requires only one or two people (such as swimming, bicycling, jogging, and racquet sports). The proxy measure for this objective is the percent of class time spent in actual physical activity. The data used to track this objective are not comparable. 1983 data show the percent of physical education class time spent being physically active for all students. The YRBS updates, for students in grades 9–12, show the percent who exercised 20 or more minutes in physical education class 3–5 times a week in 1990, and the percent who exercised 30 or more minutes in physical education class 1 or more times a week in 1991.

Table 1. Physical activity and fitness objective status

Objective	1987 baseline Original	1987 baseline Revised	1990	1991	Target 2000
1.1 **Coronary heart disease deaths (age adjusted per 100,000)**	135	[1]No change	122	– – –	100
a. Blacks (age adjusted per 100,000)	163	[1]168	158	– – –	115
1.2 **Overweight prevalence**					
People 20 years and over....................................	[2]26%	. . .	27%	28%	20%
Males..	[2]24%	. . .	27%	28%	. . .
Females..	[2]27%	. . .	27%	28%	. . .
Adolescents 12–19 years	[2]15%	. . .	– – –	– – –	15%
a. Low-income females 20 years and over	[2]37%	. . .	37%	39%	25%
b. Black females 20 years and over........................	[2]44%	. . .	42%	44%	30%
c. Hispanic females 20 years and over	. . .	[3]27%	33%	32%	25%
Mexican-American females	[4]39%	. . .	– – –	38%	. . .
Cuban females....................................	[4]34%	. . .	– – –	– – –	. . .
Puerto Rican females..............................	[4]37%	. . .	– – –	– – –	. . .
d. American Indians/Alaska Natives........................	[5]29–75%	. . .	– – –	40%	30%
e. People with disabilities.................................	[3]36%	. . .	– – –	38%	25%
f. Females with high blood pressure........................	[2]50%	. . .	– – –	– – –	41%
g. Males with high blood pressure..........................	[2]39%	. . .	– – –	– – –	35%
1.3 **Moderate physical activity**					
People 6 years and over......................................	– – –	. . .	– – –	– – –	30%
People 18–74 years					
5 or more times per week...................................	[3]22%	[3,6]No change	23%	24%	. . .
7 or more times per week...................................	[3]12%	[3,6]16%	16%	17%	. . .
1.4 **Vigorous physical activity**					
Children and adolescents 6–17 years	– – –	. . .	– – –	– – –	75%
Children and adolescents 10–17 years	[7]66%	. . .	– – –	– – –	. . .
Students in 9th–12th grade	– – –	. . .	37%	– – –	. . .
People 18 years and over.....................................	[3]12%	. . .	– – –	14%	20%
a. Lower-income people 18 years and over (annual family income less than $20,000)	[3]7%	. . .	– – –	13%	12%
1.5 **Sedentary lifestyle**					
People 6 years and over......................................	– – –	. . .	– – –	– – –	15%
People 18 years and over.....................................	[3]24%	. . .	– – –	24%	15%
a. People 65 years and over	[3]43%	. . .	– – –	29%	22%
b. People with disabilities.................................	[3]35%	. . .	– – –	30%	20%
c. Lower-income people (annual family income less than $20,000)	[3]32%	. . .	– – –	32%	17%
1.6 **Muscular strength, endurance, and flexibility**					
People 6 years and over......................................	– – –	. . .	– – –	– – –	40%
Students in 9th–12th grade					
Stretching 4 or more times per week......................	. . .	. . .	– – –	43%	. . .
Strengthening 4 or more times per week...................	. . .	. . .	– – –	37%	. . .
Weight-lifting					
People 18–64 years....................................	. . .	[8]11%	– – –	16%	. . .
1.7 **Weight loss practices among overweight people 12 years and over.**	– – –	. . .	– – –	– – –	50%
Overweight females 18 years and over	[3]30%	. . .	29%	22%	. . .
Overweight males 18 years and over........................	[3]25%	. . .	22%	19%	. . .
1.8 **Daily school physical education**					
Students in 1st–12th grade	[9]36%	. . .	– – –	– – –	50%
Students in 9th–12th grade	. . .	. . .	– – –	42%	. . .
1.9 **School physical education quality**					
All students...	[10]27%	. . .	– – –	– – –	50%
Students in 9th–12th grade	. . .	. . .	[11]33%	[12]49%	. . .
1.10 **Worksite fitness programs**					
50–99 employees	[3]14%	. . .	– – –	[13]33%	20%
100–249 employees	[3]23%	. . .	– – –	[13]47%	35%
250–749 employees	[3]32%	. . .	– – –	[13]66%	50%
750 and more employees....................................	[3]54%	. . .	– – –	[13]83%	80%
1.11 **Community fitness facilities**					
Hiking, biking, and fitness trail miles	[14]1 per 71,000 people	. . .	– – –	– – –	1 per 10,000 people

Table 1. Physical activity and fitness objective status—Con.

Objective	1987 baseline Original	1987 baseline Revised	1990	1991	Target 2000
Public swimming pools...	[14]1 per 53,000 people	. . .	- - -	- - -	1 per 25,000 people
Acres of park and recreation open space	[14]1.8 per 1,000 people	. . .	- - -	- - -	4 per 1,000 people
1.12 Clinician counseling about physical activity					
Percent of sedentary patients..................................	[15]30%	. . .	- - -	- - -	50%

[1]Data have been recomputed to reflect revised intercensal population estimates; see *Health, United States, 1992,* Appendix I.
[2]1976–80 data.
[3]1985 data.
[4]1982–84 data.
[5]1984–88 data for different tribes.
[6]Data source has been changed and data have been revised to reflect updated methodology; see Introduction.
[7]1984 data.
[8]1990 data.
[9]1984–86 data.
[10]1983 data.
[11]Percent who exercised 20 or more minutes in physical education class 3–5 times per week.
[12]Percent who exercised 30 or more minutes in physical education class 1 or more times per week.
[13]1992 data.
[14]1986 data.
[15]1988 data.

NOTE: Data sources are in table C.

Physical Activity and Fitness Objectives

1.1*: Reduce coronary heart disease deaths to no more than 100 per 100,000 people.

Duplicate objectives: 2.1, 3.1, and 15.1

> **1.1a***: Reduce coronary heart disease deaths among blacks to no more than 115 per 100,000.

Duplicate objectives: 2.1a, 3.1a, and 15.1a

1.2*: Reduce overweight to a prevalence of no more than 20 percent among people aged 20 and older and no more than 15 percent among adolescents aged 12–19.

NOTE: For people aged 20 and older, overweight is defined as body mass index (BMI) equal to or greater than 27.8 for men and 27.3 for women. For adolescents, overweight is defined as BMI equal to or greater than 23.0 for males aged 12–14, 24.3 for males aged 15–17, 25.8 for males aged 18–19, 23.4 for females aged 12–14, 24.8 for females aged 15–17, and 25.7 for females aged 18–19. The values for adolescents are the age- and sex-specific 85th percentile values of the 1976–80 National Health and Nutrition Examination Survey (NHANES II), corrected for sample variation. BMI is calculated by dividing weight in kilograms by the square of height in meters. The cut points used to define overweight approximate the 120 percent of desirable body weight definition used in the 1990 objectives.

Duplicate objectives: 2.3, 15.10, and 17.12

> **1.2a***: Reduce overweight to a prevalence of no more than 25 percent among low-income women aged 20 and older.

Duplicate objectives: 2.3a, 15.10a, and 17.12a

> **1.2b***: Reduce overweight to a prevalence of no more than 30 percent among black women aged 20 and older.

Duplicate objectives: 2.3b, 15.10b, and 17.12b

> **1.2c***: Reduce overweight to a prevalence of no more than 25 percent among Hispanic women aged 20 and older.

Duplicate objectives: 2.3c, 15.10c, and 17.12c

> **1.2d***: Reduce overweight to a prevalence of no more than 30 percent among American Indians and Alaska Natives.

Duplicate objectives: 2.3d, 15.10d, and 17.12d

> **1.2e***: Reduce overweight to a prevalence of no more than 25 percent among people with disabilities.

Duplicate objectives: 2.3e, 15.10e, and 17.12e

> **1.2f***: Reduce overweight to a prevalence of no more than 41 percent among women with high blood pressure.

Duplicate objectives: 2.3f, 15.10f, and 17.12f

> **1.2g***: Reduce overweight to a prevalence of no more than 35 percent among men with high blood pressure.

Duplicate objectives: 2.3g, 15.10g, and 17.12g

1.3*: Increase to at least 30 percent the proportion of people aged 6 and older who engage regularly, preferably daily, in light to moderate physical activity for at least 30 minutes per day.

NOTE: Light to moderate physical activity is activity that requires sustained, rhythmic muscular movements, is at least equivalent to sustained walking, and is performed at less than 60 percent of maximum heart rate for age. Maximum heart rate equals roughly 220 beats per minute minus age. Examples may include walking, swimming, cycling, and dancing; gardening and yardwork; various domestic and occupational activities; and games and other childhood pursuits.

Duplicate objectives: 15.11 and 17.13

1.4: Increase to at least 20 percent the proportion of people aged 18 and older and to at least 75 percent the proportion of children and adolescents aged 6–17 who engage in vigorous physical activity that promotes the development and maintenance of cardiorespiratory fitness 3 or more days per week for 20 or more minutes per occasion.

NOTE: Vigorous physical activities are rhythmic, repetitive physical activities that use large muscle groups at 60 percent or more of maximum heart rate for age. An exercise heart rate of 60 percent of maximum heart rate for age is about 50 percent of maximal cardiorespiratory capacity and is sufficient for cardiorespiratory conditioning. Maximum heart rate equals roughly 220 beats per minute minus age.

> **1.4a**: Increase to at least 12 percent the proportion of lower-income people aged 18 and older (annual family income less than $20,000) who engage in vigorous physical activity that promotes the development and maintenance of cardiorespiratory fitness 3 or more days per week for 20 or more minutes per occasion.

1.5: Reduce to no more than 15 percent the proportion of people aged 6 and older who engage in no leisure-time physical activity.

NOTE: For this objective, people with disabilities are people who report any limitation in activity due to chronic conditions.

> **1.5a**: Reduce to no more than 22 percent the proportion of people aged 65 and older who engage in no leisure-time physical activity.

> **1.5b**: Reduce to no more than 20 percent the proportion of people with disabilities who engage in no leisure-time physical activity.

> **1.5c**: Reduce to no more than 17 percent the proportion of lower-income people aged 18 and older (annual family income less than $20,000) who engage in no leisure-time physical activity.

1.6: Increase to at least 40 percent the proportion of people aged 6 and older who regularly perform physical activities that enhance and maintain muscular strength, muscular endurance, and flexibility.

1.7*: Increase to at least 50 percent the proportion of overweight people aged 12 and older who have adopted sound dietary practices combined with regular physical activity to attain an appropriate body weight.

Duplicate objective: 2.7:

1.8: Increase to at least 50 percent the proportion of children and adolescents in 1st–12th grade who participate in daily school physical education.

1.9: Increase to at least 50 percent the proportion of school physical education class time that students spend being physically active, preferably engaged in lifetime physical activities.

NOTE: Lifetime activities are activities that may be readily carried into adulthood because they generally need only one or two people. Examples include swimming, bicycling, jogging, and racquet sports. Also counted as lifetime activities are vigorous social activities such as dancing. Competitive group sports and activities typically played only by young children such as group games are excluded.

1.10: Increase the proportion of worksites offering employer-sponsored physical activity and fitness programs as follows:

Worksites with —	2000 target (percent)
50–99 employees	20
100–249 employees	35
250–749 employees	50
750 or more employees	80

1.11: Increase community availability and accessibility of physical activity and fitness facilities as follows:

Hiking, biking, and fitness trail miles: 1 per 10,000 people

Public swimming pools: 1 per 25,000 people

Acres of park and recreation open space: 4 per 1,000 people (250 people per managed acre)

1.12: Increase to at least 50 percent the proportion of primary care providers who routinely assess and counsel their patients regarding the frequency, duration, type, and intensity of each patient's physical activity practices.

*Duplicate objective.

References

1. Harris SS, Caspersen CJ, DeFriese GH, Estes EH. Physical activity counseling for healthy adults as a primary preventive intervention in the clinical setting. JAMA 261: 3590–8. 1989.

2. Powell KE, Caspersen CJ, Koplan JP, Ford ES. Physical activity and chronic disease. Amer J Clin Nut 49: 999–1006. 1989.

3. Salonen JT, Puska P, Tuomilehto J. Physical activity and risk of myocardial infarction, cerebral stroke and death: A longitudinal study in Eastern Finland. Amer J Epidemiol 115: 526–37. 1982.

4. Cady LD, Bischoff DP, O'Connell ER, et al. Strength and fitness and subsequent back injuries in firefighters. J Occup Med 21: 269–72. 1979.

5. Paffenbarger RS, Hyde RT, Wing AL, Hsieh CC. Physical activity, all-cause mortality, and longevity of college alumni. N Engl J Med 314: 605–13. 1986.

6. Katz S, Branch LG, Branson MH, et al. Active life expectancy. N Engl J Med 309: 1218–24. 1983.

7. Schoenborn CA. Health habits of U.S. adults, 1985: The "Alameda 7" revisited. Public Health Rep 101:571–8. 1988.

8. Stephens T, Craig CL. Fitness and activity measurement in the 1981 Canada Fitness Survey, in Thomas F. Drury, ed. Assessing physical fitness and physical activity in population-based surveys. National Center for Health Statistics. Hyattsville, Maryland: 401–32. 1989.

9. Ainsworth BE, et al. Compendium of physical activities: classification of energy costs of human physical activities. Med and Sci and Sports and Exercise 25(1):71–80. 1993.

10. Rowland ML. Reporting bias in height and weight data. Stat Bull 70(2): 2–11. 1989.

11. Rowland ML. Self-reported weight and height. Am J Clin Nutr 52: 1125–33. 1990.

Priority Area 2
Nutrition

Background and Data Summary

Dietary factors contribute substantially to preventable illness and premature death in the United States. For the majority of adults who do not smoke and do not drink excessively, what they eat is the most significant controllable risk factor affecting their long-term health (1). Five leading causes of death are associated with dietary factors: coronary heart disease, some types of cancer, stroke, noninsulin-dependent diabetes mellitus, and coronary artery disease (2). In general, once-prevalent nutrient deficiencies have been replaced by excesses and imbalances of other food components in the diet. Malnutrition still occurs in some groups of people, however, including those who are isolated or economically deprived.

Of the 21 objectives in this area, progress toward the targets has been made on five (objectives 2.1, 2.4, 2.13, 2.16, and 2.20). Coronary heart disease mortality continues to decline, although the decline is less marked among black Americans. Growth retardation among the high risk subpopulations has decreased, although data for all low income children 5 years and under are not available. More people are examining food labels when purchasing food, and an increased proportion of restaurants are offering low-fat and low-calorie selections. Additionally, the proportion of worksites with 50 or more employees that offer nutrition education and/or weight management programs for employees has increased.

Baselines have been obtained for two objectives (2.12 and 2.18). The new baseline for objective 2.12b (appropriate baby bottle feeding practices among American Indians and Alaska Natives) appears to indicate that the target of 65 percent has been exceeded. See definition of preventive bottle feeding practices (2.12) in priority area 13, duplicate objective 13.11.

Four objectives moved away from the target: cancer mortality (2.2), the

proportion of the population that is overweight (2.3), the percent of overweight people engaging in weight-loss practices (2.7), and the proportion of breastfeeding mothers (2.11). Dietary fat intake has remained stable (2.5). Progress has been mixed for the proportion of people limiting their salt and sodium intake (2.9).

Five nutrition objectives have no new data (2.6, 2.8, 2.10 excluding 2.10e, 2.15, and 2.21), and three objectives do not yet have complete baseline data (2.14, 2.17, and 2.19).

Data from the third National Health and Nutrition Examination Survey (NHANES III) will provide estimates for objectives 2.6, 2.8, and 2.10.

Figure 8. Overweight adults 20–74 years of age according to selected characteristics targeted by year 2000 objective 2.3: United States, 1991

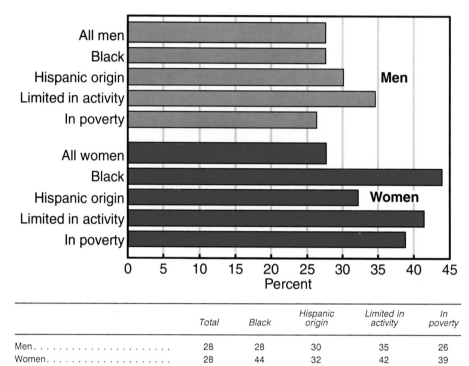

	Total	Black	Hispanic origin	Limited in activity	In poverty
Men....................	28	28	30	35	26
Women..................	28	44	32	42	39

NOTE: Overweight is defined for men as body mass index greater than or equal to 27.8 kilograms/meter and for women as 27.3 kilograms/meter. Weights and heights were self-reported. A related table in *Health, United States, 1992,* is 73.

SOURCE: Centers for Disease Control and Prevention, National Center for Health Statistics, National Health Interview Survey.

Data Issues

Comparability of Data Sources

The evaluation of trends in dietary intake is affected by food composition data base changes and food coding decisions made during or between surveys. Trend data for two nutrition objectives have been obtained from different surveys with different methodologies or changes in method administration (2.3 and 2.9). Different food composition data bases were used over time for objective 2.5, although the method was primarily the same. Data for objective 2.7 were obtained from the same survey that asked a different set of questions in different years (see discussion of duplicate objective 1.7 in priority area 1).

Tracking can also be affected by changing the population from which the survey sample is drawn. Growth retardation among low-income children (2.4) is tracked by the Pediatric Nutrition Surveillance System (PedNSS). PedNSS covered 41 States in 1988 and 46 States in 1991, with plans to expand coverage. The addition of States could affect the comparability of future results.

Proxy Measures

Objective 2.3 (overweight) and 2.5 (dietary fat intake) will be measured by NHANES III. Until these data are available, self-reported data from the National Health Interview Survey for objective 2.3 and provisional estimates from the 1989 Continuing Survey of Food Intakes of Individuals for objective 2.5 are being used for tracking. The comparability of measured overweight and self-reported overweight (2.3) is discussed in priority area 1 (duplicate objective 1.2).

Table 2. Nutrition objective status

Objective	1987 baseline Original	1987 baseline Revised	1990	1991	Target 2000
2.1 Coronary heart disease deaths (age adjusted per 100,000)	[1]135	[1,2]No change	122	- - -	100
a. Blacks (age adjusted per 100,000)	[1]163	[1,2]168	158	- - -	115
2.2 Cancer deaths (age adjusted per 100,000)	[1]133	[1,2]134	135	- - -	130
2.3 Overweight prevalence					
People 20 years and over....................................	[3]26%	. . .	27%	28%	20%
Males..	[3]24%	. . .	27%	28%	. . .
Females..	[3]27%	. . .	27%	28%	. . .
Adolescents 12–19 years	[3]15%	. . .	- - -	- - -	15%
a. Low-income females 20 years and over	[3]37%	. . .	37%	39%	25%
b. Black females 20 years and over..........................	[3]44%	. . .	42%	44%	30%
c. Hispanic females 20 years and over	. . .	[4]27%	33%	32%	25%
Mexican-American females	[5]39%	. . .	- - -	38%	. . .
Cuban females..	[5]34%	. . .	- - -	- - -	. . .
Puerto Rican females..................................	[5]37%	. . .	- - -	- - -	. . .
d. American Indians/Alaska Natives	[6]29–75%	. . .	- - -	40%	30%
e. People with disabilities	[4]36%	. . .	- - -	38%	25%
f. Females with high blood pressure	[3]50%	. . .	- - -	- - -	41%
g. Males with high blood pressure..........................	[3]39%	. . .	- - -	- - -	35%
2.4 Growth retardation among low income children 5 years and under....	[7]16%	. . .	- - -	- - -	10%
a. Low-income black children under 1 year....................	[7]15%	. . .	15%	15%	10%
b. Low-income Hispanic children under 1 year	[7]13%	. . .	9%	8%	10%
c. Low-income Hispanic children 1 year	[7]16%	. . .	12%	11%	10%
d. Low-income Asian/Pacific Islander children 1 year	[7]14%	. . .	14%	13%	10%
e. Low-income Asian/Pacific Islander children age 2–4 years.............	[7]16%	. . .	14%	12%	10%
2.5 Dietary fat intake among people 2 years and over					
Percent of calories from total fat...........................	- - -	. . .	- - -	- - -	30%
Percent of calories from saturated fat.......................	- - -	. . .	- - -	- - -	10%
People 20–74 years					
Percent of calories from total fat...........................	[3]36%	. . .	[8]36%	- - -	. . .
Percent of calories from saturated fat.......................	[3]13%	. . .	[8]13%	- - -	. . .
Females 19–50 years					
Percent of calories from total fat...........................	[4]36%	. . .	- - -	- - -	. . .
Percent of calories from saturated fat.......................	[4]13%	. . .	- - -	- - -	. . .
2.6 Daily intake of vegetables, fruits, and grain products					
Adults (number of servings)					
Vegetables and fruits..	- - -	. . .	- - -	- - -	5.0
Grain products..	- - -	. . .	- - -	- - -	6.0
Females 19–50 years (number of servings)					
Vegetables and fruits..	[9]2.5	. . .	- - -	- - -	. . .
Grain products..	[9]3.0	. . .	- - -	- - -	. . .
2.7 Weight loss practices among overweight people 12 years and over...	- - -	. . .	- - -	- - -	50%
Overweight females 18 years and over	[4]30%	. . .	29%	22%	. . .
Overweight males 18 years and over..........................	[4]25%	. . .	22%	19%	. . .
2.8 Calcium intake					
3 or more servings daily.....................................					
People 12–24 years..	- - -	. . .	- - -	- - -	50%
Males 19–24 years	[9]14%	. . .	- - -	- - -	. . .
Females 19–24 years	[9]7%	. . .	- - -	- - -	. . .
Pregnant and lactating females	[9]24%	. . .	- - -	- - -	50%
2 or more servings daily					
People 25 years and over..................................	- - -	. . .	- - -	- - -	50%
Males 25–50 years	[9]23%	. . .	- - -	- - -	. . .
Females 25–50 years	[9]15%	. . .	- - -	- - -	. . .
2.9 Salt and sodium intake					
Prepare foods without adding salt	[4]54%	. . .	- - -	- - -	65%
Adults who avoid using salt at table..........................	[4]68%	. . .	- - -	55%	80%
Adults who regularly purchase foods lower in sodium	[7]20%	. . .	- - -	36%	40%
2.10 Iron deficiency					
Children 1–4 years	- - -	. . .	- - -	- - -	3%
Children 1–2 years	[3]9%	. . .	- - -	- - -	3%

Table 2. Nutrition objective status—Con.

Objective	1987 baseline Original	1987 baseline Revised	1990	1991	Target 2000
Children 3–4 years	[3]4%	...	– – –	– – –	3%
Females of childbearing age (20–44 years)	[3]5%	...	– – –	– – –	3%
Iron deficiency prevalence					
a. Low-income children 1–2 years	[3]21%	...	– – –	– – –	10%
b. Low-income children 3–4 years	[3]10%	...	– – –	– – –	5%
c. Low-income females 20–44 years	[3]8%	...	– – –	– – –	4%
Anemia Prevalence					
d. Alaska Native children 1–5 years	[10]22–28%	...	– – –	– – –	10%
e. Black, low-income pregnant females 15–44 years (third trimester)	[7]41%	...	41%	30%	20%
2.11 Breastfeeding					
During early postpartum period	[7]54%	...	52%	53%	75%
a. Low-income mothers	[7]32%	...	35%	33%	75%
b. Black mothers	[7]25%	...	16%	26%	75%
c. Hispanic mothers	[7]51%	...	44%	52%	75%
d. American Indian/Alaska Native mothers	[7]47%	...	47%	46%	75%
At age 5–6 months	[7]21%	...	18%	18%	50%
a. Low-income mothers	[7]9%	...	8%	9%	50%
b. Black mothers	[7]8%	...	7%	7%	50%
c. Hispanic mothers	[7]16%	...	14%	16%	50%
d. American Indian/Alaska Native mothers	[7]28%	...	27%	22%	50%
2.12 Baby bottle tooth decay					
Parents and caregivers who use preventive feeding practices	...	[11]51%	– – –	– – –	75%
a. Parents and caregivers with less than high school education	...	[11]31%	– – –	– – –	65%
b. American Indian/Alaska Native parents and caregivers	...	[12]74%	– – –	– – –	65%
2.13 Use of food labels	[7]74%	...	76%	– – –	85%
2.14 Informative nutrition labeling					
Processed foods	[7]60%	...	– – –	– – –	100%
Fresh and carry-away foods	– – –	...	– – –	– – –	40%
2.15 Availability of reduced-fat processed foods	[13]2,500	...	– – –	– – –	5,000
2.16 Low-fat, low-calorie restaurant food choices	[8]70%	...	75%	– – –	90%
2.17 Nutritious school and child care food services	– – –	...	– – –	– – –	90%
2.18 Home-delivered meals for older adults	...	[11]7%	– – –	– – –	80%
2.19 Nutrition education in schools	– – –	...	– – –	– – –	75%
2.20 Worksite nutrition/weight management programs					
Nutrition education	[4]17%	...	– – –	[14]31%	50%
Weight control	[4]15%	...	– – –	[14]24%	50%
2.21 Nutrition assessment, counseling, and referral by clinicians	[7]40–50%	...	– – –	– – –	75%

[1]1987 data.
[2]Data have been recomputed to reflect revised intercensal population estimates; see *Health, United States, 1992,* Appendix I.
[3]1976–80 data.
[4]1985 data.
[5]1982–84 data.
[6]1984–88 data for different tribes.
[7]1988 data.
[8]1989 data.
[9]1985–86 data.
[10]1983–85 data.
[11]1991 data.
[12]1985–89 data.
[13]1986 data.
[14]1992 data.

NOTE: Data sources are in table C.

Nutrition Objectives

2.1*: Reduce coronary heart disease deaths to no more than 100 per 100,000 people.

Duplicate objectives: 1.1, 3.1, and 15.1

> **2.1a***: Reduce coronary heart disease deaths among blacks to no more than 115 per 100,000 people.

Duplicate objectives: 1.1a, 3.1a, and 15.1a

2.2*: Reverse the rise in cancer deaths to achieve a rate of no more than 130 per 100,000 people.

NOTE: In its publications, the National Cancer Institute age adjusts cancer death rates to the 1970 U.S. population. Using the 1970 standard, the equivalent target value for this objective would be 175 per 100,000.

Duplicate objective: 16.1

2.3*: Reduce overweight to a prevalence of no more than 20 percent among people aged 20 and older and no more than 15 percent among adolescents aged 12–19.

NOTE: For people aged 20 and older, overweight is defined as body mass index (BMI) equal to or greater than 27.8 for men and 27.3 for women. For adolescents, overweight is defined as BMI equal to or greater than 23.0 for males aged 12–14, 24.3 for males aged 15–17, 25.8 for males aged 18–19, 23.4 for females aged 12–14, 24.8 for females aged 15–17, and 25.7 for females aged 18–19. The values for adolescents are the age- and sex-specific 85th percentile values of the 1976–80 National Health and Nutrition Examination Survey (NHANES II), corrected for sample variation. BMI is calculated by dividing weight in kilograms by the square of height in meters. The cut points used to define overweight approximate the 120 percent of desirable body weight definition used in the 1990 objectives.

Duplicate objectives: 1.2, 15.10, and 17.12

> **2.3a***: Reduce overweight to a prevalence of no more than 25 percent among low-income women aged 20 and older.

Duplicate objectives: 1.2a, 15.10a, and 17.12a

> **2.3b***: Reduce overweight to a prevalence of no more than 30 percent among black women aged 20 and older.

Duplicate objectives: 1.2b, 15.10b, and 17.12b

> **2.3c***: Reduce overweight to a prevalence of no more than 25 percent among Hispanic women aged 20 and older.

Duplicate objectives: 1.2c, 15.10c, and 17.12c

> **2.3d***: Reduce overweight to a prevalence of no more than 30 percent among American Indians and Alaska Natives.

Duplicate objectives: 1.2d, 15.10d, and 17.12d

> **2.3e***: Reduce overweight to a prevalence of no more than 25 percent among people with disabilities.

Duplicate objectives: 1.2e, 15.10e, and 17.12e

> **2.3f***: Reduce overweight to a prevalence of no more than 41 percent among women with high blood pressure.

Duplicate objectives: 1.2f, 15.10f, and 17.12f

> **2.3g***: Reduce overweight to a prevalence of no more than 35 percent among men with high blood pressure.

Duplicate objectives: 1.2g, 15.10g, and 17.12g

2.4: Reduce growth retardation among low-income children aged 5 and younger to less than 10 percent.

NOTE: Growth retardation is defined as height-for-age below the fifth percentile of children in the National Center for Health Statistics' reference population.

> **2.4a**: Reduce growth retardation among low-income black children younger than age 1 to less than 10 percent.
>
> **2.4b**: Reduce growth retardation among low-income Hispanic children younger than age 1 to less than 10 percent.
>
> **2.4c**: Reduce growth retardation among low-income Hispanic children aged 1 to less than 10 percent.
>
> **2.4d**: Reduce growth retardation among low-income Asian and Pacific Islander children aged 1 to less than 10 percent.
>
> **2.4e**: Reduce growth retardation among low-income Asian and Pacific Islander children aged 2–4 to less than 10 percent.

2.5*: Reduce dietary fat intake to an average of 30 percent of calories or less and average saturated fat intake to less than 10 percent of calories among people aged 2 and older.

Duplicate objectives: 15.9 and 16.7

2.6*: Increase complex carbohydrate and fiber-containing foods in the diets of adults to five or more daily servings for vegetables (including legumes) and fruits, and to six or more daily servings for grain products.

Duplicate objective: 16.8

2.7*: Increase to at least 50 percent the proportion of overweight people aged 12 and older who have adopted sound dietary practices combined with regular physical activity to attain an appropriate body weight.

Duplicate objective: 1.7

2.8: Increase calcium intake so at least 50 percent of youth aged 12–24 and 50 percent of pregnant and lactating women consume three or more servings daily of foods rich in calcium, and at least 50 percent of people aged 25 and older consume two or more servings daily.

NOTE: The number of servings of foods rich in calcium is based on milk and milk products. A serving is considered to be 1 cup of skim milk or its equivalent in calcium (302 mg). The number of servings in this objective will generally provide approximately three-fourths of the 1989 Recommended Dietary Allowance (RDA) of calcium. The RDA is 1200 mg for people aged 12 through 24 years, 800 mg for people aged 25 and older, and 1200 mg for pregnant and lactating women.

2.9: Decrease salt and sodium intake so at least 65 percent of home meal preparers prepare foods without adding salt, at least 80 percent of people avoid using salt at the table, and at least 40 percent of adults regularly purchase foods modified or lower in sodium.

2.10: Reduce iron deficiency to less than 3 percent among children aged 1 through 4 and among women of childbearing age.

NOTE: Iron deficiency is defined as having abnormal results for two or more of the following tests: mean corpuscular volume, erythrocyte protoporphryn, and transferrin saturation. Anemia is used as an index of iron deficiency. Anemia among Alaska Native children and among pregnant women in the third trimester was defined as hemoglobin less than 11 gm/dL or hematocrit less than 33 percent. For children and pregnant women, hematology is adjusted for altitude. In pregnant and non-pregnant women, hematology is also adjusted for smoking status. The above prevalences of iron deficiency and anemia may be due to inadequate dietary iron intakes or to inflammatory conditions and infections. For anemia, genetics may also be a factor.

2.10a: Reduce iron deficiency to less than 10 percent among low-income children aged 1–2.

2.10b: Reduce iron deficiency to less than 5 percent among low-income children aged 3–4.

2.10c: Reduce iron deficiency to less than 4 percent among low-income women of childbearing age.

2.10d: Reduce the prevalence of anemia to less than 10 percent among Alaska Native children aged 1–5.

2.10e: Reduce the prevalence of anemia to less than 20 percent among black, low-income pregnant women (third trimester).

2.11*: Increase to at least 75 percent the proportion of mothers who breastfeed their babies in the early postpartum period and to at least 50 percent the proportion who continue breastfeeding until their babies are 5 to 6 months old.

Duplicate objective: 14.9

2.11a*: Increase to at least 75 percent the proportion of low-income mothers who breastfeed their babies in the early postpartum period and to at least 50 percent the proportion who continue breastfeeding until their babies are 5 to 6 months old.

Duplicate objective: 14.9a

2.11b*: Increase to at least 75 percent the proportion of black mothers who breastfeed their babies in the early postpartum period and to at least 50 percent the proportion who continue breastfeeding until their babies are 5 to 6 months old.

Duplicate objective: 14.9b

2.11c*: Increase to at least 75 percent the proportion of Hispanic mothers who breastfeed their babies in the early postpartum period and to at least 50 percent the proportion who continue breastfeeding until their babies are 5 to 6 months old.

Duplicate objective: 14.9c

2.11d*: Increase to at least 75 percent the proportion of American Indian and Alaska Native mothers who breastfeed their babies in the early postpartum period and to at least 50 percent the proportion who continue breastfeeding until their babies are 5 to 6 months old.

Duplicate objective: 14.9d

2.12*: Increase to at least 75 percent the proportion of parents and caregivers who use feeding practices that prevent baby bottle tooth decay.

Duplicate objective: 13.11

2.12a*: Increase to at least 65 percent the proportion of parents and caregivers with less than a high school education who use feeding practices that prevent baby bottle tooth decay.

Duplicate objective: 13.11a

2.12b*: Increase to at least 65 percent the proportion of American Indian and Alaska Native parents and caregivers who use feeding practices that prevent baby bottle tooth decay.

Duplicate objective: 13.11b

2.13: Increase to at least 85 percent the proportion of people aged 18 and older who use food labels to make nutritious food selections.

2.14: Achieve useful and informative nutrition labeling for virtually all processed foods and at least 40 percent of fresh meats, poultry, fish, fruits, vegetables, baked goods, and ready-to-eat carry-away foods.

2.15: Increase to at least 5,000 brand items the availability of processed food products that are reduced in fat and saturated fat.

NOTE: A brand item is defined as a particular flavor and/or size of a specific brand and is typically the consumer unit of purchase.

2.16: Increase to at least 90 percent the proportion of restaurants and institutional food service operations that offer identifiable low-fat, low-calorie food choices, consistent with the Dietary Guidelines for Americans.

2.17: Increase to at least 90 percent the proportion of school lunch and breakfast services and child care food services with menus that are consistent with the nutrition principles in the Dietary Guidelines for Americans.

2.18: Increase to at least 80 percent the receipt of home food services by people aged 65 and older who have difficulty in preparing their own meals or are otherwise in need of home-delivered meals.

2.19: Increase to at least 75 percent the proportion of the Nation's schools that provide nutrition education from preschool–12th grade, preferably as part of quality school health education.

2.20: Increase to at least 50 percent the proportion of worksites with 50 or more employees that offer nutrition education and/or weight management programs for employees.

2.21: Increase to at least 75 percent the proportion of primary care providers who provide nutrition assessment and counseling and/or referral to qualified nutritionists or dietitians.

References

1. U.S. Department of Health and Human Services. The Surgeon General's report on nutrition and health. Washington: Public Health Service. 1988.

2. U.S. Department of Health and Human Services. Healthy people 2000: National health promotion and disease prevention objectives. Washington: Public Health Service. 1991.

Priority Area 3
Tobacco

Background and Data Summary

Tobacco use is responsible for more than one of every six deaths in the United States and is the most important single preventable cause of death and disease in our society (1). Cigarette smoking accounts for about 434,000 deaths yearly (2) including 21 percent of all coronary heart disease deaths, 87 percent of all lung cancer deaths, and 82 percent of all deaths from chronic obstructive pulmonary disease (1).

Smoking contributes substantially to chronic morbidity and disability as well. For example, in 1983–85, chronic bronchitis, emphysema, and lung cancer were the main causes of activity limitation for nearly 4 per 1,000 people in the United States and accounted for nearly 3 percent of all activity limitation (3). Cigarette smoking during pregnancy accounts for 29 to 42 percent of low-birth weight babies (4). Passive or involuntary smoking also causes disease, including lung cancer in healthy nonsmokers and respiratory problems in young children and infants. The prevalence of smoking among adults decreased from 40 percent in 1965 to 26 percent in 1991; however, the decline has been substantially slower among women than among men. The prevalence of smoking also remains disproportionately high among blue-collar workers, military personnel and American Indians and Alaska Natives.

Recent data show some progress towards achieving the objectives in the tobacco priority area. Data for eight objectives (3.1, 3.3, 3.4, 3.5, 3.6, 3.11, 3.12, and 3.13) show improvements toward the year 2000 targets. This includes declining mortality from coronary heart disease (3.1). However, coronary heart disease mortality is declining more slowly among black persons; a substantial decline must occur to achieve the year 2000 target for this population. Objectives 3.2 and 3.3 address slowing the rise of deaths due to lung cancer and chronic obstructive

pulmonary disease. If the current rate of increase in chronic obstructive lung disease mortality is maintained or reduced, the target for objective 3.3 will be met. No progress was observed toward slowing the rise of lung cancer deaths (3.2); nor was progress observed for objective 3.7.

Progress was mixed regarding smokeless tobacco use among youth (3.9). Smokeless tobacco use among adolescents aged 12–17 years declined over the period 1988 to 1991, but increased slightly among young men aged 18–24 years. Data beyond

baseline were not available for five objectives (3.8, 3.10, 3.14, 3.15, and 3.16).

Data Issues

Definitions

The proportion of people aged 20–24 years who smoke cigarettes regularly is used as a proxy measure for initiation of cigarette smoking by children and youth (objective 3.5). A

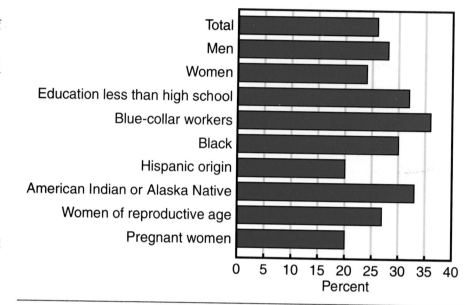

Figure 9. Current cigarette smokers among persons 20 years of age and over, according to selected characteristics targeted by year 2000 objective 3.4: United States, 1991

Characteristics	Percent
Total	26
Men	28
Women	24
Education less than high school	32
Blue-collar workers	36
Black	30
Hispanic origin	20
American Indian or Alaska Native	33
Women 18–44 years	27
Pregnant women	20

NOTE: Related tables in *Health, United States, 1992*, are 64–67.

SOURCE: Centers for Disease Control and Prevention, National Center for Health Statistics, National Health Interview Survey.

regular cigarette smoker is defined as a person who has smoked at least 100 cigarettes and who smokes currently.

The baseline for objective 3.7 (cessation of cigarette smoking early in pregnancy, with abstinence throughout pregnancy) is from a 1986 telephone interview of white women selected from the respondents to the 1985 National Health Interview Survey (NHIS) (5). Beginning with 1991, progress toward the target is being tracked using periodic supplements to the NHIS. The two surveys used different definitions for smoking before pregnancy and for the duration of quitting during pregnancy. The 1991 measure, focused on women who quit during the first trimester, is closer to the objective, but not comparable to the 1986 baseline that counted women who quit any time during pregnancy.

Comparability of Data Sources

Information on objective 3.9 (smokeless tobacco use by males 12–24 years of age) is tracked by a combination of two surveys. Males 12–17 years of age are tracked by the National Household Survey on Drug Abuse (NHSDA). In this survey smokeless tobacco use is defined as any use of snuff or chewing tobacco in the preceding month. For males 18–24 years of age information is obtained from the National Health Interview Survey. A smokeless tobacco user is someone who has used either snuff or chewing tobacco at least 20 times and who currently uses either of these substances. However, information for males 18–25 years of age is also available from the NHSDA using the same definition as for the younger age group. As measured in the NHIS the proportion of men 18–24 years of age using smokeless tobacco increased from 8.9 percent in 1987 to 9.9 percent in 1991. The proportion among men 18–25 years of age was higher and decreased from 1988 to 1991 according to the NHSDA (12.3 percent in 1988 and 11.6 percent in 1991); differences may be due to sampling error.

Table 3. Tobacco objective status

Objective	1987 baseline Original	1987 baseline Revised	1990	1991	Target 2000
3.1 Coronary heart disease deaths (age adjusted per 100,000)	135	[1]No change	122	– – –	100
a. Blacks (age adjusted per 100,000)	163	[1]168	158	– – –	115
3.2 Lung cancer deaths (age adjusted per 100,000)	37.9	[1]38.5	39.9	– – –	42
3.3 Slow the rise in chronic obstructive pulmonary disease deaths (age adjusted per 100,000)	18.7	[1]18.9	19.7	– – –	25
3.4 Cigarette smoking prevalence					
People 20 years and over.	29%	. . .	26%	26%	15%
Males.	32%	. . .	28%	28%	. . .
Females.	27%		23%	24%	. . .
a. People with high school education or less 20 years and over.	34%	. . .	31%	32%	20%
b. Blue-collar workers 20 years and over.	36%	. . .	37%	36%	20%
c. Military personnel.	[2]42%	. . .	– – –	[3]35%	20%
d. Blacks 20 years and over.	34%	. . .	27%	30%	18%
e. Hispanics 20 years and over	[4]33%	. . .	24%	20%	18%
f. American Indians/Alaska Natives	[5]42–70%	. . .	38%	33%	20%
g. Southeast Asian males.	[6]55%	. . .	[7]35%	– – –	20%
h. Females of reproductive age (18–44 years)	29%	. . .	26%	27%	12%
i. Pregnant females	[8]25%	. . .	19%	20%	10%
j. Females who use oral contraceptives.	[9]36%	. . .	[2]26%	– – –	10%
3.5 Smoking initiation by children and adolescents	30%	. . .	26%	24%	15%
a. Lower socioeconomic status people 20–24 years.	40%	. . .	35%	31%	18%
3.6 Smoking cessation attempts	[10]34%	. . .	[11]34%	39%	50%
3.7 Smoking cessation during pregnancy	[8]39%	. . .	– – –	31%	60%
a. Females with less than a high school education.	[8,12]28%	. . .	– – –	21%	45%
3.8 Children's exposure to smoke at home	[10]39%	. . .	– – –	– – –	20%
3.9 Smokeless tobacco use					
Males 12–17 years	[2]6.6%	. . .	– – –	[13]5.3%	4%
Males 18–24 years	[14]8.9%	. . .	– – –	9.9%	4%
a. American Indian/Alaska Native people 18–24 years	[15]18–64%	. . .	– – –	19.7%	10%
3.10 Tobacco-use prevention education and tobacco-free schools					
Tobacco free schools	[2]17%	. . .	– – –	– – –	100%
Tobacco use prevention curricula					
High school level.	[2]78%	. . .	– – –	– – –	100%
Middle school	[2]81%	. . .	– – –	– – –	100%
Elementary school.	[2]75%	. . .	– – –	– – –	100%
3.11 Worksite smoking policies.	– – –	. . .	– – –	– – –	75%
50 or more employees	[8]27%	. . .	– – –	[3]59%	. . .
Medium and large companies	54%	. . .	– – –	85%	. . .
3.12 Clean indoor air laws					
Number of States with laws restricting smoking in public places	[2,16]42	. . .	– – –	[16]44	[16]50
Number of States with restricted smoking in public workplaces.	[2]31	. . .	– – –	[16]35	[16]50
Number of States with laws regulating smoking in private and public worksites	[2]13	. . .	– – –	[16]16	[16]50
3.13 Laws prohibiting tobacco products sale and distribution to children 18 years and under.	[17]44	. . .	– – –	[16]48	50
3.14 Number of States with plans to reduce tobacco use	[18]12	. . .	– – –	– – –	50
3.15 Tobacco product advertising and promotion to youth	[17]Minimal	. . .	– – –	– – –	Eliminate
3.16 Cessation counseling and follow-up by clinicians					
Primary care	[10,19]52%	. . .	– – –	– – –	75%
Oral health care.	[10,20]35%	. . .	– – –	– – –	75%

[1]Data have been recomputed to reflect revised intercensal population estimates; see *Health, United States, 1992*, Appendix I.
[2]1988 data.
[3]1992 data.
[4]1982–84 data.
[5]1979–87 data.
[6]1984–88 data.
[7]Vietnamese males only.
[8]1985 data.
[9]1983 data.
[10]1986 data.

[11]1987 data.
[12]Baseline for white females 20–44 years.
[13]Used in past month.
[14]1987–88 data.
[15]1986–87 data.
[16]Includes D.C.
[17]1990 data.
[18]1989 data.
[19]Counseling more than 75 percent of smoking patients.
[20]Counseling at least 75 percent of smoking patients.

NOTE: Data sources are in table C.

Tobacco Objectives

3.1*: Reduce coronary heart disease deaths to no more than 100 per 100,000 people.

Duplicate objectives: 1.1, 2.1, and 15.1

3.1a*: Reduce coronary heart disease deaths among blacks to no more than 115 per 100,000 people.

Duplicate objectives: 1.1a, 2.1a, and 15.1a

3.2*: Slow the rise in lung cancer deaths to achieve a rate of no more than 42 per 100,000 people.

NOTE: In its publications, the National Cancer Institute age adjusts cancer death rates to the 1970 U.S. population. Using the 1970 standard, the equivalent target value for this objective would be 53 per 100,000.

Duplicate objective: 16.2

3.3: Slow the rise in deaths from chronic obstructive pulmonary disease to achieve a rate of no more than 25 per 100,000 people.

NOTE: Deaths from chronic obstructive pulmonary disease include deaths due to chronic bronchitis, emphysema, asthma, and other chronic obstructive pulmonary diseases and allied conditions.

3.4*: Reduce cigarette smoking to a prevalence of no more than 15 percent among people aged 20 and older.

NOTE: A cigarette smoker is a person who has smoked at least 100 cigarettes and currently smokes cigarettes.

Duplicate objectives: 15.12 and 16.6

3.4a*: Reduce cigarette smoking to a prevalence of no more than 20 percent among people with a high school education or less aged 20 and older.

Duplicate objectives: 15.12a and 16.6a

3.4b*: Reduce cigarette smoking to a prevalence of no more than 20 percent among blue-collar workers aged 20 and older.

Duplicate objectives: 15.12b and 16.6b

3.4c*: Reduce cigarette smoking to a prevalence of no more than 20 percent among military personnel.

Duplicate objectives: 15.12c and 16.6c

3.4d*: Reduce cigarette smoking to a prevalence of no more than 18 percent among blacks aged 20 and older.

Duplicate objectives: 15.12d and 16.6d

3.4e*: Reduce cigarette smoking to a prevalence of no more than 18 percent among Hispanics aged 20 and older.

Duplicate objectives: 15.12e and 16.6e

3.4f*: Reduce cigarette smoking to a prevalence of no more than 20 percent among American Indians and Alaska Natives.

Duplicate objectives: 15.12f and 16.6f

3.4g*: Reduce cigarette smoking to a prevalence of no more than 20 percent among Southeast Asian men.

Duplicate objectives: 15.12g and 16.6g

3.4h*: Reduce cigarette smoking to a prevalence of no more than 12 percent among women of reproductive age.

Duplicate objectives: 15.12h and 16.6h

3.4i*: Reduce cigarette smoking to a prevalence of no more than 10 percent among pregnant women.

Duplicate objectives: 15.12i and 16.6i

3.4j*: Reduce cigarette smoking to a prevalence of no more than 10 percent among women who use oral contraceptives.

Duplicate objectives: 15.12j and 16.6j

3.5: Reduce the initiation of cigarette smoking by children and youth so that no more than 15 percent have become regular cigarette smokers by age 20.

3.5a: Reduce the initiation of cigarette smoking by lower socioeconomic status youth so that no more than 18 percent have become regular cigarette smokers by age 20.

3.6: Increase to at least 50 percent the proportion of cigarette smokers aged 18 and older who stopped smoking cigarettes for at least one day during the preceding year.

3.7: Increase smoking cessation during pregnancy so that at least 60 percent of women who are cigarette smokers at the time they become pregnant quit smoking early in pregnancy and maintain abstinence for the remainder of their pregnancy.

3.7a: Increase smoking cessation during pregnancy so that at least 45 percent of women with less than a high school education who are cigarette smokers at the time they become pregnant quit smoking early in pregnancy and maintain abstinence for the remainder of their pregnancy.

3.8: Reduce to no more than 20 percent the proportion of children aged 6 and younger who are regularly exposed to tobacco smoke at home.

NOTE: Regular exposure to tobacco smoke at home is defined as the occurrence of tobacco smoking anywhere in the home on more than three days each week.

3.9: Reduce smokeless tobacco use by males aged 12–24 to a prevalence of no more than 4 percent.

NOTE: For males aged 12–17, a smokeless tobacco user is someone who has used snuff or chewing tobacco in the preceding month. For males aged 18–24, a smokeless tobacco user is someone who has used either snuff or chewing tobacco at least 20 times and who currently uses snuff or chewing tobacco.

3.9a: Reduce smokeless tobacco use by American Indian and Alaska Native youth to a prevalence of no more than 10 percent.

3.10: Establish tobacco-free environments and include tobacco use prevention in the curricula of all elementary, middle, and secondary schools, preferably as part of quality school health education.

3.11: Increase to at least 75 percent the proportion of worksites with a formal smoking policy that prohibits or severely restricts smoking at the workplace.

3.12: Enact in 50 States comprehensive laws on clean indoor air that prohibit or strictly limit smoking in the workplace and enclosed public places (including health care facilities, schools, and public transportation).

3.13: Enact and enforce in 50 States laws prohibiting the sale and distribution of tobacco products to youth younger than age 19.

NOTE: Model legislation proposed by the Department of Health and Human Services (DHHS) recommends licensure of tobacco vendors, civil money penalties and license suspension or revocation for violations, and a ban on cigarette vending machines.

3.14: Increase to 50 the number of States with plans to reduce tobacco use, especially among youth.

3.15: Eliminate or severely restrict all forms of tobacco product advertising and promotion to which youth younger than age 18 are likely to be exposed.

3.16: Increase to at least 75 percent the proportion of primary care and oral health care providers who routinely advise cessation and provide assistance and followup for all of their tobacco-using patients.

*Duplicate objective.

References

1. Office of Smoking and Health. Reducing the health consequences of smoking: 25 years of progress. A Report of the Surgeon General. Washington: U.S. Department of Health and Human Services. 1989.

2. Centers for Disease Control. Smoking-attributable mortality and years of potential life lost—United States, 1988. MMWR. 1991.

3. LaPlante, MP. Data on disability from the National Health Interview Survey, 1983–85. An InfoUse Report. Washington: U.S. National Institute on Disability and Rehabilitation Research. 1988.

4. U.S. Department of Health and Human Services. The Health Benefits of Smoking Cessation. U.S. Department of Health and Human Services, Public Health Service, Centers for Disease Control, Center for Chronic Disease Prevention and Health Promotion, Office on Smoking and Health. 1990.

5. Fingerhut LA, Kleinman JC, Kendrick JS. Smoking before, during, and after pregnancy. Am J Public Health 80: 541–4. 1990.

Priority Area 4
Alcohol and Other Drugs

Background and Data Summary

Large numbers of Americans have used illicit drugs and misused alcohol; these behaviors can have serious health and social consequences. Alcohol is implicated in nearly half of all deaths caused by motor vehicle crashes and fatal intentional injuries such as suicides and homicides (1). Alcohol is the principal contributor to cirrhosis, the ninth leading cause of death in the United States in 1990 (2, table 30). Intravenous drug users and their sexual partners are at high risk of infection with the human immunodeficiency virus.

The 1991 National Household Survey on Drug Abuse estimated that 19.5 million Americans had used marijuana in the past year, and 67.7 million had tried marijuana at least once (3). In the same year an estimated 23.7 million people had a history of cocaine use. 1991 data for objective 4.7 show that heavy alcohol use is very common among young people; 30 percent of high school seniors and 43 percent of college students had five or more drinks on one occasion in the previous 2-week period (a related table in *Health, United States* is 67).

Recent data indicate that progress is being made toward improving alcohol and other drug problems. Eight objectives (4.2, 4.3, 4.6, 4.8, 4.9, 4.10, 4.11, and 4.15) show improvement toward the year 2000 targets, and objective 4.1 has surpassed the target. Average age at first use among adolescents aged 12–17 years did not change substantially for either cigarettes or marijuana but declined markedly for alcohol (4.5). Heavy alcohol consumption has decreased among high school seniors but has increased among college students (4.7). New data were available to establish baseline information for two objectives, drug-related emergency room visits (4.4) and work sites with alcohol and other drug policies (4.14).

No new data were available for two objectives (4.13 and 4.18) in this priority area; four objectives (4.12, 4.16, 4.17, and 4.19) have no baseline data.

Data Issues

Definitions

Cirrhosis deaths are tracked in objective 4.2 as an indicator of abusive alcohol consumption. The tracking variable included all deaths coded to ICD–9 571.0–571.9. This variable is more inclusive than alcoholic liver disease and cirrhosis (571.0–571.3). Alcohol-related liver disease is underreported; a significant proportion of these deaths are coded

to less specific categories such as 571.8 and 571.9. Estimates of the proportion of all cirrhosis deaths that are alcohol-related range from 41 to 95 percent (4).

Data from the National Vital Statistics System are used to track drug-related deaths (objective 4.3). Although the objective discusses drug-related deaths, it is tracked by a category of deaths that is more accurately called "drug-induced deaths" (a related table in *Health, United States* is 28). The category includes deaths whose underlying cause was drug dependence, nondependent use of drugs, and poisoning from drugs, all of which may include medically prescribed drugs. It excludes accidents,

Figure 10. Average age of first use of cigarettes, alcohol, and marijuana by adolescents 12–17 years of age: United States, 1988–91 and year 2000 targets for objective 4.5

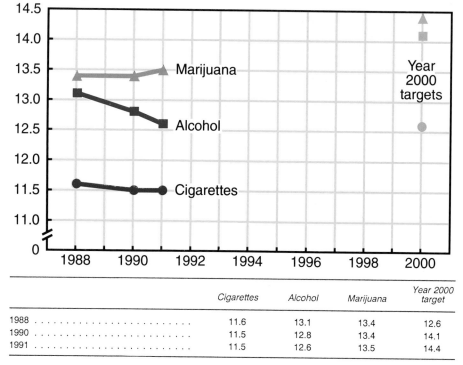

	Cigarettes	Alcohol	Marijuana	Year 2000 target
1988	11.6	13.1	13.4	12.6
1990	11.5	12.8	13.4	14.1
1991	11.5	12.6	13.5	14.4

SOURCE: National Institute for Drug Abuse, National Household Survey of Drug Abuse.

homicides, and other causes indirectly related to drug use.

Data Source Description

Alcohol-related motor vehicle crashes (4.1) are tracked using data from the Department of Transportation's Fatal Accident Reporting System (FARS). The FARS supplements death certificate data with information on the circumstances of the death to determine whether the death was alcohol related. The National Vital Statistics System does not specify alcohol-related motor vehicle crashes.

Comparability of Data Sources

Alcohol consumption among people 18–20 years of age increased from 52 percent in 1990 to 57 percent in 1991. However, because the scope of the 1991 National Household Survey on Drug Abuse, used to measure this objective, was expanded to include college students living in dormitories, the results are not comparable to previous years. When the subsample of these college students is removed from the 1991 data, the proportion of young adults using alcohol in the past month (53 percent) is only slightly higher than the 1990 figure.

Table 4. Alcohol and other drugs objective status

Objective	1987 baseline Original	1987 baseline Revised	1990	1991	Target 2000
4.1 Alcohol-related motor vehicle deaths (per 100,000)	9.8	. . .	8.9	7.9	8.5
a. American Indian/Alaska Native males	52.2	[1]40.4	– –	– – –	44.8
b. People 15–24 years	21.5	. . .	18.5	– – –	18.0
4.2 Cirrhosis deaths (age adjusted per 100,000)	9.1	[2]9.2	8.6	– – –	6.0
a. Black males	22.0	[2]22.6	20.0	– – –	12.0
b. American Indians/Alaska Natives	25.9	[1]20.5	19.8	– – –	13.0
4.3 Drug-related deaths (age adjusted per 100,000)	3.8	[2]No change	3.6	– – –	3.0
4.4 Drug abuse-related emergency room visits (per 100,000)	. . .	[3]164.9	– – –	– – –	131.9
4.5 Average age of first use (adolescents 12–17 years)					
Cigarettes	[4]11.6	. . .	11.5	11.5	12.6
Alcohol	[4]13.1	. . .	12.8	12.6	14.1
Marijuana	[4]13.4	. . .	13.4	13.5	14.4
4.6 Use in past month by children and adolescents					
Alcohol					
12–17 years	[4]25.2%	. . .	24.5%	20.3%	12.6%
18–20 years	[4]57.9%	. . .	52.3%	57.0%	29.0%
Marijuana					
12–17 years	[4]6.4%	. . .	5.2%	4.3%	3.2%
18–25 years	[4]15.5%	. . .	12.7%	13.0%	7.8%
Cocaine					
12–17 years	[4]1.1%	. . .	0.6%	0.4%	0.6%
18–25 years	[4]4.5%	. . .	2.2%	2.0%	2.3%
4.7 Heavy drinking in past 2 weeks					
High school seniors	[5]33.0%	. . .	32.2%	29.8%	28.0%
College students	[5]41.7%	. . .	41.0%	42.8%	32.0%
4.8 Alcohol consumption (gallons per capita)	2.54	. . .	[5]2.46	– – –	2.0
4.9 Perception of social disapproval by high school seniors					
Heavy use of alcohol	[5]56.4%	. . .	68.9%	67.4%	70.0%
Occasional use of marijuana	[5]71.1%	. . .	80.5%	79.4%	85.0%
Trying cocaine once or twice	[5]88.9%	. . .	91.5%	88.0%	95.0%
4.10 Perception of harm by high school seniors					
Heavy use of alcohol	[5]44.0%	. . .	47.1%	48.6%	70.0%
Occasional use of marijuana	[5]77.5%	. . .	77.8%	78.6%	90.0%
Trying cocaine once or twice	[5]54.9%	. . .	59.4%	59.4%	80.0%
4.11 Anabolic steroid use (ever used in lifetime)					
Male high school seniors	[5]4.7%	. . .	5.0%	3.6%	3.0%
4.12 Number of States with access to treatment programs	– – –	. . .	– – –	– – –	50
4.13 Alcohol and drug education in schools	– – –	. . .	– – –	– – –	100%
Provided students with some instruction	63%	. . .	– – –	– – –	. . .
Provided students with counseling	39%	. . .	– – –	– – –	. . .
Referred students for clinical assessments	23%	. . .	– – –	– – –	. . .
4.14 Worksite alcohol and drug policies					
Alcohol	. . .	[6]88%	– – –	– – –	60%
Other Drugs	. . .	[6]89%	– – –	– – –	60%
4.15 Number of States with administrative license suspension/revocation laws	[7,8]28	. . .	– – –	[8]29	[8]50
4.16 Number of States with policies to reduce minors' access to alcohol	– – –	. . .	– – –	– – –	50
4.17 Number of States with restrictions on promotion of alcohol to children and adolescents	– – –	. . .	– – –	– – –	20
4.18 Number of States with 0.04 alcohol concentration tolerance levels	[7]0	. . .	– – –	– – –	50
Number of States with 0.00 alcohol concentration tolerance levels	[7]0	. . .	– – –	– – –	50
4.19 Screening, counseling, and referral by clinicians	– – –	. . .	– – –	– – –	75%

[1]Data have been revised to include the entire U.S. American Indian/Alaska Native population; see Introduction.
[2]Data have been recomputed to reflect revised intercensal population estimates; see *Health, United States, 1992*, Appendix I.
[3]1991 data.
[4]1988 data.
[5]1989 data.
[6]1992 data.
[7]1990 data.
[8]Includes Washington, DC.

NOTE: Data sources are in table C.

Alcohol and Other Drugs Objectives

4.1: Reduce deaths caused by alcohol-related motor vehicle crashes to no more than 8.5 per 100,000 people.

> **4.1a**: Reduce deaths among American Indian and Alaska Native men caused by alcohol-related motor vehicle crashes to no more than 44.8 per 100,000.

> **4.1b**: Reduce deaths among people aged 15–24 caused by alcohol-related motor vehicle crashes to no more than 18 per 100,000.

4.2: Reduce cirrhosis deaths to no more than 6 per 100,000 people.

> **4.2a**: Reduce cirrhosis deaths among black men to no more than 12 per 100,000.

> **4.2b**: Reduce cirrhosis deaths among American Indians and Alaska Natives to no more than 13 per 100,000.

4.3: Reduce drug-related deaths to no more than 3 per 100,000 people.

4.4: Reduce drug abuse-related hospital emergency department visits by at least 20 percent.

4.5: Increase by at least 1 year the average age of first use of cigarettes, alcohol, and marijuana by adolescents aged 12–17.

4.6: Reduce the proportion of young people who have used alcohol, marijuana, and cocaine in the past month, as follows:

Substance and age	2000 target (percent)
Alcohol:	
12–17 years	12.6
18–20 years	29.0
Marijuana:	
12–17 years	3.2
18–25 years	7.8
Cocaine:	
12–17 years	0.6
18–25 years	2.3

4.7: Reduce the proportion of high school seniors and college students engaging in recent occasions of heavy drinking of alcoholic beverages to no more than 28 percent of high school seniors and 32 percent of college students.

NOTE: Recent heavy drinking is defined as having five or more drinks on one occasion in the previous 2–week period as monitored by self-reports.

4.8: Reduce alcohol consumption by people aged 14 and older to an annual average of no more than 2 gallons of ethanol per person.

4.9: Increase the proportion of high school seniors who perceive social disapproval associated with the heavy use of alcohol, occasional use of marijuana, and experimentation with cocaine, as follows:

	2000 target (percent)
Heavy use of alcohol	70
Occasional use of marijuana	85
Trying cocaine once or twice	95

NOTE: Heavy drinking is defined as having five or more drinks once or twice each weekend.

4.10: Increase the proportion of high school seniors who associate risk of physical or psychological harm with the heavy use of alcohol, regular use of marijuana, and experimentation with cocaine, as follows:

	2000 target (percent)
Heavy use of alcohol	70
Regular use of marijuana	90
Trying cocaine once or twice	80

NOTE: Heavy drinking is defined as having five or more drinks once or twice each weekend.

4.11: Reduce to no more than 3 percent the proportion of male high school seniors who use anabolic steroids.

4.12: Establish and monitor in 50 States comprehensive plans to ensure access to alcohol and drug treatment programs for traditionally underserved people.

4.13: Provide to children in all school districts and private schools primary and secondary school educational programs on alcohol and other drugs, preferably as part of quality school health education.

4.14: Extend adoption of alcohol and drug policies for the work environment to at least 60 percent of worksites with 50 or more employees.

4.15: Extend to 50 States administrative driver's license suspension/revocation laws or programs of equal effectiveness for people determined to have been driving under the influence of intoxicants.

4.16: Increase to 50 the number of States that have enacted and enforce policies, beyond those in existence in 1989, to reduce access to alcoholic beverages by minors.

4.17: Increase to at least 20 the number of States that have enacted statutes to restrict promotion of alcoholic beverages that are focused principally on young audiences.

4.18: Extend to 50 States legal blood alcohol concentration tolerance levels of .04 percent for motor vehicle drivers aged 21 and older and .00 percent for those younger than age 21.

4.19: Increase to at least 75 percent the proportion of primary care providers who screen for alcohol and other drug use problems and provide counseling and referral as needed.

*Duplicate objective.

References

1. Perrine M, Peck R, Fell J. Epidemiologic perspectives on drunk driving. In Surgeon General's workshop on drunk driving: Background papers. Washington: U.S. Department of Health and Human Services. 1989.

2. National Center for Health Statistics. Health United States, 1992 and Healthy People 2000 Review. Hyattsville, Maryland: Public Health Service. 1993.

3. National Institute on Drug Abuse. National Household Survey on Drug Abuse: Population estimates, 1991. Washington: U.S. Department of Health and Human Services. 1991.

4. National Institute on Alcohol Abuse and Alcoholism. County alcohol problem indicators 1979–85 (U.S. Alcohol Epidemiologic Data Reference Manual, vol 3, third ed.) Washington: U.S. Department of Health and Human Services. 1991.

Priority Area 5
Family Planning

Background and Data Summary

The formation and growth of families have significant public health and socio-psychological impact on society and individuals (1). Family planning, defined as the process of establishing the preferred number and spacing of children in one's family and selecting the means by which this is achieved, presupposes the importance of family and the importance of planning (2). Problems attendant to poor family planning exact a tremendous toll. Low birth weight (3), high rates of infant mortality (4), and inadequate family support (5) are some of the consequences of poor family planning.

Five of the 11 objectives in this priority area focus on the teenage population. More than three out of four young women and 85 percent of young men have had sexual intercourse by age 20. Each year, 1 out of 10 young women in this age group becomes pregnant. By age 20, approximately 40 percent of all women have been pregnant while 63 percent of black women have been pregnant. An estimated 84 percent of these teen pregnancies were unintended (2).

Updated data were available for four objectives. Objective 5.1 (adolescent pregnancy) moved away from the target, although there was a slight decline among black females. Objective 5.4 (adolescent postponement of sexual intercourse) also moved away from the target. Two objectives (5.5 and 5.6) showed mixed progress. Data from the Youth Risk Behavior Survey indicate that teenage male abstinence from sexual intercourse (5.5) increased slightly while female abstinence remained essentially unchanged. Contraceptive use (5.6) increased for high school males and females; combined (use of condom and pill) contraceptive use increased for males.

Data Issues

Comparability of Data Sources

Data used to update objective 5.4 (postponement of sexual intercourse) came from the 1990 Youth Risk Behavior Survey (YRBS). The YRBS surveys adolescents in school; it misses dropouts, who may be at a higher risk. Information from the YRBS is only available by school grade and not age; therefore, the data are not exactly comparable to the baseline. Fifteen year old adolescents are compared with 10th graders and those 17 years of age compared with 12th graders.

Data Availability

Baseline data for four objectives (5.7, 5.9, 5.10, and 5.11) came from one-time surveys. An ongoing data source has not yet been established for three of these objectives (5.9, 5.10, and 5.11); data from the National Survey of Family Growth (NSFG) will be used to monitor the fourth objective (5.7). The NSFG, the data source for many of the family planning objectives, is conducted every 3 to 4 years.

Table 5. Family planning objective status

Objective	1988 Baseline		1990	1991	Target 2000
	Original	Revised			
5.1 Adolescent pregnancy					
Females 15–17 years (per 1,000)...............................	[1]71.1	. . .	[2]74.3	– – –	50
a. Black adolescent females 15–19 years......................	[1,3]186	. . .	[2,3]184	– – –	120
b. Hispanic adolescent females 15–19 years	[1]158	. . .	– – –	– – –	105
5.2 Unintended pregnancy	56%	. . .	– – –	– – –	30%
a. Black females	78%	. . .	– – –	– – –	40%
5.3 Infertility					
Married couples with wives 15–44 years.....................	7.9%	. . .	– – –	– – –	6.5%
a. Black couples	12.1%	. . .	– – –	– – –	9%
b. Hispanic couples	12.4%	. . .	– – –	– – –	9%
5.4 Adolescents who ever had sexual intercourse					
Adolescents 15 years					
Females..	27%	. . .	[4]43%	[4]45%	15%
Males..	33%	. . .	[4]53%	[4]51%	15%
Adolescents 17 years					
Females..	50%	. . .	[5]67%	[5]65%	40%
Males..	66%	. . .	[5]76%	[5]68%	40%
5.5 Adolescent abstinence from sexual intercourse					
Ever sexually active females 15–17 years	26%	. . .	24%	25%	40%
Ever sexually active males 15–17 years.......................	. . .	33%	30%	36%	40%
5.6 Contraception use by sexually active adolescents					
Females 15–19 years					
First intercourse..	63%	. . .	– – –	– – –	90%
Recent intercourse	78%	. . .	78%	81%	90%
Oral contraception and condom use at most recent intercourse	2%	. . .	– – –	– – –	90%
High school males					
Recent intercourse	. . .	[6]78%	– – –	83%	90%
Oral contraception and condom use at most recent intercourse	. . .	[6]2.3%	– – –	3.3%	90%
Males 17–19 years					
Condom and oral contraception use at last intercourse	. . .	15%	[7]14%	– – –	90%
5.7 Failure of contraceptive method	[8]10%	. . .	– – –	– – –	5%
5.8 Family discussion of human sexuality					
People 13–18 years who have discussed sexuality with parents	[9]66%	. . .	– – –	– – –	85%
5.9 Adoption information from pregnancy counselors	[10]60%	. . .	– – –	– – –	90%
5.10 Age-appropriate preconception counseling by clinicians	– – –	. . .	– – –	– – –	60%
5.11 Clinic services for HIV and other sexually transmitted diseases	– – –	. . .	– – –	– – –	50%
Family planning clinics	[11]40%	. . .	– – –	– – –	. . .

[1]1985 data.
[2]1988 data.
[3]Adolescents other than white.
[4]10th grade students.
[5]12th grade students.
[6]1990 data.
[7]1990-91 data.
[8]1982 data.
[9]1986 data.
[10]1984 data.
[11]1989 data.

NOTE: Data sources are in table C.

Family Planning Objectives

5.1: Reduce pregnancies among girls aged 17 and younger to no more than 50 per 1,000 adolescents.

NOTE: For black and Hispanic adolescent girls, baseline data are unavailable for those aged 15–17. The targets for these two populations are based on data for women aged 15–19. If more complete data become available, a 35-percent reduction from baseline figures should be used as the target.

> **5.1a**: Reduce pregnancies among black adolescent girls aged 15–19 to no more than 120 per 1,000.

> **5.1b**: Reduce pregnancies among Hispanic adolescent girls aged 15–19 to no more than 105 per 1,000.

5.2: Reduce to no more than 30 percent the proportion of all pregnancies that are unintended.

> **5.2a**: Reduce to no more than 40 percent the proportion of all pregnancies among black women that are unintended.

5.3: Reduce the prevalence of infertility to no more than 6.5 percent.

NOTE: Infertility is the failure of couples to conceive after 12 months of intercourse without contraception.

> **5.3a**: Reduce the prevalence of infertility among black women to no more than 9 percent.

> **5.3b**: Reduce the prevalence of infertility among Hispanic couples to no more than 9 percent.

5.4*: Reduce the proportion of adolescents who have engaged in sexual intercourse to no more than 15 percent by age 15 and no more than 40 percent by age 17.

Duplicate objectives: 18.3 and 19.9

5.5: Increase to at least 40 percent the proportion of ever sexually active adolescents aged 17 and younger who have abstained from sexual activity for the previous 3 months.

5.6: Increase to at least 90 percent the proportion of sexually active, unmarried people aged 19 and younger who use contraception, especially combined method contraception that both effectively prevents pregnancy and provides barrier protection against disease.

5.7: Increase the effectiveness with which family planning methods are used, as measured by a decrease to no more than 5 percent in the proportion of couples experiencing pregnancy despite use of a contraceptive method.

5.8: Increase to at least 85 percent the proportion of people aged 10–18 who have discussed human sexuality, including values surrounding sexuality, with their parents and/or have received information through another parentally endorsed source, such as youth, school, or religious programs.

NOTE: This objective, which supports family communication on a range of vital personal health issues, will be tracked using the National Health Interview Survey, a continuing, voluntary, national sample survey of adults who report on household characteristics including such items as illnesses, injuries, use of health services, and demographic characteristics.

5.9: Increase to at least 90 percent the proportion of pregnancy counselors who offer positive, accurate information about adoption to their unmarried patients with unintended pregnancies.

NOTE: Pregnancy counselors are any providers of health or social services who discuss the management or outcome of pregnancy with a woman after she has received a diagnosis of pregnancy.

5.10*: Increase to at least 60 percent the proportion of primary care providers who provide age-appropriate preconception care and counseling.

Duplicate objective: 14.12

5.11*: Increase to at least 50 percent the proportion of family planning clinics, maternal and child health clinics, sexually transmitted disease clinics, tuberculosis clinics, drug treatment centers, and primary care clinics that screen, diagnose, treat, counsel, and provide (or refer for) partner notification services for HIV infection and bacterial sexually transmitted diseases (gonorrhea, syphilis, and Chlamydia).

Duplicate objectives: 18.13 and 19.11

*Duplicate objective.

References

1. Billy JOG, et al. Final report: Effects of sexual activity on social and psychological development. Seattle. 1986.

2. U.S. Department of Health and Human Services. Healthy people 2000: National health promotion and disease prevention objectives. Washington: Public Health Service. 1991.

3. Institute of Medicine, NAS. Preventing low birth weight. Washington. 1985.

4. Centers for Disease Control. Infant mortality marital status of mother—United States, 1983. MMWR 39(30): 521-2. 1990.

5. U.S. Congress. House select committee on children, youth, and families. U.S. children and their families: Current conditions and recent trends. Washington. 1989.

Priority Area 6
Mental Health and
Mental Disorders

Background and Data Summary

Mental health refers to an individual's ability to negotiate the daily challenges and social interactions of life without experiencing undue emotional or behavioral incapacity. Mental health and mental disorders can be affected by numerous factors ranging from biologic and genetic vulnerabilities, acute or chronic physical dysfunction, to environmental conditions and stresses.

Progress has been reported for 6 (objectives 6.1, 6.2, 6.5, 6.7, 6.8, and 6.11) of the 14 objectives in this area. Suicide (6.1), one of the most serious potential outcomes of mental disorders (1), declined slightly from the 1987 baseline. Adolescent suicide rates, while remaining stable for the past 3 years, are higher than the 1987 baseline. The suicide rate for American Indians and Alaska Natives did not change appreciably. Injurious suicide attempts among adolescents (6.2) showed a decline from the 1990 baseline and surpassed the year 2000 target of 1.8 percent. The prevalence of stress (6.5) has declined and a greater proportion of people suffering from depression (6.7) are receiving treatment.

Trends for two objectives moved away from the year 2000 targets. Funding reductions caused the small decline in the number of State clearinghouses for mental health information (6.12). More people are *not* seeking help for stress related problems (6.9). A baseline of three States was established for objective 6.10 (suicide prevention in jails). Baseline data for objectives 6.13 and 6.14 will be available in late 1993. The three remaining objectives (6.3, 6.4, and 6.6) had no new data beyond the baseline.

Data Issues

Definitions

The baseline for objective 6.3, the prevalence of mental disorders in

Figure 11. Persons 18 years and over with adverse health effects of stress in the past year: United States, 1985, 1990, and year 2000 target for objective 6.5

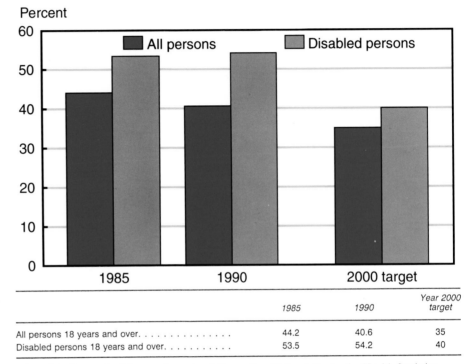

	1985	1990	Year 2000 target
All persons 18 years and over.	44.2	40.6	35
Disabled persons 18 years and over.	53.5	54.2	40

SOURCE: Centers for Disease Control and Prevention, National Center for Health Statistics, National Health Interview Survey.

children and adolescents, was revised because the diagnostic categories (2) have been expanded considerably since the establishment of the baseline (3). The target was also revised to reflect the same proportional decline sought in the original baseline. This change will affect monitoring.

Comparability of Data Sources

Several objectives will be tracked using a data source different from that used for the baseline. Objectives 6.4 (prevalence of mental disorders) and 6.7 (prevalence of depression) had baselines established by Epidemiological Catchment Area Studies, but will rely on the National Comorbidity Survey for future data.

Data to monitor progress for objective 6.2 are obtained from the Youth Risk Behavior Survey. These data reflect the number of sucide attempts in a 12-month period that required medical treatment.

Table 6. Mental health and mental disorders objective status

Objective	1987 baseline Original	1987 baseline Revised	1990	1991	Target 2000
6.1 Suicide (age adjusted per 100,000)	11.7	[1]No change	11.5	– – –	10.5
a. Adolescents 15–19 years (per 100,000)	10.3	[1]10.2	11.1	– – –	8.2
b. Males 20–34 years (per 100,000)	25.2	[1]No change	25.1	– – –	21.4
c. White males 65 years and over (per 100,000)	46.1	[1]46.7	44.4	– – –	39.2
d. American Indian/Alaska Native males (age adjusted per 100,000)	15	[2]20.1	21.0	– – –	12.8
6.2 Suicide attempts among adolescents	. . .	[3]2.1%	– – –	1.7%	1.8%
6.3 Mental disorders					
Children and adolescents 18 years and under	[4]12%	[5,6]20%	– – –	– – –	[7]17%
6.4 Mental disorders among adults	[8]12.6%	. . .	– – –	– – –	10.7%
6.5 Adverse health effects from stress	[9]42.6%	[6,9]44.2%	40.6%	– – –	35%
a. People with disabilities	[9]53.5%	. . .	54.2%	– – –	40%
6.6 Use of community support	[10]15%	. . .	– – –	– – –	30%
6.7 Treatment for depression	[11]31%	. . .	[12]36%	– – –	45%
6.8 Seeking help with problems	[9]11.1%	. . .	12.5%	– – –	20%
a. People with disabilities	[9]14.7%	. . .	17.0%	– – –	30%
6.9 Not taking steps to control stress	[9]21%	[6,9]24%	28%	– – –	5%
6.10 Number of States with suicide prevention in jails	. . .	[13]3	– – –	– – –	50
6.11 Worksite stress management programs	[9]26.6%	. . .	– – –	[13]37.0%	40%
6.12 Number of States with mutual help clearinghouses	[4]9	. . .	– – –	[13]8	25
6.13 Clinician review of patients' mental functioning	– – –	. . .	– – –	– – –	50%
6.14 Clinician review of childrens' mental functioning	– – –	. . .	– – –	– – –	75%

[1]Data have been recomputed to reflect revised intercensal population estimates; see *Health, United States, 1992*, Appendix I.
[2]Data have been revised to include the entire U.S. American Indian/Alaska Native population; see Introduction
[3]1990 data.
[4]1989 data.
[5]1988 data.
[6]Data have been revised to reflect updated methodology; see Introduction.
[7]Target has been revised to reflect proportional reduction from revised baseline.
[8]1984 data.
[9]1985 data.
[10]1986 data.
[11]1982 data.
[12]1983 data.
[13]1992 data.

NOTE: Data sources are in table C.

Mental Health and Mental Disorders Objectives

6.1*: Reduce suicides to no more than 10.5 per 100,000 people.

Duplicate objective: 7.2

> **6.1a***: Reduce suicides among youth aged 15–19 to no more than 8.2 per 100,000.

Duplicate objective: 7.2a

> **6.1b***: Reduce suicides among men aged 20–34 to no more than 21.4 per 100,000.

Duplicate objective: 7.2b

> **6.1c***: Reduce suicides among white men aged 65 and older to no more than 39.2 per 100,000.

Duplicate objective: 7.2c

> **6.1d***: Reduce suicides among American Indian and Alaska Native men in Reservation States to no more than 12.8 per 100,000.

Duplicate objective: 7.2d

6.2*: Reduce by 15 percent the incidence of injurious suicide attempts among adolescents aged 14–17.

Duplicate objective: 7.8

6.3: Reduce to less than 10 percent the prevalence of mental disorders among children and adolescents.

6.4: Reduce the prevalence of mental disorders (exclusive of substance abuse) among adults living in the community to less than 10.7 percent.

6.5: Reduce to less than 35 percent the proportion of people aged 18 and older who experienced adverse health effects from stress within the past year.

NOTE: For this objective, people with disabilities are people who report any limitation in activity due to chronic conditions.

> **6.5a**: Reduce to less than 40 percent the proportion of people with disabilities who experienced adverse health effects from stress within the past year.

6.6: Increase to at least 30 percent the proportion of people aged 18 and older with severe, persistent mental disorders who use community support programs.

6.7: Increase to at least 45 percent the proportion of people with major depressive disorders who obtain treatment.

6.8: Increase to at least 20 percent the proportion of people aged 18 and older who seek help in coping with personal and emotional problems.

> **6.8a**: Increase to at least 30 percent the proportion of people with disabilities who seek help in coping with personal and emotional problems.

6.9: Decrease to no more than 5 percent the proportion of people aged 18 and older who report experiencing significant levels of stress who do not take steps to reduce or control their stress.

6.10*: Increase to 50 the number of States with officially established protocols that engage mental health, alcohol and drug, and public health authorities with corrections authorities to facilitate identification and appropriate intervention to prevent suicide by jail inmates.

Duplicate objective: 7.18

6.11: Increase to at least 40 percent the proportion of worksites employing 50 or more people that provide programs to reduce employee stress.

6.12: Establish mutual help clearinghouses in at least 25 States.

6.13: Increase to at least 50 percent the proportion of primary care providers who routinely review with patients their patients' cognitive, emotional, and behavioral functioning and the resources available to deal with any problems that are identified.

6.14: Increase to at least 75 percent the proportion of providers of primary care for children who include assessment of cognitive, emotional, and parent-child functioning with appropriate counseling, referral, and followup, in their clinical practices.

*Duplicate objective

References

1. Centers for Disease Control. Youth suicide in the United States: 1970–80. Atlanta: Division of Epidemiology and Control. 1986.

2. American Psychiatric Association. Diagnostic and statistical manual. Third ed. 1980.

3. Costello EJ, et al. Psychiatric disorders and pediatric primary care: Prevalence of risk factors. 1988.

Priority Area 7
Violent and Abusive Behavior

Background and Data Summary

Violent and abusive behaviors continue to be major causes of death, injury, and stress in the United States. Suicide and homicide have resulted in over 50,000 deaths annually between 1985 and 1990 (table 30) (1) and victims of violence have exceeded 2 million persons annually (2). Violence creates extensive physical costs and emotional consequences for society (3). The widespread nature of these consequences may indicate that violence has become a routine part of social interaction in many domestic settings (4). It may also become a mode of behavior adopted by future generations raised in such settings (5). For these reasons, an area that has historically been the responsibility of the fields of law enforcement and social services has become a national public health priority.

Three of the 18 objectives (7.2, 7.7, and 7.8) in this priority area progressed toward the year 2000 targets. Suicides (7.2) have declined slightly for the total population; however, rates for some population subgroups have increased or remained the same. Rates of adolescent suicide (aged 15–19 years) have remained stable in 1988, 1989 and 1990, but are higher than the 1987 baseline. Suicide rates for American Indians and Alaska Natives have not changed appreciably from the 1987 baseline (see introduction). Rates of rape and attempted rape (7.7) have dropped and the target has been surpassed. Rape reporting, however, remains a sensitive issue, subject to a range of social and contextual influences (6). Injurious suicide attempts by adolescents (7.8) declined from the 1990 baseline and surpassed the year 2000 target. These data were obtained from the Youth Risk Behavior Survey and reflect suicide attempts in a 12-month period that required medical attention.

Movement away from the targets was reported for three objectives: homicides (7.1), weapon-related

Figure 12. Death rates for homicide among black males 15–34 years of age: United States, 1987–90 and year 2000 target for objective 7.1

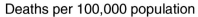
Deaths per 100,000 population

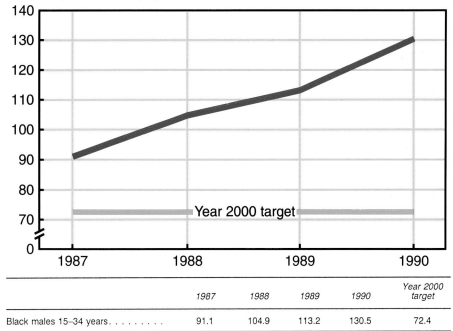

	1987	1988	1989	1990	Year 2000 target
Black males 15–34 years.........	91.1	104.9	113.2	130.5	72.4

NOTE: Death rates are age adjusted. ICD codes differ from similar categories published in *Health, United States* and elsewhere. See table A for specific codes. Related tables in *Health, United States, 1992,* are 28, 30, and 43.

SOURCE: Centers for Disease Control and Prevention, National Center for Health Statistics, National Vital Statistics System.

deaths (7.3), and assault injuries (7.6). The homicide rate for black males aged 15–34 years increased 43 percent between 1987 and 1990. Almost all of this increase is due to a sharp rise in firearm homicides (nonfirearm homicides were unchanged over the period), and it may be associated with increased violence related to drug trafficking. Weapon carrying has increased among young people (7).

The increase in weapon carrying appears linked to the increase in deaths from firearms (7.3). This rate increased by 12 percent from the 1987 baseline. In contrast, the rate of deaths from knives has remained stable for the past 4 years. The rate of injuries from crimes involving assaultive behavior (rape, robbery, and assault) rose to 11 per 1,000 in 1991.

Baseline data were established for five of the objectives (7.8, 7.9, 7.10, 7.13, and 7.18). Data to update progress were not available for three objectives (7.4, 7.5, and 7.15); these data are expected within the next 2 years. Five objectives remain without baseline data, although these should be established in the next 2 years as well (7.11, 7.12, 7.14, 7.16, and 7.17).

Data Issues

Data Availability

Four objectives without baselines (7.11, 7.14, 7.16, and 7.17) relate to children and violence prevention. Baseline data on these objectives will be available in 1994.

Table 7. Violent and abusive behavior objective status

Objective	1987 baseline Original	1987 baseline Revised	1990	1991	Target 2000
7.1 Homicide (age adjusted per 100,000)	8.5	[1]No change	10.1	– – –	7.2
a. Children 3 years and under (per 100,000)	3.9	[1]No change	4.4	– – –	3.1
b. Spouses 15–34 years (per 100,000)	1.7	. . .	[2]1.5	– – –	1.4
c. Black males 15–34 years (per 100,000)	90.5	[1]91.1	130.5	– – –	72.4
d. Hispanic males 15–34 years (per 100,000)	53.1	[1]41.3	47.8	– – –	42.5
e. Black females 15–34 years (per 100,000)	20.0	[1]20.2	22.1	– – –	16.0
f. American Indians/Alaska Natives (age adjusted per 100,000)	14.1	[3]11.2	10.7	– – –	11.3
7.2 Suicide (age adjusted per 100,000)	11.7	[1]No change	11.5	– – –	10.5
a. Adolescents 15–19 years (per 100,000)	10.3	[1]10.2	11.1	– – –	8.2
b. Males 20–34 years (per 100,000)	25.2	[1]No change	25.1	– – –	21.4
c. White males 65 years and over (per 100,000)	46.1	[1]46.7	44.4	– – –	39.2
d. American Indian/Alaska Native males (age adjusted per 100,000)	15	[3]20.1	21.0	– – –	[1]10.4
7.3 Weapon-related violent deaths (age adjusted per 100,000)	14.8	[1]No change	16.5	– – –	12.6
Firearms (age adjusted per 100,000)	12.9	[1]13.0	14.6	– – –	. . .
Knives (age adjusted per 100,000)	1.9	[1]1.8	1.8	– – –	. . .
7.4 Child abuse and neglect (per 1,000)	[4]25.2	. . .	– – –	– – –	less than 25.2
Incidence of types of maltreatment					
a. Physical abuse	[4]5.7	. . .	– – –	– – –	less than 5.7
b. Sexual abuse	[4]2.5	. . .	– – –	– – –	less than 2.5
c. Emotional abuse	[4]3.4	. . .	– – –	– – –	less than 3.4
d. Neglect	[4]15.9	. . .	– – –	– – –	less than 15.9
7.5 Partner abuse (per 1,000)	[5]30.0	. . .	– – –	– – –	27.0
7.6 Assault injuries (per 100,000)	[4]11.1	[4,6]9.7	10.3	11.0	[7]8.7
7.7 Rape and attempted rape (per 100,000)	[4]120	. . .	100	– – –	108
Incidence of rape and attempted rape					
a. Females 12–34 years	[4]250	. . .	206	– – –	225
7.8 Suicide attempts among adolescents	. . .	[8]2.1%	– – –	1.7%	1.8%
7.9 Physical fighting among adolescents 14–17 years (incidents per 100 students per month)	. . .	[9]137	– – –	– – –	110
7.10 Weapon-carrying by adolescents 14–17 years (incidents per 100 students per month)	. . .	[9]107	– – –	– – –	86
7.11 Inappropriate storage of weapons	– – –	. . .	– – –	– – –	20% reduction
7.12 Emergency room protocols for victims of violence	– – –	. . .	– – –	– – –	90%
7.13 Number of States with child death review systems	. . .	[9]33	– – –	– – –	45
7.14 Number of States that follow-up abused children	– – –	. . .	– – –	– – –	30
7.15 Battered women turned away from shelters	40%	. . .	– – –	– – –	10%
7.16 Conflict resolution education in schools	– – –	. . .	– – –	– – –	50%
7.17 Comprehensive violence prevention programs	– – –	. . .	– – –	– – –	80%
7.18 Number of States with suicide prevention in jails	. . .	[10]3	– – –	– – –	50

[1]Data have been recomputed to reflect revised intercensal population estimates; see *Health, United States, 1992*, Appendix I.
[2]1989 data.
[3]Data have been revised to include the entire U.S. American Indian/Alaska Native population; see Introduction.
[4]1986 data.
[5]1985 data.
[6]Baseline has been revised to reflect updated methodology.
[7]Target has been revised to reflect proportional reduction from revised baseline.
[8]1990 data.
[9]1991 data.
[10]1992 data.

NOTE: Data sources are in table C.

Violent and Abusive Behavior Objectives

7.1: Reduce homicides to no more than 7.2 per 100,000 people.

> **7.1a**: Reduce homicides among children aged 3 and younger to no more than 3.1 per 100,000 children.

> **7.1b**: Reduce homicides among spouses aged 15–34 to no more than 1.4 per 100,000.

> **7.1c**: Reduce homicides among black men aged 15–34 to no more than 72.4 per 100,000.

> **7.1d**: Reduce homicides among Hispanic men aged 15–34 to no more than 42.5 per 100,000.

> **7.1e**: Reduce homicides among black women aged 15–34 to no more than 16.0 per 100,000.

> **7.1f**: Reduce homicides among American Indians and Alaska Natives in Reservation States to no more than 11.3 per 100,000.

7.2*: Reduce suicides to no more than 10.5 per 100,000 people.

Duplicate objective: 6.1

> **7.2a***: Reduce suicides among youth aged 15–19 to no more than 8.2 per 100,000.

Duplicate objective: 6.1a

> **7.2b***: Reduce suicides among men aged 20–34 to no more than 21.4 per 100,000.

Duplicate objective: 6.1b

> **7.2c***: Reduce suicides among white men aged 65 and older to no more than 39.2 per 100,000.

Duplicate objective: 6.1c

> **7.2d***: Reduce suicides among American Indian and Alaska Native men in Reservation States to no more than 12.8 per 100,000.

Duplicate objective: 6.1d

7.3: Reduce weapon-related violent deaths to no more than 12.6 per 100,000 people from major causes.

7.4: Reverse to less than 25.2 per 1,000 children the rising incidence of maltreatment of children younger than age 18.

> **7.4a**: Reverse to less than 5.7 per 1,000 children the rising incidence of physical abuse of children younger than age 18.

> **7.4b**: Reverse to less than 2.5 per 1,000 children the rising incidence of sexual abuse of children younger than age 18.

> **7.4c**: Reverse to less than 3.4 per 1,000 children the rising incidence of emotional abuse of children younger than age 18.

> **7.4d**: Reverse to less than 15.9 per 1,000 children the rising incidence of neglect of children younger than age 18.

7.5: Reduce physical abuse directed at women by male partners to no more than 27 per 1,000 couples.

7.6: Reduce assault injuries among people aged 12 and older to no more than 10 per 1,000.

7.7: Reduce rape and attempted rape of women aged 12 and older to no more than 108 per 100,000 women.

7.7a: Reduce rape and attempted rape of women aged 12–34 to no more than 225 per 100,000.

7.8*: Reduce by 15 percent the incidence of injurious suicide attempts among adolescents aged 14–17.

Duplicate objective: 06.02

7.9: Reduce by 20 percent the incidence of physical fighting among adolescents aged 14–17.

7.10: Reduce by 20 percent the incidence of weapon-carrying by adolescents aged 14–17.

7.11: Reduce by 20 percent the proportion of people who possess weapons that are inappropriately stored and therefore dangerously available.

7.12: Extend protocols for routinely identifying, treating, and properly referring suicide attempters, victims of sexual assault, and victims of spouse, elder, and child abuse to at least 90 percent of hospital emergency departments.

7.13: Extend to at least 45 States implementation of unexplained child death review systems.

7.14: Increase to at least 30 the number of States in which at least 50 percent of children identified as neglected or physically or sexually abused receive physical and mental evaluation with appropriate followup as a means of breaking the intergenerational cycle of abuse.

7.15: Reduce to less than 10 percent the proportion of battered women and their children turned away from emergency housing due to lack of space.

7.16: Increase to at least 50 percent the proportion of elementary and secondary schools that teach nonviolent conflict resolution skills, preferably as a part of quality school health education.

7.17: Extend coordinated, comprehensive violence prevention programs to at least 80 percent of local jurisdictions with populations over 100,000.

7.18*: Increase to 50 the number of States with officially established protocols that engage mental health, alcohol and drug, and public health authorities with corrections authorities to facilitate identification and appropriate intervention to prevent suicide by jail inmates.

Duplicate objective: 6.10

*Duplicate objective.

References

1. National Center for Health Statistics. Health, United States, 1992. Hyattsville, Maryland: Public Health Service. 1993.

2. Harlow CW. Injuries from crime. Washington: Department of Justice. 1989.

3. Block R. The fear of crime. Princeton. 1977.

4. Strauss MA. Violence and homicide antecedents. Bull N Y AcadMed 62: 446–62. 1986.

5. Widom CS. The Cycle of violence. Science 244: 160–6. 1989.

6. Bureau of Justice Statistics. The crime of rape. Washington. 1985.

7. Rivara FP. Traumatic deaths among children in the U.S.: Currently available prevention strategies. Pediatrics 75(3):456–62. 1985.

Priority Area 8
Educational and
Community-Based
Programs

Background and Data Summary

Community-based interventions attempt to reach groups of people outside of traditional health care settings. Many of these programs are community-based, designed for people who meet in diverse settings, such as students within a school, employees at a worksite, or members of civic or religious groups. Other programs are planned to be community-wide. These health promotion programs can reach large numbers of people with intensive and effective interventions; in addition, they are relatively easy to implement. While community-based programs may address a single risk factor or health problem, many programs are starting to take a more comprehensive, and often more positive, approach to health and well-being. Community-based programs also increasingly recognize the importance of addressing the social and physical environment in which behavior occurs.

Of the 14 Educational and Community-Based Programs objectives, 4 are progressing toward the year 2000 targets (objectives 8.3, 8.6, 8.9, and 8.12), while none are moving away from the targets. New baselines were established this year for three objectives (8.1, 8.2, and 8.14). Baselines for the remaining seven objectives are not yet available.

Data Issues

Years of Healthy Life

The concept of increasing years of healthy life is one of the three *Healthy People 2000* goals, and is included as three specific objectives (8.1, 17.1, and 21.1). See the introduction to the *Healthy People 2000 Review* for a discussion of years of healthy life.

Figure 13. Percent of worksites offering health promotion activities: United States, 1985, 1992, and year 2000 target for objective 8.6

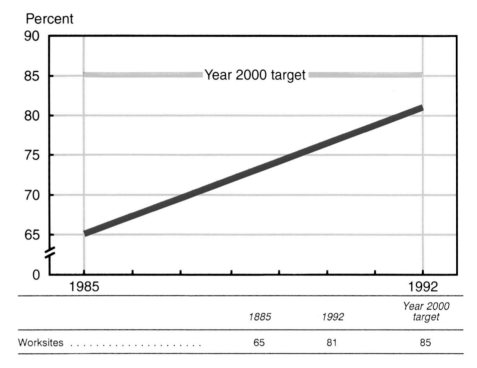

	1885	1992	Year 2000 target
Worksites	65	81	85

SOURCE: Office of the Assistant Secretary for Health, Office of Disease Prevention and Health Promotion.

Data Source Description

Objectives 8.2 (completion of high school) and 8.3 (preschool child development programs) and their targets are consistent with the National Education Goals for these areas. The data used to track these objectives come from the National Center for Education Statistics.

Data Availability

Objective 8.9 addresses the proportion of people aged 10 years and older who have discussed any of several health-related issues with family members in the last month. Until a broader variable is available,
progress is being measured by the percent of 9th–12th graders engaging in family discussions about HIV/AIDS. Similarly, objective 8.14, which focuses on the proportion of people served by effective local health departments, is being monitored by the proportion of health departments carrying out the core functions of public health.

Because of the nature of many of the objectives, this chapter poses as significant a challenge in obtaining relevant data to measure progress as any *Healthy People 2000* priority area. A concerted effort will be made over the decade to locate complete data sources for those objectives that are only being partially measured.

Table 8. Educational and community based programs objective status

Objective	Baseline Original	Baseline Revised	1990	1991	Target 2000
8.1 **Years of healthy life**	[1]62.0	[2,3]64.0	– – –	– – –	65
a. Blacks	[1]56.0	[2,3]No change	– – –	– – –	60
b. Hispanics	[1]62.0	[2,3,4]64.8	– – –	– – –	65
c. People 65 years and over[5]	[1]12.0	[2,3]11.9	– – –	– – –	14
8.2 **Completion of high school**					
People 19–20 years	[6]79%	[2,3]83%	– – –	– – –	90%
8.3 **Preschool child development programs**					
Eligible children 4 years afforded opportunity to enroll in Head Start ...	[2]47%	...	– – –	55%	100%
Disabled children 3–5 years enrolled in preschool	– – –	...	– – –	56%	100%
8.4 **Schools with quality school health education**	– – –	...	– – –	– – –	75%
8.5 **Health promotion in postsecondary institutions**					
Percent of higher education institutions offering health promotion activities	[7]20%	...	– – –	– – –	50%
8.6 **Worksite health promotion activities**					
Worksites with 50 or more employees	[8]65%	...	– – –	[9]81%	85%
Medium and large companies having a wellness program	[8]63%	...	– – –	– – –	...
8.7 **Hourly workers in health promotion activities**	– – –	...	– – –	– – –	20%
8.8 **Health promotion programs for older adults**	– – –	...	– – –	– – –	90%
8.9 **Family discussion of health issues-ages 10 years and over**	...	...	– – –	– – –	75%
Among 9th–12th grade students engaging in family discussion of HIV/AIDS	...	[10]54%	53%	61%	...
8.10 **Number of States with community health programs for 40 percent of the population**	– – –	...	– – –	– – –	40%
8.11 **Counties with programs for racial/ethnic minority groups**	– – –	...	– – –	– – –	50%
8.12 **Hospital-based patient education and community health promotion**					
Patient education programs					
Community hospitals	[11]66%	[3,12]68%	86%	– – –	90%
Health maintenance organizations	– – –	...	– – –	– – –	90%
Health education classes	...	...	[12]75%	– – –	...
Nutrition counseling	...	...	[12]85%	– – –	...
Community health promotion					
Community hospitals	[10]60%	...	77%	– – –	90%
8.13 **Television partnerships with community organizations for health promotion**	– – –	...	– – –	– – –	75%
8.14 **Effective public health systems**					
Local health departments reporting					
Health assessment	...	...	– – –	– – –	90%
Behavioral risk assessment	...	[2]33%	– – –	– – –	...
Morbidity data	...	[2]49%	– – –	– – –	...
Reportable disease	...	[2]87%	– – –	– – –	...
Vital records and statistics	...	[2]64%	– – –	– – –	...
Surveillance chronic disease	...	[2]55%	– – –	– – –	...
Surveillance communicable disease	...	[2]92%	– – –	– – –	...
Policy development functions and services					
Health code development and enforcement	...	[2]59%	– – –	– – –	...
Health planning	...	[2]57%	– – –	– – –	...
Health assurance					
Health education	...	[2]74%	– – –	– – –	...
Child health	...	[2]84%	– – –	– – –	...
Immunizations	...	[2]92%	– – –	– – –	...
Prenatal care	...	[2]59%	– – –	– – –	...
Primary care	...	[2]22%	– – –	– – –	...

[1]1980 data.
[2]1990 data.
[3]Data have been revised to reflect updated methodology; see Introduction.
[4]Estimated based on preliminary data
[5]Years of healthy life remaining at age 65.
[6]1989 data for people 20–21 years.
[7]1989–90 data.
[8]1985 data.

[9]1992 data.
[10]1989 data.
[11]1987 data.
[12]1988 data.

NOTE: Data sources are in table C.

Educational and Community-Based Programs Objectives

8.1*: Increase years of healthy life to at least 65 years.

NOTE: Years of healthy life is a summary measure of health that combines mortality (quantity of life) and morbidity and disability (quality of life) into a single measure. For people aged 65 and older, active life-expectancy, a related summary measure, also will be tracked.

Duplicate objectives: 17.1 and 21.1

> **8.1a***: Increase years of healthy life among black persons to at least 60 years.

Duplicate objectives: 17.1a and 21.1a

> **8.1b***: Increase years of healthy life among Hispanics to at least 65 years.

Duplicate objectives: 17.1b and 21.1b

> **8.1c***: Increase years of healthy life among people aged 65 and older to at least 14 years remaining at age 65.

Duplicate objectives: 17.1c and 21.1c

8.2: Increase the high school graduation rate to at least 90 percent, thereby reducing risks for multiple problem behaviors and poor mental and physical health.

NOTE: This objective and its target are consistent with the National Education Goal to increase high school graduation rates.

8.3: Achieve for all disadvantaged children and children with disabilities access to high quality and developmentally appropriate preschool programs that help prepare children for school, thereby improving their prospects with regard to school performance, problem behaviors, and mental and physical health.

NOTE: This objective and its target are consistent with the National Education Goal to increase school readiness and its objective to increase access to preschool programs for disadvantaged and disabled children.

8.4: Increase to at least 75 percent the proportion of the Nation's elementary and secondary schools that provide planned and sequential kindergarten–12th grade quality school health education.

8.5: Increase to at least 50 percent the proportion of postsecondary institutions with institution wide health promotion programs for students, faculty, and staff.

8.6: Increase to at least 85 percent the proportion of workplaces with 50 or more employees that offer health promotion activities for their employees, preferably as part of a comprehensive employee health promotion program.

8.7: Increase to at least 20 percent the proportion of hourly workers who participate regularly in employer-sponsored health promotion activities.

8.8: Increase to at least 90 percent the proportion of people aged 65 and older who had the opportunity to participate during the preceding year in at least one organized health promotion program through a senior center, lifecare facility, or other community-based setting that serves older adults.

8.9: Increase to at least 75 percent the proportion of people aged 10 and older who have discussed issues related to nutrition, physical activity, sexual behavior, tobacco, alcohol, other drugs, or safety with family members on at least one occasion during the preceding month.

8.10: Establish community health promotion programs that separately or together address at least three of the Healthy People 2000 priorities and reach at least 40 percent of each State's population.

8.11: Increase to at least 50 percent the proportion of counties that have established culturally and linguistically appropriate community health promotion programs for racial and ethnic minority populations.

NOTE: This objective will be tracked in counties in which a racial or ethnic group constitutes more than 10 percent of the population.

8.12: Increase to at least 90 percent the proportion of hospitals, health maintenance organizations, and large group practices that provide patient education programs, and to at least 90 percent the proportion of community hospitals that offer community health promotion programs addressing the priority health needs of their communities.

8.13: Increase to at least 75 percent the proportion of local television network affiliates in the top 20 television markets that have become partners with one or more community organizations around one of the health problems addressed by the Healthy People 2000 objectives.

8.14: Increase to at least 90 percent the proportion of people who are served by a local health department that is effectively carrying out the core functions of public health.

NOTE: The core functions of public health have been defined as assessment, policy development, and assurance. Local health department refers to any local component of the public health system, defined as an administrative and service unit of local or State government concerned with health and carrying some responsibility for the health of a jurisdiction smaller than a State.

*Duplicate objective.

Priority Area 9
Unintentional
Injuries

Background and Data Summary

Unintentional injuries are the fourth leading cause of death in the United States, accounting for more than 90,000 deaths annually (table 30) (1). They are a major cause of disabilities and hospitalization and have significant impact on health care costs (2). For example, the National Highway Traffic Safety Administration has estimated that motor vehicle crashes alone cost the United States $75 billion annually (3). The 22 objectives in this area focus on a wide range of mechanical, legislative, and educational means to reduce the occurrence of these events.

Progress toward the year 2000 targets was made on 11 objectives (9.1, 9.2, 9.3, 9.5, 9.6, 9.8, 9.9, 9.12, 9.13, 9.14, and 9.17). In a few cases (9.3, 9.8, and 9.9), the year 2000 target has been equaled or surpassed. Much of this progress is in areas related to motor vehicle fatalities, injuries, and use of vehicle occupant restraints (9.3, 9.9, and 9.12). This improvement may be attributable to reduction in the amount of driving and alcohol consumption during the recent economic slowdown. The recent increases in the number of States with seat belt laws, helmet laws (4), and programs targeting drivers under the influence of alcohol (5) also contributed to the declines in these areas. The national rate of residential fire deaths (9.6) and all special populations monitored as subobjectives show declining rates. These improvements may be associated with increased use of smoke detectors (9.17).

The hospitalization rates for hip fractures (9.7) and spinal cord injuries (9.10) increased, indicating movement away from the year 2000 target. Baseline data were established for objective 9.16. Objectives 9.4, 9.15, and 9.22 did not change. Data to monitor progress was unavailable for two objectives (9.11 and 9.19), and three objectives (9.18, 9.20, and 9.21) still require baseline data.

Figure 14. Number of States with laws requiring safety belt and motorcycle helmet use for all ages: United States, 1989–91 and year 2000 target for objective 9.14

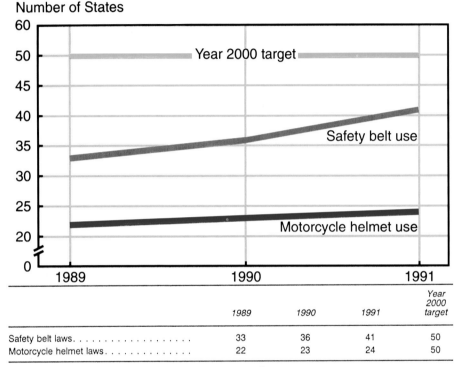

	1989	1990	1991	Year 2000 target
Safety belt laws	33	36	41	50
Motorcycle helmet laws	22	23	24	50

SOURCE: National Highway Traffic Safety Administration.

Data Issues

Data Source Description

Data for objective 9.3 (motor vehicle crash deaths) are crude rates from the Fatal Accident Reporting System (FARS). See the introduction for a discussion of crude and age-adjusted rates and priority area 4 for a description of FARS. The rates for 9.3d (American Indian and Alaska Natives) are age-adjusted data from the National Vital Statistics System.

Table 9. Unintentional injuries objective status

Objective	1987 baseline Original	1987 baseline Revised	1990	1991	Target 2000
9.1 **Unintentional injury deaths (age adjusted per 100,000)**.......	34.5	[1]34.7	32.5	---	29.3
a. American Indians/Alaska Natives (age adjusted per 100,000) ...	82.6	[2]66.0	59.0	---	66.1
b. Black males (age adjusted per 100,000)....................	64.9	[1]68.0	62.4	---	51.9
c. White males (age adjusted per 100,000)...................	53.6	[1]49.8	46.4	---	42.9
9.2 **Unintentional injury hospitalizations (per 100,000)**...........	[3,4]887	[3–5]832	[4]780	[4]764	754
9.3 **Motor vehicle crash-related deaths**					
Per 100 million vehicle miles traveled (VMT)....................	2.4		2.1	1.9	1.9
Age adjusted per 100,000 people	18.8	[5]19.2	17.9	16.3	16.8
a. Children 14 years and under (per 100,000)	6.2	...	5.3	---	5.5
b. People 15–24 years (per 100,000).......................	36.9	...	33.3	---	33
c. People 70 years and over (per 100,000)	22.6	...	23.9	---	20
d. American Indians/Alaska Natives (age adjusted per 100,000) ...	46.8	[2]37.7	33.2	---	39.2
e. Motorcyclist (per 100 million VMT).......................	40.9	...	33.8	---	33.0
(per 100,000)	1.7		1.3	---	1.5
f. Pedestrians (per 100,000)	3.1	[5]2.8	2.6	---	2.7
9.4 **Fall-related deaths (age adjusted per 100,000)**...............	2.7	No change	2.7	---	2.3
a. People 65–84 years (per 100,000)........................	18.0	[1]18.1	17.8	---	14.4
b. People 85 years and over (per 100,000)..................	131.2	[1]133.0	143.1	---	105.0
c. Black males 30–69 years (per 100,000)...................	8.0	[1]8.1	6.8	---	5.6
9.5 **Drowning deaths (age adjusted per 100,000)**................	2.1	No change	1.9	---	1.3
a. Children aged 4 and under (per 100,000).................	4.2	[1]4.3	3.4	---	2.3
b. Males 15–34 years (per 100,000)	4.5	No change	4.0	---	2.5
c. Black males (age adjusted per 100,000).................	6.6	No change	5.0	---	3.6
9.6 **Residential fire deaths (age adjusted per 100,000)**	1.5	[1]1.7	1.5	---	1.2
a. Children 4 years and under (per 100,000)	4.4	[1]4.5	3.5	---	3.3
b. People 65 years and over (per 100,000).................	4.4	[1]4.9	4.1	---	3.3
c. Black males (age adjusted per 100,000).................	5.7	[1]6.4	5.2	---	4.3
d. Black females (age adjusted per 100,000)..............	3.4	[1]3.3	2.7	---	2.6
e. Residential fire deaths caused by smoking.............	17%	[5]26%	[6]17%	---	5%
9.7 **Hip fractures among older adults (per 100,000)**..............	[3]714	...	776	814	607
a. White females 85 years and over..........................	[3]2,721	...	3,075	3,791	2,177
9.8 **Nonfatal poisoning (per 100,000)**	[7]103	[5,7]108	76	---	88
a. Among children 4 years and under	[7]650	[5,7]648	729	---	520
9.9 **Nonfatal head injuries (per 100,000)**	[3]125	[3,5]118	110	104	106
9.10 **Nonfatal spinal cord injuries (per 100,000)**	[3]5.9	[3,5]5.3	4.4	6.4	5.0
a. Males..	[3]8.9	[3,5]9.6	6.9	9.8	7.1
9.11 **Secondary disabilities associated with head and spinal cord injuries**					
Head injuries (per 100,000)	[7]20.0	...	---	---	16.0
Spinal cord injuries (per 100,000)	[7]3.2	...	---	---	2.6
9.12 **Motor vehicle occupant protection systems**	[3]42%	...	49%	59%	85%
a. Children 4 years and under	[3]84%	...	84%	85%	95%
9.13 **Helmet use by motorcyclists and bicyclists**					
Motorcyclists..	[3]60%	...	60%	62%	80%
Bicyclists..	[3]8%	...	---	5–10%	50%
9.14 **Safety belt and helmet use laws**					
Number of States with safety belt laws[7]......................	[6]33	...	36	41	50
Number of States with Motorcycle Helmet Use Laws[8]	[6]22	...	23	24	50
9.15 **Number of States with handgun design to protect children**	[6]0	...	0	---	50
9.16 **Fire suppression sprinkler installation (number of localities)**...	...	[6]700	---	---	2,000
9.17 **Residences with smoke detectors**	[6]81%	...	82%	---	100%
9.18 **Injury prevention instruction in schools.**....................	---	...	---	---	50%
9.19 **Protective equipment in sporting and recreation events**	---	...	---	---	100%
National Collegiate Athletic Association					
Football	[3]Required	...	---	---	...
Hockey...............................	[3]Required	...	---	---	...
Lacrosse	[3]Required	...	---	---	...
High school football	[3]Required	...	---	---	...
Amateur boxing.............................	[3]Required	...	---	---	...
Amateur ice hockey	[3]Required	...	---	---	...

Table 9. Unintentional injuries objective status—Con.

Objective	1987 baseline Original	1987 baseline Revised	1990	1991	Target 2000
9.20 Number of States with design standards for roadway safety	– – –	. . .	– – –	– – –	30
9.21 Injury prevention counseling by primary care providers	– – –	. . .	– – –	– – –	50%
9.22 Number of States with linked emergency medical services and trauma systems	2	. . .	[6]2	– – –	50

[1]Data have been recomputed to reflect revised intercensal population estimates; see *Health, United States, 1992*, Appendix I.
[2]Data have been revised to include the entire U.S. American Indian/Alaska Native population; see Introduction.
[3]1988 data.
[4]Data include unintentional and intentional injuries and injuries where the intent was not known.
[5]Data have been revised to reflect updated methodology; see Introduction.
[6]1989 data.
[7]1986 data.
[8]DC also has a safety belt law.
[9]DC and Puerto Rico also have motorcycle helmet laws.

NOTE: Data sources are in table C.

Unintentional Injuries Objectives

9.1: Reduce deaths caused by unintentional injuries to no more than 29.3 per 100,000 people.

> **9.1a**: Reduce deaths among American Indians and Alaska Natives caused by unintentional injuries to no more than 66.1 per 100,000 people.

> **9.1b**: Reduce deaths among black males caused by unintentional injuries to no more than 51.9 per 100,000 people.

> **9.1c**: Reduce deaths among white males caused by unintentional injuries to no more than 42.9 per 100,000.

9.2: Reduce nonfatal unintentional injuries so that hospitalizations for this condition are no more than 754 per 100,000 people.

9.3: Reduce deaths caused by motor vehicle crashes to no more than 1.9 per 100 million vehicle miles traveled and 16.8 per 100,000 people.

> **9.3a**: Reduce deaths among children aged 14 and younger caused by motor vehicle crashes to no more than 5.5 per 100,000.

> **9.3b**: Reduce deaths among youth aged 15–24 caused by motor vehicle crashes to no more than 33 per 100,000.

> **9.3c**: Reduce deaths among people aged 70 and older caused by motor vehicle crashes to no more than 20 per 100,000.

> **9.3d**: Reduce deaths among American Indians and Alaska Natives caused by motor vehicle crashes to no more than 39.2 per 100,000.

> **9.3e**: Reduce deaths among motorcyclists caused by motor vehicle crashes to no more than 33 per 100 million vehicle miles traveled and 1.5 per 100,000.

> **9.3f**: Reduce deaths among pedestrians caused by motor vehicle crashes to no more than 2.7 per 100,000.

9.4: Reduce deaths from falls and fall-related injuries to no more than 2.3 per 100,000 people.

> **9.4a**: Reduce deaths among people aged 65–84 from falls and fall-related injuries to no more than 14.4 per 100,000.

> **9.4b**: Reduce deaths among people aged 85 and older from falls and fall-related injuries to no more than 105 per 100,000.

> **9.4c**: Reduce deaths among black men aged 30–69 from falls and fall-related injuries to no more than 5.6 per 100,000.

9.5: Reduce drowning deaths to no more than 1.3 per 100,000 people.

> **9.5a**: Reduce drowning deaths among children aged 4 and younger to no more than 2.3 per 100,000.

> **9.5b**: Reduce drowning deaths among men aged 15–34 to no more than 2.5 per 100,000.

> **9.5c**: Reduce drowning deaths among black males to no more than 3.6 per 100,000.

9.6: Reduce residential fire deaths to no more than 1.2 per 100,000 people.

> **9.6a**: Reduce residential fire deaths among children aged 4 and younger to no more than 3.3 per 100,000.

> **9.6b**: Reduce residential fire deaths among people aged 65 and older to no more than 3.3 per 100,000.

> **9.6c**: Reduce residential fire deaths among black males to no more than 4.3 per 100,000.

9.6d: Reduce residential fire deaths among black females to no more than 2.6 per 100,000.

9.6e: Reduce residential fire deaths from residential fires caused by smoking to no more than 5 percent.

9.7: Reduce hip fractures among people aged 65 and older so that hospitalizations for this condition are no more than 607 per 100,000 people.

9.7a: Reduce hip fractures among white women aged 85 and older so that hospitalizations for this condition are no more than 2,177 per 100,000.

9.8: Reduce nonfatal poisoning to no more than 88 emergency department treatments per 100,000 people.

9.8a: Reduce nonfatal poisoning among children aged 4 and younger to no more than 520 emergency department treatments per 100,000.

9.9: Reduce nonfatal head injuries so that hospitalizations for this condition are no more than 106 per 100,000 people.

9.10: Reduce nonfatal spinal cord injuries so that hospitalizations for this condition are no more than 5.0 per 100,000 people.

9.10a: Reduce nonfatal spinal cord injuries among males so that hospitalizations for this condition are no more than 7.1 per 100,000.

9.11: Reduce the incidence of secondary disabilities associated with injuries of the head and spinal cord to no more than 16 and 2.6 per 100,000 people, respectively.

NOTE: Secondary disabilities are defined as those medical conditions secondary to traumatic head or spinal cord injury that impair independent and productive lifestyles.

9.12: Increase use of occupant protection systems, such as safety belts, inflatable safety restraints, and child safety seats, to at least 85 percent of motor vehicle occupants.

9.12a: Increase use of occupant protection systems, such as safety belts, inflatable safety restraints, and child safety seats, to at least 95 percent of motor vehicle occupants aged 4 and younger.

9.13: Increase use of helmets to at least 80 percent of motorcyclists and at least 50 percent of bicyclists.

9.14: Extend to 50 States laws requiring safety belt and motorcycle helmet use for all ages.

9.15: Enact in 50 States laws requiring that new handguns be designed to minimize the likelihood of discharge by children.

9.16: Extend to 2,000 local jurisdictions the number whose codes address the installation of fire suppression sprinkler systems in those residences at highest risk for fires.

9.17: Increase the presence of functional smoke detectors to at least one on each habitable floor of all inhabited residential dwellings.

9.18: Provide academic instruction on injury prevention and control, preferably as part of quality school health education, in at least 50 percent of public school systems (grades K–12).

9.19*: Extend requirement of the use of effective head, face, eye, and mouth protection to all organizations, agencies, and institutions sponsoring sporting and recreation events that pose risks of injury.

Duplicate objective: 13.16

9.20: Increase to at least 30 the number of States that have design standards for signs, signals, markings, lighting, and other characteristics of the roadway environment to improve the visual stimuli and protect the safety of older drivers and pedestrians.

9.21: Increase to at least 50 percent the proportion of primary care providers who routinely provide age appropriate counseling on safety precautions to prevent unintentional injury.

9.22: Extend to 50 States emergency medical service and trauma systems linking prehospital, hospital, and rehabilitation services in order to prevent trauma deaths and long-term disability.

*Duplicate objective.

References

1. National Center for Health Statistics. Health, United States, 1992. Hyattsville, Maryland: Public Health Service. 1993.

2. Rice DP, et al. Cost of injury in the United States: A report to Congress, 1989. San Francisco. 1989.

3. National Highway Traffic Safety Administration. The economic cost of society of motor vehicle accidents. Washington. 1987.

4. National Highway Traffic Safety Administration. The effectiveness of motorcyle helmets in preventing fatalities. Washington. 1989.

5. National Highway Traffic Safety Administration. Fatal accident reporting system, 1987. Washington. 1987.

Priority Area 10
Occupational Safety and Health

Background and Data Summary

Work-related injuries and deaths are an important public health problem. Although work-related deaths have declined slightly from a 1983–87 average of 6 per 100,000 workers to a rate of 4.3 in 1990, work-related injuries remain above the 1983–87 average of 7.7 per 100 (8.3 in 1990 (1) and 7.9 in 1991 (2)). The leading cause of occupational deaths is motor vehicle accidents (3); reductions in this area are, in part, a consequence of increased legislation and enforcement of seat belt laws.

Some specific professions (such as mining, construction, farming and nursing) have higher levels of mortality and morbidity, due to physical and environmental demands (4). Work-related deaths for some of these groups have declined from the 1983–87 averages. Mine-worker deaths dropped to 17.3 per 100,000 in 1989 which is below the year 2000 target (21 per 100,000). Data on mine-workers were not available for 1990, but rates for construction workers and transportation workers declined. The rate for farm workers increased to a level of 23.8 per 100,000 in 1990; there was no concomitant increase in work-related injuries among farm workers during this time period. Many work-related deaths and injuries are among younger, newer workers, who may require safety training and other initiatives to further reduce work-related mortality and morbidity (5).

Five of the 15 objectives in this priority area moved toward the year 2000 targets (10.1, 10.5, 10.6, 10.10, and 10.13). The new baseline established for objective 10.6 (worksite mandates for use of occupant protection systems) surpassed the year 2000 target. Since seat belt use is a component of this objective, the achievement of the target level is probably a result of increased legislation and enforcement of State seat belt laws.

Figure 15. Death rates for work-related injuries among full-time workers according to selected occupations: United States, 1983–90, and year 2000 targets for objective 10.1

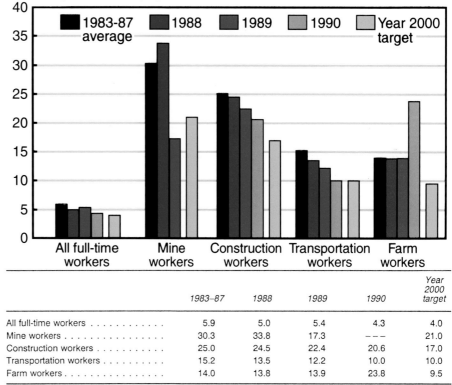

Deaths per 100,000 population

	1983–87	1988	1989	1990	Year 2000 target
All full-time workers	5.9	5.0	5.4	4.3	4.0
Mine workers	30.3	33.8	17.3	– – –	21.0
Construction workers	25.0	24.5	22.4	20.6	17.0
Transportation workers	15.2	13.5	12.2	10.0	10.0
Farm workers	14.0	13.8	13.9	23.8	9.5

NOTE: Death rates are crude rates. Related tables in *Health, United States, 1992,* are 46, 47, and 75. The data in tables 46, 47, and 75 are age-adjusted.

SOURCE: Bureau of Labor Statistics, Annual Summary of Occupational Injuries and Illnesses.

Two objectives (10.2, nonfatal occupation-related injuries and 10.4, occupational skin disorders) remained relatively stable between 1988 and 1991, but were higher than the 1987 baseline. Objective 10.3 (cumulative trauma disorders) continued to increase between 1987 and 1991. Occupational lead exposure (10.8) increased considerably, but the number of States reporting also increased from 7 to 10.

Baselines were established for objectives 10.9 (hepatitis immunization), 10.12 (health and safety programs), and 10.14 (State safety and health programs for small businesses). Three objectives (10.7, 10.11, and 10.15) remain without baseline data; the data is expected in mid-1993.

Data Issues

Description of Data Source

Work-related injury deaths (10.1) are tracked by the Bureau of Labor Statistics (BLS) of the Department of Labor (1). These data are compiled from a survey of employer logs of deaths among current employees. The rates are crude rates and may differ from age-adjusted rates calculated by

NIOSH and shown in other tables in Health United States.

The data are based on surveys; thus they do not capture all occupational deaths. While occupational deaths are a relatively rare event, comparisons of BLS data with other data sources suggest that there is considerable underreporting in the survey (6). Some of the disparity is attributable to differences in the reporting of unintentional injuries which occur on the job as "work-related" (7). To address this problem, BLS will begin using the Census of Fatal Occupational Injuries (CFOI) to report 1992 work-related mortality. As this reporting mechanism will employ multiple sources to capture work-related deaths, the rates will probably increase.

Table 10. Occupational safety and health objective status

Objective	1987 baseline Original	1987 baseline Revised	1990	1991	Target 2000
10.1 Work-related injury deaths (per 100,000)	[1]6	. . .	4.3	– – –	4
a. Mine workers.	[1]30.3	. . .	[2]17.3	– – –	21
b. Construction workers	[1]25.0	. . .	20.6	– – –	17
c. Transportation workers.	[1]15.2	. . .	10.0	– – –	10
d. Farm workers	[1]14.0	. . .	23.8	– – –	9.5
10.2 Nonfatal work-related injuries (per 100)	7.7	. . .	8.3	7.9	6
a. Construction workers	14.9	. . .	14.1	12.8	10
b. Nursing and personal care workers.	12.7	. . .	15.4	15.0	9
c. Farm workers	12.4	. . .	12.3	11.1	8
d. Transportation workers.	8.3	. . .	8.4	9.1	6
e. Mine workers.	8.3	. . .	8.1	7.1	6
10.3 Cumulative trauma disorders (per 100,000)	100	. . .	241	297	60
a. Manufacturing industry workers	355	. . .	867	– – –	150
b. Meat product workers.	3,920	. . .	8,245	– – –	2,000
10.4 Occupational skin disorders (per 100,000)	64	. . .	79	77	55
10.5 Hepatitis B infections among occupationally exposed workers (number of cases).	6,200	[3]3,090	1,258	2,576	1,250
10.6 Worksite occupant protection system mandates	. . .	[4]82.4%	– – –	– – –	75%
10.7 Occupational noise exposure	– – –	. . .	– – –	– – –	15%
10.8 Occupational lead exposure	[5]4,804	. . .	4,531	[6]7,842	0
10.9 Hepatitis B immunizations among occupationally exposed workers . . .	. . .	[2]37%	– – –	– – –	90%
10.10 Number of States with occupational health and safety plans	[2]10	. . .	– – –	[4]32	50
10.11 Number of States with occupational lung disease exposure standards.	– – –	. . .	– – –	– – –	50
10.12 Worksite health and safety programs.	. . .	[4]63.8%	– – –	– – –	70%
10.13 Worksite back injury prevention and rehabilitation programs.	[7]28.6%	. . .	– – –	[4]32.5%	50%
10.14 Number of States with programs for small business safety and health.	. . .	[8]26	– – –	– – –	50
10.15 Clinician assessment of occupational health exposures.	– – –	. . .	– – –	– – –	75%

[1]1983–1987 average.
[2]1989 data.
[3]Data have been revised to reflect updated methodology; see Introduction.
[4]1992 data.
[5]1988 data in seven States.
[6]1992 data in 10 States.
[7]1985 data.
[8]1991 data.

NOTE: Data sources are in table C.

Occupational Safety and Health Objectives

10.1: Reduce deaths from work-related injuries to no more than 4 per 100,000 full-time workers.

> **10.1a**: Reduce deaths among mine workers from work-related injuries to no more than 21 per 100,000 full-time workers.

> **10.1b**: Reduce deaths among construction workers from work-related injuries to no more than 17 per 100,000 full-time workers.

> **10.1c**: Reduce deaths among transportation workers from work-related injuries to no more than 10 per 100,000 full-time workers.

> **10.1d**: Reduce deaths among farm workers from work-related injuries to no more than 9.5 per 100,000 full-time workers.

10.2: Reduce work-related injuries resulting in medical treatment, lost time from work, or restricted-work activity to no more than 6 cases per 100 full-time workers.

> **10.2a**: Reduce work-related injuries among construction workers resulting in medical treatment, lost time from work,or restricted-work activity to no more than 10 cases per 100 full-time workers.

> **10.2b**: Reduce work-related injuries among nursing and personal care workers resulting in medical treatment, lost time from work, or restricted-work activity to no more than 9 cases per 100 full-time workers.

> **10.2c**: Reduce work-related injuries among farm workers resulting in medical treatment, lost time from work, or restricted-work activity to no more than 8 cases per 100 full-time workers.

> **10.2d**: Reduce work-related injuries among transportation workers resulting in medical treatment, lost time from work, or restricted-work activity to no more than 6 cases per 100 full-time workers.

> **10.2e**: Reduce work-related injuries among mine workers resulting in medical treatment, lost time from work, or restricted-work activity to no more than 6 cases per 100 full-time workers.

10.3: Reduce cumulative trauma disorders to an incidence of no more than 60 cases per 100,000 full-time workers.

> **10.3a**: Reduce cumulative trauma disorders among manufacturing industry workers to an incidence of no more than 150 cases per 100,000 full-time workers.

> **10.3b**: Reduce cumulative trauma disorders among meat product workers to an incidence of no more than 2,000 cases per 100,000 full-time workers.

10.4: Reduce occupational skin disorders or diseases to an incidence of no more than 55 per 100,000 full-time workers.

10.5*: Reduce hepatitis B infections among occupationally exposed workers to an incidence of no more than 1,250 cases.

Duplicate objective: 20.3e

10.6: Increase to at least 75 percent the proportion of worksites with 50 or more employees that mandate employee use of occupant protection systems, such as seatbelts, during all work-related motor vehicle travel.

10.7: Reduce to no more than 15 percent the proportion of workers exposed to average daily noise levels that exceed 85 dBA.

10.8: Eliminate exposures that result in workers having blood lead concentrations greater than 25 ug/dL of whole blood.

10.9*: Increase hepatitis B immunization levels to 90 percent among occupationally exposed workers.

Duplicate objective: 20.11

10.10: Implement occupational safety and health plans in 50 States for the identification, management, and prevention of leading work-related diseases and injuries within the State.

10.11: Establish in 50 States exposure standards adequate to prevent the major occupational lung diseases to which their worker populations are exposed (byssinosis, asbestosis, coal workers' pneumoconiosis, and silicosis).

10.12: Increase to at least 70 percent the proportion of worksites with 50 or more employees that have implemented programs on worker health and safety.

10.13: Increase to at least 50 percent the proportion of worksites with 50 or more employees that offer back injury prevention and rehabilitation programs.

10.14: Establish in 50 States either public health or labor department programs that provide consultation and assistance to small businesses to implement safety and health programs for their employees.

10.15: Increase to at least 75 percent the proportion of primary care providers who routinely elicit occupational health exposures as a part of patient history and provide relevant counseling.

*Duplicate objective.

References

1. Department of Labor. Annual survey of occupational injuries and illnesses. Washington. 1990.

2. Department of Labor. Survey of Occupational Injuries and Illnesses: 1991. Washington. 1992.

3. National Safety Council. Accident Facts. Chicago, Illinois. 1988.

4. Bureau of Labor Statistics. Annual survey of occupational injuries and illnesses. Washington. 1988.

5. National Institute for Occupational Safety and Health. National traumatic occupational fatalities: 1980–86. September 1989.

6. Department of Labor. Monthly Labor Review. September 1992.

7. National Institute of Occupational Safety and Health. National Traumatic Occupational Facilities, 1980–85. March 1989.

Priority Area 11
Environmental
Health

Background and Data Summary

Environmental factors play a fundamental role in health and disease. One of the most famous public health interventions to control disease (cholera) succeeded through control of a contaminated public water supply (1). Despite this historic and other more recent successes, the etiology linking toxic exposure to disease is not well documented (2). The monitoring of public exposure to toxins and research into the relationship of toxic exposure to health and disease are important due to the increasing public and commercial use of hazardous substances (3).

Research may clarify current ambiguity about exposure thresholds. Dioxin continues to be the focus of research (4), but lead has been shown to have toxic effects at even lower exposure levels than originally believed (5,6). Research will aid priority setting among environmental and public health interventions.

The 16 objectives in this priority area cover a broad range of exposure media, including air, water, soil, and groundwater. They also include a variety of sources, such as radon, toxic chemicals, waterborne disease, and lead. Five of the objectives (11.3, 11.5, 11.7, 11.12, and 11.13) showed some progress towards the year 2000 targets. Two (11.12, and 11.13) relate to radon; despite extensive publicity about radon during the late 1980's and early 1990's, the rate of progress on these objectives is minimal.

Two objectives (11.1 and 11.9) showed movement away from the year 2000 targets. Asthma morbidity (11.1) increased slightly and the proportion of people who receive water that meets safe drinking water standards (11.9) decreased slightly from the 1989 baseline. Baseline data were established for objective 11.14 (health risks from hazardous waste); updated information shows an increase in the number of National Priorities List (NPL) sites, health assessments and the number of sites with public health concerns. This objective is discussed further in the data issues section. Baseline data were also established for objective 11.11.

Data to assess progress were not available for six objectives (11.2, 11.4, 11.6, 11.8, 11.10, and 11.15). Two of these, blood lead levels (11.4) and programs to recycle waste (11.15), have received considerable public attention during recent years. Objective 11.16, State monitoring plans for tracking sentinel diseases, remains without baseline.

Data Issues

Definitions

The list of toxic agents used to monitor objective 11.7 (toxic agent releases) has been revised by the Agency for Toxic Substances and Disease Registry (ATSDR) and Environmental Protection Agency's EPA and will be revised annually by the two agencies. This will pose problems in data comparability. The ATSDR is exploring ways to provide continued monitoring of this objective.

Objective 11.14 (health risks from hazardous waste sites) is currently tracked using the number of sites on the National Priorities List (NPL), the number of health assessments conducted at these sites, and the number of sites with public health concerns or hazards. No numeric target was identified in the original publication of *Healthy People 2000*.

The number of NPL sites, assessments, and sites with public health concerns frequently change

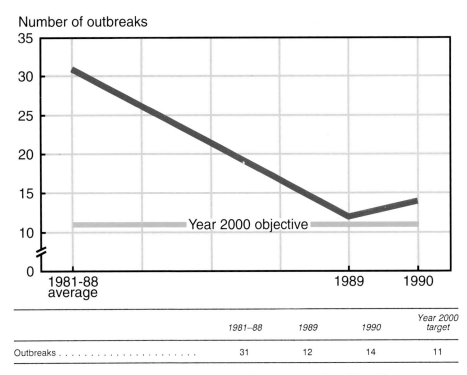

Figure 16. Outbreaks of waterborne disease: United States, 1981–88 average, 1989, 1990, and year 2000 target for objective 11.3

Number of outbreaks

	1981–88	1989	1990	Year 2000 target
Outbreaks	31	12	14	11

SOURCE: Centers for Disease Control and Prevention, Waterborne Surveillance System.

and will probably continue to increase due to the identification of additional sites and the duration of time required to clean up NPL sites (3). Additionally, EPA is currently revising its method of NPL site identification and prioritization, so future additions to the NPL list may be based on different criteria. The comparability of the indicators being used to track this objective will be reviewed when these changes are implemented.

Of critical importance to monitoring progress for this objective is a measure of those sites which posed a health concern or hazard in the past but have subsequently been remediated. With the addition of this information, a ratio of sites which posed threats but have been remediated to sites which pose a threat could be used to track this objective. A target for the year 2000 could then be derived using estimates of required time for clean up and EPA workload data. The ATSDR is currently exploring mechanisms to address these issues.

Table 11. Environmental health objective status

Objective	1988 Baseline Original	1988 Baseline Revised	1990	1991	Target 2000
11.1 Asthma hospitalizations (per 100,000)	[1]188	...	192	196	160
a. Blacks and other nonwhites	[1]334	...	340	349	265
b. Children 14 years and under	[1]284	...	308	339	225
11.2 Mental retardation (per 1,000 school aged children)	[2]2.7	...	---	---	2
11.3 Waterborne diseases (number of outbreaks)	[3]31	...	14	---	11
a. People served by community water systems	[3]13	...	---	---	6
11.4 Blood lead levels exceeding 15 & 25 mg/dL	[4]3 million & 234,000	...	---	---	500,000 & 0
a. Inner-city low-income black children	[4]234,900 & 36,700	...	---	---	75,000 & 0
11.5 People in counties meeting criteria air pollutants	49.7%	...	[5]69.4%	65.3%	85%
Ozone	53.6%	...	74.2%	72.0%	85%
Carbon monoxide	87.8%	...	91.1%	92.0%	85%
Nitrogen dioxide	96.6%	...	96.5%	96.5%	85%
Sulfur dioxide	99.3%	...	99.4%	98.0%	85%
Particulates	89.4%	...	92.3%	91.4%	85%
Lead	99.3%	...	97.8%	94.1%	85%
Total (any of above pollutants)	49.7%	...	69.4%	65.3%	85%
11.6 Radon testing	[5]Less than 5%	...	---	---	40%
a. Homes with smokers and former smokers	---	...	---	---	50%
b. Homes with children	---	...	---	---	50%
11.7 Toxic agent releases					
DHHS list of carcinogens (billion pounds)	0.32	...	[5]0.30	---	0.24
ATSDR list of the most toxic chemicals (billion pounds)					
200 substances	2.62	...	[5]2.40	---	2.60
250 substances	...	3.70	[5]3.30	---	...
11.8 Solid waste (average pounds per person per day)	4.0	...	---	---	3.6
11.9 People receiving safe drinking water	74%	...	73%	---	85%
11.10 Contaminated surface water	25%	...	---	---	15%
11.11 Homes tested for lead-based paint	...	[6,7]5%	---	---	50%
11.12 Number of States with construction standards to minimize radon concentrations	[5]1	...	3	---	35
11.13 Disclosure of lead and radon concentrations (number of States)					
Disclosure of lead	[5]2	...	2	5	30
Disclosure of radon	[5]1	...	3	5	30
11.14 Significant health risks from hazardous waste sites (Indicators)					
Sites on list	[8]1,082	...	---	[9]1,357	...
Health assessments conducted	[8]1,000	...	---	[9]1,422	...
Sites with public health concerns/hazards	...	[8]124	---	[9]254	...
11.15 Counties with programs for recyclable materials and household hazardous waste	[1]850 programs in 41 States	...	---	---	75%
11.16 Number of States that track sentinel environmental diseases	---	...	---	---	35

[1]1987 data.
[2]1985–88 data.
[3]1981–88 data.
[4]1984 data.
[5]1989 data.
[6]1991 data.
[7]Data represent proportion of people with homes built before 1950 who report that their paint has been analyzed for lead content.
[8]1990 data.
[9]1992 data.

NOTE: Data sources are in table C.

Environmental Health Objectives

11.1: Reduce asthma morbidity, as measured by a reduction in asthma hospitalizations to no more than 160 per 100,000 people.

> **11.1a**: Reduce asthma morbidity among blacks and other nonwhites, as measured by a reduction in asthma hospitalizations to no more than 265 per 100,000 people.

> **11.1b**: Reduce asthma morbidity among children, as measured by a reduction in asthma hospitalizations to no more than 225 per 100,000 people.

11.2*: Reduce the prevalence of serious mental retardation among school-aged children to no more than 2 per 1,000 children.

Duplicate objective: 17.8

11.3: Reduce outbreaks of waterborne disease from infectious agents and chemical poisoning to no more than 11 per year.

NOTE: Community water systems are public or investor-owned water systems that serve large or small communities, subdivisions, or trailer parks with at least 15 service connections or 25 year-round residents.

> **11.3a**: Reduce outbreaks of waterborne disease from infectious agents and chemical poisoning among people served by community water systems to no more than 6 per year.

11.4: Reduce the prevalence of blood lead levels exceeding 15 ug/dL and 25 ug/dL among children aged 6 months–5 years to no more than 500,000 and zero, respectively.

> **11.4a**: Reduce the prevalence of blood lead levels exceeding 15 ug/dL and 25 ug/dL among inner-city low-income black children (annual family income less than $6,000 in 1984 dollars) to no more than 75,000 and zero, respectively.

11.5: Reduce human exposure to criteria air pollutants, as measured by an increase to at least 85 percent in the proportion of people who live in counties that have not exceeded any Environmental Protection Agency standard for air quality in the previous 12 months.

NOTE: An individual living in a county that exceeds an air quality standard may not actually be exposed to unhealthy air. Of all criteria air pollutants, ozone is the most likely to have fairly uniform concentrations throughout an area. Exposure is to criteria air pollutants in ambient air. Due to weather fluctuations, multi-year averages may be the most appropriate way to monitor progress toward this objective.

11.6: Increase to at least 40 percent the proportion of homes in which homeowners/occupants have tested for radon concentrations and that have either been found to pose minimal risk or have been modified to reduce risk to health.

> **11.6a**: Increase to at least 50 percent the proportion of homes with smokers and former smokers in which homeowners/ occupants have tested for radon concentrations and that have either been found to pose minimal risk or have been modified to reduce risk to health.

> **11.6b**: Increase to at least 50 percent the proportion of homes with children in which homeowners/occupants have tested for radon concentrations and that have either been found to pose minimal risk or have been modified to reduce risk to health.

11.7: Reduce human exposure to toxic agents by confining total pounds of toxic agents released into the air, water, and soil each year to no more than:

> 0.24 billion pounds of those toxic agents included on the Department of Health and Human Services list of carcinogens.

2.6 billion pounds of those toxic agents included on the Agency for Toxic Substances and Disease Registry list of the most toxic chemicals.

11.8: Reduce human exposure to solid waste-related water, air, and soil contamination, as measured by a reduction in average pounds of municipal solid waste produced per person each day to no more than 3.6 pounds.

11.9: Increase to at least 85 percent the proportion of people who receive a supply of drinking water that meets the safe drinking water standards established by the Environmental Protection Agency.

NOTE: Safe drinking water standards are measured using Maximum Contaminant Level (MCL) standards set by the Environmental Protection Agency which define acceptable levels of contaminants. See objective 11.3 for definition of community water systems.

11.10: Reduce potential risks to human health from surface water, as measured by a decrease to no more than 15 percent in the proportion of assessed rivers, lakes, and estuaries that do not support beneficial uses, such as fishing and swimming.

NOTE: Designated beneficial uses, such as aquatic life support, contact recreation (swimming), and water supply, are designated by each State and approved by the Environmental Protection Agency. Support of beneficial use is a proxy measure of risk to human health, as many pollutants causing impaired water uses do not have human health effects (for example, siltation and impaired fish habitat).

11.11: Perform testing for lead-based paint in at least 50 percent of homes built before 1950.

11.12: Expand to at least 35 the number of States in which at least 75 percent of local jurisdictions have adopted construction standards and techniques that minimize elevated indoor radon levels in those new building areas locally determined to have elevated radon levels.

NOTE: Since construction codes are frequently adopted by local jurisdictions rather than States, progress toward this objective also may be tracked using the proportion of cities and counties that have adopted such construction standards.

11.13: Increase to at least 30 the number of States requiring that prospective buyers be informed of the presence of lead-based paint and radon concentrations in all buildings offered for sale.

11.14: Eliminate significant health risks from National Priority List hazardous waste sites, as measured by performance of clean-up at these sites sufficient to eliminate immediate and significant health threats as specified in health assessments completed at all sites.

NOTE: The Comprehensive Environmental Response, Compensation, and Liability Act of 1980 required the Environmental Protection Agency to develop criteria for determining priorities among hazardous waste sites and to develop and maintain a list of these priority sites. The resulting list is called the National Priorities List (NPL).

11.15: Establish programs for recyclable materials and household hazardous waste in at least 75 percent of counties.

11.16: Establish and monitor in at least 35 States plans to define and track sentinel environmental diseases.

NOTE: Sentinel environmental diseases include lead poisoning, other heavy metal poisoning (e.g., cadmium, arsenic, and mercury), pesticide poisoning, carbon monoxide poisoning, heatstroke, hypothermia, acute chemical poisoning, methemoglobinemia, and respiratory diseases triggered by environmental factors (e.g., asthma).

*Duplicate objective.

References

1. Lilienfield AM, Lilienfield DE. Foundations of epidemiology. New York: 1980.

2. National Research Council. Toxicity testing: Strategies to determine needs and priorities. Washington: 1984.

3. Environmental Protection Agency. Environmental progress and challenges: EPA's update. Washington: 1988.

4. Roberts L. Research news. October 1991.

5. National Institute of Environmental Health Sciences. Symposium on lead blood pressure relationships, environmental health perspectives. Washington: 1988.

6. Department of Health and Human Services. Strategic plan for the elimination of childhood lead poisoning. Washington: Public Health Service. 1990.

Priority Area 12
Food and Drug Safety

Background and Data Summary

The development of systems to protect consumers from dangers posed by unapproved food additives, pesticides, food contaminants, and drugs has been a major public health accomplishment. Despite effective food and drug safety procedures, this country still experiences outbreaks of foodborne diseases and incidents of therapeutic drug-related illness and death. Foodborne disease outbreaks sometimes result from failures in protective systems, but are more often the result of improper food handling. Salmonella enteritidis, Campylobacter jejuni, Escherichia coli 0157:H7, and Listeria monocytogenes are four of the most common foodborne pathogens in the United States, based on numbers of reported cases and the severity of illness. Children, the very old, and people with immunological deficiencies are at increased risk of infection and death resulting from infection.

Older adults, who use more prescription and nonprescription medicines than younger people, are at increased risk of suffering adverse drug reactions. The physiological changes associated with increasing age and particular diseases and conditions may alter the effects of drugs. In addition, use of multiple medications increases the risk of an adverse outcome.

The food and drug safety priority area contains six objectives that address reductions in foodborne diseases and precautions to reduce adverse medication interactions, especially among older people. Reported outbreaks of infections due to Salmonella enteritidis fell from 77 outbreaks in 1989 to 68 outbreaks in 1991 (objective 12.2). Data beyond baseline information are not available for three objectives (12.1, 12.3, and 12.4) and baseline levels still need to be established for two objectives (12.5 and 12.6) Objective 12.5 seeks to increase the proportion of pharmacies and other dispensers of prescription

medications that use linked systems to warn of potential adverse drug reactions. The Omnibus Budget Reconciliation Act of 1990 provides statutorial impetus for States to move toward this objective. Fifteen States currently plan to install point-of-sale, electronic drug claims processing sytems in all their pharmacies that serve the Medicaid population by January 1994 (1).

Data Issues

Data Source Descriptions

Various surveillance systems of the Centers for Disease Control and Prevention (CDC), including the Salmonella Surveillance System, the

Campylobacter Surveillance System, and the Bacterial Meningitis Surveillance System are used to monitor progress for objectives 12.1 and 12.2. The Salmonella Surveillance System is a passive laboratory-based system that uses reports from 49 States, the Food and Drug Administration, and the Department of Agriculture. This system measures the incidence of infection from salmonella species (12.1) and the number of outbreaks caused by Salmonella enteritidis (12.2). Many factors, including the intensity of surveillance, the severity of the illness, access to medical care, and association with a recognized outbreak, affect whether the infection will be reported. Reporting is incomplete; the incidence of

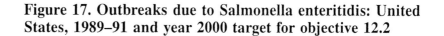

Figure 17. Outbreaks due to Salmonella enteritidis: United States, 1989–91 and year 2000 target for objective 12.2

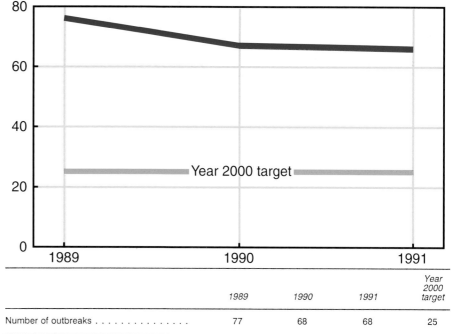

Number of outbreaks

	1989	1990	1991	Year 2000 target
Number of outbreaks	77	68	68	25

SOURCE: Centers for Disease Control and Prevention, National Center for Infectious Diseases, Salmonella Surveillance System.

salmonellosis is substantially underreported.

The Campylobacter Surveillance System is also a passive system that receives weekly reports of laboratory isolates of campylobacter. The number of participating States has increased each year. Surveillance mechanisms, including laboratory isolation procedures, vary from State to State. These issues must be taken into account when interpreting trends in campylobacter incidence.

The incidence of foodborne Listeria monocytogenes is measured using the Bacterial Meningitis Surveillance System. This is an active, laboratory-based surveillance system conducted in six States; it counts all cases of bacterial meningitis and other invasive bacterial diseases caused by the five most common pathogens causing bacterial meningitis, including Listeria monocytogenes. The participating surveillance areas represent several regions throughout the country and a population of 33.5 million, 14 percent of the U.S. population.

A surveillance system to track the incidence of E. Coli 0157:H7 is not available. Estimates of the incidence of cases of this disease are obtained from special studies (2,3). A survey of State public health laboratories conducted by CDC in 1989 demonstrated that E. Coli 0157:H7 has been detected in most areas of the United States (4). Laboratory methods varied from State to State; improved surveillance data are needed to determine trends in incidence.

Table 12. Food and drug safety objective status

Objective	Baseline 1987	1990	1991	Target 2000
12.1 **Foodborne infections (cases per 100,000)**				
Salmonella species	18	---	---	16
Campylobacter jejuni	50	---	---	25
Escherichia coli 0157:H7	8	---	---	4
Listeria monocytogenes	0.7	---	---	0.5
12.2 *Salmonella enteriditis* outbreaks	[1]77	68	68	25
12.3 **Refrigeration and cutting board practices**				
For refrigeration of perishable foods	[2]70%	---	---	75%
For washing cutting boards with soap	[2]66%	---	---	75%
For washing utensils with soap	[2]55%	---	---	75%
12.4 **Food protection standards (proportion of States)**				
Institutional food operations currently using FDA's model codes	[3]20%	---	---	70%
Using "Unicode"	[3]0%	---	---	70%
12.5 **Pharmacies with linked systems**	---	---	---	75%
12.6 **Providers reviewing medication for older patients**	---	---	---	75%

[1]1989 data.
[2]1988 data.
[3]1990 data.

NOTE: Data sources are in table C.

Food and Drug Safety Objectives

12.1: Reduce infections caused by key foodborne pathogens to incidences of no more than:

Disease	2000 target (per 100,000)
Salmonella species	16
Campylobacter	25
Escherichia coli 0157:H7	4
Listeria monocytogenes	0.5

12.2: Reduce outbreaks of infections due to Salmonella enteritidis to fewer than 25 outbreaks yearly.

12.3: Increase to at least 75 percent the proportion of households in which principal food preparers routinely refrain from leaving perishable food out of the refrigerator for over 2 hours and wash cutting boards and utensils with soap after contact with raw meat and poultry.

12.4: Extend to at least 70 percent the proportion of States and territories that have implemented model food codes for institutional food operations and to at least 70 percent the proportion that have adopted the new uniform food protection code ("Unicode") that sets recommended standards for regulation of all food operations.

12.5: Increase to at least 75 percent the proportion of pharmacies and other dispensers of prescription medications that use linked systems to provide alerts to potential adverse drug reactions among medications dispensed by different sources to individual patients.

12.6: Increase to at least 75 percent the proportion of primary care providers who routinely review with their patients aged 65 and older all prescribed and over-the-counter medicines taken by their patients each time a new medication is prescribed.

References

1. Unpublished data. Telephone survey of Medicaid pharmacy program representatives. Health Care Financing Adminstration Medicaid Bureau. 1992.

2. MacDonald KL, O'Leary MJ, Cohen ML, et al. Escherichia coli 0157:H7, an emerging gastrointestinal pathogen: Results of a one-year, prospective, population-based study. JAMA 259: 3567–70. 1988.

3. Ostroff SM, Kobayashi JM, Lewis JH. Infections with Escherichia coli 0157:H7 in Washington State: The first year of statewide disease surveillance. JAMA 262: 355–9. 1989.

4. Ostroff SM, Hopkins DP, Tauxe RV, et al. Surveillance of Escherichia coli 0157:H7 isolation and confirmation, United States, 1988. MMWR 40(SS-1):1–5. 1991.

Priority Area 13
Oral Health

Background and Data Summary

Oral diseases are among the most common health problems in the United States. Even though the overall prevalence of dental caries among school-aged children has declined steadily since the 1940's, half of them have had at least some decay in their permanent teeth (1). Among people aged 40–44 years, an average of more than 30 tooth surfaces have been affected by decay (1). Periodontal diseases are also a chronic problem. For example, 40 to 50 percent of adults (1) and 60 percent of 15-year olds experience gingival infections (2). Despite a steady decline in tooth loss over the past several decades, 36 percent of people 65 years of age and over have lost all of their natural teeth (3). Expenditures for dental care are projected to reach $40 billion in 1992 (4). In 1989 dental visits or problems resulted in 148 hours missed from work per 100 employed people, 117 hours missed from school per 100 school-aged children, and 17 days with restricted activity per 100 people among the total U.S. population (5).

Progress has been made toward achievement of oral health objectives. Small improvements were observed in the proportion of 8- and 14-year olds who had received dental sealants (objective 13.8) and there have been small increases in the proportion of adults who have had a regular dental visit in the preceding year (13.14). Complete tooth loss (13.4) is less common in older adults overall, although there has been no change among those with lower incomes. Oral cancer mortality rates (13.7) have decreased modestly among men and women aged 45–74 years.

Objective 13.12, regarding the proportion of children who have visited a dentist in the past year, is moving away from the target. Recent data beyond the baseline are not available for nine objectives in this priority area. However, for two of these objectives (13.1 and 13.2) recent data are available for the subobjectives targeting American

Indians and Alaska Natives. These data show mixed results. Information on dental caries among 6–8 year-old children are not comparable to baseline, which showed prevalence separately for primary and permanent teeth. Among 15 year-olds, prevalence of dental caries declined slightly. Untreated dental caries increased among 6–8 year-olds and declined among 15 year-olds.

New data are available to establish baselines for objective 13.11 and the subobjectives on the proportion of parents and caregivers who use feeding practices that prevent baby bottle tooth decay. For the total population and for caregivers with less than a high school

education, feeding practices that prevent baby bottle tooth decay were determined for children aged 6–23 months who had ever used a bottle. The preventive feeding practices included children no longer using a bottle and children not given a bottle at bedtime (excluding bottles with plain water) in the past 2 weeks. Although new data were not available for topical and systemic fluoride use among people in areas without fluoridated water (13.10), data are provided that show the proportion of people using these products in the United States overall. Baseline data on oral examination and services requirements for institutions other than nursing facilities (13.13) are not yet available.

Figure 18. Percent of persons 65 years and over who have lost all of their natural teeth: United States, 1986–91 and year 2000 targets for objective 13.4

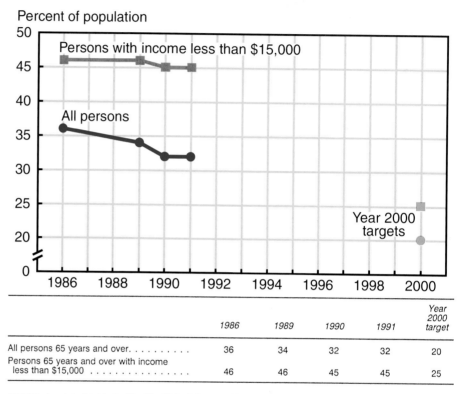

NOTE: A related table in *Health, United States, 1992,* is 82.

SOURCE: Centers for Disease Control and Prevention, National Center for Health Statistics, National Health Interview Survey.

	1986	1989	1990	1991	Year 2000 target
All persons 65 years and over.	36	34	32	32	20
Persons 65 years and over with income less than $15,000	46	46	45	45	25

Data Issues

Proxy Measures

Nationally representative data on topical or systemic fluoride use among people not receiving optimally fluoridated public water are not readily obtainable. It is difficult to identify a national sample of people who are not served by a fluoridated water system. Survey interview methods are limited because many people cannot accurately state the fluoridation status of their water supply. For example, in the 1990 National Health Interview Survey (NHIS), 21 percent of respondents believed that the purpose of water fluoridation was to purify water and 17 percent did not know the reason (6). Presumably, these people and possibly others would also not correctly identify whether their water supply was fluoridated. For this reason, additional baseline data for this objective is use of fluoridated products among all U.S. residents. The measurement of use of fluoride products among people without fluoridated water is estimated from the 1989 NHIS data and information on water fluoridation patterns in the United States.

Comparability of Data Sources

Information on the proportion of 5 year old children and adults aged 35 years and older who visited a dentist in the past 12 months (13.12 and 13.14, respectively) is obtained from supplements to the NHIS. In 1986 and 1989 these data were obtained from a knowledgeable respondent who provided information for all people in the household. The question on dental visits in the past 12 months followed questions about dental visits and problems in the past 2 weeks. The question on visits in the past 2 weeks was not included in the 1991 survey. These may have differentially affected recall about visits in the past 12 months. Among adults, a person sampled from each family provided information only for himself or herself and not others in the household in the 1991 survey.

Table 13. Oral health objective status

Objective	1986–87 baseline Original	1986–87 baseline Revised	1990	1991	Target 2000
13.1 Dental caries					
Children 6–8 years	53%	...	---	---	35%
Adolescents 15 years	78%	...	---	---	60%
a. Children 6–8 years whose parents have less than high school education	70%	...	---	---	45%
b. American Indian/Alaska Native children 6–8 years					
Primary or permanent teeth	---	...	---	88%	45%
Primary teeth	[1]92%	...	---	---	...
Permanent teeth	[1]52%	...	---	---	...
c. Black children 6–8 years	61%	...	---	---	40%
d. American Indian/Alaska Native adolescents 15 years					
Permanent teeth	[1]93%	...	---	91%	70%
13.2 Untreated dental caries					
Children 6–8 years	27%	...	---	---	20%
a. Children whose parents have less than a high school education	43%	...	---	---	30%
b. American Indian/Alaska Native children	[1]64%	...	---	70%	35%
c. Black children	38%	...	---	---	25%
d. Hispanic children	[2]36%	...	---	---	25%
Adolescents 15 years	23%	...	---	---	15%
a. Adolescents whose parents have less than a high school education	41%	...	---	---	25%
b. American Indian/Alaska Native adolescents	[1]84%	...	---	59%	40%
c. Black adolescents	38%	...	---	---	20%
d. Hispanic adolescents	[2]31–47%	...	---	---	25%
13.3 No tooth loss					
People 35–44 years	[3]31%	...	---	---	45%
13.4 Complete tooth loss					
People 65 years and over	[4]36%	...	32%	32%	20%
a. Low-income people (annual family income less than $15,000)	[4]46%	...	45%	45%	25%
13.5 Gingivitis					
People 35–44 years	[3]42%	...	---	---	30%
a. Low-income people (annual family income less than $12,000)	[3]50%	...	---	---	35%
b. American Indians/Alaska Natives	[1]95%	...	---	96%	50%
c. Hispanics	---	...	---	---	50%
Mexican Americans	[2]74%	...	---	---	...
Cubans	[2]79%	...	---	---	...
Puerto Ricans	[2]82%	...	---	---	...
13.6 Periodontal diseases					
People 35–44 years	[3]24%	...	---	---	15%
13.7 Oral cancer deaths					
Males 45–74 years (per 100,000)	[5]12.1	[5,6]13.6	13.4	---	10.5
Females 45–74 years (per 100,000)	[5]4.1	[5,6]4.8	4.6	---	4.1
13.8 Protective sealants					
Children 8 years	11%	...	[7]17%	---	50%
Adolescents 14 years	8%	...	[7]13%	---	50%
13.9 Water fluoridation					
People served by optimally fluoridated water	[7]62%	[7,8]61%	---	---	75%
13.10 Topical and systemic fluorides					
People in nonfluoridated areas who use fluoride	[7]50%	...	---	---	85%
US-wide data people using:					
Toothpaste containing fluoride	...	[4]94%	---	---	...
Fluoride mouthrinse					
Children and adolescents 6–17 years	...	[7]22.0%	---	---	...
People 18 years and over	...	[7]7.7%	---	---	...
Fluoride supplements					
Children and adolescents 2–16	...	[7]10.3%	---	---	...

Table 13. Oral health objective status—Con.

Objective	1986–87 baseline Original	1986–87 baseline Revised	1990	1991	Target 2000
13.11 Baby bottle tooth decay					
Parents and caregivers who use preventive feeding practices	. . .	[9]51%	– – –	– – –	75%
a. Parents and caregivers with less than high school education	. . .	[9]31%	– – –	– – –	65%
b. American Indian/Alaska Native parents and caregivers	. . .	[10]74%	– – –	– – –	65%
13.12 Oral health screening, referral, and follow-up					
Children 5 years who visited the dentist in the past year	[4]66%	. . .	[7]60%	63%	90%
13.13 Oral health care at institutional facilities	– – –	. . .	– – –	– – –	100%
Nursing facilities	[11]Required	. . .	– – –	– – –	. . .
Federal prisons	– – –	. . .	– – –	– – –	. . .
Nonfederal prisons	– – –	. . .	– – –	– – –	. . .
Juvenile homes	– – –	. . .	– – –	– – –	. . .
Detention facilities	– – –	. . .	– – –	– – –	. . .
13.14 Regular dental visits					
People 35 years and over	[4]54%	. . .	[7]55%	58%	70%
a. Edentulous people	[4]11%	. . .	[7]13%	13%	50%
b. People 65 years and over	[4]42%	. . .	[7]43%	47%	60%
13.15 Oral health care for infants with cleft lip and/or palate					
Number of States with existing systems for recording and referring infants	[12]25	. . .	– – –	– – –	40
13.16 Protective equipment in sporting and recreation events	– – –	. . .	– – –	– – –	100%
National Collegiate Athletic Association					
Football	[12]Required	. . .	– – –	– – –	. . .
Hockey	[12]Required	. . .	– – –	– – –	. . .
Lacrosse	[12]Required	. . .	– – –	– – –	. . .
High school football	[12]Required	. . .	– – –	– – –	. . .
Amateur boxing	[12]Required	. . .	– – –	– – –	. . .
Amateur ice hockey	[12]Required	. . .	– – –	– – –	. . .

[1]1983–84 data.
[2]1982–84 data.
[3]1985–86 data.
[4]1986 data.
[5]1987 data.
[6]Data have been recomputed to reflect revised intercensal population estimates; see *Health, United States, 1992*, Appendix I.
[7]1989 data.
[8]Data have been revised. Original data were estimated based on preliminary analyses; see introduction.
[9]1991 data.
[10]1985-89 data.
[11]1990 data.
[12]1988 data.

NOTE: Data sources are in table C.

Oral Health Objectives

13.1: Reduce dental caries (cavities) so that the proportion of children with one or more caries (in permanent or primary teeth) is no more than 35 percent among children aged 6–8 and no more than 60 percent among adolescents aged 15.

> **13.1a**: Reduce dental caries (cavities) so that the proportion of children with one or more caries (in permanent or primary teeth) is no more than 45 percent among children aged 6–8 whose parents have less than high school education.

> **13.1b**: Reduce dental caries (cavities) so that the proportion of children with one or more caries (in permanent or primary teeth) is no more than 45 percent among American Indian and Alaska Native children aged 6–8.

> **13.1c**: Reduce dental caries (cavities) so that the proportion of children with one or more caries (in permanent or primary teeth) is no more than 40 percent among black children aged 6–8.

> **13.1d**: Reduce dental caries (cavities) so that the proportion of adolescents with one or more caries (in permanent teeth) is no more than 70 percent among American Indian and Alaska Native adolescents aged 15.

13.2: Reduce untreated dental caries so that the proportion of children with untreated caries (in permanent or primary teeth) is no more than 20 percent among children aged 6–8 and no more than 15 percent among adolescents aged 15.

> **13.2a**: Reduce untreated dental caries so that the proportion of lower socioeconomic status children (those whose parents have less than a high school education) with untreated dental caries (in permanent or primary teeth) is no more than 30 percent among children aged 6–8 and no more than 25 percent among adolescents aged 15.

> **13.2b**: Reduce untreated dental caries so that the proportion of American Indian and Alaska Native children with untreated caries (in permanent or primary teeth) is no more than 35 percent among children aged 6–8 and no more than 40 percent among adolescents aged 15.

> **13.2c**: Reduce untreated dental caries so that the proportion of black children with untreated caries (in permanent or primary teeth) is no more than 25 percent among children aged 6–8 and no more than 20 percent among adolescents aged 15.

> **13.2d**: Reduce untreated dental caries so that the proportion of Hispanic children with untreated caries (in permanent or primary teeth) is no more than 25 percent among children aged 6–8 and no more than 25 percent among adolescents aged 15.

13.3: Increase to at least 45 percent the proportion of people aged 35–44 who have never lost a permanent tooth due to dental caries or periodontal diseases.

NOTE: Never lost a permanent tooth is having 28 natural teeth exclusive of third molars.

13.4: Reduce to no more than 20 percent the proportion of people aged 65 and older who have lost all of their natural teeth.

13.4a: Reduce to no more than 25 percent the proportion of low-income people (annual family income less than $15,000) aged 65 and older who have lost all of their natural teeth.

13.5: Reduce the prevalence of gingivitis among people aged 35–44 to no more than 30 percent.

13.5a: Reduce the prevalence of gingivitis among low-income people (annual family income less than $12,500) aged 35–44 to no more than 35 percent.

13.5b: Reduce the prevalence of gingivitis among American Indians and Alaska Natives aged 35–44 to no more than 50 percent.

13.5c: Reduce the prevalence of gingivitis among Hispanics aged 35–44 to no more than 50 percent.

13.6: Reduce destructive periodontal diseases to a prevalence of no more than 15 percent among people aged 35–44.

NOTE: Destructive periodontal disease is one or more sites with 4 millimeters or greater loss of tooth attachment.

13.7: Reduce deaths due to cancer of the oral cavity and pharynx to no more than 10.5 per 100,000 men aged 45–74 and 4.1 per 100,000 women aged 45–74.

13.8: Increase to at least 50 percent the proportion of children who have received protective sealants on the occlusal (chewing) surfaces of permanent molar teeth.

NOTE: Progress toward this objective will be monitored based on prevalence of sealants in children at ages 8 and 14, when first and second molars, respectively are erupted.

13.9: Increase to at least 75 percent the proportion of people served by community water systems providing optimal levels of fluoride.

NOTE: Optimal levels of fluoride are determined by the mean maximum daily air temperature over a 5-year period and range between 0.7 and 1.2 parts of fluoride per one million parts of water (ppm).

13.10: Increase use of professionally or self-administered topical or systemic (dietary) fluorides to at least 85 percent of people not receiving optimally fluoridated public water.

13.11*: Increase to at least 75 percent the proportion of parents and caregivers who use feeding practices that prevent baby bottle tooth decay.

Duplicate objective: 2.12

13.11a*: Increase to at least 65 percent the proportion of parents and caregivers with less than a high school education who use feeding practices that prevent baby bottle tooth decay.

Duplicate objective: 2.12a

13.11b*: Increase to at least 65 percent the proportion of American Indian and Alaska Native parents and caregivers who use feeding practices that prevent baby bottle tooth decay.

Duplicate objective: 2.12b

13.12: Increase to at least 90 percent the proportion of all children entering school programs for the first time who have received an oral health screening, referral, and followup for necessary diagnostic, preventive, and treatment services.

NOTE: School programs include Head Start, prekindergarten, kindergarten, and first grade.

13.13: Extend to all long-term institutional facilities the requirement that oral examinations and services be provided no later than 90 days after entry into these facilities.

NOTE: Long term institutional facilities include nursing homes, prisons, and juvenile homes, and detention facilities.

13.14: Increase to at least 70 percent the proportion of people aged 35 and older using the oral health care system during each year.

> **13.14a**: Increase to at least 50 percent the proportion of edentulous people using the oral health care system during each year.

> **13.14b**: Increase to at least 60 percent the proportion of people aged 65 and older using the oral health care system during each year.

13.15: Increase to at least 40 the number of States that have an effective system for recording and referring infants with cleft lips and/or palates to craniofacial anomaly teams.

13.16*: Extend requirement of the use of effective head, face, eye, and mouth protection to all organizations, agencies, and institutions sponsoring sporting and recreation events that pose risk of injury.

Duplicate objective: 9.19

*Duplicate objective

References

1. National Institute of Dental Research. The oral health of United States adults. The National Survey of Oral Health in U.S. Employed Adults and Seniors: 1985–86. Bethesda, Maryland: U.S. Department of Health and Human Services. 1987.

2. National Institute of Dental Research. The oral health of United States children. The National Survey of Dental Caries in U.S. School Children, 1986–87. Bethesda, Maryland: U.S. Department of Health and Human Services. 1989.

3. Jack SS, Bloom B. Use of dental services and dental health, United States, 1986. National Center for Health Statistics. Vital Health Stat 10(165). 1988.

4. U.S. Department of Commerce. U.S. industrial outlook '92. Washington: U.S. Department of Commerce. 1992.

5. Gift HC, Reisine ST, Larach DC. The social impact of dental problems and visits. Am J Public Health 82:1663–8. 1992.

6. Centers for Disease Control. Knowledge of the purpose of community water fluoridation – United States, 1990. MMWR 14:919–27. 1992.

Priority Area 14
Maternal and Infant Health

Background and Data Summary

Improving the health of mothers and infants is a national challenge. Of every 1,000 babies born in the United States each year, about 9 die before their first birthday (1). Although the infant mortality rate in the United States continues to decline and has reached an all-time low, in recent years the pace of progress has slowed Important measures of increased risk of infant death, such as incidence of low birth weight and receipt of prenatal care, show little or no recent improvement. The mortality rate for black infants is twice the rate for white infants, and there is evidence that this difference is increasing (2).

Of the 16 Maternal and Infant Health objectives for the total population, 7 moved toward the year 2000 targets (objectives 14.1, 14.2, 14.6, 14.7, 14.8, 14.10, and 14.15); 5 moved away from the targets (14.3, 14.4, 14.5, 14.9, and 14.11). Data to update progress for the remaining four objectives are not yet available. For some objectives, even though the overall objective is showing progress, the picture for minority racial subgroups is less encouraging. For example, although the overall infant, neonatal, and postneonatal mortality rates are declining (objective 14.1, 14.1d, and 14.1g), postneonatal rates among black infants (14.1h) are not improving. Further reductions in infant mortality and morbidity will require a focus on strategies to modify the behaviors and lifestyles that affect birth outcomes.

Data Issues

Definitions

In 1989 NCHS changed the method for tabulating race for live births, assigning to the infant the race of mother rather than using the previous, more complicated algorithm for race of child. This change affects the natality data by race in this chapter. In addition, because live

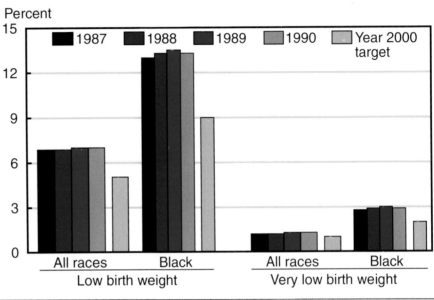

Figure 19. Proportion of live births that are low birth weight and are very low birth weight by race of mother: United States, 1987–90 and year 2000 targets for objective 14.5

	1987	1988	1989	1990	Year 2000 target
Low birth weight (All races)	6.9	6.9	7.0	7.0	5
Low birth weight (Black)	13.0	13.3	13.5	13.3	9
Very low birth weight (All races)	1.2	1.2	1.3	1.3	1
Very low birth weight (Black)	2.8	2.9	3.0	2.9	2

NOTE: Related tables in *Health, United States, 1992,* are 8, 11, and 12. See definition of birth weight in *Health, United States, 1992,* Appendix II.

SOURCE: Centers for Disease Control and Prevention, National Center for Health Statistics, National Vital Statistics System.

births comprise the denominator of infant (including neonatal and postneonatal), maternal mortality, and fetal death rates, these rates are also affected. These changes are described in the technical notes and in greater detail in a 1991 NCHS publication (3).

Quantitatively, the change in the basis for tabulating live births by race results in more births to the white population and fewer births to the black population and other races. Because of changes in the denominators, infant mortality rates (14.1), fetal death rates (14.2), and maternal mortality rates (14.3) under the new classification tend to be

lower for white infants and higher for infants of other races than they would be when computed by the previous method. Conversely, natality measures such as percent low birth weight (14.5) and percent receiving early care (14.11) tend to be higher for white births and lower for births of other races.

The special target populations for racial subgroups in this priority area are being monitored with the "new" data by race of mother. Therefore, the original baselines (by race of child) for these racial subgroups have been recomputed by race of mother to allow comparable trend comparisons.

Studies indicate that infant mortality for minorities other than blacks from the annual vital statistics files have been seriously underestimated (4). Therefore, infant mortality (objective 14.1) for American Indians and Alaska Natives and for Puerto Ricans is being monitored through data from the Linked Infant Birth and Infant Death Files, which categorizes deaths by the race of mother as reported on the birth certificate.

Table 14. Maternal and infant health objective status

Objective	1987 baseline Original	1987 baseline Revised	1990	1991	Target 2000
14.1 Infant mortality (per 1,000 live births)	10.1	. . .	9.2	[1]8.9	7
a. Blacks	17.9	[2]18.8	18.0	– – –	11
b. American Indians/Alaska Natives	[3]12.5	[2,3]13.4	[4]13.0	– – –	8.5
c. Puerto Ricans	[3]12.9	. . .	[4]9.9	– – –	8
d. Neonatal mortality	6.5	. . .	5.8	[1]5.5	4.5
e. Neonatal mortality among blacks	11.7	[2]12.3	11.6	– – –	7
f. Neonatal mortality among Puerto Ricans	[3]8.6	. . .	[4]6.7	– – –	5.2
g. Postneonatal mortality	3.6	. . .	3.4	[1]3.4	2.5
h. Postneonatal mortality among blacks	6.1	[2]6.4	6.4	– – –	4
i. Postneonatal mortality among American Indians/Alaska Natives	[3]6.5	[2,3]7.0	[4]6.8	– – –	4
j. Postneonatal mortality among Puerto Ricans	[3]4.3	. . .	[4]3.2	– – –	2.8
14.2 Fetal deaths (per 1,000 live births plus fetal deaths)	7.6	. . .	7.5	– – –	5
a. Blacks	12.8	[2]13.5	13.7	– – –	7.5
14.3 Maternal mortality (per 100,000 live births)	6.6	. . .	8.2	– – –	3.3
a. Blacks	14.2	[2]14.9	22.4	– – –	5
14.4 Fetal alcohol syndrome (per 1,000 live births)	0.22	. . .	0.41	– – –	0.12
a. American Indians/Alaska Natives	4.0	. . .	5.2	– – –	2.0
b. Blacks	0.8	. . .	1.4	– – –	0.4
14.5 Low birth weight	6.9%	. . .	7.0%	– – –	5%
Very low birth weight	1.2%	. . .	1.3%	– – –	1%
a. Low-birth weight blacks	12.7%	[2]13.0%	13.3%	– – –	9%
b. Very-low birth weight blacks	2.7%	[2]2.8%	2.9%	– – –	2%
14.6 Recommended weight gain during pregnancy	[5]67%	[5,6]68%	[7]75%	– – –	85%
14.7 Severe complications of pregnancy (per 100 deliveries)	22	. . .	18	18	15
14.8 Cesarean delivery (per 100 deliveries)	24.4	. . .	23.5	23.5	15
a. Primary (first time) cesarean delivery	17.4	. . .	16.8	17.1	12
b. Repeat cesarean deliveries (among woman with previous cesarean delivery)	91.2	. . .	79.6	75.8	65
14.9 Breastfeeding					
During early postpartum period	[7]54%	. . .	52%	53%	75%
a. Low-income mothers	[7]32%	. . .	35%	33%	75%
b. Black mothers	[7]25%	. . .	16%	26%	75%
c. Hispanic mothers	[7]51%	. . .	44%	52%	75%
d. American Indian/Alaska Native mothers	[7]47%	. . .	47%	46%	75%
At 5–6 months	[7]21%	. . .	18%	18%	50%
a. Low-income mothers	[7]9%	. . .	8%	9%	50%
b. Black mothers	[7]8%	. . .	7%	7%	50%
c. Hispanic mothers	[7]16%	. . .	14%	16%	50%
d. American Indian/Alaska Native mothers	[7]28%	. . .	27%	22%	50%
14.10 Alcohol, tobacco, and drug use during pregnancy					
Abstinence from					
Tobacco	[8]75%	. . .	79%	80%	90%
Alcohol	– – –	. . .	[7]79%	– – –	Increase by 20%
Cocaine	– – –	. . .	[7]99%	– – –	Increase by 20%
Marijuana	– – –	. . .	[7]98%	– – –	Increase by 20%
14.11 Prenatal care in the first trimester (percent of live births)	76.0%	. . .	75.8%	– – –	90%
a. Blacks	61.1%	[2]60.8%	60.6%	– – –	90%
b. American Indians/Alaska Natives	60.2%	[2]57.6%	57.9%	– – –	90%
c. Hispanics	61.0%	. . .	60.2%	– – –	90%

Table 14. Maternal and infant health objective status—Con.

Objective	1987 baseline		1990	1991	Target 2000
	Original	Revised			
14.12 Age-appropriate preconception counseling by clinicians	---	...	---	---	60%
14.13 Counseling on detection of fetal abnormalities...................	...	[7]29%	---	---	90%
14.14 Pregnant women and infants receiving risk-appropriate care.......	---	...	---	---	90%
14.15 Newborn screening and treatment					
Screened by State-sponsored programs for genetic disorders and other conditions	---	...	---	---	95%
Testing positive for disease and receiving appropriate treatment.......	---	...	---	---	90%
Sickle cell screening.....................................	[9]33%	...	[10]89%	---	...
Black infants	[9]57%	...	[11]77%	---	...
Newborns diagnosed positive for sickle cell anemia receiving treatment.	---	...	95%	---	...
Galactosemia screening (38 states).........................	70%	...	97%	---	...
Newborns diagnosed positive for galactosemia receiving treatment	---	...	100%	---	...
14.16 Babies receiving primary care................................	---	...	---	---	90%

[1]Provisional data.
[2]Data have been revised to reflect the change in tabulating births from the race of the child to the race of the mother; see *Health, United States, 1992*, Appendix I.
[3]1984 data.
[4]1987 data.
[5]1980 data for married females who had a full-term live birth and prenatal care.
[6]Data have been revised to reflect updated methodology; see Introduction.
[7]1988 data.
[8]1985 data.
[9]Based on 20 States reporting.
[10]Based on 43 States reporting.
[11]Based on 9 States reporting.

NOTE: Data sources are in table C.

Maternal and Infant Health Objectives

14.1: Reduce the infant mortality rate to no more than 7 per 1,000 live births.

NOTE: Infant mortality is deaths of infants under 1 year; neonatal mortality is deaths of infants under 28 days; and postneonatal mortality is deaths of infants aged 28 days up to 1 year.

> **14.1a**: Reduce the infant mortality rate among blacks to no more than 11 per 1,000 live births.

> **14.1b**: Reduce the infant mortality rate among American Indians and Alaska Natives to no more than 8.5 per 1,000 live births.

> **14.1c**: Reduce the infant mortality rate among Puerto Ricans to no more than 8 per 1,000 live births.

> **14.1d**: Reduce the neonatal mortality rate to no more than 4.5 per 1,000 live births.

> **14.1e**: Reduce the neonatal mortality rate among blacks to no more than 7 per 1,000 live births.

> **14.1f**: Reduce the neonatal mortality rate among Puerto Ricans to no more than 5.2 per 1,000 live births.

> **14.1g**: Reduce the postneonatal mortality rate to no more than 2.5 per 1,000 live births.

> **14.1h**: Reduce the postneonatal mortality rate among blacks to no more than 4 per 1,000 live births.

> **14.1i**: Reduce the postneonatal mortality rate among American Indians and Alaska Natives to no more than 4 per 1,000 live births.

> **14.1j**: Reduce the postneonatal mortality rate among Puerto Ricans to no more than 2.8 per 1,000 live births.

14.2: Reduce the fetal death rate (20 or more weeks of gestation) to no more than 5 per 1,000 live births plus fetal deaths.

> **14.2a**: Reduce the fetal death rate (20 or more weeks of gestation) among blacks to no more than 7.5 per 1,000 live births plus fetal deaths.

14.3: Reduce the maternal mortality rate to no more than 3.3 per 100,000 live births.

NOTE: The objective uses the maternal mortality rate as defined by the National Center for Health Statistics. However, if other sources of maternal mortality data are used, a 50-percent reduction in maternal mortality is the intended target.

> **14.3a**: Reduce the maternal mortality rate among black women to no more than 5 per 100,000 live births.

14.4: Reduce the incidence of fetal alcohol syndrome to no more than 0.12 per 1,000 live births.

> **14.4a**: Reduce the incidence of fetal alcohol syndrome among American Indians and Alaska Natives to no more than 2 per 1,000 live births.

> **14.4b**: Reduce the incidence of fetal alcohol syndrome among blacks to no more than 0.4 per 1,000 live births.

14.5: Reduce low birth weight to an incidence of no more than 5 percent of live births and very low birth weight to no more 1 percent of live births.

NOTE: Low birth weight is weight at birth of less than 2,500 grams; very low birth weight is weight at birth of less than 1,500 grams.

> **14.5a**: Reduce low birth weight among blacks to an incidence of no more than 9 percent of live births and very low birth weight to no more 2 percent of live births.

14.6: Increase to at least 85 percent the proportion of mothers who achieve the minimum recommended weight gain during their pregnancies.

NOTE: Recommended weight gain is pregnancy weight gain recommended in the 1990 National Academy of Science's report, Nutrition During Pregnancy.

14.7: Reduce severe complications of pregnancy to no more than 15 per 100 deliveries.

NOTE: Severe complications of pregnancy will be measured using hospitalizations due to pregnancy-related complications.

14.8: Reduce the cesarean delivery rate to no more than 15 per 100 deliveries.

14.8a: Reduce the primary (first time) cesarean delivery rate to no more than 12 per 100 deliveries.

14.8b: Reduce the repeat cesarean delivery rate to no more than 65 per 100 deliveries among women who had a previous cesarean delivery.

14.9*: Increase to at least 75 percent the proportion of mothers who breastfeed their babies in the early postpartum period and to at least 50 percent the proportion who continue breastfeeding until their babies are 5 to 6 months old.

Duplicate objective: 2.11

14.9a*: Increase to at least 75 percent the proportion of low-income mothers who breastfeed their babies in the early postpartum period and to at least 50 percent the proportion who continue breastfeeding until their babies are 5 to 6 months old.

Duplicate objective: 2.11a

14.9b*: Increase to at least 75 percent the proportion of black mothers who breastfeed their babies in the early postpartum period and to at least 50 percent the proportion who continue breastfeeding until their babies are 5 to 6 months old.

Duplicate objective: 2.11b

14.9c*: Increase to at least 75 percent the proportion of Hispanic mothers who breastfeed their babies in the early postpartum period and to at least 50 percent the proportion who continue breastfeeding until their babies are 5 to 6 months old.

Duplicate objective: 2.11c

14.9d*: Increase to at least 75 percent the proportion of American Indian and Alaska Native mothers who breastfeed their babies in the early postpartum period and to at least 50 percent the proportion who continue breastfeeding until their babies are 5 to 6 months old.

Duplicate objective: 2.11d

14.10: Increase abstinence from tobacco use by pregnant women to at least 90 percent and increase abstinence from alcohol, cocaine, and marijuana by pregnant women by at least 20 percent.

14.11: Increase to at least 90 percent the proportion of all pregnant women who receive prenatal care in the first trimester of pregnancy.

14.11a: Increase to at least 90 percent the proportion of pregnant black women who receive prenatal care in the first trimester of pregnancy.

14.11b: Increase to at least 90 percent the proportion of pregnant American Indian and Alaska Native women who receive prenatal care in the first trimester of pregnancy.

14.11c: Increase to at least 90 percent the proportion of pregnant Hispanic women who receive prenatal care in the first trimester of pregnancy.

14.12*: Increase to at least 60 percent the proportion of primary care providers who provide age-appropriate preconception care and counseling.

Duplicate objective: 05.10

14.13: Increase to at least 90 percent the proportion of women enrolled in prenatal care who are offered screening and counseling on prenatal detection of fetal abnormalities.

NOTE: This objective will be measured by tracking use of maternal serum alpha-feto protein screening tests.

14.14: Increase to at least 90 percent the proportion of pregnant women and infants who receive risk-appropriate care.

NOTE: This objective will be measured by tracking the proportion of very low-birth weight infants (less than 1,500 grams) born in facilities covered by a neonatologist 24 hours a day.

14.15: Increase to at least 95 percent the proportion of newborns screened by State-sponsored programs for genetic disorders and other disabling conditions and to 90 percent the proportion of newborns testing positive for disease who receive appropriate treatment.

NOTE: As measured by the proportion of infants served by programs for sickle cell anemia and galactosemia. Screening programs should be appropriate for State demographic characteristics.

14.16: Increase to at least 90 percent the proportion of babies aged 18 months and younger who receive recommended primary care services at the appropriate intervals.

*Duplicate objective.

References

1. National Center for Health Statistics. Births, marriages, divorces, and deaths for 1991. Monthly vital statistics report; vol 40 no 12. Hyattsville, Maryland: Public Health Service. 1992.

2. National Center for Health Statistics. Advance report of final mortality statistics, 1990. Monthly vital statistics report; vol 40 no 8, suppl 2. Hyattsville, Maryland: Public Health Service. 1993.

3. National Center for Health Statistics. Advance report of final natality statistics, 1989. Monthly vital statistics report; vol 40 no 8, suppl. Hyattsville, Maryland: Public Health Service. Dec 1991.

4. Hahn, RA, Mulinare J, Teutsh SM. Inconsistencies in coding of race and ethnicity between birth and death in U.S. infants: A new look at infant mortality, 1983 through 1985. JAMA 267:259–263. 1992

Priority Area 15
Heart Disease and Stroke

Background

Over the past 15 years the death rate for cardiovascular disease has declined dramatically: 35 percent for all cardiovascular disease, 40 percent for coronary heart disease, and more than 50 percent for stroke. Even so, cardiovascular diseases—primarily coronary heart disease and stroke—kill nearly as many Americans as all other diseases combined (1). Cardiovascular disease is also among the leading causes of disability (2). The major modifiable risk factors for cardiovascular disease are high blood pressure, high blood cholesterol, and cigarette smoking. Other important risk factors are obesity, physical inactivity, and diabetes mellitus. Approximately 26 percent of adults have high blood pressure (3). Overall, black persons have a higher prevalence of high blood pressure than white persons. About 60 million adults have high blood cholesterol requiring medical advice and intervention (4,5). Twenty-six percent of adults are current cigarette smokers (See chapter 3, Tobacco).

Of 17 objectives in the heart disease and stroke priority area, data for nine objectives show improvements toward meeting the year 2000 targets (objectives 15.1, 15.2, 15.4, 15.5, 15.11, 15.12, 15.13, 15.14, and 15.17). Mortality due to coronary heart disease (15.1) and stroke (15.2) declined from the 1987 baseline through 1990 in the population as a whole; however, for both causes of death, black persons have much higher mortality rates and the decline in mortality over the same time period was much less substantial. A small improvement in the proportion of adults who have ever had their blood cholesterol checked was noted for the period 1988 to 1991 (15.14). Information is not available regarding the proportion of adults who have had their cholesterol checked in the preceding 5 years as specified in the objective. New baseline data were obtained for

one objective (15.16). Self-reported data for proxy tracking of objective 15.10 (proportion of the population that is overweight) indicate movement away from the target. The rate of end stage renal disease (15.3) is also moving away from the target. Data on dietary fat intake (15.9) showed no change. Recent data are not available for three objectives (15.6, 15.7, and 15.8). Baseline data are needed for objective 15.15.

Data Issues

Definitions

Objective 15.4 addresses the proportion of people with hypertension whose blood pressure is

under control. High blood pressure is defined as blood pressure greater than 140/90 mm Hg. The estimates used to track this objective define control as using antihypertensive medication only and do not include nonpharmacologic treatments (such as weight loss, low sodium diets or restriction of alcohol) as a method of keeping blood pressure under control. The 1976–80 baseline is from the second National Health and Nutrition Examination Survey (NHANES II), which covered people 18–74 years of age; 1988–91 preliminary data from the NHANES III are for people 18 years and over. The 1982–84 baseline originally published in *Healthy People 2000* (2) from the Seven States Study, representing the medians of data from selected States, will no longer be used for tracking this objective. In

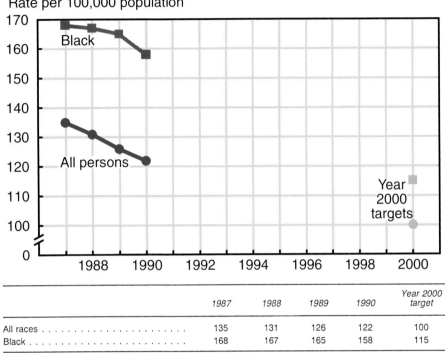

Figure 20. Age-adjusted death rates for coronary heart disease: United States, 1987–90 and year 2000 targets for objective 15.1

Rate per 100,000 population

	1987	1988	1989	1990	Year 2000 target
All races	135	131	126	122	100
Black	168	167	165	158	115

NOTE: Death rates are age adjusted. ICD codes differ from similar categories published in *Health, United States* and elsewhere. See table A for specific codes. Related tables in *Health, United States, 1992,* are 28 and 35 for diseases of heart.

SOURCE: Centers for Disease Control and Prevention, National Center for Health Statistics, National Vital Statistics System.

1976–80, among all people with high blood pressure (whether aware or unaware of their conditon), only 11 percent were on medication and had their condition under control; 1988–91 preliminary data indicate that 21 percent of people with hypertension had their condition under control. Among people being treated for hypertension, 33 percent were controlling their high blood pressure in 1976–80; the proportion has increased to 43 percent based on 1988–91 preliminary data.

Objective 15.5 refers to people with high blood pressure who are aware of their condition defined by self-reported data and not blood pressure measurement. Data from the National Health Interview Survey (NHIS) are used to measure progress towards increasing the proportion of people with high blood pressure who are taking action to help control their blood pressure. People with high blood pressure are defined as those who report being told that they had high blood pressure on two or more occasions by a doctor or other health professional. Respondents with a history of high blood pressure were asked whether they used the following methods to control blood pressure: taking medication, dieting to lose weight, cutting down on salt, and exercising.

Comparability of Data Sources

Objective 15.13 addresses blood pressure screening and whether people know if their blood pressure is normal or high. Data for the 1985 baseline and for 1990 show the proportion of people 18 years of age and over who had their blood pressure measured within the preceding 2 years by a health professional or other trained observer and who can state the diastolic and systolic values of the measure. The proportion of adults 18 years and over who had their blood pressure checked within the previous 2 years and who could state whether their blood pressure was high, normal, or low was 86 percent in 1990 and 85 percent in 1991. This measure is not available for the 1985 baseline.

Objective 15.14, proportion of people who have had their blood cholesterol checked within the preceding 5 years, has been tracked with three different surveys. The baseline data are from the 1988 Health and Diet Survey; 1990 data are from the Cholesterol Awareness Survey; and 1991 data are from the NHIS. Data from these three surveys indicate that the percent of the population who have ever had their blood cholesterol measured is increasing. However, these differences may be due in part to survey differences.

Data Availability

Objectives 15.6, 15.7, and 15.8, which address mean serum cholesterol level, high blood cholesterol prevalence, and awareness of a high blood cholesterol condition, will be measured by the NHANES III. Data from the first 3 years of this survey will be available in mid-1993.

Proxy Measures

Objectives 15.9 (dietary fat intake) and 15.10 (overweight) will be measured by the NHANES III. Provisional estimates from the 1989 Continuing Survey of Food Intakes for Individuals for objective 15.9 and self-reported data from the NHIS for objective 15.10 are being used to track these objectives until NHANES III data are available.

See priority area 1 for a discussion of self-reported height and weight (15.10), as well as light to moderate physical activity (15.11).

Table 15. Heart disease and stroke objective status

Objective	1987 baseline Original	1987 baseline Revised	1990	1991	Target 2000
		[1]No			
15.1 Coronary heart disease deaths (age adjusted per 100,000)	135	change	122	---	100
a. Blacks (age adjusted per 100,000)	163	[1]168	158	---	115
15.2 Stroke deaths (age adjusted per 100,000).......................	30.3	[1]30.4	27.7	---	20.0
a. Blacks (age adjusted per 100,000)	51.2	[1]52.5	48.4	---	27.0
15.3 End-stage renal disease (per 100,000).........................	13.9	[2]14.4	18.4	---	13.0
a. Blacks	32.4	[2]34.0	43.0	---	30.0
15.4 Controlled high blood pressure[3]					
People with high blood pressure 18 years and over.................	[4,5]11%	...	[6]21%	---	50%
a. Males with high blood pressure...................................	[3]6%	...	[6]16%	---	40%
15.5 Taking action to control blood pressure					
People 18 years and over...	[7]79%	...	80%	---	90%
a. White hypertensive males 18–34 years	[7]51%	...	54%	---	80%
b. Black hypertensive males 18–34 years	[7]63%	...	56%	---	80%
15.6 Mean serum cholesterol level (mg/dL)					
People 20–74 years...	[4]213	...	---	---	200
15.7 High blood cholesterol prevalence					
People 20–74 years...	[4]27%	...	---	---	20%
15.8 Awareness of high blood cholesterol condition					
Adults with high blood cholesterol.................................	[8]30%	...	---	---	60%
15.9 Dietary fat intake among people 2 years and over					
People 2 years and over					
Percent of calories from total fat.................................	---	...	---	---	30%
Percent of calories from saturated fat............................	---	...	---	---	10%
People 20–74 years					
Percent of calories from total fat.................................	[4]36%	...	[9]36%	---	...
Percent of calories from saturated fat............................	[4]13%	...	[9]13%	---	...
Females 19–50 years					
Percent of calories from total fat.................................	[7]36%	...	---	---	...
Percent of calories from saturated fat............................	[7]13%	...	---	---	...
15.10 Overweight prevalence					
People 20 years and over...	[4]26%	...	27%	28%	20%
Males..	[4]24%	...	27%	28%	...
Females..	[4]27%	...	27%	28%	...
Adolescents 12–19 years	[4]15%	...	---	---	15%
a. Low-income females 20 years over...............................	[4]37%	...	37%	39%	25%
b. Black females 20 years and over................................	[4]44%	...	42%	44%	30%
c. Hispanic females 20 years and over	...	[6]27%	33%	32%	25%
Mexican-American females	[10]39%	...	---	38%	...
Cuban females	[10]34%	...	---	---	...
Puerto Rican females	[10]37%	...	---	---	...
d. American Indians/Alaska Natives	[11]29–75%	...	---	40%	30%
e. People with disabilities.......................................	[6]36%	...	---	38%	25%
f. Females with high blood pressure..............................	[3]50%	...	---	---	41%
g. Males with high blood pressure................................	[3]39%	...	---	---	35%
15.11 Moderate physical activity					
People 6 years and over..	---	...	---	---	30%
People 18–74 years					
		[7,12]No			
5 or more times per week..	[7]22%	change	23%	24%	...
7 or more times per week..	[7]12%	[7,12]16%	16%	17%	...
15.12 Cigarette smoking prevalence					
People 20 years and over...	29%	...	26%	26%	15%
Males..	32%	...	28%	28%	...
Females..	27%	...	23%	24%	...
a. People with high school education or less					
20 years and over	34%	...	31%	32%	20%
b. Blue-collar workers 20 years and over..........................	36%	...	37%	36%	20%
c. Military personnel	[13]42%	...	---	[14]35%	20%
d. Blacks 20 years and over.......................................	34%	...	27%	30%	18%
e. Hispanics 20 years and over	[10]33%	...	24%	20%	18%

Table 15. Heart disease and stroke objective status—Con.

Objective	1987 baseline Original	Revised	1990	1991	Target 2000
f. American Indians/Alaska natives	[15]42–70%	. . .	38%	33%	20%
g. Southeast Asian males	[11]55%	. . .	[16]35%	– – –	20%
h. Females of reproductive age (18–44 years)	29%	. . .	26%	27%	12%
i. Pregnant females	[7]25%	. . .	19%	20%	10%
j. Females who use oral contraceptives	[17]36%	. . .	[13]26%	– – –	10%
15.13 Knowledge of blood pressure values					
People 18 years and over	[7]61%	. . .	67%	– – –	90%
15.14 Blood cholesterol checked in past 5 years					
People 18 years and over	– – –	. . .	– – –	– – –	75%
Ever checked	[13]59%	. . .	65%	63%	. . .
Within past 2 years	52%	. . .	– – –	50%	. . .
15.15 Primary care providers who provide appropriate therapy for high blood cholesterol	– – –	. . .	– – –	– – –	75%
15.16 Worksite blood pressure/cholesterol education programs					
High blood pressure and/or cholesterol activity	[14]35%	. . .	– – –	– – –	50%
High blood pressure activity	[7]16.5%	. . .	– – –	– – –	. . .
Nutrition education activity	[7]16.8%	. . .	– – –	– – –	. . .
15.17 Laboratory accuracy in cholesterol measurement	[5]53%	. . .	[18]84%	– – –	90%

[1]Data have been recomputed to reflect revised intercensal population estimates; see *Health, United States, 1992*, Appendix I.
[2]Data have been revised. Original data were estimated based on preliminary analyses; see Introduction.
[3]The published 1982–84 Seven States Study baseline of 24 percent of adults 18 years and over with hypertension who are controlling their high blood pressure will not be used for tracking.
[4]1976–80 data.
[5]People 18–74 years.
[6]1988–91 provisional estimates from NHANES III for people 18 years and over.
[7]1985 data.
[8]Data source for updates has changed; previously published tracking data will be replaced.
[9]1989 data.
[10]1982–84 data.
[11]1984–88 data.
[12]Data source has been changed and data have been revised to reflect updated methodology; see Introduction.
[13]1988 data.
[14]1992 data.
[15]1979–87 data.
[16]Vietnamese males only.
[17]1983 data.
[18]1987 data.

NOTE: Data sources are in table C.

Heart Disease and Stroke Objectives

15.1*: Reduce coronary heart disease deaths to no more than 100 per 100,000 people.

Duplicate objectives: 1.1, 2.1, and 3.1

> **15.1a***: Reduce coronary heart disease deaths among blacks to no more than 115 per 100,000 people.

Duplicate objectives: 1.1a, 2.1a, and 3.1a

15.2: Reduce stroke deaths to no more than 20 per 100,000 people.

> **15.2a**: Reduce stroke deaths among blacks to no more than 27 per 100,000.

15.3: Reverse the increase in end-stage renal disease (requiring maintenance dialysis or transplantation) to attain an incidence of no more than 13 per 100,000.

> **15.3a**: Reverse the increase in end-stage renal disease (requiring maintenance dialysis or transplantation) among black persons to attain an incidence of no more than 30 per 100,000.

15.4: Increase to at least 50 percent the proportion of people with high blood pressure whose blood pressure is under control.

**NOTE: People with high blood pressure have blood pressure equal to or greater than 140 mm Hg systolic and/or 90 mm Hg diastolic and/or take antihypertensive medication. Blood pressure control is defined as maintaining a blood pressure less than 140 mm Hg systolic and 90 mm Hg diastolic. Nonpharmacologic treatment (e.g., through weight loss, low sodium diets, or restriction of alcohol) is not included.

> **15.4a**: Increase to at least 40 percent the proportion of men with high blood pressure whose blood pressure is under control.

15.5: Increase to at least 90 percent the proportion of people with high blood pressure who are taking action to help control their blood pressure.

**NOTE: Self-reported data are used for this objective. People with high blood pressure are defined as people who have been told that they have high blood pressure on two or more occasions by a doctor or other health professional. Actions to control blood pressure include taking medication, dieting to lose weight, cutting down on salt, and exercising.

> **15.5a**: Increase to at least 80 percent the proportion of white hypertensive men aged 18–34 who are taking action to help control their blood pressure.

> **15.5b**: Increase to at least 80 percent the proportion of black hypertensive men aged 18–34 who are taking action to help control their blood pressure.

15.6: Reduce the mean serum cholesterol level among adults to no more than 200 mg/dL.

15.7: Reduce the prevalence of blood cholesterol levels of 240 mg/dL or greater to no more than 20 percent among adults.

15.8: Increase to at least 60 percent the proportion of adults with high blood cholesterol who are aware of their condition and are taking action to reduce their blood cholesterol to recommended levels.

NOTE: "High blood cholesterol" means a level that requires diet and, if necessary, drug treatment. Action to control high blood cholesterol include keeping medical appointments, making recommended dietary changes (e.g., reducing saturated fat, total fat, and dietary cholesterol), and, if necessary, taking prescribed medication.

15.9*: Reduce dietary fat intake to an average of 30 percent of calories or less and average saturated fat intake to less than 10 percent of calories among people aged 2 and older.

Duplicate objectives: 2.5 and 16.7

15.10*: Reduce overweight to a prevalence of no more than 20 percent among people aged 20 and older and no more than 15 percent among adolescents aged 12–19.

NOTE: For people aged 20 and older, overweight is defined as body mass index (BMI) equal to or greater than 27.8 for men and 27.3 for women. For adolescents, overweight is defined as BMI equal to or greater than 23.0 for males aged 12–14, 24.3 for males aged 15–17, 25.8 for males aged 18–19, 23.4 for females aged 12–14, 24.8 for females aged 15–17, and 25.7 for females aged 18–19. The values for adolescents are the age- and gender-specific 85th percentile values of the 1976–80 National Health and Nutrition Examination Survey (NHANES II), corrected for sample variation. BMI is calculated by dividing weight in kilograms by the square of height in meters. The cut points used to define overweight approximate the 120 percent of desirable body weight definition used in the 1990 objectives.

Duplicate objectives: 1.2, 2.3, and 17.12

> **15.10a***: Reduce overweight to a prevalence of no more than 25 percent among low-income women aged 20 and older.

Duplicate objectives: 1.2a, 2.3a, and 17.12a

> **15.10b***: Reduce overweight to a prevalence of no more than 30 percent among black women aged 20 and older.

Duplicate objectives: 1.2b, 2.3b, and 17.12b

> **15.10c***: Reduce overweight to a prevalence of no more than 25 percent among Hispanic women aged 20 and older.

Duplicate objectives: 1.2c, 2.3c, and 17.12c

> **15.10d***: Reduce overweight to a prevalence of no more than 30 percent among American Indians and Alaska Natives.

Duplicate objectives: 1.2d, 2.3d, and 17.12d

> **15.10e***: Reduce overweight to a prevalence of no more than 25 percent among people with disabilities.

Duplicate objectives: 1.2e, 2.3e, and 17.12e

> **15.10f***: Reduce overweight to a prevalence of no more than 41 percent among women with high blood pressure aged 20 and older.

Duplicate objectives: 1.2f, 2.3f, and 17.12f

> **15.10g***: Reduce overweight to a prevalence of no more than 35 percent among men with high blood pressure aged 20 and older.

Duplicate objectives: 1.2g, 2.3g, and 17.12g

15.11*: Increase to at least 30 percent the proportion of people aged 6 and older who engage regularly, preferably daily, in light to moderate physical activity for at least 30 minutes per day.

NOTE: Light to moderate physical activity requires sustained, rhythmic muscular movements, is at least equivalent to sustained walking, and is performed at less than 60 percent of maximum heart rate for age. Maximum heart rate equals roughly 220 beats per minute minus age. Examples may include walking, swimming, cycling, dancing, gardening and yard work, various domestic and occupational activities, and games and other childhood pursuits.

Duplicate objectives: 1.3 and 17.13

15.12*: Reduce cigarette smoking to a prevalence of no more than 15 percent among people aged 20 and older.

NOTE: A cigarette smoker is a person who has smoked at least 100 cigarettes and currently smokes cigarettes.

Duplicate objectives: 3.4 and 16.6

15.12a*: Reduce cigarette smoking to a prevalence of no more than 20 percent among people aged 20 and older with a high school education or less.

Duplicate objectives: 3.4a and 16.6a

15.12b*: Reduce cigarette smoking to a prevalence of no more than 20 percent among blue-collar workers aged 20 and older.

Duplicate objectives: 3.4b and 16.6b

15.12c*: Reduce cigarette smoking to a prevalence of no more than 20 percent among military personnel.

Duplicate objectives: 3.4c and 16.6c

15.12d*: Reduce cigarette smoking to a prevalence of no more than 18 percent among blacks aged 20 and older.

Duplicate objectives: 3.4d and 16.6d

15.12e*: Reduce cigarette smoking to a prevalence of no more than 18 percent among Hispanics aged 20 and older.

Duplicate objectives: 3.4e and 16.6e

15.12f*: Reduce cigarette smoking to a prevalence of no more than 20 percent among American Indians and Alaska Natives.

Duplicate objectives: 3.4f and 16.6f

15.12g*: Reduce cigarette smoking to a prevalence of no more than 20 percent among Southeast Asian men.

Duplicate objectives: 3.4g and 16.6g

15.12h*: Reduce cigarette smoking to a prevalence of no more than 12 percent among women of reproductive age.

Duplicate objectives: 3.4h and 16.6h

15.12i*: Reduce cigarette smoking to a prevalence of no more than 10 percent among pregnant women.

Duplicate objectives: 3.4i and 16.6i

15.12j*: Reduce cigarette smoking to a prevalence of no more than 10 percent among women who use oral contraceptives.

Duplicate objectives: 3.4j and 16.6j

15.13: Increase to at least 90 percent the proportion of adults who have had their blood pressure measured within the preceding 2 years and can state whether their blood pressure was normal or high.

NOTE: A blood pressure measurement within the preceding 2 years refers to a measurement by a health professional or other trained observer.

15.14: Increase to at least 75 percent the proportion of adults who have had their blood cholesterol checked within the preceding 5 years.

15.15: Increase to at least 75 percent the proportion of primary care providers who initiate diet and, if necessary, drug therapy at levels of blood cholesterol consistent with current management guidelines for patients with high blood cholesterol.

NOTE: Current treatment recommendations are outlined in detail in the Report of the Expert Panel on the Detection, Evaluation, and Treatment of High Blood Cholesterol in Adults, released by the National Cholesterol Education Program in 1987. Guidelines appropriate for children are currently being established. Treatment recommendations are likely to be refined over time. Thus, for the year 2000, "current" means whatever recommendations are then in effect.

15.16: Increase to at least 50 percent the proportion of worksites with 50 or more employees that offer high blood pressure and/or cholesterol education and control activities to their employees.

15.17: Increase to at least 90 percent the proportion of clinical laboratories that meet the recommended accuracy standard for cholesterol measurement.

*Duplicate objective.

**Updated from original note in *Healthy People 2000.*

References

1. National Center for Health Statistics. Health, United States, 1992. Hyattsville, Maryland: Public Health Service. 1993.

2. U.S. Department of Health and Human Services. Healthy people 2000: National health promotion and disease prevention objectives for the nation. Washington: Public Health Service. 1991.

3. Unpublished data from the National Health and Nutrition Examination Survey III.

4. National Heart, Lung, and Blood Institute. Fifth report of the joint national committee on detection, evaluation, and treatment of high blood pressure. Joint National Committee V. U.S. Department of Health and Human Services. 1993.

5. Sempos C, Fulwood R, Haines C, et al. The prevalence of high blood cholesterol levels among adults in the United States. JAMA 262: 45–52. 1989.

6. Sempos, C, et. al. Divergence of the recent trends in coronary mortality for the four major race-sex groups in the United States. Am J Public Health 78: 1422-7. 1988.

Priority Area 16
Cancer

Background and Data Summary

Cancer accounts for nearly one out of every four deaths in the United States (1). Cancer is not one disease, but a constellation of more than 1,000 different diseases, each characterized by the uncontrolled growth and spread of abnormal cells. Of the 250 million Americans now living, about 75 million will eventually have cancer. While the incidence of cancer has increased in the past two decades, death rates for those under 55 have fallen. More people are surviving cancer now than several decades ago (2). Research has demonstrated that many cancers can be prevented or, if detected and treated at early stages, cured.

Recent data indicate that progress toward the year 2000 objectives has been made for three of the objectives (16.5, 16.6, and 16.10) in this priority area. The trends in the overall cancer death rate (16.1) and the breast cancer death rate (16.3) are moving away from the target, while lung cancer mortality (16.2) is rising at a rate, which at its current pace, would not meet the target before the year 2000. Two objectives (16.4 and 16.7) show no change from the baseline figures. Complete data were unavailable to update progress for the remaining eight objectives.

Data Issues

Age-Adjusted Death Rates

The death rates shown in objectives 16.1–16.5 have been age-adjusted to the 1940 U.S. population. (See Appendix II for more information on age-adjusted rates.) The National Cancer Institute age adjusts cancer deaths to the 1970 U.S. population. When the 1970 standard population is used, the equivalent baseline, interim, and target rates are all somewhat higher than those generated using the 1940 population.

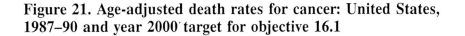

Figure 21. Age-adjusted death rates for cancer: United States, 1987–90 and year 2000 target for objective 16.1

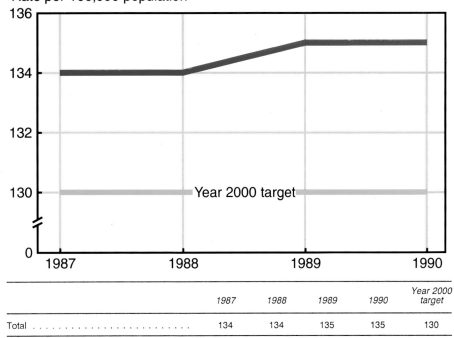

Rate per 100,000 population

	1987	1988	1989	1990	Year 2000 target
Total	134	134	135	135	130

NOTE: Related tables in *Health, United States, 1992*, are 28–31, 37–39, and 50.

SOURCE: Centers for Disease Control and Prevention, National Center for Health Statistics, National Vital Statistics System.

Data Availability

Only partial data were available to update progress for several objectives. For objective 16.11 (the proportion of women receiving a clinical breast exam and a mammogram), the 1991 data from the National Health Interview Survey (NHIS) report mammogram only. Similarly, the 1991 data on Pap smears (16.12) are for women with a uterine cervix who have had a Pap test in the past 12 months. Data on ever receiving a Pap test and receiving a Pap test in the preceding 1–3 years were not obtained in the 1991 survey. Complete data to measure objectives 16.11 and 16.12 will be available from the 1993 NHIS.

Table 16. Cancer objective status

Objective	1987 baseline Original	1987 baseline Revised	1990	1991	Target 2000
16.1 Cancer deaths (age adjusted per 100,000)	133	[1]134	135	– – –	130
16.2 Lung cancer deaths (age adjusted per 100,000)..................	37.9	[1]38.5	39.9	– – –	42.0
16.3 Breast cancer deaths (age adjusted per 100,000)	22.9	[1]23.0	23.1	– – –	20.6
16.4 Cervical cancer deaths (age adjusted per 100,000)	2.8	[1]No change	2.8	– – –	1.3
16.5 Colorectal cancer deaths (age adjusted per 100,000)	14.4	[1]14.7	13.8	– – –	13.2
16.6 Cigarette smoking prevalence					
People 20 years and over...................................	29%	. . .	26%	26%	15%
Males....................................	32%	. . .	28%	28%	. . .
Females................................	27%	. . .	23%	24%	. . .
a. People with high school education or less					
20 years and over	34%	. . .	31%	32%	20%
b. Blue-collar workers 20 years and over..........................	36%	. . .	37%	36%	20%
c. Military personnel..................................	[2]42%	. . .	– – –	[3]35%	20%
d. Blacks 20 years and over.............................	34%	. . .	27%	30%	18%
e. Hispanics 20 years and over	[4]33%	. . .	24%	20%	18%
f. American Indians/Alaska Natives..............................	[5]42–70%	. . .	38%	33%	20%
g. Southeast Asian males................................	[6]55%	. . .	[7]35%	– – –	20%
h. Females of reproductive age (18–44 years).................	29%	. . .	26%	27%	12%
i. Pregnant females	[8]25%	. . .	19%	20%	10%
j. Females who use oral contraceptives..........................	[9]36%	. . .	[2]26%	– – –	10%
16.7 Dietary fat intake among people 2 years and over					
People 2 years and over					
Percent of calories from total fat................................	– – –	. . .	– – –	– – –	30%
Percent of calories from saturated fat............................	– – –	. . .	– – –	– – –	10%
People 20–74 years					
Percent of calories from total fat................................	[10]36%	. . .	[11]36%	– – –	. . .
Percent of calories from saturated fat............................	[10]13%	. . .	[11]13%	– – –	. . .
Females 19–50 years					
Percent of calories from total fat................................	[8]36%	. . .	– – –	– – –	. . .
Percent of calories from saturated fat............................	[8]13%	. . .	– – –	– – –	. . .
16.8 Daily intake of vegetables, fruits, and grain products					
Adults (number of servings)					
Vegetables and fruits................................	– – –	. . .	– – –	– – –	5
Grain products...................................	– – –	. . .	– – –	– – –	6
Women aged 19–50 (number of servings)					
Vegetables and fruits................................	[8]2.5	. . .	– – –	– – –	. . .
Grain products...................................	[8]3.0	. . .	– – –	– – –	. . .
16.9 Actions to reduce sun exposure	– – –	. . .	– – –	– – –	60%
16.10 Tobacco, diet, and cancer screening and counseling by clinicians ..	[12,13]52%	. . .	[11,13]96%	– – –	75%
16.11 Breast examination and mammogram					
Females 40 years and over (ever received)........................	36%	. . .	60%	– – –	80%
Females 50 years and over (preceding 1–2 years)..................	25%	. . .	47%	[14]54%	60%
Ever received					
a. Hispanic females 40 years and over........................	20%	. . .	52%	– – –	80%
b. Low-income females 40 years and over					
(annual family income less than $10,000)	22%	. . .	41%	– – –	80%
c. Females 40 years and over with less than high school education ...	23%	. . .	45%	– – –	80%
d. Females 70 years and over.............................	25%	. . .	48%	– – –	80%
e. Black females 40 years and over	28%	. . .	53%	– – –	80%
Received within preceding 2 years					
a. Hispanic females 50 years and over........................	18%	. . .	42%	[14]54%	60%
b. Low-income females 50 years and over					
(annual family income less than $10,000)	15%	. . .	31%	[14]39%	60%
c. Females 50 years and over with less than high school education ...	16%	. . .	34%	[14]40%	60%
d. Females 70 years and over.............................	18%	. . .	37%	[14]45%	60%
e. Black females 50 years and over	19%	. . .	42%	[14]48%	60%
16.12 Pap test					
Ever received	88%	. . .	– – –	– – –	95%
Received within preceding 3 years	75%	. . .	– – –	[15]59%	85%

Table 16. Cancer objective status—Con.

Objective	1987 baseline		1990	1991	Target 2000
	Original	Revised			
Ever received					
a. Hispanic females 18 years and over............................	75%	. . .	— — —	— — —	95%
b. Females 70 years and over..................................	76%	. . .	— — —	— — —	95%
c. Females 18 years and over with less than high school education . . .	79%	. . .	— — —	— — —	95%
d. Low-income females 18 years and over (annual family income less than $10,000)	80%	. . .	— — —	— — —	95%
Received within preceding 3 years					
a. Hispanic females 18 years and over............................	66%	. . .	— — —	[15]58%	80%
b. Females 70 years and over..................................	44%	. . .	— — —	[15]33%	70%
c. Females 18 years and over with less than high school education . . .	58%	. . .	— — —	[15]45%	75%
d. Low-income females 18 years and over (annual family income less than $10,000)	64%	. . .	— — —	[15]50%	80%
16.13 Fecal occult blood test and proctosigmoidoscopy					
Received fecal occult blood testing within preceding 2 years	27%	. . .	— — —	— — —	50%
Ever received proctosigmoidoscopy	25%	. . .	— — —	— — —	40%
People 65 years and over with routine checkup in past 2 years who had a fecal blood test.....................................	. . .	. . .	— — —	36%	. . .
16.14 Oral, skin, and digital rectal examinations					
People 50 years and over (during past year)	27%	. . .	— — —	— — —	40%
16.15 Pap test quality					
Monitoring cytology laboratory..................................	— — —	. . .	— — —	— — —	100%
16.16 Mammogram facilities certified by American College of Radiology..	[16]18– 21%	. . .	— — —	— — —	80%

[1]Data have been recomputed to reflect revised intercensal population estimates; see *Health, United States, 1992*, Appendix I.
[2]1988 data.
[3]1992 data.
[4]1982-84 data.
[5]1979–87 data.
[6]1984–88 data.
[7]Vietnamese males only.
[8]1985 data.
[9]1983 data.
[10]1976–80 data.
[11]1989 data.
[12]1985–86 data.
[13]Data reflect tobacco screening and counseling only.
[14]Mammogram only.
[15]Females with uterine cervix who had a Pap test in past 12 months.
[16]1990 data.

NOTE: Data sources are in table C.

Cancer Objectives

16.1*: Reverse the rise in cancer deaths to achieve a rate of no more than 130 per 100,000 people.

NOTE: In its publications the National Cancer Institute age adjusts cancer death rates to the 1970 U.S. population. Using the 1970 standard, the equivalent target value for this objective would be 175 per 100,000.

Duplicate objective: 2.2

16.2*: Slow the rise in lung cancer deaths to achieve a rate of no more than 42 per 100,000 people.

NOTE: In its publications the National Cancer Institute age adjusts cancer death rates to the 1970 U.S. population. Using the 1970 standard, the equivalent target value for this objective would be 53 per 100,000.

Duplicate objective: 3.2

16.3: Reduce breast cancer deaths to no more than 20.6 per 100,000 women.

NOTE: In its publications the National Cancer Institute age adjusts cancer death rates to the 1970 U.S. population. Using the 1970 standard, the equivalent target value for this objective would be 25.2 per 100,000.

16.4: Reduce deaths from cancer of the uterine cervix to no more than 1.3 per 100,000 women.

NOTE: In its publications the National Cancer Institute age adjusts cancer death rates to the 1970 U.S. population. Using the 1970 standard, the equivalent target value for this objective would be 1.5 per 100,000.

16.5: Reduce colorectal cancer deaths to no more than 13.2 per 100,000 people.

NOTE: In its publications the National Cancer Institute age adjusts cancer death rates to the 1970 U.S. population. Using the 1970 standard, the equivalent target value for this objective would be 18.7 per 100,000.

16.6*: Reduce cigarette smoking to a prevalence of no more than 15 percent among people aged 20 and older.

NOTE: A cigarette smoker is a person who has smoked at least 100 cigarettes and currently smokes cigarettes.

Duplicate objectives: 3.4 and 15.12

> **16.6a***: Reduce cigarette smoking to a prevalence of no more than 20 percent among people aged 20 and older with a high school education or less.

Duplicate objectives: 3.4a and 15.12a

> **16.6b***: Reduce cigarette smoking to a prevalence of no more than 20 percent among blue-collar workers aged 20 and older.

Duplicate objectives: 3.4b and 15.12b

> **16.6c***: Reduce cigarette smoking to a prevalence of no more than 20 percent among military personnel.

Duplicate objectives: 3.4c and 15.12c

> **16.6d***: Reduce cigarette smoking to a prevalence of no more than 18 percent among blacks aged 20 and older.

Duplicate objectives: 3.4d and 15.12d

> **16.6e***: Reduce cigarette smoking to a prevalence of no more than 18 percent among Hispanics aged 20 and older.

Duplicate objectives: 3.4e and 15.12e

16.6f*: Reduce cigarette smoking to a prevalence of no more than 20 percent among American Indians and Alaska Natives.

Duplicate objectives: 3.4f and 15.12f

16.6g*: Reduce cigarette smoking to a prevalence of no more than 20 percent among Southeast Asian men.

Duplicate objectives: 3.4g and 15.12g

16.6h*: Reduce cigarette smoking to a prevalence of no more than 12 percent among women of reproductive age.

Duplicate objectives: 3.4h and 15.12h

16.6i*: Reduce cigarette smoking to a prevalence of no more than 10 percent among pregnant women.

Duplicate objectives: 3.4i and 15.12i

16.6j*: Reduce cigarette smoking to a prevalence of no more than 10 percent among women who use oral contraceptives.

Duplicate objectives: 3.4j and 15.12j

16.7*: Reduce dietary fat intake to an average of 30 percent of calories or less and average saturated fat intake to less than 10 percent of calories among people aged 2 and older.

NOTE: The inclusion of a saturated fat target in this objective should not be interpreted as evidence that reducing only saturated fat will reduce cancer risk. Epidemiologic and experimental animal studies suggest that the amount of fat consumed rather than the specific type of fat can influence the risk of some cancers.

Duplicate objectives: 2.5 and 15.9

16.8*: Increase complex carbohydrate and fiber-containing foods in the diets of adults to five or more daily servings for vegetables (including legumes) and fruits, and to six or more daily servings for grain products.

Duplicate objective: 2.6

16.9: Increase to at least 60 percent the proportion of people of all ages who limit sun exposure, use sunscreens and protective clothing when exposed to sunlight, and avoid artificial sources of ultraviolet light (e.g. sun lamps, tanning booths).

16.10: Increase to at least 75 percent the proportion of primary care providers who routinely counsel patients about tobacco use cessation, diet modification, and cancer screening recommendations.

16.11: Increase to at least 80 percent the proportion of women aged 40 and older who have ever received a clinical breast examination and a mammogram, and to at least 60 percent those aged 50 and older who have received them within the preceding 1 to 2 years.

16.11a: Increase to at least 80 percent the proportion of Hispanic women aged 40 and older who have ever received aclinical breast examination and a mammogram, and to at least 60 percent those aged 50 and older who have received them within the preceding 1 to 2 years.

16.11b: Increase to at least 80 percent the proportion of low-income (annual family income less than $10,000) women aged 40 and older who have ever received a clinical breast examination and a mammogram, and to at least 60 percent those aged 50 and older who have received them within the preceding 1 to 2 years.

16.11c: Increase to at least 80 percent the proportion of women with less than a high school education aged 40 and older who have ever received a clinical breast examination and a mammogram, and to at least 60 percent those aged 50 and older who have received them within the preceding 1 to 2 years.

16.11d: Increase to at least 80 percent the proportion of women aged 70 and older who have ever received a clinical breast examination and a mammogram, and to at least 60 percent those who have received them within the preceding 1 to 2 years.

16.11e: Increase to at least 80 percent the proportion of black women aged 40 and older who have ever received a clinical breast examination and a mammogram, and to at least 60 percent those aged 50 and older who have received them within the preceding 1 to 2 years.

16.12: Increase to at least 95 percent the proportion of women aged 18 and older with uterine cervix who have ever received a Pap test, and to at least 85 percent those who received a Pap test within the preceding 1 to 3 years.

16.12a: Increase to at least 95 percent the proportion of Hispanic women aged 18 and older with uterine cervix who have ever received a Pap test, and to at least 80 percent those who received a Pap test within the preceding 1 to 3 years.

16.12b: Increase to at least 95 percent the proportion of women aged 70 and older with uterine cervix who have ever received a Pap test, and to at least 70 percent those who received a Pap test within the preceding 1 to 3 years.

16.12c: Increase to at least 95 percent the proportion of women aged 18 and older with less than a high school education with uterine cervix who have ever received a Pap test, and to at least 75 percent those who received a Pap test within the preceding 1 to 3 years.

16.12d: Increase to at least 95 percent the proportion of low-income women (annual family income less than $10,000) aged 18 and older with uterine cervix who have ever received a Pap test, and to at least 80 percent those who received a Pap test within the preceding 1 to 3 years.

16.13: Increase to at least 50 percent the proportion of people aged 50 and older who have received fecal occult blood testing within the preceding 1 to 2 years, and to at least 40 percent those who have ever received proctosigmoidoscopy.

16.14: Increase to at least 40 percent the proportion of people aged 50 and older visiting a primary care provider in the preceding year who have received oral, skin, and digital rectal examinations during one such visit.

16.15: Ensure that Pap tests meet quality standards by monitoring and certifying all cytology laboratories.

16.16: Ensure that mammograms meet quality standards by monitoring and certifying at least 80 percent of mammography facilities.

*Duplicate objective.

References

1. National Center for Health Statistics. Advance report of final mortality statistics, 1990. Monthly vital statistics report; vol 41 no 7, suppl. Hyattsville, Maryland: Public Health Service. 1993.

2. National Cancer Institute. Cancer control objectives for the nation: 1985–2000. Bethesda, Maryland: National Cancer Institute Monographs. 2(1986). 1986.

Priority Area 17
Diabetes and
Chronic Disabling
Conditions

Background and Data Summary

As the population of the United States grows older, the problems posed by chronic and disabling conditions increasingly demand the Nation's attention. Chronic conditions such as heart disease, cancer, stroke, and lung and liver disease are joined in importance by other chronic and disabling conditions, such as diabetes, arthritis, deformities or orthopedic impairments, hearing and visual impairments, and mental retardation.

Disability, defined by a limitation of the ability to perform major activities caused by chronic conditions, affected about 10 percent of Americans in 1991 (1). Over 30 million people have functional limitations that interfere with their daily activities, and about 10 million have limitations that prevent them from working, attending school, or maintaining a household. The underlying impairments most often responsible for these conditions are arthritis, heart disease, back conditions, lower extremity impairments, and intervertebral disk disorders (2). For those under age 18 years the most frequent causes of activity limitation are asthma, mental retardation, mental illness, and hearing and speech impairments.

Five objectives (17.7, 17.11, 17.13, 17.14, and 17.19) are moving toward the year 2000 targets. Six (17.2, 17.4, 17.5, 17.6, 17.10, 17.12) are moving away from the targets. People with self-care problems (17.3) showed no changed for the total noninstitutionalized population. Diabetes-related mortality (17.9) also showed no change for the total population, although the black and American Indian subobjectives are moving away from the targets. As with a number of other Healthy People 2000 priority areas, missing data is a problem: for the remaining seven objectives, four have no baseline and three have no data beyond the baseline.

Figure 22. Limitation of major activity caused by chronic conditions, according to selected characteristics targeted by year 2000 objective 17.2: United States, 1991

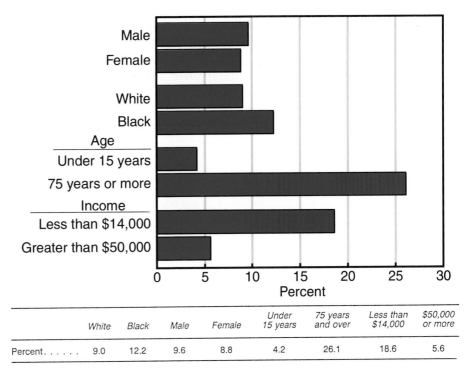

	White	Black	Male	Female	Under 15 years	75 years and over	Less than $14,000	$50,000 or more
Percent......	9.0	12.2	9.6	8.8	4.2	26.1	18.6	5.6

NOTE: A related table in *Health, United States,* 1992, is 61.

SOURCE: Centers for Disease Control and Prevention, National Center for Health Statistics, National Health Interview Survey.

Objective 17.19 calls for the voluntary establishment of policies or programs for the hiring of people with disabilities. Since this objective was created, Congress has passed the Americans with Disabilities Act of 1990 that prohibits all employers from discriminating against "a qualified disabled individual because of the disability in regard to job application procedures, hiring, advancement . . . (3)." As a result, this objective has been achieved via legislation.

Data Issues

Years of Healthy Life

Years of Healthy Life (17.1) is discussed in the introduction.

Data Availability

The 1984–85 baseline figures for 17.3 were derived by combining estimates for the noninstitutionalized population from the National Health Interview Survey with data for the nursing home population from the National Nursing Home Survey. At the present time, only data for the noninstitutionalized population are available to update progress.

Proxy Measures

See priority area 1 (Physical Activity and Fitness) for a discussion of self-reported height and weight (17.12), as well as light to moderate physical activity (17.13).

Table 17. Diabetes and chronic disabling conditions objective status

Objective	1987 baseline Original	1987 baseline Revised	1990	1991	Target 2000
17.1 Years of healthy life	[1]62.0	[2,3]64.0	– – –	– – –	65
a. Blacks	[1]56.0	No change	– – –	– – –	60
b. Hispanics	[1]62.0	[2,3,4]64.8	– – –	– – –	65
c. People 65 years and over[5]	[1]12.0	[2,3]11.9	– – –	– – –	14
17.2 Limitation in activity due to chronic conditions	9.4%	...	9.3%	9.6%	8%
a. Low-income people (annual family income less than $10,000)	18.9%	...	19.2%	19.6%	15%
b. American Indians/Alaska Natives	[6]13.4%	...	[7]12.3%	[8]12.0%	11%
c. Blacks	11.2%	...	10.7%	11.0%	9%
17.3 People with self care problems (per 1,000)					
People 65 years and over	[9]111	...	– – –	– – –	90
Non-institutionalized population	[10]77	...	[11]77	– – –	...
a. People 85 years and over	[9]371	...	– – –	– – –	325
Non-institutionalized population	[10]223	...	[11]204	– – –	...
17.4 Percent of people with asthma with activity limitation	[12]19.4%	...	[7]20.4%	[8]21.8%	10%
17.5 Activity limitation due to chronic back conditions (per 1,000)	[12]21.9	...	[7]23.7	[8]25.1	19.0
17.6 Significant hearing impairment (per 1,000)	[12]88.9	...	[7]89.5	[8]89.7	82.0
a. People 45 years and over	[12]203	...	[7]206	[8]206	180
17.7 Significant visual impairment (per 1,000)	[12]34.5	...	[7]32.5	[8]31.7	30.0
a. People 65 years and over	[12]87.7	...	[7]81.8	[8]78.0	70.0
17.8 Mental retardation (per 1,000 school aged children)	[13]2.7	...	– – –	– – –	2.0
17.9 Diabetes-related deaths (age adjusted per 100,000)	[11]38	[11,14]No change	38	– – –	34
a. Blacks (age adjusted per 100,000)	[11]65	[11,14]67	71	– – –	58
b. American Indians/Alaska Natives (age adjusted per 100,000)	[11]54	[11,14]46	53	– – –	48
17.10 Diabetes-related complications					
People with diabetes					
End-stage renal disease (ESRD) (per 1,000)	[15]1.5	...	[16]2.0	– – –	1.4
Blindness (per 1,000)	2.2	...	2.5	– – –	1.4
Lower extremity amputation (per 1,000)	[15]8.2	...	8.3	– – –	4.9
Perinatal mortality (among infants of females with established diabetes)	5%	...	– – –	– – –	2%
Major congenital malformations	8%	...	– – –	– – –	4%
ESRD due to diabetes (per 1,000)					
a. Blacks with diabetes	[17]2.2	...	[16]3.1	– – –	2.0
b. American Indians/Alaska Natives with diabetes	[17]2.1	...	[12]2.2	– – –	1.9
Lower extremity amputations due to diabetes					
c. Blacks with diabetes (per 1,000)	[18]10.2	[15]8.8	8.2	– – –	6.1
17.11 Diabetes incidence and prevalence					
Total population (per 1,000)					
Incidence of diabetes	[1]2.9	[2,12]No change	[7]2.6	– – –	2.5
Prevalence of diabetes	[1]28	[2,12]No change	[7]26	– – –	25
Special populations-prevalence of diabetes (per 1,000)					
a. American Indians/Alaska Natives	[15]69	...	67	63	62
b. Puerto Ricans	[19]55	...	– – –	– – –	49
c. Mexican Americans	[19]54	...	– – –	– – –	49
d. Cuban Americans	[19]36	...	– – –	– – –	32
e. Blacks	[12]36	...	[7]35	– – –	32
17.12 Overweight prevalence					
People 20 years and over	[20]26%	...	27%	28%	20%
Males	[20]24%	...	27%	28%	...
Females	[20]27%	...	27%	28%	...
Adolescents 12–19 years	[20]15%	...	– – –	– – –	15%
a. Low-income females 20 years and over	[20]37%	...	37%	39%	25%
b. Black females 20 years and over	[20]44%	...	42%	44%	30%
c. Hispanic females 20 years and over	...	[21]27%	33%	32%	25%
Mexican-American females	[19]39%	...	– – –	38%	...
Cuban females	[19]34%	...	– – –	– – –	...
Puerto Rican females	[19]37%	...	– – –	– – –	...
d. American Indians/Alaska Natives	[22]29–75%	...	– – –	40%	30%

Table 17. Diabetes and chronic disabling conditions objective status

Objective	1987 baseline Original	1987 baseline Revised	1990	1991	Target 2000
e. People with disabilities.............................	[10]36%	. . .	– – –	38%	25%
f. Females with high blood pressure...................	[20]50%	. . .	– – –	– – –	41%
g. Males with high blood pressure	[20]39%	. . .	– – –	– – –	35%
17.13 Moderate physical activity					
People 6 years and over.............................	– – –	. . .	– – –	– – –	30%
People 18–74 years					
5 or more times per week........................	[21]22%	[21,23]No change	23%	24%	. . .
7 or more times per week........................	[21]12%	[21,23]16%	16%	17%	. . .
17.14 Patient education for people with chronic and disabling conditions . .	– – –	. . .	– – –	– – –	40%
a. People with diabetes	[24]32% (classes) [24]68% (counseling)	. . .	[16]33.1%	39%	75%
b. People with asthma	– – –	. . .	– – –	9%	50%
17.15 Clinician assessment of childhood development	– – –	. . .	– – –	– – –	80%
17.16 Earlier detection of significant hearing impairment in children (average age in months)	24–30	. . .	– – –	27	12
17.17 Clinician assessment of cognitive and other functioning in older adults	– – –	. . .	– – –	– – –	60%
17.18 Providers who counsel about estrogen replacement therapy	– – –	. . .	– – –	– – –	90%
17.19 Employment of people with disabilities					
Percent of worksites with voluntary policy	[1]37%	. . .	[25]100%	[25]100%	75%
17.20 Service systems for children with or at risk of chronic and disabling conditions (number of States)	– – –	. . .	– – –	– – –	50

[1]1980 data.
[2]Data have been revised to reflect updated methodology; see Introduction.
[3]1990 data.
[4]Estimate based on preliminary data.
[5]Years of healthy life remaining at age 65.
[6]1983–85 data.
[7]1988–90 data.
[8]1989–91 data.
[9]1984–85 data.
[10]1984 data.
[11]1986 data.
[12]1986–88 data.
[13]1985–88 data.
[14]Data have been recomputed to reflect revised intercensal population estimates; see *Health, United States, 1992*, Appendix I.
[15]1987 data.
[16]1989 data.
[17]1983–86 data.
[18]1984–87 data.
[19]1982–84 data.
[20]1976–80 data.
[21]1985 data.
[22]1984–88 data.
[23]Data source has been changed and data have been revised to reflect updated methodology; see Introduction.
[24]1983–84 data.
[25]Achieved through passage of the Americans with Disabilitites Act of 1990.

NOTE: Data sources are in table C.

Diabetes and Chronic Disabling Conditions Objectives

17.1*: Increase years of healthy life to at least 65 years.

NOTE: Years of healthy life is a summary measure of health that combines mortality (quantity of life) and morbidity and disability (quality of life) into a single measure. For people aged 65 and older, active life-expectancy, a related summary measure, also will be tracked.

Duplicate objectives: 8.1 and 21.1

17.1a*: Increase years of healthy life among blacks to at least 60 years.

Duplicate objectives: 8.1a and 21.1a

17.1b*: Increase years of healthy life among Hispanics to at least 65 years.

Duplicate objectives: 8.1b and 21.1b

17.1c*: Increase years of healthy life among people aged 65 and older to at least 14 more years of healthy life.

Duplicate objectives: 8.1c and 21.1c

17.2: Reduce to no more than 8 percent the proportion of people who experience a limitation in major activity due to chronic conditions.

NOTE: Major activity refers to the usual activity for one's age-sex group whether it is working, keeping house, going to school, or living independently. Chronic conditions are defined as conditions that either (1) were first noticed 3 or more months ago, or (2) belong to a group of conditions such as heart disease and diabetes, which are considered chronic regardless of when they began.

17.2a: Reduce to no more than 15 percent the proportion of low-income people (annual family income of less than $10,000 in 1988) who experience a limitation in major activity due to chronic conditions.

17.2b: Reduce to no more than 11 percent the proportion of American Indians and Alaska Natives who experience a limitation in major activity due to chronic conditions.

17.2c: Reduce to no more than 9 percent the proportion of blacks who experience a limitation in major activity due to chronic conditions.

17.3: Reduce to no more than 90 per 1,000 people the proportion of all people aged 65 and older who have difficulty in performing two or more personal care activities, thereby preserving independence.

NOTE: Personal care activities are bathing, dressing, using the toilet, getting in and out of bed or chair, and eating.

Duplicate objective: Age-related objective for people aged 65 and older

17.3a: Reduce to no more than 300 per 1,000 people the proportion of all people aged 85 and older who have difficulty in performing two or more personal care activities, thereby preserving independence.

Duplicate objective: Age-related objective for people aged 65 and older

17.4: Reduce to no more than 10 percent the proportion of people with asthma who experience activity limitation.

NOTE: Activity limitation refers to any self-reported limitation in activity attributed to asthma.

17.5: Reduce activity limitation due to chronic back conditions to a prevalence of no more than 19 per 1,000 people.

NOTE: Chronic back conditions include intervertebral disk disorders, curvature of the back or spine, and other self-reported chronic back impairments such as

permanent stiffness or deformity of the back or repeated trouble with the back. Activity limitation refers to any self-reported limitation in activity attributed to a chronic back condition.

17.6: Reduce significant hearing impairment to a prevalence of no more than 82 per 1,000 people.

NOTE: Hearing impairment covers the range of hearing deficits from mild loss in one ear to profound loss in both ears. Generally, inability to hear sounds at levels softer (less intense) than 20 decibels (dB) constitutes abnormal hearing. Significant hearing impairment is defined as having hearing thresholds for speech poorer than 25 dB. However, for this objective, self-reported hearing impairment (that is, deafness in one or both ears or any trouble hearing in one or both ears) will be used as a proxy measure for significant hearing impairment.

> **17.6a**: Reduce significant hearing impairment among people aged 45 and older to a prevalence of no more than 180 per 1,000.

17.7: Reduce significant visual impairment to a prevalence of no more than 30 per 1,000 people.

NOTE: Significant visual impairment is generally defined as a permanent reduction in visual acuity and/or field of vision that is not correctable with eyeglasses or contact lenses. Severe visual impairment is defined as inability to read ordinary news print even with corrective lenses. For this objective, self-reported blindness in one or both eyes and other self-reported visual impairments (that is, any trouble seeing with one or both eyes even when wearing glasses or color blindness) will be used as a proxy measure for significant visual impairment.

> **17.7a**: Reduce significant visual impairment among people aged 65 and older to a prevalence of no more than 70 per 1,000.

17.8*: Reduce the prevalence of serious mental retardation in school-aged children to no more than 2 per 1,000 children.

NOTE: Serious mental retardation is defined as an Intelligence Quotient (I.Q.) less than 50. This includes individuals defined by the American Association of Mental Retardation as profoundly retarded (I.Q. of 20 or less), severely retarded (I.Q. of 21–35), and moderately retarded (I.Q. of 36–50).

Duplicate objective: 11.2

17.9: Reduce diabetes-related deaths to no more than 34 per 100,000.

> **17.9a**: Reduce diabetes-related deaths among blacks to no more than 58 per 100,000.

> **17.9b**: Reduce diabetes-related deaths among American Indians and Alaska Natives to no more than 48 per 100,000.

17.10: Reduce the most severe complications of diabetes as follows:

Complications among people with diabetes:	2000 target
End-stage renal disease	1.4 per 1,000
Blindness	1.4 per 1,000
Lower extremity amputation	4.9 per 1,000
Perinatal mortality[1]	2 percent
Major congenital malformation	4 percent

[1]Among infants of women with established diabetes

NOTE: End-stage renal disease (ESRD) is defined as requiring dialysis or transplantation and is limited to ESRD due to diabetes. Blindness refers to blindness due to diabetic eye disease.

> **17.10a**: Reduce end-stage renal disease due to diabetes among black persons with diabetes to no more than 2 per 1,000.

> **17.10b**: Reduce end-stage renal disease due to diabetes among American Indians and Alaska Natives with diabetes to no more than 1.9 per 1,000.

17.10c: Reduce lower extremity amputations due to diabetes among blacks with diabetes to no more than 6.1 per 1,000.

17.11: Reduce diabetes to an incidence of no more than 2.5 per 1,000 people and a prevalence of no more than 25 per 1,000 people.

17.11a: Reduce diabetes among American Indians and Alaska Natives to a prevalence of no more than 62 per 1,000.

17.11b: Reduce diabetes among Puerto Ricans to a prevalence of no more than 49 per 1,000.

17.11c: Reduce diabetes among Mexican Americans to a prevalence of no more than 49 per 1,000.

17.11d: Reduce diabetes among Cuban Americans to a prevalence of no more than 32 per 1,000.

17.11e: Reduce diabetes among blacks to a prevalence of no more than 32 per 1,000.

17.12*: Reduce overweight to a prevalence of no more than 20 percent among people aged 20 and older and no more than 15 percent among adolescents aged 12–19.

NOTE: For people aged 20 and older, overweight is defined as body mass index (BMI) equal to or greater than 27.8 for men and 27.3 for women. For adolescents, overweight is defined as BMI equal to or greater than 23.0 for males aged 12–14, 24.3 for males aged 15–17, 25.8 for males aged 18–19, 23.4 for females aged 12–14, 24.8 for females aged 15–17, and 25.7 for females aged 18–19. The values for adolescents are the age- and gender-specific 85th percentile values of the 1976–80 National Health and Nutrition Examination Survey (NHANES II), corrected for sample variation. BMI is calculated by dividing weight in kilograms by the square of height in meters. The cut points used to define overweight approximate the 120 percent of desirable body weight definition used in the 1990 objectives.

Duplicate objectives: 1.2, 2.3, and 15.10

17.12a*: Reduce overweight to a prevalence of no more than 25 percent among low-income women aged 20 and older.

Duplicate objectives: 1.2a, 2.3a, and 15.10a

17.12b*: Reduce overweight to a prevalence of no more than 30 percent among black women aged 20 and older.

Duplicate objectives: 1.2b, 2.3b, and 15.10b

17.12c*: Reduce overweight to a prevalence of no more than 25 percent among Hispanic women aged 20 and older.

Duplicate objectives: 1.2c, 2.3c, and 15.10c

17.12d*: Reduce overweight to a prevalence of no more than 30 percent among American Indians and Alaska Natives.

Duplicate objectives: 1.2d, 2.3d, and 15.10d

17.12e*: Reduce overweight to a prevalence of no more than 25 percent among people with disabilities.

Duplicate objectives: 1.2e, 2.3e, and 15.10e

17.12f*: Reduce overweight to a prevalence of no more than 41 percent among women with high blood pressure aged 20 and older.

Duplicate objectives: 1.2f, 2.3f, and 15.10f

17.12g*: Reduce overweight to a prevalence of no more than 35 percent among men with high blood pressure aged 20 and older.

Duplicate objectives: 1.2g, 2.3g, and 15.10g

17.13*: Increase to at least 30 percent the proportion of people aged 6 and older who engage regularly, preferably daily, in light to moderate physical activity for at least 30 minutes per day.

NOTE: Light to moderate physical activity requires sustained, rhythmic muscular movements, is at least equivalent to sustained walking, and is performed at less than 60 percent of maximum heart rate. Maximum heart rate equals roughly 220 beats per minute minus age. Examples may include walking, swimming, cycling, dancing, gardening and yardwork, various domestic and occupational activities, and games and other childhood pursuits.

Duplicate objectives: 1.3 and 15.11

17.14: Increase to at least 40 percent the proportion of people with chronic and disabling conditions who receive formal patient education including information about community and self-help resources as an integral part of the management of their condition.

> **17.14a**: Increase to at least 75 percent the proportion of people with diabetes who receive formal patient education including information about community and self-help resources as an integral part of the management of their condition.

> **17.14b**: Increase to at least 50 percent the proportion of people with asthma who receive formal patient education including information about community and self-help resources as an integral part of the management of their condition.

17.15: Increase to at least 80 percent the proportion of providers of primary care for children who routinely refer or screen infants and children for impairments of vision, hearing, speech and language, and assess other developmental milestones as part of well-child care.

17.16: Reduce the average age at which children with significant hearing impairment are identified to no more than 12 months.

17.17: Increase to at least 60 percent the proportion of providers of primary care for older adults who routinely evaluate people aged 65 and older for urinary incontinence and impairments of vision, hearing, cognition, and functional status.

17.18: Increase to at least 90 percent the proportion of perimenopausal women who have been counseled about the benefits and risks of estrogen replacement therapy (combined with progestin, when appropriate) for prevention of osteoporosis.

17.19: Increase to at least 75 percent the proportion of worksites with 50 or more employees that have a voluntarily established policy or program for the hiring of people with disabilities.

NOTE: Voluntarily established policies and programs for the hiring of people with disabilities are encouraged for worksites of all sizes. This objective is limited to worksites with 50 or more employees for tracking purposes.

17.20: Increase to 50 the number of States that have service systems for children with or at risk of chronic and disabling conditions, as required by Public Law 101–239.

NOTE: Children with or at risk of chronic and disabling conditions, often referred to as children with special health care needs, include children with psychosocial as well as physical problems. This population encompasses children with a wide variety of actual or potential disabling conditions, including children with or at risk for cerebral palsy, mental retardation, sensory deprivation, developmental disabilities, spina bifida, hemophilia, other genetic disorders, and health-related educational and behavioral problems. Service systems for such children are organized networks of comprehensive, community-based, coordinated, and family-centered services.

*Duplicate objective.

References

1. National Center for Health Statistics. Unpublished data from the National Health Interview Survey.

2. LaPlante MP. Data on disability from the National Health Interview Survey, 1983–85. An Info Use Report. Washington: National Institute on Disability and Rehabilitation Research. 1988.

3. Americans with Disabilities Act of 1990. Public Law 101–336, 101st Congress. Washington: July 26, 1990.

Priority Area 18
HIV Infection

Background and Data Summary

An estimated 1 million people in the United States are infected with the human immunodeficiency virus (HIV) (1). By the end of 1993, a projected total of 390,000 to 480,000 cases of AIDS will have been reported (1). This projection is based on the case definition used prior to the latest revision in January 1993. Although antimicrobial treatment extends survival, no treatment is yet available to prevent death among people with acquired immunodeficiency syndrome (AIDS). HIV and AIDS are a growing threat to the health of the nation and will continue to make major demands on health and social services systems for decades.

Data beyond baseline are available for 5 of the 14 objectives in this priority area. The first two objectives (18.1 and 18.2) aim to slow the rise in the number of AIDS cases and the prevalence of HIV infection. In 1991 the number of new AIDS cases reported was about 10 percent higher than the 1989 baseline figure (18.1). This pattern was similar for special population subgroups. At the current rate of increase, the number of cases for the total and special populations will exceed the year 2000 targets. The prevalence of HIV infection among the total population is still estimated at 400 per 100,000 people, showing no change from the baseline in 1989 (18.2). National data are not available regarding seroprevalence among men who have sex with men or among intravenous drug users. Data from the 1990 Youth Risk Behavior Survey on the history of sexual intercourse among adolescents show a worsening situation (18.3). The same survey shows the proportion of sexually active, teenage females whose partners used condoms at the last sexual intercourse (18.4a) increased since 1988, but a decrease in the proportion of sexually active, teenage males who use condoms (18.4b). Data for objective 18.7 on the risk of transfusion-transmitted HIV infection show an improvement toward the

Figure 23. Annual incidence of diagnosed AIDS cases according to selected characteristics targeted by year 2000 objective 18.1: United States, 1989–91

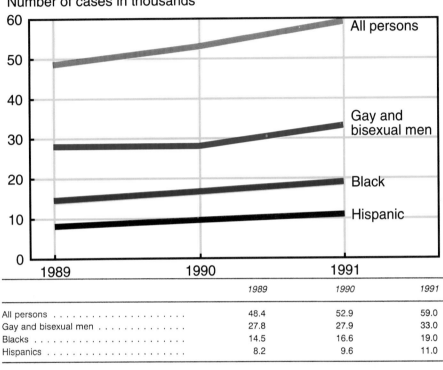

Number of cases in thousands

	1989	1990	1991
All persons	48.4	52.9	59.0
Gay and bisexual men	27.8	27.9	33.0
Blacks	14.5	16.6	19.0
Hispanics	8.2	9.6	11.0

NOTE: Related tables in *Health, United States, 1992*, are 53–58.

SOURCE: Centers for Disease Control and Prevention, National Center for Health Statistics, National Center for Infectious Diseases.

year 2000 goal. Recent data are available to establish a baseline for objective 18.12 on the proportion of cities with outreach programs to contact drug abusers and deliver HIV risk reduction messages.

Data Issues

Definition

In January 1993 a new AIDS case definition was implemented for the AIDS Surveillance System (2). The new definition adds pulmonary tuberculosis, recurrent pneumonia, and invasive cervical cancer to the list of diseases that indicate that AIDS has fully developed among HIV-infected people. In addition, the new definition includes HIV-infected

people with a CD4 cell count below 200 cells per microliter of blood, regardless of whether those persons have opportunistic infections, neoplasms, or any other symptoms of HIV infection. It is expected that the expanded definition could increase cases reported in 1993 by approximately 75 percent.

Data Source Description

Data on the annual number of diagnosed AIDS cases are available from the AIDS Surveillance System of the Centers for Disease Control. Completeness of reporting varies by geographic region and patient population. Recent research shows that the completeness of reporting was 92 percent for hospitalized patients diagnosed with AIDS through 1988 (3). The data for monitoring the objective are adjusted for delayed and incomplete reporting (1).

Data Availability

No national data are available that directly measure HIV seroprevalence among the general population or that provide nationally representative estimates for high risk groups such as men who have sex with men and intravenous drug users. Estimates of the prevalence of HIV infection in the U.S. population as a whole are based on mathematical models using back calculation, a statistical method that estimates the number of prior HIV infections that would account for the number of AIDS cases that have subsequently occurred (1).

Information on the proportion infected among various high risk groups has been obtained from seroprevalence studies conducted in clinical settings as part of a sentinel surveillance system conducted by CDC in collaboration with State and local health departments (4). The surveillance system covers various clinical settings in selected metropolitan areas. Seroprevalence estimates for men who have sex with men are based on anonymous surveys conducted in sexually transmitted disease (STD) clinics. For intravenous drug users, estimates are based on surveys among drug users entering treatment programs. Clients attending STD clinics and drug treatment programs are not representative of all persons with these high risk behaviors. In addition, there is considerable geographic variation in seroprevalence in both groups. For these reasons, data beyond baseline are not presented here on HIV seroprevalence levels in high risk groups.

National estimates of the total number of intravenous drug users are needed to properly measure progress towards meeting objective 18.5, which addresses the proportion of intravenous drug users in treatment. Enumeration of intravenous drug users is difficult because of the illegality of the behavior. In addition, surveys such as the National Household Survey on Drug Abuse will miss an unknown proportion of intravenous drug users who are homeless, institutionalized, or difficult to locate. The 1991 National Household Survey on Drug Abuse estimated there were approximately one million people who had used needles to inject illicit drugs in the past year (5).

Comparability of Data Sources

The 1990 Youth Risk Behavior Survey (YRBS) provides the most recent information on the proportion of sexually active teenagers who used condoms during last sexual intercourse (18.4a and 18.4b). The YRBS is a school-based survey and so does not include teenagers who are not in school and at higher risk. The data presented are for students in the 9th–12th grades; for most students, ages ranged from 14–17 years. These data are not directly comparable to the baseline, which shows condom use among young men and women aged 15–19 years.

Objective 18.3 (adolescent postponement of sexual intercourse) is discussed in priority area 5.

Table 18. HIV objective status

Objective	1989 baseline		1990	1991	Target 2000
	Original	Revised			
18.1 AIDS (number of diagnosed cases per year)	44,000–50,000	[1]48,400	52,900	[2]59,000	98,000
a. Gay and bisexual males	26,000–28,000	[1]27,800	27,900	[2]33,000	48,000
b. Blacks	14,000–15,000	[1]14,500	16,600	[2]19,000	37,000
c. Hispanics	7,000–8,000	[1]8,200	9,600	[2]11,000	18,000
18.2 HIV infection (per 100,000)	400	...	400	– – –	800
a. Homosexual males	2,000–42,000	...	– – –	– – –	20,000
b. Intravenous drug abusers	30,000–40,000	...	– – –	– – –	40,000
c. Females giving birth to live-born infants	150	...	150	– – –	100
18.3 Adolescents who ever had sexual intercourse					
Adolescents 15 years					
Females	[3]27%	...	[4]43%	[4]45%	15%
Males	[3]33%	...	[4]53%	[4]51%	15%
Adolescents 17 years					
Females	[3]50%	...	[5]67%	[5]65%	40%
Males	[3]66%	...	[5]76%	[5]68%	40%
18.4 Condom use at last sexual intercourse					
Sexually active unmarried females 15–44 years	[3]19%	...	– – –	– – –	50%
a. Sexually active females 15–19 years	[3]26%	...	[6]40%	[6]38%	60%
b. Sexually active males 15–19 years	[3]57%	...	[6]49%	[6]54%	75%
c. Intravenous drug abusers	– – –	...	– – –	– – –	60%
18.5 IV-drug abusers in treatment	11%	...	– – –	– – –	50%
18.6 IV-drug abusers using uncontaminated drug paraphernalia	[7]25–30%	[1,8]30.8%	– – –	– – –	50%
18.7 Risk of transfusion-transmitted HIV infection (units of blood)	1 per 40,000–150,000	...	1 per 225,000	...	1 per 250,000
18.8 Testing for HIV infection (HIV infected people)	15%	...	– – –	– – –	80%
18.9 Clinician counseling to prevent HIV and other sexually transmitted disease	[9]10%	...	– – –	– – –	75%
a. Providers practicing in high incidence areas	– – –	...	– – –	– – –	90%
18.10 HIV education in schools					
Students in grades 4th–12th	66%	...	– – –	– – –	95%
18.11 HIV education in colleges and universities	– – –	...	– – –	– – –	90%
18.12 Outreach programs for drug abusers (cities with populations greater than 100,000)	...	[8]35%	– – –	– – –	90%
18.13 Clinic services for HIV and other sexually transmitted diseases	– – –	...	– – –	– – –	50%
Family planning clinics	40%	...	– – –	– – –	...
18.14 Occupational exposure to HIV	– – –	...	– – –	– – –	100%

[1]Data have been revised. Original data were estimated based on preliminary analysis; see Introduction.
[2]Estimated from first half of 1991.
[3]1988 data.
[4]10th grade students.
[5]12th grade students.
[6]9th–12th grade students.
[7]1989 data.
[8]1991 data.
[9]1987 data.

NOTE: Data sources are in table C.

HIV Infection Objectives

18.1: Confine annual incidence of diagnosed AIDS cases to no more than 98,000 cases.

NOTE: Targets for this objective are equal to upper bound estimates of the incidence of diagnosed AIDS cases projected for 1993.

    18.1a: Confine annual incidence of diagnosed AIDS cases among gay and bisexual men to no more than 48,000 cases.

    18.1b: Confine annual incidence of diagnosed AIDS cases among blacks to no more than 37,000 cases.

    18.1c: Confine annual incidence of diagnosed AIDS cases among Hispanics to no more than 18,000 cases.

18.2: Confine the prevalence of HIV infection to no more than 800 per 100,000 people.

    18.2a: Confine the prevalence of HIV infection among homosexual men to no more than 20,000 per 100,000 homosexual men.

    18.2b: Confine the prevalence of HIV infection among intravenous drug abusers to no more than 40,000 per 100,000 intravenous drug abusers.

    18.2c: Confine the prevalence of HIV infection among women giving birth to live-born infants to no more than 100 per 100,000.

18.3*: Reduce the proportion of adolescents who have engaged in sexual intercourse to no more than 15 percent by age 15 and no more than 40 percent by age 17.

Duplicate objectives: 5.4 and 19.9

18.4*: Increase to at least 50 percent the proportion of sexually active, unmarried people who used a condom at last sexual intercourse.

NOTE: Strategies to achieve this objective must be undertaken sensitively to avoid indirectly encouraging or condoning sexual activity among teens who are not yet sexually active.

Duplicate objective: 19.10

    18.4a*: Increase to at least 60 percent the proportion of sexually active, unmarried young women aged 15–19 whose partners used a condom at last sexual intercourse.

Duplicate objective: 19.10a

    18.4b*: Increase to at least 75 percent the proportion of sexually active, unmarried young men aged 15–19 who used a condom at last sexual intercourse.

Duplicate objective: 19.10b

    18.4c*: Increase to at least 60 percent the proportion of intravenous drug abusers who used a condom at last sexual intercourse.

Duplicate objective: 19.10c

18.5: Increase to at least 50 percent the estimated proportion of all intravenous drug abusers who are in drug abuse treatment programs.

18.6: Increase to at least 50 percent the estimated proportion of intravenous drug abusers not in treatment who use only uncontaminated drug paraphernalia ("works").

18.7: Reduce to no more than 1 per 250,000 units of blood and blood components the risk of transfusion-transmitted HIV infection.

18.8: Increase to at least 80 percent the proportion of HIV-infected people who have been tested for HIV infection.

18.9*: Increase to at least 75 percent the proportion of primary care and mental health care providers who provide age-appropriate counseling on the prevention of HIV and other sexually transmitted diseases.

NOTE: Primary care providers include physicians, nurses, nurse practitioners, and physician assistants. Areas of high AIDS and sexually transmitted disease incidence are cities and States with incidence rates of AIDS cases, HIV seroprevalence, gonorrhea, or syphilis that are at least 25 percent above the national average.

Duplicate objective: 19.14

> **18.9a***: Increase to at least 90 percent the proportion of primary care and mental health care providers who practice in areas of high AIDS and sexually transmitted disease incidence, who provide age appropriate counseling on the prevention of HIV and other sexually transmitted diseases.

Duplicate objective: 19.14a

18.10: Increase to at least 95 percent the proportion of schools that have age-appropriate HIV education curricula for students in 4th–12th grade, preferably as part of quality school health education.

18.11: Provide HIV education for students and staff in at least 90 percent of colleges and universities.

18.12: Increase to at least 90 percent the proportion of cities with populations over 100,000 that have outreach programs to contact drug abusers (particularly intravenous drug abusers) to deliver HIV risk reduction messages.

NOTE: HIV risk reduction messages include messages about reducing or eliminating drug use, entering drug treatment, disinfection of injection equipment if still injecting drugs, and safer sex practices.

18.13*: Increase to at least 50 percent the proportion of family planning clinics, maternal and child health clinics, sexually transmitted disease clinics, tuberculosis clinics, drug treatment centers, and primary care clinics that screen, diagnose, treat, counsel, and provide (or refer for) partner notification services for bacterial sexually transmitted diseases (gonorrhea, syphilis, and chlamydia).

Duplicate objectives: 5.11 and 19.11

18.14: Extend to all facilities where workers are at risk for occupational transmission of HIV regulations to protect workers from exposure to blood borne infections, including HIV infection.

NOTE: The Occupational Safety and Health Administration (OSHA) is expected to issue regulations requiring worker protection from exposure to blood borne infections, including HIV, during 1991. Implementation of the OSHA regulations would satisfy this objective.

*Duplicate objective.

References

1. Centers for Disease Control. Estimates of HIV prevalence and projected AIDS cases: Summary of a workshop, October 31–November 1, 1989. MMWR 39: 110–19. 1990.

2. Centers for Disease Control. 1993 revised classification system for HIV infection and expanded surveillance case definition for AIDS among adolescents and adults. MMWR 41(No RR-17): 1–19, 1992.

3. Rosenblum L, Buehler JW, Morgan MW, et al. The completeness of AIDS case reporting, 1988: A multisite collaborative surveillance project. Am J Public Health 82: 1495–9. 1992.

4. Centers for Disease Control. National HIV serosurveillance summary, vol 2. Results through 1990. No HIV/NCID/11–91/011. Atlanta, Georgia: U.S. Department of Health and Human Services. 1991.

5. National Institute on Drug Abuse. National Household Survey on Drug Abuse: Population estimates 1991. No (ADM)92–1887. Washington: U.S. Department of Health and Human Services. 1992.

Priority Area 19
Sexually Transmitted Diseases

Background and Data Summary

In 1989, excluding infection with the human immunodeficiency virus (HIV), almost 12 million cases of sexually transmitted diseases were reported, 86 percent of them in people aged 15–29 years (1). By age 21, approximately one of every five young people has required treatment for a sexually transmitted disease (2). Women and children suffer a disproportionate amount of the sexually transmitted disease burden, with pelvic inflammatory disease, sterility, ectopic pregnancy, blindness, cancer associated with human papilloma virus, fetal and infant deaths, birth defects, and mental retardation among the most serious complications. Ethnic and racial minorities also shoulder a disproportionate share of the sexually transmitted disease burden, experiencing higher rates of disease and disability than the population as a whole. The total societal cost of sexually transmitted diseases exceeds $3.5 billion annually, with the cost of pelvic inflammatory disease (PID) and PID-associated ectopic pregnancy and infertility alone exceeding $2.6 billion (2).

Results toward achieving the sexually transmitted disease objectives are mixed. Data to monitor progress are available for 9 of the 15 objectives. For four objectives, trends are in a positive direction; recent data show reduced incidence of gonorrhea (objective 19.1), nongonococcal urethritis (19.2), primary and secondary syphilis (19.3), and pelvic inflammatory disease (19.6) compared with baseline rates. The incidence of primary and secondary syphilis has increased among black persons, in contrast to a decrease in the population as a whole. A worsening situation has been seen for three objectives. The incidence of congenital syphilis (19.4), the number of sexually transmitted hepatitis B cases (19.7), and percent of adolescents having sexual intercourse

(19.9) have increased and are moving away from the year 2000 targets. The annual number of first physician office visits for genital herpes increased from the 1988 baseline, while first physician office visits for genital warts decreased (19.5). The proportion of sexually active teenage females whose partners used condoms at their last sexual intercourse (19.10a) has increased compared with baseline data, showing an improvement toward the year 2000 target. However, a reverse trend was seen among teenage males (19.10b). Data subsequent to baseline measures are unavailable for six objectives (19.8, 19.11–19.15). In addition,

baseline data are not yet available for two subobjectives: condom use among intravenous drug users (19.10c) and counseling on HIV and STD prevention by providers practicing in high incidence areas (19.14a).

Data Issues

Definition

In January 1988 CDC issued new guidelines for classifying and reporting cases of congenital syphilis. The new definition is more useful for public health surveillance; the previous definition involved physical

Figure 24. Annual incidence of gonorrhea, according to selected characteristics: United States, 1989–91 and year 2000 targets for objective 19.1

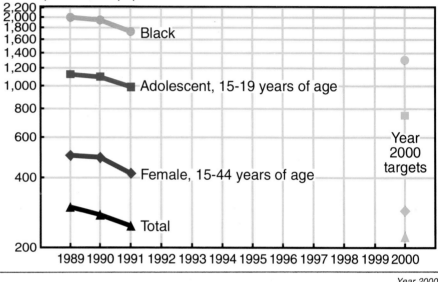

Cases per 100,000 population

	1989	1990	1991	Year 2000 target
Total	300	278	249	225
Black	1,990	1,938	1,720	1,300
Adolescent 15–19 years	1,123	1,098	991	750
Female 15–44 years	501	493	419	290

NOTE: Related table in *Health, United States, 1992*, is 52.

SOURCE: Centers for Disease Control and Prevention, National Center for Prevention Services, Gonorrhea Surveillance System.

examination, laboratory and radiographic results, and follow-up serological data (3). Follow-up information was often difficult to obtain and led to delayed and underreporting. In addition, the clinical criteria excluded stillbirths to mothers with untreated syphilis. The new surveillance guidelines provide criteria that can be obtained soon after delivery. The new case definition includes criteria for presumptive and confirmed cases of syphilis in infants and children and includes stillbirths. A presumptive case includes all infants whose mothers have untreated or inadequately treated syphilis at delivery (4). Thus, an increased number of cases will be reported using the new guidelines. The new case reporting criteria were fully implemented by States in 1991. The data presented for objective 19.4 on the incidence of congenital syphilis per 100,000 live births in 1989 and 1990 have been adjusted to reflect the expected rate if the new case definition had been used in all States.

Comparability of Data Sources

The history of sexual intercourse among adolescents (19.9) is discussed in priority area 5. Condom use at last sexual intercourse (19.10) is discussed in priority area 18.

Table 19. Sexually transmitted diseases objective status

Objective	1988 baseline		1990	1991	Target 2000
	Original	Revised			
19.1 Gonorrhea (per 100,000)	[1]300	...	278	249	225
a. Blacks	[1]1,990	...	1,938	1,720	1,300
b. Adolescents 15–19 years	[1]1,123	...	1,098	991	750
c. Females 15–44 years	[1]501	...	493	419	290
19.2 Nongonococcal urethritis (per 100,000)	215	...	[1]200	170	170
19.3 Primary and secondary syphilis (per 100,000)	[1]18.1	...	20.1	17.3	10
a. Blacks	[1]118	...	143	124	65
19.4 Congenital syphilis (per 100,000 live births)	[1]100.0	...	78.3	103.4	50
19.5 Annual number of first time consultations[2]					
Genital herpes	167,000	[3]163,000	[1]172,000	285,000	142,000
Genital warts	451,000	[3]290,000	[1]275,000	282,000	385,000
19.6 Pelvic inflammatory disease incidence (per 100,000)					
Females 15–44 years	311	...	261	234	250
19.7 Sexually transmitted Hepatitis B (number of cases)	[4]58,300	[4,5]47,593	47,881	58,393	30,500
19.8 Repeat gonorrhea infection	[4]20%	...	– – –	– – –	15%
19.9 Adolescents who ever had sexual intercourse					
Adolescents 15 years					
Females	27%	...	[6]43%	[6]45%	15%
Males	33%	...	[6]53%	[6]51%	15%
Adolescents 17 years					
Females	50%	...	[7]67%	[7]65%	40%
Males	66%	...	[7]76%	[7]68%	40%
19.10 Condom use at last sexual intercourse					
Sexually active unmarried females 15– 44 years	19%	...	– – –	– – –	50%
a. Sexually active females 15–19 years	25%	[8]26%	[9]40%	[9]38%	60%
b. Sexually active males 15–19 years	57%	...	[9]49%	[9]54%	75%
c. Intravenous drug abusers	– – –	...	– – –	– – –	60%
19.11 Clinic services for HIV and other sexually transmitted diseases	– – –	...	– – –	– – –	50%
Family planning clinics	[1]40%	...	– – –	– – –	...
19.12 Sexually transmitted disease education in schools	95%	...	– – –	– – –	100%
19.13 Correct management of sexually transmitted disease cases by primary care providers	70%	...	– – –	– – –	90%
19.14 Clinician counseling to prevent HIV and other sexually transmitted diseases	[4]10%	...	– – –	– – –	75%
a. Providers practicing in high incidence areas	– – –	...	– – –	– – –	90%
19.15 Partner notification of exposure to sexually transmitted diseases					
Patients with bacterial sexually transmitted diseases	20%	...	– – –	– – –	50%

[1]1989 data.
[2]As measured by first time visits to physicians' offices.
[3]Data have been revised to reflect updated methodology; see Introduction.
[4]1987 data.
[5]Data have been revised. Original data were estimated based on preliminary analyses; see Introduction.
[6]10th grade students.
[7]12th grade students.
[8]Baseline was revised due to error in original publication.
[9]9th–12th grade students.

NOTE: Data sources are in table C.

Sexually Transmitted Diseases Objectives

19.1: Reduce gonorrhea to an incidence of no more than 225 cases per 100,000 people.

> **19.1a**: Reduce gonorrhea among blacks to an incidence of no more than 1,300 cases per 100,000.

> **19.1b**: Reduce gonorrhea among adolescents aged 15–19 to no more than 750 cases per 100,000.

> **19.1c**: Reduce gonorrhea among women aged 15–44 to no more than 290 cases per 100,000.

19.2: Reduce Chlamydia trachomatis infections, as measured by a decrease in the incidence of nongonococcal urethritis to no more than 170 cases per 100,000 people.

19.3: Reduce primary and secondary syphilis to an incidence of no more than 10 cases per 100,000 people.

> **19.3a**: Reduce primary and secondary syphilis among blacks to an incidence of no more 65 cases per 100,000.

19.4: Reduce congenital syphilis to an incidence of no more than 50 cases per 100,000 live births.

19.5: Reduce genital herpes and genital warts, as measured by a reduction to 142,000 and 385,000, respectively, in the annual number of first-time consultations with a physician for the conditions.

19.6: Reduce the incidence of pelvic inflammatory disease, as measured by a reduction in hospitalizations for pelvic inflammatory disease to no more than 250 per 100,000 women aged 15–44.

19.7*: Reduce sexually transmitted hepatitis B infection to no more than 30,500 cases.

Duplicate objectives: 20.03b and 20.03c, combined

19.8: Reduce the rate of repeat gonorrhea infection to no more than 15 percent within the previous year.

NOTE: As measured by a reduction in the proportion of gonorrhea patients who, within the previous year, were treated for a separate case of gonorrhea.

19.9*: Reduce the proportion of adolescents who have engaged in sexual intercourse to no more than 15 percent by age 15 and no more than 40 percent by age 17.

Duplicate objectives: 5.4 and 18.3

19.10*: Increase to at least 50 percent the proportion of sexually active, unmarried people who used a condom at last sexual intercourse.

Duplicate objective: 18.4

> **19.10a***: Increase to at least 60 percent the proportion of sexually active, unmarried young women aged 15–19 whose partner used a condom at last sexual intercourse.

Duplicate objective: 18.4a

> **19.10b***: Increase to at least 75 percent the proportion of sexually active, unmarried young men aged 15–19 who used a condom at last sexual intercourse.

Duplicate objective: 18.4b

> **19.10c***: Increase to at least 60 percent the proportion of intravenous drug abusers who used a condom at last sexual intercourse.

Duplicate objective: 18.4c

19.11*: Increase to at least 50 percent the proportion of family planning clinics, maternal and child health clinics, sexually transmitted disease clinics, tuberculosis clinics, drug treatment centers, and primary care clinics that screen, diagnose, treat, counsel, and provide (or refer for) partner notification services for bacterial sexually transmitted diseases (gonorrhea, syphilis, and chlamydia).

Duplicate objectives: 5.11 and 18.13

19.12: Include instruction in sexually transmitted disease transmission prevention in the curricula of all middle and secondary schools, preferably as part of quality school health education.

NOTE: Strategies to achieve this objective must be undertaken sensitively to avoid indirectly encouraging or condoning sexual activity among teens who are not yet sexually active.

19.13: Increase to at least 90 percent the proportion of primary care providers treating patients with sexually transmitted diseases who correctly manage cases, as measured by their use of appropriate types and amounts of therapy.

19.14*: Increase to at least 75 percent the proportion of primary care and mental health care providers who provide age-appropriate counseling on the prevention of HIV and other sexually transmitted diseases.

NOTE: Primary care providers include physicians, nurses, nurse practitioners, and physician assistants. Areas of high AIDS and sexually transmitted disease incidence are cities and States with incidence rates of AIDS cases, HIV seroprevalence, gonorrhea, or syphilis that are at least 25 percent above the national average.

Duplicate objective: 18.9

> **19.14a***: Increase to at least 90 percent the proportion of primary care and mental health care providers who practice in areas of high AIDS and sexually transmitted disease incidence who provide age appropriate counseling on the prevention of HIV and other sexually transmitted diseases.

Duplicate objective: 18.9a

19.15: Increase to at least 50 percent the proportion of all patients with bacterial sexually transmitted diseases (gonorrhea, syphilis, and chlamydia) who are offered provider referral services.

NOTE: Provider referral (previously called contact tracing) is the process whereby health department personnel directly notify the sexual partners of infected individuals of their exposure to an infected individual.

*Duplicate objective.

References

1. Centers for Disease Control. Division of STD/HIV prevention annual report, 1989. Atlanta, Georgia: U.S. Department of Health and Human Services. 1990.

2. Washington AE, Arno PS, Brooks MA. The economic costs of pelvic inflammatory disease. JAMA 255: 1735–8. 1986.

3. Kaufman RE, Jones OG, Blount JH, Wiesner PJ. Questionnaire survey of reported early congenital syphilis: Problems in diagnosis, prevention, and treatment. Sex Transm Dis 4: 135–9. 1977.

4. Zenker P. New case definition for congenital syphilis reporting. Sex Transm Dis 18: 44–5. 1991.

Priority Area 20
Immunization and
Infectious Diseases

Background and Data Summary

The reduction in incidence of infectious diseases is a significant public health achievement of this century. Much of this progress is a result of improvements in basic hygiene, food production and handling, and water treatment. The development and widespread use of vaccines has been instrumental in reducing the incidence of many infectious diseases. For others, antimicrobial agents have greatly reduced illness and death. Despite the progress that has been made, infectious diseases remain an important cause of illness and death in the United States. The very young, older adults, and members of minority groups are at increased risk for many infectious diseases. Each of the causative agents of infectious diseases, even those that are currently rare, pose a potential threat of recurrence or development of resistance to current treatment. For example, susceptibility to active tuberculosis among persons infected with HIV has contributed to an increase in the number of tuberculosis cases after a steady decline since the 1950's (1). Outbreaks of multiple drug-resistant tuberculosis cases have occurred in recent years. A number of newly recognized infectious diseases have emerged. Recent examples include Legionnaires' Disease, toxic shock syndrome, Lyme disease, and the wide spectrum of diseases associated with the human immunodeficiency virus (HIV).

Recent data indicate mixed results regarding trends toward achieving the year 2000 objectives in the immunization and infectious diseases priority area. For 3 of the 19 objectives (20.3, 20.13, and 20.15) there is progress toward achieving the year 2000 targets. This includes an overall reduction in the incidence of viral hepatitis (20.3). The target for hepatitis C has been surpassed. Among the special population targets

Figure 25. Annual incidence of tuberculosis, according to race and ethnicity: United States, 1988–91 and year 2000 targets for objective 20.4

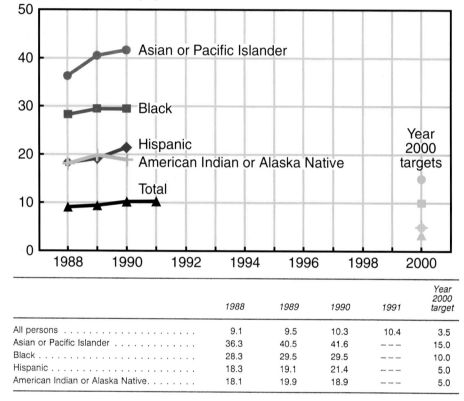

Cases per 100,000 population

	1988	1989	1990	1991	Year 2000 target
All persons	9.1	9.5	10.3	10.4	3.5
Asian or Pacific Islander	36.3	40.5	41.6	---	15.0
Black	28.3	29.5	29.5	---	10.0
Hispanic	18.3	19.1	21.4	---	5.0
American Indian or Alaska Native	18.1	19.9	18.9	---	5.0

NOTE: A related table in *Health, United States, 1992*, is table 52.

SOURCE: Centers for Disease Control and Prevention, Center for Prevention Services.

for hepatitis B, a dramatic reduction in the number of cases has occurred among intravenous drug users, surpassing the number targeted for the year 2000. However, hepatitis B cases have increased among heterosexually active people and men who have sex with men.

Five objectives (20.2, 20.4, 20.9, 20.12, and 20.18) are moving away from the target. These include increased morbidity from various infectious diseases, including pneumonia and influenza (20.2), tuberculosis (20.4), and middle ear infections among children (20.9). Mixed results are shown for four

other objectives (20.1, 20.6, 20.10, and 20.11). Cases of many vaccine-preventable diseases increased since baseline, although declines were observed for mumps and pertussis (20.1). Although the number of measles cases in 1991 was considerably higher than the number reported in 1988, the 1991 data show a decline from the number of cases reported in 1989 and 1990. Hepatitis A reported among international travelers has declined, while malaria and typhoid cases have increased (20.6). Restricted activity related to pneumonia decreased among children less than 5 years old but increased among those 65 years and older (20.10). New data are available to establish baseline measures for three objectives (20.5, 20.8, and 20.16). Data are not yet available to establish baseline measures for three objectives (20.14, 20.17, and 20.19) or to provide a measure after baseline for one objective (20.7).

Data Issues

Data Source Description

The National Notifiable Disease Surveillance System (NNDSS) is the data source for tracking cases of vaccine-preventable diseases (20.1). Interim data from this system are routinely published in the Morbidity and Mortality Weekly Report. Final data, used to track objective 20.1, are published in the Annual Summary of Notifiable Diseases (2). Detailed epidemiologic analyses of data from NNDSS are sometimes published in special surveillance reports. Data in these reports may not agree exactly with reports published in the Morbidity and Mortality Weekly Report because of differences in timing or refinements in case definition. The NNDSS is the data source for specific disease surveillance systems, such as the Viral Hepatitis Surveillance System and the Tuberculosis Morbidity Data System (20.3 and 20.4). In the case of the Viral Hepatitis Surveillance System, the data are corrected for underreporting.

Definition

Epidemic-related pneumonia and influenza deaths are defined as those that are above the normal yearly fluctuations of mortality. The data cannot be obtained directly from published mortality figures. Each year expected numbers of pneumonia and influenza deaths are calculated through a cyclical regression model using data for previous years but excluding data for the periods when mortality was known to be raised by influenza epidemics (3). Epidemic-related deaths are defined as those that exceed by 1.645 standard deviations the expected number based on the model.

Comparability of Data Sources

Recent data on immunization levels among children less than 2 years old are not directly comparable with the baseline data (20.11). The revised baseline was obtained from the 1985 United States Immunization Survey and shows the range of antigen-specific vaccination levels at the time of interview among children 2 years old. The specific immunization levels were 54 percent for polio, 61 percent for measles-containing vaccines, and 64 percent for diphtheria-tetanus-pertussis (DTP). The 1991 figure of 37 percent, obtained from the National Health Interview Survey (NHIS), represents the proportion of children 2 years of age who are fully immunized for measles-mumps-rubella (MMR), polio, and DTP at the time of interview. The antigen-specific immunization levels were 52 percent for polio, 67 percent for DTP and 80 percent for MMR (a related table in *Health, United States, 1992*, is 51, which shows data for 1–4 year-olds).

The NHIS may have underestimated immunization levels among 2 year old children for whom shot records were not available at time of interview. Among 52 percent of white respondents and 40 percent of respondents of all other races who either had shot records or who reported that the child had never received a vaccination, 56 percent of 2 year old children were fully immunized for polio, MMR, and DTP at the time of interview. Among the same group of respondents, 47 percent of the 2 year olds were fully immunized by their second birthday.

Table 20. Immunization and infectious diseases objective status

Objective	1987 baseline Original	1987 baseline Revised	1990	1991	Target 2000
20.1 Vaccine-preventable diseases (number of cases)					
Diphtheria among people 25 years and under	[1]1	...	2	2	0
Tetanus among people 25 years and under	[1]3	...	6	4	0
Polio (wild-type virus)	[1]0	...	0	0	0
Measles	[1]3,058	...	26,527	9,411	0
Rubella	[1]225	...	1,125	1,401	0
Congenital Rubella Syndrome	[1]6	...	11	47	0
Mumps	[1]4,866	...	5,292	4,264	500
Pertussis	[1]3,450	...	4,570	2,719	1,000
20.2 Epidemic-related pneumonia and influenza deaths among older adults (per 100,000)	[2]9.1	...	[3]12.0	– – –	7.3
20.3 Viral hepatitis (cases per 100,000)					
Hepatitis B (HBV)	63.5	...	50.6	42.6	40.0
Hepatitis A	31.0	[4]33.0	37.9	29.0	23.0
Hepatitis C	18.3	...	13.1	8.3	13.7
HBV Cases (number of cases)					
a. Intravenous drug abusers	30,000	[4]44,348	17,615	12,666	22,500
b. Heterosexually active people	33,000	[4]33,995	33,971	43,795	22,000
c. Homosexual males	25,300	[4]13,598	13,840	14,598	8,500
d. Children of Asians/Pacific Islanders	8,900	[4]10,817	8,807	7,514	1,800
e. Occupationally exposed workers	6,200	[4]3,090	1,258	2,576	1,250
f. Infants	3,500	[4]3,863	3,003	2,235	550
New Carriers					
g. Alaska Natives	15	...	15	15	1
20.4 Tuberculosis (cases per 100,000)	[1]9.1	...	10.3	10.4	3.5
a. Asians/Pacific Islanders	[1]36.3	...	41.6	– – –	15.0
b. Blacks	[1]28.3	...	29.5	– – –	10.0
c. Hispanics	[1]18.3	...	21.4	– – –	5.0
d. American Indians/Alaska Natives	[1]18.1	...	18.9	– – –	5.0
20.5 Surgical wound and nosocomial infections					
Surgical wound infection rates (per 100 operations)					
Low risk patients	...	[5]1.1	– – –	– – –	1.0
Medium-low risk patients	...	[5]3.2	– – –	– – –	2.9
Medium-high risk patients	...	[5]6.3	– – –	– – –	5.7
High risk patients	...	[5]14.4	– – –	– – –	13.0
Device-associated nosocomial infection rates (per 1,000 device-days)					
Bloodstream Infections					
Medical/Coronary ICUs	...	[5]6.9	– – –	– – –	6.2
Surgical/Medical-Surgical ICUs	...	[5]5.3	– – –	– – –	4.8
Pediatric ICUs	...	[5]11.4	– – –	– – –	10.3
Urinary Tract Infections					
Medical/Coronary ICUs	...	[5]10.7	– – –	– – –	9.6
Surgical/Medical-Surgical ICUs	...	[5]7.6	– – –	– – –	6.8
Pediatric ICUs	...	[5]5.8	– – –	– – –	5.2
Pneumonia					
Medical/Coronary ICUs	...	[5]12.8	– – –	– – –	11.5
Surgical/Medical-Surgical ICUs	...	[5]17.6	– – –	– – –	15.8
Pediatric ICUs	...	[5]4.7	– – –	– – –	4.2
20.6 Illness among international travelers (number of cases)					
Typhoid fever	280		386	351	140
Hepatitis A	1,280	[4]4,475	3,962	3,730	640
Malaria	2,000	[4]932	[6]1,102	1,021	1,000
20.7 Bacterial meningitis (per 100,000)	[7]6.3	[4,7]6.5	– – –	– – –	4.7
a. Alaska Natives	33	...	– – –	17	8
20.8 Diarrhea among children in child care centers					
Children 0–6 years	...	[8]32%	– – –	– – –	24%
Children 0–3 years	...	[8]38%	– – –	– – –	28%
20.9 Ear infections among children (restricted activity days per 100 children)	131	[9]135.4	125.0	155.7	105.0

Table 20. Immunization and infectious diseases objective status — Con.

Objective	1987 baseline		1990	1991	Target 2000
	Original	Revised			
20.10 Pneumonia-related illness (restricted activity days per 100 people)					
People 65 years and over	48.0	[8]19.1	46.2	78.5	38.0
Children 4 years and under	27.0	[8]29.4	51.3	24.1	24.0
20.11 Immunization (percent immunized)					
Basic immunization series among children					
Children 2 years and under	[10]70–80%	[9,11]54–64%	– – –	[12]37%	90%
Children in licensed child care facilities	94%	[9,13]94–95%	[13]94–96%	[13]94–96%	95%
Children in kindergarten through post-secondary education institutions	97%	[9,13]97–98%	[13]97–98%	[13]96–98%	95%
Pneumococcal pneumonia and influenza immunizations					
Institutionalized chronically ill people or older people	– – –	. . .	– – –	– – –	80%
Non-institutionalized high risk populations	[10]10–20%	[9,14]14–30%	– – –	[15]16%	60%
Hepatitis B immunizations					
Infants of antigen-positive mothers	. . .	[9]40%	– – –	– – –	90%
Occupationally exposed workers	. . .	[6]37%	– – –	– – –	90%
IV-drug users in drug treatment programs	– – –	. . .	– – –	– – –	50%
Homosexual males	– – –	. . .	– – –	– – –	50%
20.12 Post exposure rabies treatments (number)	18,000	. . .	– – –	18,800	9,000
20.13 Immunization laws (number of States)	[16,17]10	[6,9]10–49	– – –	[18]34–50	50
20.14 Provision of immunizations by clinicians	– – –	. . .	– – –	– – –	90%
20.15 Financial barriers to immunization					
Employment-based insurance plans that provide coverage for immunizations					
Conventional insurance plans	[6]45%	. . .	47%	– – –	100%
Preferred Provider Organization plans	[6]62%	. . .	65%	– – –	100%
Health Maintenance Organization plans	[6]98%	. . .	98%	– – –	100%
20.16 Public health department provision of immunizations	. . .	[16]37–70%	– – –	– – –	90%
20.17 Local health programs to identify tuberculosis	– – –	. . .	– – –	– – –	90%
20.18 Preventive therapy for tuberculosis (percent of infected persons completing therapy)	66.3%	. . .	63.0%	– – –	85%
20.19 Laboratory capability for influenza diagnosis					
Tertiary care hospitals	– – –	. . .	– – –	– – –	85%
Secondary care hospitals and HMOs	– – –	. . .	– – –	– – –	50%

[1]1988 data.

[2]1980–87 data.

[3]1986–88 data.

[4]Data have been revised. Original data were estimated based on preliminary analysis; see Introduction.

[5]1986–90 data.

[6]1989 data.

[7]1986 data.

[8]1991 data.

[9]Data have been revised to reflect updated methodology; see Introduction.

[10]1985 data.

[11]1985 data; range of antigen-specific immunization levels among 2 year old children (see text).

[12]Proportion of 2 year old children who have received all the recommended doses of diptheria-tetanus-pertussis, measles-mumps-rubella, and polio (see text).

[13]Range of antigen-specific immunization levels.

[14]1989 data; among people 65 years and over, 14 percent received pneumococcal vaccine and 30 percent received influenza vaccine.

[15]Proportion of people 65 years and over who received both pneumococcal and influenza vaccines; 21 percent received pneumoccal vaccine and 42 percent received influenza vaccine.

[16]1990 data.

[17]Includes Washington, DC.

[18]1992 data.

NOTE: Data sources are in table C.

Immunization and Infectious Diseases Objectives

20.1: Reduce indigenous cases of vaccine-preventable diseases as follows:

Disease	2000 target
Diphtheria among people aged 25 and younger	0
Tetanus among people aged 25 and younger	0
Polio (wild-type virus)	0
Measles (indigenous)	0
Rubella	0
Congenital Rubella Syndrome	0
Mumps	500
Pertussis	1,000

20.2: Reduce epidemic-related pneumonia and influenza deaths among people aged 65 and older to no more than 7.3 per 100,000 people.

NOTE: Epidemic-related pneumonia and influenza deaths are those that occur above and beyond the normal yearly fluctuations of mortality. Because of the extreme variability in epidemic-related deaths from year to year, the target is a 3-year average.

20.3*: Reduce viral hepatitis as follows:

Hepatitis B (HBV): 40 per 100,000 people
Hepatitis A: 23 per 100,000 people
Hepatitis C: 13.7 cases per 100,000 people

Duplicate objectives: 19.07, 10.5

> **20.3a**: Reduce Hepatitis B (HBV) among intravenous drug abusers to no more than 22,500 cases per 100,000.

> **20.3b***: Reduce Hepatitis B (HBV) among heterosexually active people to no more than 22,000 cases per 100,000.

Duplicate objective: 19.7

> **20.3c***: Reduce Hepatitis B (HBV) among homosexual men to no more than 8,500 cases per 100,000.

Duplicate objective: 19.7

> **20.3d**: Reduce Hepatitis B (HBV) among children of Asian and Pacific Islanders to no more than 1,800 cases per 100,000.

> **20.3e***: Reduce Hepatitis B (HBV) among occupationally exposed workers to no more than 1,250 cases per 100,000.

Duplicate objective: 10.5

> **20.3f**: Reduce Hepatitis B (HBV) among infants to no more than 550 new carriers per 100,000.

> **20.3g**: Reduce Hepatitis B (HBV) among Alaska Natives to no more than 1 case per 100,000.

20.4: Reduce tuberculosis to an incidence of no more than 3.5 cases per 100,000 people.

> **20.4a**: Reduce tuberculosis among Asians and Pacific Islanders to an incidence of no more than 15 cases per 100,000.

> **20.4b**: Reduce tuberculosis among blacks to an incidence of no more than 10 cases per 100,000.

> **20.4c**: Reduce tuberculosis among Hispanics to an incidence of no more than 5 cases per 100,000.

> **20.4d**: Reduce tuberculosis among American Indians and Alaska Natives to an incidence of no more than 5 cases per 100,000.

20.5: Reduce by at least 10 percent the incidence of surgical wound infections and no socomial infections in intensive care patients.

20.6: Reduce selected illness among international travelers as follows:

Typhoid fever: 140 cases
Hepatitis A: 640 cases
Malaria: 1,000 cases

20.7: Reduce bacterial meningitis to no more than 4.7 cases per 100,000 people.

20.7a: Reduce bacterial meningitis among Alaska Natives to no more than 8 cases per 100,000 people.

20.8: Reduce infectious diarrhea by at least 25 percent among children in licensed child care centers and children in programs that provide an Individualized Education Program (IEP) or Individualized Health Plan (IHP).

20.9: Reduce acute middle ear infections among children aged 4 and younger, as measured by days of restricted activity or school absenteeism, to no more than 105 days per 100 children.

20.10: Reduce pneumonia-related days of restricted activity as follows:

38 days per 100 people aged 65 and older.
24 days per 100 children aged 4 and younger.

20.11: Increase immunization levels as follows:

Basic immunization series among children under age 2: at least 90 percent.

Basic immunization series among children in licensed child care facilities and kindergarten through post-secondary education institutions: at least 95 percent.

Pneumococcal pneumonia and influenza immunization among institutionalized chronically ill or older people: at least 80 percent.

Pneumococcal pneumonia and influenza immunization among noninstitutionalized, high-risk populations, as defined by the Immunization Practices Advisory Committee: at least 60 percent.

Hepatitis B immunization among high-risk populations, including infants of surface antigen-positive mothers to at least 90 percent; occupationally exposed workers to at least 90 percent; IV-drug users in drug treatment programs to at least 50 percent; and homosexual men to at least 50 percent.

Duplicate objective for occupationally exposed workers: 10.9

20.12: Reduce postexposure rabies treatments to no more than 9,000 per year.

20.13: Expand immunization laws for schools, preschools, and day care settings to all States for all antigens.

20.14: Increase to at least 90 percent the proportion of primary care providers who provide information and counseling about immunizations and offer immunizations as appropriate for their patients.

20.15: Improve the financing and delivery of immunizations for children and adults so that virtually no American has a financial barrier to receiving recommended immunizations.

20.16: Increase to at least 90 percent the proportion of public health departments that provide adult immunization for influenza, pneumococcal disease, hepatitis B, tetanus, and diphtheria.

20.17: Increase to at least 90 percent the proportion of local health departments that have ongoing programs for actively identifying cases of tuberculosis and latent infection in populations at high risk for tuberculosis.

NOTE: Local health department refers to any local component of the public health system, defined as an administrative and service unit of local or State government concerned with health and carrying some responsibility for the health of a jurisdiction smaller than a State.

20.18: Increase to at least 85 percent the proportion of people found to have tuberculosis infection who completed courses of preventive therapy.

20.19: Increase to at least 85 percent the proportion of tertiary care hospital laboratories and to at least 50 percent the proportion of secondary care hospital and health maintenance organization laboratories possessing technologies for rapid viral diagnosis of influenza.

*Duplicate objective

References

1. Jereb JA, Kelly GD, Dooley SW, et al. Tuberculosis morbidity in the United States: Final data, 1990. MMWR 40(SS-3) :23–7. 1991.

2. Centers for Disease Control. Summary of notifiable diseases, United States, 1990. MMWR 39(53). 1991.

3. Lui K-J, Kendal AP. Impact of influenza epidemics on mortality in the United States from October 1972 to May 1985. Am J Public Health 77: 712–6. 1987.

Priority Area 21
Clinical Preventive Services

Background and Data Summary

Clinical preventive services are those disease prevention and health promotion services—immunizations, screening for early detection of disease or risk factors, and patient counseling—that are delivered to individuals in a health care setting. The U.S. Clinical Preventive Services Task Force, a panel of prevention experts appointed by the U.S. Public Health Service, has reviewed the full range of scientific literature on clinical preventive services and developed scientifically sound recommendations for specific services based on age, gender, and other risk factors (1).

Preventive services for specific diseases and health-related behaviors are addressed in other priority areas of *Healthy People 2000*. For example, receipt of pap smears, clinical breast exams, and mammography are addressed in the cancer priority area. The objectives in this priority area support those objectives by considering clinical preventive services as a complete package and addressing barriers that impede access to and use of these services.

Data are available for only two objectives (21.3 and 21.8) to assess trends towards meeting the eight Clinical Preventive Services objectives, although recent data are available to establish baseline measures for four other objectives (21.2, 21.4, 21.5, and 21.7). Data from the 1991 NHIS on the proportion of people who have a specific source of ongoing primary care show a slight decline from the 1986 baseline for the population as a whole and for Hispanics and people with low incomes (21.3). Over the same time period, the proportion of black persons who had a specific source of primary care did not change. In 1991 the proportion of black persons who had a specific source of care was similar to that in the population as a whole, whereas the proportion was lower among Hispanics and

low-income people. Information on degrees awarded to minorities in the health professions for the academic year 1990–91 show slight improvements toward meeting the year 2000 target (21.8). The baseline for 21.1 has been revised. No baseline has been established for 21.6.

Data Issues

Years of Healthy Life

See the introduction for a discussion of years of healthy life.

Definition

Receipt of all of the screening and immunization services and at least one of the counseling services, at the appropriate interval, and as recommended by the U.S. Preventive Services Task Force is considered in objective 21.2. The recommendations vary by age, gender, and risk group; several of the objective's special population targets correspond to age groups specified by the Task Force. Questions to establish receipt of clinical preventive services among

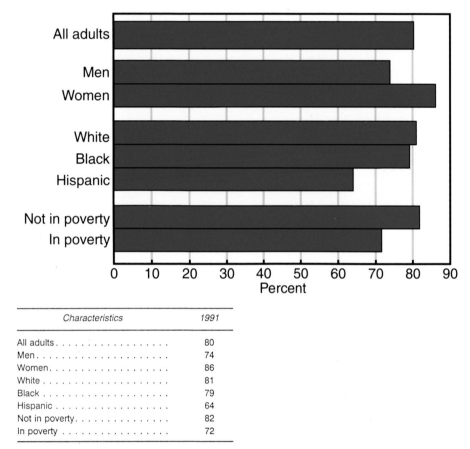

Figure 26. Adults with a usual source of medical care, according to selected characteristics related to year 2000 objective 21.3: United States, 1991

Characteristics	1991
All adults	80
Men	74
Women	86
White	81
Black	79
Hispanic	64
Not in poverty	82
In poverty	72

NOTE: Related tables in *Health, United States, 1992*, are 78–81.

SOURCE: Centers for Disease Control and Prevention, National Center for Health Statistics, National Health Interview Survey.

persons 19 years of age and over were included in the Health Promotion and Disease Prevention Supplement of the 1991 NHIS and were used to establish a baseline for this objective. The supplement provides information on all of the recommended immunizations and screening components, including the history, physical examination, and laboratory and diagnostic recommendations; counseling services and specific recommendations for high risk groups are not addressed. Information was obtained on the interval since last routine check-up by a medical doctor or other health care professional and receipt of several of the recommended services at the last check-up. Questions on receipt of other recommended services, namely immunizations, pap tests, clinical breast examinations, and mammograms were asked separately. For these, respondents of appropriate age and gender were asked whether they had received the service within a specific interval, usually the interval recommended by the Task Force.

The proportion of people receiving the minimum set of recommended services at the appropriate interval is quite low; among people 65 years of age and over, no one received the complete set of preventive services. However, much larger proportions of people have received components of the recommended services, for example the history, physical examination, laboratory diagnostic procedures, and immunizations. The measure for older people may be influenced by the way the information is obtained in the NHIS supplement. Older people are likely to have more frequent visits to health professionals for various health problems, which should increase the likelihood of receiving preventive services. However, complete preventive services may not be received at the last regular check-up as specified in some of the NHIS questions.

In 1989, 16 percent of the U.S. population less than 65 years old did not have health care coverage, neither private insurance, Medicare, Medicaid, nor a military plan. This measure is used to establish a baseline for objective 21.4, financial barriers to receiving recommended clinical preventive services. However,

this only provides a partial measure for the objective since many health insurance plans do not provide full coverage for preventive health care. In 1988, 41 percent of employer-sponsored health insurance plans covered adult physical examinations, 56 percent covered well baby care, and 69 percent covered preventive diagnostic tests (2).

In 1990 people who indicated emergency rooms as the usual place they went if they were sick or needed advice about their health were included as having a usual source of care, whereas they were not included in 1991. In 1990, 0.6 percent of all people who had a usual source of care as defined above indicated a hospital emergency room as their usual source (3). This objective will continue to be monitored with the NHIS; emergency rooms as a usual source of care will be excluded from the estimates.

Comparability of Data Sources

Baseline data on the proportion of people who have a specific source of ongoing primary care were obtained from a survey conducted by the Robert Wood Johnson Foundation (4). Recent information for this objective is available from the NHIS. Some differences in this measure between the baseline and more recent years may be accounted for by differences in survey methods.

Table 21. Clinical preventive services objective status

Objective	Baseline Original	Baseline Revised	1990	1991	Target 2000
21.1 Years of healthy life	[1]62.0	[2,3]64.0	---	---	65
a. Blacks	[1]56.0	[2,3]No change	---	---	60
b. Hispanics	[1]62.0	[2,3,4]64.8	---	---	65
c. People 65 years and over	[1]12.0	[2,3,5]11.9	---	---	[4]14
21.2 Receipt of recommended services	...	[6,7]2%	---	---	50%
a. Infants up to 24 months	...	---	---	---	90%
b. Children 2–12 years	...	---	---	---	80%
c. Adolescents 13–18 years	...	---	---	---	50%
d. People 19–39 years	...	[6]3%	---	---	40%
e. People 40–64 years	...	[6]2%	---	---	40%
f. People 65 years and over	...	[6]0%	---	---	40%
g. Low-income people	...	[6,7]2%	---	---	50%
h. Blacks	...	[6,7]3%	---	---	50%
i. Hispanics	...	[6,7]2%	---	---	50%
j. Asians/Pacific Islanders	...	[6,7]3%	---	---	50%
k. American Indians/Alaska Natives	...	[6,7]3%	---	---	70%
l. People with disabilities	...	[6,7]1%	---	---	80%
21.3 Access to primary care (percent with source of care)	[8]82%	...	77%	80%	95%
a. Hispanics	[8]70%	...	64%	64%	95%
b. Blacks	[8]80%	...	75%	79%	95%
c. Low-income people	[8]80%	...	71%	72%	95%
21.4 Financial barriers to receipt of clinical preventive services	---	...	---	---	0%
Proportion without health care coverage					
People under 65 years	...	[9]16%	---	---	...
21.5 Clinical preventive services from publicly funded programs (proportion of eligible people)	---	...	---	---	90%
Federal programs					
Screening	...	[10]10–100%	---	---	...
Counseling	...	[10]40–100%	---	---	...
Immunizations	...	[10]10–96%	---	---	...
21.6 Provision of recommended services by primary care providers	---	...	---	---	50%
21.7 Local health department assurance of access to essential clinical preventive service					
Proportion of people served	---	...	---	---	90%
Proportion of local health departments providing:					
Health education	...	[11]74%	---	---	...
Child health	...	[11]84%	---	---	...
Immunizations	...	[11]92%	---	---	...
Prenatal care	...	[11]59%	---	---	...
Primary care	...	[11]22%	---	---	...
21.8 Racial/ethnic minority representation in the health professions					
Degrees Awarded To:					
Blacks	[12]5.0%	...	---	[13]5.7%	8.0%
Hispanics	[12]3.0%	...	---	[13]4.3%	6.4%
American Indians/Alaska Natives	[12]0.3%	...	---	[13]0.4%	0.6%

[1]1980 data.
[2]1990 data.
[3]Data have been revised to reflect updated methodology; see Introduction.
[4]Estimate based on preliminary data.
[5]Years of healthy life remaining at age 65.
[6]1991 data.
[7]Among people 19 years and over.
[8]1986 data.
[9]1989 data.
[10]1991–92 data.
[11]1990 data.
[12]1985–86 data.
[13]Academic year 1990–91.

NOTE: Data sources are in table C.

Clinical Preventive Services Objectives

21.1*: Increase years of healthy life to at least 65 years.

NOTE: Years of healthy life is a summary measure of health that combines mortality (quantity of life) and morbidity and disability (quality of life) into a single measure. For people aged 65 and older, active life-expectancy, a related summary measure, also will be tracked.

Duplicate objectives: 8.1 and 17.1

21.1a*: Increase years of healthy life among blacks to at least 60 years.

Duplicate objectives: 8.1 and 17.1a

21.1b*: Increase years of healthy life among Hispanics to at least 65 years.

Duplicate objectives: 8.1b and 17.1b

21.1c*: Increase years of healthy life among people aged 65 and older to at least 14 years remaining.

Duplicate objectives: 8.1c and 17.1c

21.2: Increase to at least 50 percent the proportion of people who have received, as a minimum within the appropriate interval, all of the screening and immunization services and at least one of the counseling services appropriate for their age and gender as recommended by the U.S. Preventive Services Task Force.

21.2a: Increase to at least 90 percent the proportion of infants up to 24 months who have received, as a minimum within the appropriate interval, all of the screening and immunization services and at least one of the counseling services appropriate for their age and gender as recommended by the U.S. Preventive Services Task Force.

21.2b: Increase to at least 80 percent the proportion of children aged 2–12 who have received, as a minimum within the appropriate interval, all of the screening and immunization services and at least one of the counseling services appropriate for their age and gender as recommended by the U.S. Preventive Services Task Force.

21.2c: Increase to at least 50 percent the proportion of adolescents aged 13–18 who have received, as a minimum within the appropriate interval, all of the screening and immunization services and at least one of the counseling services appropriate for their age and gender as recommended by the U.S. Preventive Services Task Force.

21.2d: Increase to at least 40 percent the proportion of adults aged 19–39 who have received, as a minimum within the appropriate interval, all of the screening and immunization services and at least one of the counseling services appropriate for their age and gender as recommended by the U.S. Preventive Services Task Force.

21.2e: Increase to at least 40 percent the proportion of adults aged 40–64 who have received, as a minimum within the appropriate interval, all of the screening and immunization services and at least one of the counseling services appropriate for their age and gender as recommended by the U.S. Preventive Services Task Force.

21.2f: Increase to at least 40 percent the proportion of adults aged 65 and older who have received, as a minimum within the appropriate interval, all of the screening and immunization services and at least one of the counseling services appropriate for their age and gender as recommended by the U.S. Preventive Services Task Force.

21.2g: Increase to at least 50 percent the proportion of low-income people who have received, as a minimum within the appropriate interval, all of the screening and immunization services and at least one of the counseling services appropriate for their age and gender as recommended by the U.S. Preventive Services Task Force.

21.2h: Increase to at least 50 percent the proportion of blacks who have received, as a minimum within the appropriate interval, all of the screening and immunization services and at least one of the counseling services appropriate for their age and gender as recommended by the U.S. Preventive Services Task Force.

21.2i: Increase to at least 50 percent the proportion of Hispanics who have received, as a minimum within the appropriate interval, all of the screening and immunization services and at least one of the counseling services appropriate for their age and gender as recommended by the U.S. Preventive Services Task Force.

21.2j: Increase to at least 50 percent the proportion of Asians and Pacific Islanders who have received, as a minimum within the appropriate interval, all of the screening and immunization services and at least one of the counseling services appropriate for their age and gender as recommended by the U.S. Preventive Services Task Force.

21.2k: Increase to at least 70 percent the proportion of American Indians and Alaska Natives who have received, as a minimum within the appropriate interval, all of the screening and immunization services and at least one of the counseling services appropriate for their age and gender as recommended by the U.S. Preventive Services Task Force.

21.2l: Increase to at least 80 percent the proportion of people with disabilities who have received, as a minimum within the appropriate interval, all of the screening and immunization services and at least one of the counseling services appropriate for their age and gender as recommended by the U.S. Preventive Services Task Force.

21.3: Increase to at least 95 percent the proportion of people who have a specific source of ongoing primary care for coordination of their preventive and episodic health care.

21.3a: Increase to at least 95 percent the proportion of Hispanics who have a specific source of ongoing primary care for coordination of their preventive and episodic healthcare.

21.3b: Increase to at least 95 percent the proportion of blacks who have a specific source of ongoing primary care for coordination of their preventive and episodic health care.

21.3c: Increase to at least 95 percent the proportion of low-income people who have a specific source of ongoing primary care for coordination of their preventive and episodic health care.

21.4: Improve financing and delivery of clinical preventive services so that virtually no American has a financial barrier to receiving, at a minimum, the screening, counseling, and immunization services recommended by the U.S. Preventive Services Task Force.

21.5: Assure that at least 90 percent of people for whom primary care services are provided directly by publicly funded programs are offered, at a minimum, the screening, counseling, and immunization services recommended by the U.S. Preventive Services Task force.

NOTE: Publicly funded programs that provide primary care services directly include federally funded programs such as the Maternal and Child Health Program, Community and Migrant Health Centers, and the Indian Health Service as well as primary care service settings funded by State and local governments. This objective does not include services covered indirectly through the Medicare and Medicaid programs.

21.6: Increase to at least 50 percent the proportion of primary care providers who provide their patients with the screening, counseling, and immunization services recommended by the U.S. Preventive Services Task Force.

21.7: Increase to at least 90 percent the proportion of people who are served by a local health department that assesses and assures access to essential clinical preventive services.

NOTE: Local health department refers to any local component of the public health system, defined as an administrative and service unit of local or State government concerned with health and carrying some responsibility for the health of a jurisdiction smaller than a State.

21.8: Increase the proportion of all degrees in the health professions and allied and associated health profession fields awarded to members of underrepresented racial and ethnic minority groups as follows:

	2000 Target (percent)
Blacks	8.0
Hispanics	6.4
American Indians and Alaska Natives	0.6

*Duplicate objective.

References

1. U.S. Preventive Services Task Force. Guide to clinical preventive services: An assessment of the effectiveness of 169 interventions. Report of the U.S. Preventive Services Task Force. Baltimore, Maryland: Williams and Wilkins. 1989.

2. Health Insurance Association of America. Research bulletin: A profile of employer-sponsored group health insurance. Washington: The Association. 1989.

3. Unpublished data, 1990 National Health Interview Survey.

4. The Robert Wood Johnson Foundation. Access to health care in the United States: Results of a 1986 survey. Special Report Number Two/1987. Princeton, New Jersey: The Foundation. 1987.

Priority Area 22
Surveillance and
Data Systems

Public health surveillance is the systematic collection, analysis, and use of health information. Surveillance is essential to understanding the health status of a population and planning effective prevention programs. The Institute of Medicine identified this assessment activity as one of the core functions of public health (1).

Surveillance is critical in all health agencies: federal, State, and local. State and local data are needed to assess health needs and to implement and evaluate community health programs. Achievement of the year 2000 objectives depends in part on our ability to monitor and compare progress toward the objectives at all levels of government.

We must also be able to measure the health status of special populations. Morbidity, mortality, health behaviors, access to and use of health services vary markedly by age, race, gender, and socio-economic status. Therefore, many of the objectives throughout Healthy People 2000 are targeted toward racial and ethnic minorities, elderly people, and people with chronic disabilities.

Some important health issues could not be addressed in the year 2000 objectives since national data to accurately characterize the problems were unavailable. The lack of data at the State and local levels are even greater concerns. Thus, several objectives in priority area 22 are directed toward enhancing data systems in States and communities. Similarly, objectives address the identification of and response to data gaps related to minorities and other special populations.

The first part of objective 22.1, development of Health Status Indicators, has been achieved. The consensus set of 18 indicators was published in July 1991 (2). National data for the Health Status Indicators were published in October 1992 (3). A summary of the national data for the Health Status Indicators is shown in table D. The achievement of the other part of this objective will be measured by tracking the use of the indicators by State and local health departments.

Work has begun on the remainder of the objectives in priority area 22. Objective 22.2 is close to being achieved. The Centers for Disease Control and Prevention (CDC) has expanded its role in supporting State assessment activities related to the year 2000 objectives. As this *Healthy People 2000 Review* demonstrates, the Department of Health and Human Services is committed to tracking the course of each priority area.

Table 22. Surveillance and data systems objective status

Objective	1989 baseline Original	1989 baseline Revised	1990	1991	Target 2000
22.1 Health status indicators					
Develop	...	[1]Indicators selected	– – –	– – –	...
Establish use (number of States)	– – –	...	– – –	– – –	40
Monitoring some indicators	...	[2]48	– – –	– – –	...
Providing HSI data to local health departments	...	[2]36	– – –	– – –	...
22.2 National data sources	[3]77%	...	– – –	[2]99%	100%
a. State level data for at least two-thirds of the objectives (number of States)	23	[1]22	– – –	[2]26	35
22.3 Comparable data collection procedures					
Federal, State, and local agencies	...	[3]12%	– – –	[2]14%	100%
22.4 Gaps in health data					
Identify	– – –	...	– – –	– – –	100%
Establish mechanisms to meet needs	– – –	...	– – –	– – –	100%
22.5 Periodic analysis and publication of data (number of States)	20	...	– – –	– – –	50
a. Analysis for racial and ethnic groups (number of States)	...	[2,4]19	– – –	– – –	25
22.6 Number of States with data transfer systems	30	...	– – –	– – –	50
National Electronic Telecommunications System for Surveillance (NETSS)	...	[2]50	– – –	– – –	...
Public Health Laboratory Information System (PHLIS)	...	[2]37%	– – –	– – –	...
22.7 Timely release of national data	– – –	...	– – –	– – –	100%
1991–92 data	...	[2]38%	– – –	– – –	...
1990 data	...	[2]23%	– – –	– – –	...

[1]1991 data.
[2]1992 data.
[3]1990 data.
[4]27 States have at least one racial/ethnic group comprising at least 10 percent of their population; 19 published vital statistics data for these racial/ethnic groups.

NOTE: Data sources are in table C.

Surveillance and Data Systems Objectives

22.1: Develop a set of health status indicators appropriate for Federal, State, and local health agencies, and establish use of the set in at least 40 States.

22.2: Identify, and create where necessary, national data sources to measure progress toward each of the year 2000 national health objectives.

    22.2a: Identify, and create where necessary, State level data for at least two-thirds of the objectives in at least 35 States.

22.3: Develop and disseminate among Federal, State, and local agencies procedures for collecting comparable data for each of the year 2000 national health objectives and incorporate these into Public Health Service data collection systems.

22.4: Develop and implement a national process to identify significant gaps in the nation's disease prevention and health promotion data, including data for racial and ethnic minorities, people with low incomes, and people with disabilities, and establish mechanisms to meet these needs.

NOTE: Disease prevention and health promotion data include disease status, risk factors, and services receipt data. Public health problems include such issue areas as HIV infection, domestic violence, mental health, environmental health, occupational health, and disabling conditions.

22.5: Implement in all States periodic analysis and publication of data needed to measure progress toward objectives for at least 10 of the priority areas of the national health objectives.

NOTE: Periodic is at least once every 3 years. Objectives include, at a minimum, one from each objectives category: health status, risk reduction, and services and protection.

    22.5a: Implement in at least 25 States periodic analysis and publication of data needed to measure State progress toward the national health objectives for each racial or ethnic group that makes up at least 10 percent of the State population.

22.6: Expand in all States systems for the transfer of health information related to the national health objectives among Federal, State, and local agencies.

NOTE: Information related to the national health objectives includes State and national level baseline data, disease prevention and health promotion evaluation results, and data generated to measure progress.

22.7: Achieve timely release of national surveillance and survey data needed by health professionals and agencies to measure progress toward the national health objectives.

NOTE: Timely release (publication of provisional or final data or public use data tapes) should be based on the use of the data, but is at least within one year of the end of data collection.

References

1. Institute of Medicine. The future of public health. Washington: National Academy Press. 1988.

2. Centers for Disease Control. Consensus set of health indicators for the general assessment of community health status, United States. MMWR 40(27) 449–51. 1991.

3. Klein RJ, Hawk SA. Health status indicators: Definitions and national data. Statistical notes; vol 1 no 3. Hyattsville, Maryland: National Center for Health Statistics. 1992.

Table A. Priority area lead agencies

Priority area	Lead agency
01 Physical Activity and Fitness	President's Council on Physical Fitness and Sports
02 Nutrition	National Institutes of Health Food and Drug Administration
03 Tobacco	Centers for Disease Control and Prevention
04 Alcohol and Other Drugs	Substance Abuse and Mental Health Services Administration
05 Family Planning	Office of Population Affairs
06 Mental Health and Mental Disorders	Substance Abuse and Mental Health Services Administration
07 Violent and Abusive Behavior	Centers for Disease Control and Prevention
08 Educational and Community-Based Programs	Centers for Disease Control and Prevention Health Resources and Services Administration
09 Unintentional Injuries	Centers for Disease Control and Prevention
10 Occupational Safety and Health	Centers for Disease Control and Prevention
11 Environmental Health	National Institutes of Health Centers for Disease Control and Prevention
12 Food and Drug Safety	Food and Drug Administration
13 Oral Health	National Institutes of Health Centers for Disease Control and Prevention
14 Maternal and Infant Health	Health Resources and Services Administration
15 Heart Disease and Stroke	National Institutes of Health
16 Cancer	National Institutes of Health
17 Diabetes and Chronic Disabling Conditions	National Institutes of Health Centers for Disease Control and Prevention
18 HIV Infection	National AIDS Program Office
19 Sexually Transmitted Diseases	Centers for Disease Control and Prevention
20 Immunization and Infectious Diseases	Centers for Disease Control and Prevention
21 Clinical Preventive Services	Health Resources and Services Administration Centers for Disease Control and Prevention
22 Surveillance and Data Systems	Centers for Disease Control and Prevention

Table B. Mortality objective cause-of-death categories

Objective number	Healthy People 2000 — Cause of death[1]	Healthy People 2000 — ICD-9 identifying codes	Mortality tabulation lists — Cause of death	Mortality tabulation lists — ICD-9 identifying codes
1.1	Coronary Heart Disease	410–414, 402, 429.2	Diseases of heart	390–398, 402, 404–429, 410–414
1.1a	[Blacks]			
2.1	See 1.1			
2.1a	See 1.1a			
2.2	Cancer (all sites)	140–208	Malignant neoplasms, including neoplasms of lymphatic hematopoietic tissues	(Same as HP2000)
3.1	See 1.1			
3.1a	See 1.1a			
3.2	Lung cancer	162.2–162.9	Malignant neoplasms of trachea, bronchus and lung	162
3.3	Chronic obstructive pulmonary disease	490–496	Chronic obstructive pulmonary diseases and allied conditions	(Same as HP2000)
4.1	Alcohol-related motor vehicle crashes	E810–E819[2]	No comparable category	...
4.1a	[American Indians/Alaska Natives]			
4.1b	[Ages 15–24]			
4.2	Cirrhosis	571	Chronic liver disease and cirrhosis	(Same as HP2000)
4.2a	[Black males]			
4.2b	[American Indians/Alaska Natives]			
4.3	Drug-related deaths	292, 304, 305.2–305.9, E850–E858, E950.0–E950.5, E962.0, E980.0–E980.5	Drug induced causes	(Same as HP2000)
6.1	Suicides	E950–E959	(Same as HP2000)	(Same as HP2000)
6.1a	[Ages 15–19]			
6.1b	[Males 20–34]			
6.1b	[White males 65 and older]			
6.1c	[American Indian/Alaska Native males]			
7.1	Homicides	E960–E969	Homicide and legal intervention	E960–E978
7.1a	[Children 0–3]			
7.1b	[Spouses 15–34]			
7.1c	[Black males 15–34]			
7.1d	[Hispanic males 15–34]			
7.1e	[Black females 15–34]			
7.1f	[American Indians/Alaska Natives]			
7.2	See 6.1			
7.2a	See 6.1a			
7.2b	See 6.1b			
7.2c	See 6.1c			
7.2d	See 6.1d			

Table B. Mortality objective cause-of-death categories—Con.

Objective number	Healthy People 2000		Mortality tabulation lists	
	Cause of death[1]	ICD–9 identifying codes	Cause of death	ICD–9 identifying codes
7.3	Firearm injuries	E922.0–E922.3, E922.8–E922.9, E955.0–E955.4, E965.0–E965.4, E970, E985.0–E985.4	No comparable category	…
	Knife injuries	E920.3, E956, E966, E986, E974	No comparable category	…
9.1	Unintentional injuries	E800–E949	Accidents and adverse effects	(Same as HP2000)
9.1a	[American Indians/Alaska Natives]			
9.1b	[Black males]			
9.1c	[White males]			
9.3	Motor vehicle crashes	E810–E825	Motor vehicle accidents	(Same as HP2000)
9.3a	[Ages 14 and younger]			
9.3b	[Ages 15–24]			
9.3c	[Ages 70 and older]			
9.3d	[American Indians/Alaska Natives]			
9.3e	[Motorcyclists]			
9.3f	[Pedestrians]			
9.4	Falls and fall-related injuries	E880–E888	Accidental falls	(Same as HP2000)
9.4a	[Ages 65–84]			
9.4b	[Ages 85+]			
9.4c	[Black males 30–69]			
9.5	Drowning	E830, E832, E910	Accidental drowning and submersion	E910
9.5a	[Ages 0–4]			
9.5b	[Males 15–34]			
9.5c	[Black males]			
9.6	Residential fires	E890–E899	Accidents caused by fire and flames (place of accident-home)	(Same as HP2000)
9.6a	[Ages 0–4]			
9.6b	[Ages 65 and older]			
9.6c	[Black males]			
9.6d	[Black females]			
10.1	Work-related injuries[3]	E800–E999	No comparable category	…
10.1a	[Mine workers]			
10.1b	[Construction workers]			
10.1c	[Transportation workers]			
10.1d	[Farm workers]			
13.7	Cancer of the oral cavity and pharynx	140–149	Malignant neoplasms of lip, oral cavity, and pharynx	(Same as HP2000)
14.3	Maternal mortality	630–676	Complications of pregnancy, childbirth, and the puerperium or maternal mortality	(Same as HP2000)
14.3a	[Blacks]			

No.	Category	ICD code	Description	HP2000
15.1	See 1.1			
15.1a	See 1.1a			
15.2	Stroke	430–438	Cerebrovascular diseases	(Same as HP2000)
15.2a	[Blacks]	See 2.2		
16.1	See 2.2			
16.2	See 3.2			
16.3	Breast cancer in women	174	Malignant neoplasm of female breast	(Same as HP2000)
16.4	Cancer of the uterine cervix	180	Malignant neoplasm of cervix uteri	(Same as HP2000)
16.5	Colorectal cancer	153.0–154.3, 154.8, 159.0	Malignant neoplasms of colon, rectum, rectosigmoid junction, and anus	153, 154
16.5	Colorectal cancer	153.0–154.3, 154.8, 159.0	Malignant neoplasms of colon, rectum, rectosigmoid junction, and anus	153, 154
17.9	Diabetes-related deaths[3]	250	Diabetes mellitus[1]	(Same as HP2000)
17.9a	[Blacks]			
17.9b	[American Indians/Alaska Natives]			
20.2	Epidemic-related pneumonia and influenza deaths for ages 65 and over	480–487	No comparable category	. . .

[1]*Healthy People 2000* uses multiple-cause-of-death data.
[2]Includes only those deaths assigned to E810–E819 that were alcohol related; see Priority Area 4, Alcohol and Other Drugs.
[3]Unless otherwise specified, *Healthy People 2000* uses underlying-cause-of-death data.

Table C. Data sources for the Healthy People 2000 objectives and subobjectives

[*Indicates duplicate objective]

Priority area	Objective number	Data source
Physical Activity	1.1*, 1.1a	National Vital Statistics System, CDC, NCHS.
	1.2*, 1.2a,b	Baseline: National Health and Nutrition Examination Survey, CDC, NCHS.
		Updates: National Health Interview Survey, CDC, NCHS.
	1.2c	Baseline: Hispanic Health and Nutrition Examination Survey, CDC, NCHS.
		Updates: National Health Interview Survey, CDC, NCHS.
	1.2d	Baseline: Indian Health Service, Office of Planning, Evaluation, and Legislation, Program Statistics Division.
		Updates: National Health Interview Survey, CDC, NCHS.
	1.2e	National Health Interview Survey, CDC, NCHS.
	1.2f,g	National Health and Nutrition Examination Survey, CDC, NCHS.
	1.3*	Original baseline: Behavioral Risk Factor Surveillance System, CDC, NCCDPHP.
		National Health Interview Survey, CDC, NCHS.
	1.4	Baseline: For ages 10–17, National Children and Youth Fitness Study I, OASH, ODPHP.
		Updates: For grades 9–12, Youth Risk Behavior Survey, CDC, NCCDPHP.
		For ages 18 and over, National Health Interview Survey, CDC, NCHS.
	1.4a	National Health Interview Survey, CDC, NCHS.
	1.5, 1.5a–c	National Health Interview Survey, CDC, NCHS.
	1.6	National Health Interview Survey, CDC, NCHS.
		Youth Risk Behavior Survey, CDC, NCCDPHP
	1.7*	National Health Interview Survey, CDC, NCHS.
	1.8	Baseline for grades 5–12: National Children and Youth Fitness Study I, OASH, ODPHP.
		Baseline for grades 1–4: National Children and Youth Fitness Study II, OASH, ODPHP.
		Update: Youth Risk Behavior Survey, CDC, NCCDPHP.
	1.9	Baseline: Siedentop D. *Developing Teaching Skills in Physical Education.* Palo Alto, Ca. Mayfield. 1983.
		Update: Youth Risk Behavior Survey, CDC, NCCDPHP.
	1.10	National Survey of Worksite Health Promotion Activities, OASH, ODPHP.
	1.11	Baseline: McDonald BL. and Cordell HK. *Local Opportunities for Americans: Final Report of the Municipal and County Park and Recreation Study,* Alexandria, Va: National Recreation and Park Association, 1988.
	1.12	Baseline: 1988 American College of Physicians Membership Survey of Prevention Practices in Adult Medicine.
		Updates: Primary Care Providers Survey, OASH, ODPHP.
Nutrition	2.1*, 2.1a	National Vital Statistics System, CDC, NCHS.
	2.2*	National Vital Statistics System, CDC, NCHS.
	2.3*, 2.3a,b	Baseline: National Health and Nutrition Examination Survey, CDC, NCHS.
		Updates: National Health Interview Survey, CDC, NCHS.
	2.3c	Baseline: Hispanic Health and Nutrition Examination Survey, CDC, NCHS.
		Updates: National Health Interview Survey, CDC, NCHS.
	2.3d	Baseline: Indian Health Service, Office of Planning, Evaluation, and Legislation, Program Statistics Division.
		Updates: National Health Interview Survey, CDC, NCHS.
	2.3e	National Health Interview Survey, CDC, NCHS.
	2.3f,g	National Health and Nutrition Examination Survey, CDC, NCHS.
	2.4, 2.4a–e	Pediatric Nutrition Surveillance System, CDC, NCCDPHP.

Table C. Data sources for the Healthy People 2000 objectives and subobjectives—Con.

[*Indicates duplicate objective]

Priority area	Objective number	Data source
	2.5*	Baseline: National Health and Nutrition Examination Survey, CDC, NCHS. Continuing Survey of Food Intakes by Individuals, USDA. 1989 Update: Continuing Survey of Food Intakes by Individuals, USDA.
	2.6*	Continuing Survey of Food Intakes by Individuals, USDA.
	2.7*	National Health Interview Survey, CDC, NCHS.
	2.8	Baseline: Continuing Survey of Food Intakes by Individuals, USDA. National Health and Nutrition Examination Survey III (Future).
	2.9	1985 Baseline: Continuing Survey of Food Intakes by Individuals, USDA. 1988 Baseline: Health and Diet Survey, FDA. 1991 Updates: National Health Interview Survey, CDC, NCHS.
	2.10, 2.10a–c	National Health and Nutrition Examination Survey, CDC, NCHS.
	2.10d	Survey of American Indians/Alaska Natives, CDC and Indian Health Service, Office of Planning, Evaluation, and Legislation, Program Statistics Division.
	2.10e	Pregnancy Nutrition Surveillance System, CDC, NCCDPHP.
	2.11*	Ross Laboratories Mothers Survey.
	2.11a–d	Pediatric Nutrition Surveillance System, CDC, NCCDPHP.
	2.12*. 2.12a	National Health Interview Survey, CDC, NCHS.
	2.12b	Baseline: 1990 Baby Bottle Tooth Decay 5-Year Evaluation Report, Indian Health Service, Dental Services Branch.
	2.13	Health and Diet Survey, FDA.
	2.14	Food Label and Package Survey, FDA. Fresh Fruit and Produce Survey, FDA (Future).
	2.15	Nielsen Company National Scantrack.
	2.16	Survey of Chain Operators, National Restaurant Association.
	2.17	School Nutrition Dietary Assessment, USDA (Future).
	2.18	National Health Interview Survey, CDC, NCHS.
	2.19	National Survey of School Health Education Activities, CDC, NCCDPHP (Future).
	2.20	National Survey of Worksite Health Promotion Activities, OASH, ODPHP.
	2.21	Primary Care Providers Survey, OASH, ODPHP.
Tobacco	3.1*, 3.1a	National Vital Statistics System, CDC, NCHS.
	3.2*	National Vital Statistics System, CDC, NCHS.
	3.3	National Vital Statistics System, CDC, NCHS.
	3.4*, 3.4a,b,d,h,i	National Health Interview Survey, CDC, NCHS.
	3.4c	Worldwide Survey of Substance Abuse and Health Behaviors Among Military Personnel, DOD, OASD.
	3.4e	Baseline: Hispanic Health and Nutrition Examination Survey CDC, NCHS. Updates: National Health Interview Survey, CDC, NCHS.
	3.4f	Baseline: CDC, 1987. Updates: National Health Interview Survey, CDC, NCHS.
	3.4g	Baseline: Local Surveys. Update: Jenkins CH. Cancer risks and prevention practices among Vietnamese refugees. Western J of Med 153:34-9. 1990.
	3.4j	Behavioral Risk Factor Surveillance System, CDC, NCCDPHP.
	3.5,3.5a	National Health Interview Survey, CDC, NCHS.

Table C. Data sources for the Healthy People 2000 objectives and subobjectives — Con.

[*Indicates duplicate objective]

Priority area	Objective number	Data source
	3.6	Baseline: Adult Use of Tobacco Survey, CDC, NCCDPHP. Updates: National Health Interview Survey, CDC, NCHS.
	3.7, 3.7a	National Health Interview Survey, CDC, NCHS.
	3.8	Baseline: Adult Use of Tobacco Survey, CDC, NCCDPHP. Updates: National Health Interview Survey, CDC, NCHS (Future).
	3.9	For males 18–24 years of age, National Health Interview Survey, CDC, NCHS. For males 12–17 years of age, National Household Survey on Drug Abuse, SAMHSA.
	3.9a	Baseline: National Medical Expenditure Survey of American Indians/Alaska Natives, PHS, NCHSR. Updates: National Health Interview Survey, CDC, NCHS.
	3.10	National Survey of School Districts' Nonsmoking Policies, NSBA, ACS, ALA, and AHA.
	3.11	For worksites with 50 or more employees, National Survey of Worksite Health Promotion Activities, OASH, ODPHP. For medium and large companies, Nationwide Survey on Smoking in the Workplace, CDC, OSH; Bureau of National Affairs; American Society for Personnel Administration.
	3.12	Baseline: State Legislative Action on Tobacco Issues, PHF. Updates: Office on Smoking and Health Legislative Tracking, CDC, NCCDPHP.
	3.13	Baseline: Association of State and Territorial Health Officals Reporting System: Cancer and Cardiovascular Diseases Survey, PHF. Updates: Office on Smoking and Health Legislative Tracking, CDC, NCCDPHP.
	3.14	Baseline: Association of State and Territorial Health Officials Reporting System: Cancer and Cardiovascular Diseases Survey, PHF; Updates: Association of State and Territorial Health Officials Survey of State Tobacco Prevention and Control Activities (Future); Office on Smoking and Health Legislative Tracking, CDC, NCCDPHP (Future).
	3.15	Baseline: Federal Trade Commission data reported by Office on Smoking and Health, CDC, NCCDPHP. Updates: Association of State and Territorial Health Officials Reporting System: Cancer and Cardiovascular Diseases Survey, PHF (Future).
	3.16	Baseline for Internists: Wells, et al. *Physicians Practice Study*, AJPH 76:1009–13. 1986. Baseline for dentists: Secker-Walker, et al. *Statewide Survey of Dentists' Smoking Cessation Advice*. JADA 118:37–40. 1989. Updates: Primary Care Providers Survey, OASH, ODPHP (Future).
Alcohol and Other Drugs	4.1, 4.1a–b	Fatal Accident Reporting System, NHTSA.
	4.2, 4.2a–b	National Vital Statistics System, CDC, NCHS. Indian Health Service Administrative Statistics, IHS.
	4.3	National Vital Statistics System, CDC, NCHS.
	4.4	Drug Abuse Warning Network, SAMHSA, OAS.
	4.5	National Household Survey of Drug Abuse, SAMHSA, OAS.
	4.6	National Household Survey of Drug Abuse, SAMHSA, OAS.
	4.7	Monitoring the Future (High School Senior Survey), NIH, NIDA.

Table C. Data sources for the Healthy People 2000 objectives and subobjectives—Con.

[*Indicates duplicate objective]

Priority area	Objective number	Data source
	4.8	Alcohol Epidemiology Data System, NIH, NIAAA.
	4.9	Monitoring the Future (High School Senior Survey), NIH, NIDA.
	4.10	Monitoring the Future (High School Senior Survey), NIH, NIDA.
	4.11	Monitoring the Future (High School Senior Survey), NIH, NIDA.
	4.12	State Substance Abuse Services Plans, SAMHSA, CSAT (Future).
	4.13	*Report to Congress and the White House on the Nature and Effectiveness of Federal, State, and Local Drug Prevention Education Programs.* U.S. Department of Education. 1987.
	4.14	National Survey of Worksite Health Promotion Activities, OASH, ODPHP.
	4.15	Office of Alcohol and State Programs, NHTSA.
	4.16	Substance Abuse Block Grant Program, SAMHSA, CSAP, CSAT (Future).
	4.17	Substance Abuse Block Grant Program, SAMHSA, CSAP, CSAT (Future).
	4.18	Office of Alcohol and State Programs, NHTSA (Future).
	4.19	Primary Care Providers Survey, OASH, ODPHP (Future).
Family Planning	5.1, 5.1a,b	Abortion Provider Survey, Alan Guttmacher Institute. 1989. National Vital Statistics System, CDC, NCHS. National Survey of Family Growth, CDC, NCHS.
	5.2, 5.2a	Baseline: National Survey of Family Growth, CDC, NCHS. Updates: National Survey of Family Growth, Telephone Reinterview. CDC, NCHS (Future). Pregnancy Risk Assessment Monitoring System, CDC (Future).
	5.3, 5.3a,b	Baseline: National Survey of Family Growth, CDC, NCHS. Updates: National Survey of Family Growth, Telephone Reinterview, CDC, NCHS (Future).
	5.4*	Baseline: National Survey of Family Growth, CDC, NCHS. National Survey of Adolescent Males, NIH, NICHD. Updates: Youth Risk Behavior Survey, CDC, NCCDPHP.
	5.5	Baseline: National Survey of Family Growth, CDC, NCHS. Youth Risk Behavior Survey, CDC, NCCDPHP.
	5.6	Baseline: National Survey of Family Growth, CDC, NCHS. Youth Risk Behavior Survey, CDC, NCCDPHP. National Survey of Adolescent Males, NIH, NICHHD.
	5.7	Baseline: Forrest, TD and Singh S. Public Sector Savings Resulting from Expenditures for Contraceptive Services. *Family Planning Perspectives* 22(1):6–15. 1990. Updates: National Survey of Family Growth, CDC, NCHS (Future). Pregnancy Risk Assessment Monitoring System, CDC, NCCDPHP (Future). National Survey of Adolescent Males, NIH, NICHHD (Future).
	5.8	Baseline: Planned Parenthood Federation of America, Inc., 1986. Update: National Survey of Family Growth, CDC, NCHS (Future). National Survey of Adolescent Males, NIH, NICHHD (Future). National Health Interview Survey, CDC, NCHS (Future).
	5.9	Baseline: Mech EB. Unpublished. 1984. Orientation of Pregnancy Counselors Toward Adoption.
	5.10*	Primary Care Providers Survey, OASH, ODPHP.

Table C. Data sources for the Healthy People 2000 objectives and subobjectives—Con.

[*Indicates duplicate objective]

Priority area	Objective number	Data source
	5.11*	National Questionnaire on Provision of STD and HIV Services by Family Planning Clinics, PHS, OPA.
Mental Health and Mental Disorders	6.1*, 6.1a–d	National Vital Statistics System, CDC, NCHS. Indian Health Service, Office of Planning, Evaluation, and Legislation, Program Statistics Division.
	6.2*	Youth Risk Behavior Survey, CDC, NCCDPHP.
	6.3	Baseline (revised): Bird HR. Estimates of the prevalence of childhood maladjustment in a community survey in Puerto Rico. Archives of Gen Psychiatry 45:1120–26. 1988.
		Costello EJ, et al. Psychiatric disorders in pediatric primary care: Prevalence risk factors. Archives of Gen Psychiatry 45:1107–16. 1988
		Updates: Child Epidemiologic Catchment Area Studys, NIH, NIMH (Future).
	6.4	Baseline: Epidemiologic Catchment Area Study, NIH, NIMH.
		Updates: National Comorbidity Study, NIH, NIMH (Future).
		National Health and Nutrition Examination Survey, CDC, NCHS. (Future).
	6.5, 6.5a	National Health Interview Survey, CDC, NCHS.
	6.6	National Institute of Mental Health Community Support Program Client Follow-Up Study, SAMHSA.
	6.7	Baseline: Epidemiologic Catchment Area Study, NIH NIMH.
		Updates: National Comorbidity Survey NIH, NIMH (Future).
	6.8, 6.8a	National Health Interview Survey, CDC, NCHS.
	6.9	"Prevention Index," Rodale Press, Inc.
	6.10*	National Center on Institutions and Alternatives. CDC, NCIPC.
	6.11	National Survey of Worksite Health Promotion Activities, OASH, ODPHP.
	6.12	Baseline: National Council of Self-Help Clearinghouses and Public Health.
		Updates: National Network of Mutual Help Centers (Future).
	6.13	Primary Care Providers Survey, OASH, ODPHP.
	6.14	Primary Care Providers Survey, OASH, ODPHP.
Violent and Abusive Behavior	7.1, 7.1a–e	National Vital Statistics System, CDC, NCHS.
	7.1f	Indian Health Service, Office of Planning, Evaluation, and Legislation, Program Statistics Division.
	7.2*, 7.2a–c	National Vital Statistics System, CDC, NCHS.
	7.2d	Indian Health Service, Office of Planning, Evaluation, and Legislation, Program Statistics Division.
	7.3	National Vital Statistics System, CDC, NCHS.
	7.4, 7.4a–d	National Incidence of Child Abuse and Neglect Survey, Office of Human Development, NCCAN.
	7.5	National Family Violence Survey, NIH, NIMH.
		National Crime Survey, Department of Justice, Bureau of Justice Statistics.
	7.6	National Crime Survey, Department of Justice, Bureau of Justice Statistics.
	7.7, 7.7a	National Crime Survey, Department of Justice, Bureau of Justice Statistics.
	7.8*	Youth Risk Behavior Survey, CDC, NCCDPHP.
	7.9	Youth Risk Behavior Survey, CDC, NCCDPHP.
	7.10	Youth Risk Behavior Survey, CDC, NCCDPHP.
	7.11	National Health Interview Survey, CDC, NCHS (Future).

Table C. Data sources for the Healthy People 2000 objectives and subobjectives—Con.

[*Indicates duplicate objective]

Priority area	Objective number	Data source
	7.12	Joint Accreditation Survey, Joint Commission on the Accreditation of Healthcare Organizations (Future). American Hospital Association. American Medical Association (Future).
	7.13	Baseline: Annual 50 State Survey, National Committee for Prevention of Child Abuse. Update: National Incidence of Child Abuse and Neglect Survey, Office of Human Development, NCCAN (Future).
	7.14	Annual 50 State Survey, National Committtee for Prevention of Child Abuse (Future). National Incidence of Child Abuse and Neglect Survey, Office of Human Development, NCCAN (Future).
	7.15	Domestic Violence Statistical Survey, National Coalition Against Domestic Violence.
	7.16	National Survey of School Health Education Activities, CDC, NCCDPHP (Future).
	7.17	National Committee for Prevention of Child Abuse (Future). CDC, NCIPC (Future).
	7.18*	National Center on Institutions and Alternatives, CDC, NCIPC.
Educational and Community-Based Programs	8.1*, 8.1a–c	National Health Interview Survey, CDC, NCHS. National Vital Statistics System, CDC, NCHS.
	8.2	National Center for Education Statistics, National Education Goals Panel.
	8.3	Head Start Bureau: Administration on Children, Youth, and Families; Administration for Children and Families. National Center for Education Statistics, National Education Goals Panel.
	8.4	National Survey of School Health Education Activities, CDC, NCCDPHP.
	8.5	Health Promotion on Campus Survey and Directory, American College Health Association.
	8.6	Baseline: Health Research Institute Biennial Survey, Health Research Institute. Baseline and Updates: National Survey of Worksite Health Promotion Activities, OASH, ODPHP.
	8.7	National Health Interview Survey, CDC, NCHS (Future).
	8.8	Catalog of Local Health Promotion Programs, National Elder Care Institute on Health Promotion, American Association of Retired Persons. State Units of Aging Reporting System, National Association of State Units of Aging.
	8.9	Baseline: Youth Risk Behavior Survey, CDC, NCCDPHP. Updates: National Health Interview Survey, CDC, NCHS (Future).
	8.10	American Hospital Association Annual Survey (Community Health Promotion Section). Public Health Impact Data Base, PHF.
	8.11	Community Demonstration Projects Review, PHS, OMH. Health Education Resource Management System, IHS. Hispanic Chronic Disease Prevention Project, National Coalition of Hispanic Health and Human Services Organizations. Bilingual Service Delivery Project, Association of State and Territorial Health Officals.
	8.12	Annual Survey of Hospitals, American Hospital Association. HMO Industry Profile, Group Health Association of America, Inc.

Table C. Data sources for the Healthy People 2000 objectives and subobjectives—Con.

[*Indicates duplicate objective]

Priority area	Objective number	Data source
	8.13	Survey to be developed and administered by a private or voluntary partner, in cooperation with ODPHP.
	8.14	National Profile of Local Health Departments, National Association of County Health Officials.
		Profile of State and Territorial Public Health Systems, CDC, ASTHO.
		State Mortality and Morbidity Data, CDC.
		National Vital Statistics System, CDC, NCHS.
Unintentional injuries	9.1, 9.1a–c	National Vital Statistics System, CDC, NCHS.
	9.2	National Hospital Discharge Survey, CDC, NCHS.
	9.3, 9.3a–c,e,f	Fatal Accident Reporting System, DOT, NHTSA.
	9.3d	Indian Health Service, Office of Planning, Evaluation, and Legislation, Program Statistics Division.
	9.4, 9.4a–c	National Vital Statistics System, CDC, NCHS.
	9.5, 9.5a–c	National Vital Statistics System, CDC, NCHS.
	9.6, 9.6a–d	National Vital Statistics System, CDC, NCHS.
	9.6e	National Fire Incident Reporting System, FEMA, US Fire Administration.
	9.7, 9.7a	National Hospital Discharge Survey, CDC, NCHS.
	9.8, 9.8a	National Electronic Injury Surveillance System, Consumer Product Safety Commission, Directorate for Epidemiology.
	9.9	National Hospital Discharge Survey, CDC, NCHS.
	9.10, 9.10a	National Hospital Discharge Survey, CDC, NCHS.
	9.11	National Head and Spinal Cord Injury Survey, NIH, NINCDS.
	9.12, 9.12a	Baseline: 19 Cities Survey, DOT, NHTSA.
		Updates: Population weighted State surveys, DOT, NHTSA.
		Youth Risk Behavior Survey, CDC, NCCDPHP (Future).
		National Health Interview Survey, CDC, NCHS (Future).
	9.13	Baseline: 19 Cities Survey, DOT, NHTSA.
		Updates: Youth Risk Behavior Survey, CDC, NCCDPHP.
	9.14	DOT, NHTSA.
	9.15	CDC, NCIPC.
	9.16	Baseline: FEMA, US Fire Administration.
		Updates: International Association of Fire Chiefs (Future).
	9.17	FEMA, US Fire Administration.
	9.18	CDC, NCCDPHP.
	9.19*	CDC, NCPS.
		NIH, NIDR.
	9.20	DOT, FHA.
	9.21	Primary Care Providers Survey, OASH, ODPHP.
	9.22	CDC, NCIPC.
Occupational Safety and Health	10.1, 10.1a–d	Annual Survey of Occupational Injuries and Illnesses, DOL, BLS.
	10.2, 10.2a,b	Annual Survey of Occupational Injuries and Illnesses, DOL, BLS.
	10.3	Annual Survey of Occupational Injuries and Illnesses, DOL, BLS.
	10.4	Annual Survey of Occupational Injuries and Illnesses, DOL, BLS.
	10.5*	Viral Hepatitis Surveillance System, CDC, NCID.
	10.6	National Survey of Worksite Health Promotion Activities, OASH, ODPHP.
	10.7	Occupational Hearing Conservation Database, CDC, NIOSH (Future).
	10.8	Adult Elevated Blood Lead Level Registries, CDC, NIOSH.
	10.9*	Regulatory Impact Analysis of OSHA Final Rule on Occupational Exposure to Bloodborne Pathogens, DOL, OSHA, ORA.

Table C. Data sources for the Healthy People 2000 objectives and subobjectives — Con.

[*Indicates duplicate objective]

Priority area	Objective number	Data source
	10.10	Association of State and Territorial Health Officials Reporting System: Unintentional Injuries Survey, PHF.
	10.11	CDC, NIOSH (Future).
	10.12	National Survey of Worksite Health Promotion Activities, OASH, ODPHP.
	10.13	National Survey of Worksite Health Promotion Activities, OASH, ODPHP.
	10.14	CDC, NIOSH.
	10.15	Primary Care Providers Survey, OASH, ODPHP (Future).
Environmental Health	11.1, 11.1a,b	National Hospital Discharge Survey, CDC, NCHS.
	11.2*	Metropolitan Atlanta Development Disabilities Study, CDC, NCEH.
	11.3, 11.3a	Waterborne Surveillance System, CDC, NCEH.
	11.4, 11.4a	National Health and Nutrition Examination Survey, CDC, NCHS. CDC State-Based Surveillance for Childhood Lead Poisoning. State & Local Childhood Lead Prevention Programs.
	11.5	National Air Quality and Emissions Trends Report, EPA.
	11.6, 11.6a,b	Baseline: OPA, OAR, Office of Radiation Programs. Updates: National Health Interview Survey, CDC, NCHS (Future).
	11.7	Toxic Chemical Release Inventory, EPA, OPPTS. ATSDR List of Priority Hazardous Substances. DHHS Annual Report on Carcinogens.
	11.8	Baseline: Characterization of Municipal Solid Waste in the United States: 1990 Update, EPA. Updates: EPA, Office of Solid Waste and Emergency Response. EPA, Office of Pollution Prevention.
	11.9	EPA Federal Reporting Data Base. EPA, Office of Ground Water and Drinking Water.
	11.10	National Water Quality Inventory, EPA, Office of Water.
	11.11	National Health Interview Survey, CDC, NCHS.
	11.12	Environmental Law Institute.
	11.13	Alliance to End Childhood Lead Poisioning.
	11.14	National Priorities List, EPA, OSWER.
	11.15	Federal Environmental Progress and Challenges, EPA's Updates.
	11.16	CDC, NCEH.
Food and Drug Safety	12.1	Bacterial Meningitis Surveillance System, CDC, NCID. Campylocacter Surveillance System, CDC, NCID. Salmonella Surveillance System, CDC, NCID.
	12.2	Salmonella Surveillance System, CDC, NCID.
	12.3	Diet–Health Knowledge Survey, USDA, ASFCS.
	12.4	Inspectional Standardization of Institutional Food Service Regulatory Officials, FDA, ORO. Listing of Confirmed Code Adoptions by Local, State, and National Jurisdictions, CFSAN, FDA.
	12.5	Food and Drug Administration.
	12.6	Primary Care Providers Survey, OASH, ODPHP.
Oral Health	13.1, 13.1c	National Survey of Dental Caries in U.S. School Children, 1986–1987, NIH, NIDR.
	13.1a	North Carolina Oral Health School Survey, North Carolina Division of Dental Health, University of North Carolina School of Public Health.
	13.1b,d	Survey of Oral Health, 1983–1984, Indian Health Service, Dental Services Branch. Update: 1991 Oral Health Status and Treatment Needs Survey of American Indians/Alaska Natives, Indian Health Service, Dental Services Branch.

Table C. Data sources for the Healthy People 2000 objectives and subobjectives—Con.

[*Indicates duplicate objective]

Priority area	Objective number	Data source
	13.2, 13.2c	Baseline: National Survey of Dental Caries in U.S. School Children, 1986–1987, NIH, NIDR.
	13.2a	Baseline: North Carolina Oral Health School Survey, North Carolina Division of Dental Health, University of North Carolina School of Public Health.
	13.2b	Baseline: Survey of Oral Health, 1983–1984, Indian Health Service, Dental Services Branch.
	13.2d	Baseline: Hispanic Health and Nutrition Examination Survey, CDC, NCHS. Update: 1991 Oral Health Status and Treatment Needs Survey of American Indians/Alaska Natives, Indian Health Service, Dental Services Branch.
	13.3	Baseline: National Survey of Oral Health in U.S. Employed Adults and Seniors, 1985–1986, NIH, NIDR.
	13.4, 13.4a	Baseline: National Health Interview Survey, CDC, NCHS.
	13.5, 13.5a	National Survey of Oral Health in U.S. Employed Adults and Seniors, 1985–1986, NIH, NIDR.
	13.5b	Baseline: Survey of Oral Health, 1983–1984, Indian Health Service, Dental Services Branch. Update: 1991 Oral Health Status and Treatment Needs Survey of American Indians/Alaska Natives, Indian Health Service, Dental Services Branch.
	13.5c	Baseline: Hispanic Health and Nutrition Examination Survey, CDC, NCHS.
	13.6	Baseline: National Survey of Oral Health in U.S. Employed Adults and Seniors, 1985–1986, NIH, NIDR.
	13.7	National Vital Statistics System, CDC, NCHS.
	13.8	Baseline: National Survey of Dental Caries in U.S. School Children, 1986–1987, NIH, NIDR. Updates: National Health Interview Survey, CDC, NCHS.
	13.9	CDC, NCPS.
	13.10	National Health Interview Survey, CDC, NCHS.
	13.11*, 13.11a	National Health Interview Survey, CDC, NCHS.
	13.11b	Baseline: 1990 Baby Bottle Tooth Decay 5-Year Evaluation Report, Indian Health Service, Dental Services Branch.
	13.12	National Health Interview Survey (1986, 1989, 1991), CDC, NCHS.
	13.13	Health Care Financing Administration. National Commission on Correctional Health Care (Future).
	13.14	National Health Interview Survey (1986, 1989, 1991), CDC, NCHS.
	13.15	Baseline: State Public Health Dentists Survey, Illinois State Health Department.
	13.16*	CDC, NCPS. NIH, NIDR.
Maternal and Infant Health	14.1, 14.1a–j	National Vital Statistics System, CDC, NCHS.
	14.2, 14.2a	National Vital Statistics System, CDC, NCHS.
	14.3, 14.3a	National Vital Statistics System, CDC, NCHS.
	14.4, 14.4a,b	Births Defects Monitoring System, CDC, NCEH.
	14.5, 14.5a,b	National Vital Statistics System, CDC, NCHS.
	14.6	Baseline: National Natality Survey, CDC, NCHS. Updates: National Maternal and Infant Health Survey, CDC, NCHS. National Vital Statistics System, CDC, NCHS.
	14.7	National Hospital Discharge Survey, CDC, NCHS.
	14.8, 14.8a,b	National Hospital Discharge Survey, CDC, NCHS.
	14.9*	Ross Laboratories Mother Survey.
	14.9a–d	Pediatric Nutrition Surveillance System, CDC, NCCDPHP.

Table C. Data sources for the Healthy People 2000 objectives and subobjectives—Con.

[*Indicates duplicate objective]

Priority area	Objective number	Data source
	14.10	Baseline: National Health Interview Survey, CDC, NCHS. Updates: National Maternal and Infant Health Survey, CDC, NCHS. National Vital Statistics System, CDC, NCHS. National Health Interview Survey, CDC, NCHS.
	14.11, 14.11a–c	National Vital Statistics System, CDC, NCHS.
	14.12*	Primary Care Providers Survey, OASH, ODPHP.
	14.13	College of American Pathologists. Foundation for Blood Research.
	14.14	Annual Report to Congress Summarizing State Reports required under title V under the MCH Block Grant, MCHB, HRSA.
	14.15	Council of Regional Networks for Genetic Services.
	14.16	Primary Care Providers Survey, OASH, ODPHP.
Heart Disease and Stroke	15.1*, 15.1a	National Vital Statistics System, CDC, NCHS.
	15.2, 15.2a	National Vital Statistics System, CDC, NCHS.
	15.3, 15.3a	End Stage Renal Disease Medicare Reimbursement Data, HCFA, Bureau of Data Management and Strategy.
	15.4	National Health and Nutrition Examination Survey, CDC, NCHS.
	15.4a	Baseline: 1982–89 Seven States Study, NIH. Updates: National Health and Nutrition Examination Survey, CDC, NCHS (Future).
	15.5, 15.5a,b	National Health Interview Survey, CDC, NCHS.
	15.6	National Health and Nutrition Examination Survey, CDC, NCHS.
	15.7	National Health and Nutrition Examination Survey, CDC, NCHS.
	15.8	Baseline: Health and Diet Survey, FDA. Update: National Health and Nutrition Examination Survey, CDC, NCHS (Future).
	15.9*	Baseline: National Health and Nutrition Examination Survey, CDC, NCHS. Continuing Survey of Food Intakes by Individuals, USDA. 1989 Update: Continuing Survey of Food Intakes by Individuals, USDA.
	15.10*, 15.10a,b	Baseline: National Health and Nutrition Examination Survey, CDC, NCHS. Updates: National Health Interview Survey, CDC, NCHS.
	15.10c	Baseline: Hispanic Health and Nutrition Examination Survey, CDC, NCHS. Updates: National Health Interview Survey, CDC, NCHS.
	15.10d	Baseline: Indian Health Service, Office of Planning, Evaluation, and Legislation, Program Statistics Division. Updates: National Health Interview Survey, CDC, NCHS.
	15.10e	National Health Interview Survey, CDC, NCHS.
	15.10f,g	National Health and Nutrition Examination Survey, CDC, NCHS.
	15.11*	National Health Interview Survey, CDC, NCHS. Original baseline: Behavioral Risk Factor Surveillance System, CDC, NCCDPHP.
	15.12, 15.12a,b,d,h,i	National Health Interview Survey, CDC, NCHS.
	15.12c	Worldwide Survey of Substance Abuse and Health Behaviors Among Military Personnel, DoD, OASD.
	15.12e	Baseline: Hispanic Health and Nutrition Examination Survey, CDC, NCHS. Updates: National Health Interview Survey, CDC, NCHS.
	15.12f	Baseline: CDC, 1987. Updates: National Health Interview Survey, CDC, NCHS.

Table C. Data sources for the Healthy People 2000 objectives and subobjectives—Con.

[*Indicates duplicate objective]

Priority area	Objective number	Data source
	15.12g	Baseline: Local Surveys. Update: Jenkins CH. Cancer risks and prevention practices among Vietnamese refugees. Western J of Med 153:34–9. 1990.
	15.12j	Behavioral Risk Factor Surveillance System, CDC, NCCDPHP.
	15.13	National Health Interview Survey, CDC, NCHS.
	15.14	Baseline: Health and Diet Survey, FDA. 1990 Update: Cholesterol Awareness Survey, NHLBI, NIH. 1991 Update: National Health Interview Survey, CDC, NCHS.
	15.15	Primary Provider Care Survey, OASH, ODPHP (Future).
	15.16	National Survey of Worksite Health Promotion Activities, OASH, ODPHP.
	15.17	Comprehensive Chemistry Survey of Laboratories Using Enzymatic Methods, College of American Pathologists.
Cancer	16.1*	National Vital Statistics System, CDC, NCHS.
	16.2*	National Vital Statistics System, CDC, NCHS.
	16.3	National Vital Statistics System, CDC, NCHS.
	16.4	National Vital Statistics System, CDC, NCHS.
	16.5	National Vital Statistics System, CDC, NCHS.
	16.6*, 16.6a,b,d,h,i	National Health Interview Survey, CDC, NCHS.
	16.6c	Worldwide Survey of Substance Abuse and Health Behaviors Among Military Personnel, DoD, OASD.
	16.6e	Baseline: Hispanic Health and Nutrition Examination Survey, CDC, NCHS. Updates: National Health Interview Survey, CDC, NCHS.
	16.6f	Baseline: CDC, 1987. Updates: National Health Interview Survey, CDC, NCHS.
	16.6g	Baseline: Local Surveys. Update: Jenkins CH. Cancer risks and prevention practices among Vietnamese refugees. Western J of Med 153:34–9. 1990.
	16.6j	Behavioral Risk Factor Surveillance System, CDC, NCCDPHP.
	16.7*	Baseline: National Health and Nutrition Examination Survey, CDC, NCHS. Continuing Survey of Food Intakes by Individuals, USDA. 1989 Update: Continuing Survey of Food Intakes by Individuals, USDA.
	16.8*	Continuing Survey of Food Intakes by Individuals, USDA.
	16.9	National Health Interview Survey. CDC, NCHS.
	16.10	Baseline: Wells, et al, 1986 Updates: 1989 Survey of Physician's Attitudes and Practices in Early Cancer Detection, NCI. Primary Care Providers Survey, OASH, ODPHP (Future).
	16.11, 16.11a–d	National Health Interview Survey, CDC, NCHS.
	16.12, 16.12a–d	National Health Interview Survey, CDC, NCHS.
	16.13	National Health Interview Survey, CDC, NCHS.
	16.14	National Health Interview Survey, CDC, NCHS.
	16.15	National Cancer Institute, Division of Cancer Prevention and Control Surveillance Progam.
	16.16	American College of Radiology.
Diabetes and Chronic Disabling Conditions	17.1*, 17.1a–c	National Vital Statistics System, CDC, NCHS. National Health Interview Survey, CDC, NCHS.
	17.2, 17.2a–c	National Health Interview Survey, CDC, NCHS.
	17.3, 17.3a	Baseline: National Health Interview Survey, CDC, NCHS. National Nursing Home Survey, CDC, NCHS. Updates: National Health Interview Survey, CDC, NCHS.

Priority area	Objective number	Data source
	17.4	National Health Interview Survey, CDC, NCHS.
	17.5	National Health Interview Survey, CDC, NCHS.
	17.6, 17.6a	National Health Interview Survey, CDC, NCHS.
	17.7, 17.7a	National Health Interview Survey, CDC, NCHS.
	17.8*	Metropolitan Atlanta Developmental Disabilities Study, CDC, NCEH.
	17.9, 17.9a,b	National Vital Statistics System, CDC, NCHS.
	17.10	Massachusetts Blind Registry, Massachusetts Commission on the Blind.
		Health Care Financing Administration, Bureau of Data Management and Strategy.
		National Health Interview Survey, CDC, NCHS.
		National Hospital Discharge Survey, CDC, NCHS.
	17.10a,b,c	Health Care Financing Administration Bureau of Data Management and Strategy National Hospital Discharge Survey
		National Hospital Discharge Survey, CDC, NCHS.
		Program Statistics, PHS, IHS.
	17.11, 17.11e	National Health Interview Survey, CDC, NCHS.
	17.11a	Ambulatory Utilization Data, Indian Health Service.
	17.11b–d	Baseline: Hispanic Health and Nutrition Examination Survey, CDC, NCHS.
	17.12*, 17.12a,b	Baseline: National Health and Nutrition Examination Survey, CDC, NCHS.
		Updates: National Health Interview Survey, CDC, NCHS.
	17.12c	Baseline: Hispanic Health and Nutrition Examination Survey, CDC, NCHS.
		Updates: National Health Interview Survey, CDC, NCHS.
	17.12d	Baseline: Indian Health Service, Office of Planning Evaluation and Legislation, Program Statistics Division.
		Updates: National Health Interview Survey, CDC, NCHS.
	17.12e	National Health Interview Survey, CDC, NCHS.
	17.12f,g	National Health and Nutrition Examination Survey, CDC, NCHS.
	17.13*	Original baseline: Behavioral Risk Factor Surveillance System, CDC, NCCDPHP.
		National Health Interview Survey, CDC, NCHS.
	17.14, 17.14a,b	Baseline: Halpern M. The impact of diabetes education in Michigan. Diabetes 38(2):151A, 1989.
		Updates: National Health Interview Survey, CDC, NCHS.
	17.15	Primary Care Providers Survey, OASH, ODPHP.
	17.16	Baseline: Annual Survey of Hearing Impaired Children and Youth, Commission on Education of the Deaf.
		Updates: National Health Interview Survey, CDC, NCHS.
	17.17	Primary Care Providers Survey, OASH, ODPHP.
	17.18	National Health Interview Survey, CDC, NCHS (Future).
	17.19	Baseline: Survey of Persons with Disability, International Center for the Disabled.
	17.20	Annual Report to Congress summarizing State reports required under Title V MCH Block Grant, MCHB, HRSA.
HIV Infection	18.1,18.1a–c	AIDS Surveillance System, CDC, NCID.
	18.2, 18.2a–c	CDC, NCID.
	18.3*	Baseline: National Survey of Family Growth, CDC, NCHS.
		National Survey of Adolescent Males, NIH, NICHD.
		Updates: Youth Risk Behavior Survey, CDC, NCCDPHP.
	18.4*	National Survey of Family Growth, CDC, NCHS.
	18.4a	Baseline: National Survey of Family Growth, CDC, NCHS.
		Updates: Youth Risk Behavior Survey, CDC, NCCDPHP.
	18.4b	Baseline: National Survey of Adolescent Males, NIH, NICHD.
		Updates: Youth Risk Behavior Survey, CDC, NCCDPHP.

Table C. Data sources for the Healthy People 2000 objectives and subobjectives — Con.

[*Indicates duplicate objective]

Priority area	Objective number	Data source
	18.4c	None.
	18.5	SAMHSA.
	18.6	National AIDS Demonstration Research Program, NIH, NIDA.
	18.7	CDC, NCID.
	18.8	HIV Counseling and Testing Data Sites System, CDC, NCPS.
	18.9	Baseline: Primary Care Physician Survey of Sexual History-taking and Counseling Practices, Lewis CE and Freeman HE. Western Journal of Medicine, 147: 165–7. 1987.
		Updates: Primary Care Providers Survey, OASH, ODPHP
	18.9a	Primary Care Providers Survey, OASH, ODPHP.
	18.10	AIDS education: Public school programs require more student information and teacher training, GAO, 1990.
	18.11	American College Health Association (Future).
	18.12	CDC, NCPS.
	18.13	National Questionnaire on Provision of STD and HIV Services by Family Planning Clinics, PHS, OPA.
	18.14	OSHA.
Sexually Transmitted Diseases	19.1, 19a–c	Sexually Transmitted Disease Surveillance System, CDC, NCPS.
	19.2	National Disease and Therapeutic Index, IMS America, Ltd.
	19.3, 19.3a	Sexually Transmitted Disease Surveillance System, CDC, NCPS.
	19.4	Sexually Transmitted Disease Surveillance System, CDC, NCPS.
	19.5	National Disease and Therapeutic Index, IMS America, Ltd.
	19.6	National Hospital Discharge Survey, CDC, NCHS.
	19.7*	Viral Hepatitis Surveillance System, CDC, NCID.
	19.8	Sexually Transmitted Disease Surveillance System, CDC, NCPS.
	19.9*	Baseline: National Survey of Family Growth, CDC, NCHS. National Survey of Adolescent Males, NIH, NICHD. Updates: Youth Risk Behavior Survey, CDC, NCCDPHP.
	19.10*	National Survey of Family Growth, CDC, NCHS.
	19.10a	Baseline: National Survey of Family Growth, CDC, NCHS. Updates: Youth Risk Behavioral Survey, CDC, NCCDPHP.
	19.10b	Baseline: National Survey of Adolescent Males, NIH, NICHD. Updates: Youth Risk Behavioral Survey, CDC, NCCDPHP.
	19.10c	None.
	19.11*	National Questionnaire on Provision of STD and HIV Services by Family Planning Clinics, PHS, OPA.
	19.12	Baseline: Risk and Responsibility: Teaching Sex Education in America's Schools Today, Survey of Large School Districts on Sex and AIDS Education, Alan Guttmacher Institute, New York. 1989.
	19.13	National Disease and Theraeutic Index, IMS Americas, Ltd.
	19.14*	Baseline: Primary Care Physician Survey of Sexual History-taking and Counseling Practices, Lewis CE and Freeman HE. Western Journal of Medicine, 147: 165–7. 1987. Updates: Primary Care Providers Survey, OASH, ODPHP.
	19.14a	Primary Care Providers Survey, OASH, ODPHP.
	19.15	Sexually Transmitted Disease Surveillance System, CDC, NCPS.

Table C. Data sources for the Healthy People 2000 objectives and subobjectives—Con.

[*Indicates duplicate objective]

Priority area	Objective number	Data source
Immunization and Infectious Diseases	20.1	National Notifiable Disease Surveillance System, CDC, EPO.
	20.2	CDC, NCID and NCHS.
	20.3*, 20.3a–g	Viral Hepatitis Surveillance System, CDC, NCID.
	20.4, 20.4a–d	Tuberculosis Morbidity Data, CDC, NCPS.
	20.5	National Nosocomial Infection Surveillance System, CDC, NCID.
	20.6	Malaria Surveillance System, CDC, NCID. Typhoid Surveillance System, CDC, NCID. Viral Hepatitis Surveillance System, CDC, NCID.
	20.7, 20.7a	Bacterial Meningitis Surveillance System, CDC, NCID.
	20.8	National Health Interview Survey, CDC, NCHS.
	20.9	National Health Interview Survey, CDC, NCHS.
	20.10	National Health Interview Survey, CDC, NCHS.
	20.11	United States Immunization Survey, CDC, NCPS. State Immunization Survey, CDC, NCPS. National Health Interview Survey, CDC, NCHS. Perinatal Hepatitis B Screening Grant Program, CDC, NCID. Regulatory Impact Analysis of OSHA Final Rule on Occupational Exposure to Bloodborne Pathogens, DOL, OSHA, ORA.
	20.12	Rabies Vaccine and Immune Globulin Manufacturers Sales Data, CDC, NCID.
	20.13	Survey of Immunization Laws, CDC, NCPS.
	20.14	Primary Care Providers Survey, OASH, ODPHP.
	20.15	Health Insurance Association of America Employer Survey, Health Insurance Association of America.
	20.16	Immunization Grant Program Profiles, CDC, NCPS.
	20.17	Tuberculosis Screening and Preventive Therapy Summary Reports, CDC, NCPS.
	20.18	Tuberculosis Program Management Report Data on Completion of Preventive Therapy, CDC, NCPS.
	20.19	Survey of Laboratories using Rapid Viral Diagnosis of Influenza, CDC, NCID.
Clinical Preventive Services	21.1, 21.1(a–c)	National Health Interview Survey, CDC, NCHS. National Vital Statistics System, CDC, NCHS.
	21.2, 21.2d–l	National Health Interview Survey, CDC, NCHS.
	21.2a–c	National Health Interview Survey, CDC, NCHS (Future).
	21.3, 21.3a–c	Baseline: 1986 Access to Health Care Survey, Robert Wood Johnson Foundation. Updates: National Health Interview Survey, CDC, NCHS.
	21.4	National Health Interview Survey, CDC, NCHS.
	21.5	BHCDA Survey, HRSA, OPEL. Survey of Federal Programs, HRSA, OPEL.
	21.6	Primary Care Providers Survey, OASH, ODPHP.
	21.7	National Profile of Local Health Departments, National Association of County Health Officials.
	21.8	Minorities and Women in the Health Fields, HRSA, BHP.
Surveillance and Data Systems	22.1	CDC, NCHS.
	22.2	Baseline: ODPHP (National data); Public Health Foundation (State data). Updates: CDC, NCHS.
	22.3	CDC, NCHS.
	22.4	Subcommittee on State and Community Health Statistics, NCVHS (Future).
	22.5	Public Health Foundation.
	22.6	CDC, IRMO, and NCHS.
	22.7	CDC.

Table D. Health Status Indicators

Health status indicators	1990
Race/ethnicity-specific infant mortality as measured by the rate (per 1,000 live births) of deaths among infants under one year of age.	9.2
White	7.6
Black	18.0
American Indian	13.0 (data are for 1987)
Chinese	7.3 "
Japanese	6.2 "
Filipino	6.6 "
Other Asian or Pacific Islander	7.9 "
Hispanic origin	8.2 "
Total deaths per 100,000 population. (ICD–9 nos. 0–E999)[1]	520.2
Motor vehicle crash deaths per 100,000 population. (ICD–9 nos. E810–E825)[1]	18.5
Work-related injury deaths per 100,000 population.	2.3
Suicides per 100,000 population. (ICD–9 nos. E950–E959)[1]	11.5
Homicides per 100,000 population. (ICD–9 nos. E960–E978)[1]	10.2
Lung cancer deaths per 100,000 population. (ICD–9 no. 162)[1]	39.9
Female breast cancer deaths per 100,000 women. (ICD–9 no. 174)[1]	23.1
Cardiovascular disease deaths per 100,000 population. (ICD–9 nos. 390–448)[1]	189.8
Reported incidence (per 100,000 population) of acquired immunodeficiency syndrome.	18.1 (data are for 1992)
Reported incidence (per 100,000 population) of measles.	3.8 (data are for 1991)
Reported incidence (per 100,000 population) of tuberculosis.	10.4 "
Reported incidence (per 100,000 population) of primary and secondary syphilis	17.3 "
Prevalence of low birth weight as measured by the percentage of live born infants weighing under 2,500 grams at birth.	7.0
Births to adolescents (ages 10-17 years) as a percentage of total live births	4.7
Prenatal care as measured by the percentage of mothers delivering live infants who did not receive care during the first trimester of pregnancy.	24.2
Childhood poverty, as measured by the proportion of children under 15 years of age living in families at or below the poverty level.	21.4
Proportion of persons living in counties exceeding U.S. Environmental Protection Agency standards for air quality during the previous year.	32

[1]Age adjusted to the 1940 population.

Index to Health, United States, 1992 Detailed Tables

(**Numbers refer to table numbers**)

A

	Table
Abortion	13–15
Abortions per 100 live births	13
Age	13
Deaths, abortion-related	15
Gestation	14,15
Location of facility	14
Marital status	13
Number of abortions	14,15
Previous induced abortions	14
Previous live births	13
Race	13
Type of procedure	14
Acute conditions, incidence	62
AIDS, see HIV/AIDS.	
Air pollution	74
Alcohol consumption	66,67,69
Adults	69
Education	67
High school seniors	67
Hispanic origin	66,69
Race	66,67,69
Youths and young adults	66
Ambulatory care, see Dental visits; Hospital utilization, outpatient visits; Hospital utilization, surgery, outpatient; Physician utilization.	
American Indian population	
AIDS cases	53
AIDS deaths	54
Birth weight, low	8,19
Births, number	7
Death rates, all causes and selected causes	31
Deaths, number, selected causes	30
Dental students	105
Education of mother	9
Infant mortality	18,19
Medical students	105,106
Nursing students	105
Optometry students	105
Pharmacy students	105
Podiatry students	105
Population, resident	1

A—Con.

	Table
American Indian population—Con.	
Prenatal care	9
Teenage mothers	10
Unmarried mothers	10
Veterinary students	105
Asian population	
AIDS cases	53
AIDS deaths	54
Birth weight, low	8,19
Births, number	7
Death rates, all causes and selected causes	31
Deaths, number, selected causes	30
Dental students	105
Education of mother	9
Infant mortality	18,19
Medical students	105,106
Nursing students	105
Optometry students	105
Pharmacy students	105
Podiatry students	105
Population, resident	1
Prenatal care	9
Teenage mothers	10
Unmarried mothers	10
Veterinary students	105

B

	Table
Bed-disability days	62
Age	62
Birth control, see Contraception.	
Births	3–12
Age of mother	3,6
Birth rates	3
Birth weight, low	8,11, 12,19
Completed fertility rates	5
Education of mother	9
Expected births	6
Fertility rates	4
Geographic division and State	11,12
Hispanic origin of mother	7–10
Live-birth order	4,5
Number of live births	3,7
Prenatal care	9
Provisional data, most recent year	3,4
Teenage mothers	10
Unmarried mothers	10
Black population	
AIDS cases	53,55
AIDS deaths	54,56
Alcohol consumption	66,67,69

B—Con.

	Table
Black population—Con.	
Birth rates	3
Birth weight, low	8,11, 12,19
Births, number	3,7
Blood pressure, elevated	70
Cancer incidence rates	59
Cancer survival, 5-year relative	60
Cholesterol, elevated serum	72
Cigarette smoking	64–67
Cocaine use	66–68
Contraception	16,17
Death rates, all causes	28,31,34, 48
Death rates, selected causes	28,31, 35–45
Deaths, number, selected causes	30
Dental students	105
Dental visits	82
Education of mother	9
Expected births	6
Fertility rates	4
Fetal mortality	24
Health, self-assessment of	63
Health insurance	135,136
Hospital utilization	83
Hypertension	71
Infant mortality	18–23
Life expectancy	27
Limitation of activity	61
Marijuana use	66,67
Medical students	105,106
Nursing home utilization	91
Nursing students	105
Optometry students	105
Overweight	73
Pharmacy students	105
Physician utilization	78–81
Podiatry students	105
Population, resident	1
Poverty level, persons and families below	2
Prenatal care	9
Region, death rates	32
Teenage mothers	10
Unmarried mothers	10
Urbanization, death rates	32
Veterinary students	105
Years of potential life lost	29
Blood pressure, elevated	70,71
Hypertension	71

C	Table
Cancer (see also Deaths; Hospital utilization)	59,60
Incidence rates	59
Survival, 5-year relative	60
Cerebrovascular disease, see Deaths; Hospital utilization, diagnoses.	
Chancroid	52
Chickenpox (varicella)	52
Chiropractors	97,104
Employees, in offices of	97
Schools	104
Students	104
Cholesterol, elevated serum	72
Cigarette smoking	64–67
Age	64
Education	65,67
High school seniors	67
Hispanic origin	66
Youths and young adults	66
Cocaine use	66–68
Age	66,68
Education	67
Emergency room episodes	68
High school seniors	67
Hispanic origin	68
Youths and young adults	66
Communicable diseases, see Diseases, notifiable.	
Consumer Price Index	118,119
Medical care components	119
Contraception	16,17
Age	16
Marital status	17

D	
Deaths (see also Abortion; HIV/AIDS; Infant mortality; Life expectancy)	28–50
Age	31,33–46, 48,50
Alcohol-induced	28
All causes	28–31,34, 48,49
Atherosclerosis	28,30,49
Cancer, all sites	28–31,37, 49,50
Cancer, breast	28,29,39, 49
Cancer, colorectal	28,29

D–Con.	Table
Deaths–Con.	
Cancer, prostate	28,29
Cancer, respiratory system	28,29,38, 49
Cause-of-death ranking	30,49
Cerebrovascular disease (stroke)	28–31,36, 49,50
Chronic liver disease and cirrhosis	28–30,49
Chronic obstructive pulmonary disease	28–30,49
Diabetes mellitus	28–30,49
Drug-induced	28
Educational attainment	33
External causes	28
Firearm injuries	45
Heart disease	28–31,35, 50
Hispanic origin	31
HIV	31,40
Homicide and legal intervention	28–31,43, 49
Ischemic heart disease	28,29,49
Maternal mortality	41
Motor vehicle crashes	28,29,31, 42,49
Natural causes	28
Nephritis, nephrotic syndrome, nephrosis	28,30,49
Number of deaths	30,46,47
Occupational diseases	46
Occupational injuries	47
Pneumonia and influenza	28–30,49
Provisional data, most recent year	48–50
Race	28–45,48
Region	32
Septicemia	28,30,49
Sex	28–38,40, 42–45,48
Suicide	28–31,44, 49
Unintentional injuries	28–30,49
Urbanization	32
Years of potential life lost	29
Dental visits	82
Dentists	97,101, 104–106
Employees in offices of	97
Geographic region	101
Schools	104
Students	104–106
Diphtheria	51,52
Disability days, see Bed-disability days; Restricted-activity days.	

D–Con.	Table
Drug use, see Alcohol consumption; Cigarette smoking; Cocaine use; Marijuana use.	

E	
Elderly population	
Acute conditions, incidence	62
Alcohol consumption	69
Bed-disability days	62
Blood pressure, elevated	70
Cholesterol, elevated serum	72
Cigarette smoking	64
Death rates, all causes	31,34,48
Deaths or death rates, selected causes	31,35–40, 42–46,50
Dental visits	82
Health, self-assessment of	63
Health insurance	136
Hospital utilization	83,84, 86–89
Hypertension	71
Life expectancy at age 65	26,27
Limitation of activity	61
Medicaid	136,141, 142
Medicare	136–140
Mental health care utilization	95,96
Nursing home expenditures	116, 125–127, 134
Nursing home utilization	91,92, 126,127
Nursing homes	113
Overweight	73
Physician utilization	78–81
Population, resident	1
Restricted-activity days	62
Expenditures, national health (see also Consumer Price Index; Health research and development; HIV/AIDS, expenditures by Federal agency; Hospital expenses; Medicaid; Medicare; Mental health expenditures;	

E—Con. | *Table*

Expenditures, national
health—Con.
Nursing home
expenditures;
Physician expenditures;
Public health
expenditures;
Veterans medical care) .. 114–117,
122–125,
131,132
Amount in billions 114,
122–124
Amount per capita 114,115,
122,123,
132
Factors affecting
growth............... 117
Federal government 114,123
Geographic division and
State 132
International 115
Out-of-pocket payments.. 123–125
Percentage of gross
domestic product....... 114,115
Personal health care..... 117,123,
132
Source of funds 122,123,
125,131
State and local
government............ 114,123
Type of expenditure 116
Type of payer........... 124

F

Fertility rates, see Births.
Fetal mortality 20,24

G

Gonorrhea............... 52
Gross Domestic Product.... 114

H

Health expenditures, national,
see Expenditures,
national health.
Health insurance (see also
Health maintenance
organizations;
Medicaid;
Medicare)............. 135,136
65 years of age and
older 136
Under 65 years of age ... 135
Health maintenance
organizations........... 137

H—Con. | *Table*

Health research and
development (see also
HIV/AIDS) 128,129
Federal funding, by
agency............... 129
Source of funds 128
Health, self-assessment of .. 63
Hepatitis 52
Hispanic origin population
AIDS cases............ 53,55
AIDS deaths 54,56
Alcohol consumption 66,69
Birth weight, low........ 8,19
Births, number.......... 7
Cigarette smoking 66
Cocaine use 66,68
Death rates, all causes
and selected causes..... 31
Dental students 105
Education of mother..... 9
Infant mortality 18,19
Marijuana use 66
Medical students........ 105,106
Nursing students 105
Optometry students 105
Pharmacy students 105
Podiatry students........ 105
Population, resident 1
Poverty level, persons
and families below........ 2
Prenatal care 9
Teenage mothers........ 10
Unmarried mothers 10
Veterinary students...... 105
HIV/AIDS............... 28–31,40,
49,53–58,
85,130
Age 31,40,53,
54,85
AIDS cases............ 53,55,57
Death rates 28,31,40,
49
Deaths, number........ 30,54,56,
58
Expenditures by Federal
agency and activity 130
Geographic division and
State 57,58
Hispanic origin 31,53–56
Hospital utilization 85
Provisional mortality
data, most recent year .. 49
Race 28–31,40,
53–56
Rank as cause of death .. 30,49
Sex................... 28–31,40,
53–56
Transmission category ... 55,56
Years of potential life
lost.................. 29

H—Con. | *Table*

Hospital employees (see also
Mental health
resources)............. 97,102,
112,120
Full-time employees 102,112,
120
Geographic division and
State 112
Number employed in
hospitals 97
Occupation............. 102
Hospital expenses (see also
Consumer Price Index;
Medicaid; Medicare) 116,
119–121,
125,133
Amount in billions 125
Amount per capita 133
Employee costs 120
Geographic division and
State 133
Inpatient care expenses .. 120,121
Ownership type 121
Size of hospital 121
Source of funds 125
Hospital utilization (see also
Medicaid; Medicare;
Veterans medical care)..... 83–90
Admissions............. 90
Average length of stay...... 83–85,87,
90
Days of care............ 83–86
Diagnoses, selected...... 85–87
Diagnostic and other
nonsurgical procedures.. 89
Discharges for
inpatients 83–87
Family income 83
Geographic region....... 83,84
Outpatient visits 90
Ownership type 90
Race 83
Residence within/
outside MSA 83
Sex................... 83,84,
86–89
Size of hospital 90
Surgery, inpatient 88
Surgery, outpatient 90
Hospitals (see also
Hospital employees;
Mental health resources;
Nursing homes)......... 107,108,
110,111
Beds.................. 107,108
Beds per 1,000
population 110
Geographic division and
State 110,111
Long-term hospitals 108

H—Con.	Table
Hospitals—Con.	
Number of hospitals	107,108
Occupancy rate	107,108, 111
Ownership type	107,108
Short-stay hospitals......	107,110, 111
Size of hospital	107
Hypertension, see	
Blood pressure, elevated.	

I

	Table
Immunizations, see	
Vaccinations.	
Infant mortality (see also	
Fetal mortality)	18–23,25
Birth cohort data........	18,19
Birth weight	19
Feto-infant mortality.....	25
Geographic division and	
State	21–23
Hispanic origin	18,19
International	25
Neonatal mortality	18,20,22
Perinatal mortality	20
Postneonatal mortality ...	18,20,23, 25
Provisional data, most	
recent year	20
Race	18–23
Inpatient care, see	
Hospital utilization;	
Mental health care	
utilization;	
Nursing home utilization.	
International health, see	
Expenditures;	
Infant mortality;	
Life expectancy.	

L

	Table
Life expectancy...........	26,27
International	26
Provisional data, most	
recent year	27
Race	27
Limitation of activity	61

M

	Table
Malignant neoplasms, see	
Cancer.	
Marijuana use............	66,67
Education.............	67
High school seniors......	67
Youths and young	
adults...............	66

M—Con.	Table
Maternal mortality, see	
Deaths.	
Measles (Rubeola).........	51,52
Medicaid (see also	
Health insurance)	125,141, 142
Basis of eligibility	141
Expenditures	125
Type of service	142
Medical doctors, see	
Physicians.	
Medicare (see also	
Health insurance)	125, 138–140
Age, race, and sex.......	139
Enrollment............	138,139
Expenditures	125,138
Geographic region or	
division	139,140
Hospital utilization	140
Payments	139,140
Persons served per 1,000	
enrollees	139
Type of service	138,140
Mental health care	
utilization	93–96
Additions	93,95,96
Age	95,96
Diagnosis, primary	96
Inpatient days and	
episodes	94
Race and sex	95
Type of service	93
Mental health	
expenditures	144,145
Organization type	144
State mental health	
agency...............	145
Mental health resources	103,108, 109
Beds.................	108,109
Long-term psychiatric	
hospitals	108
Patient care staff........	103
MMR (Measles, Mumps,	
Rubella).................	51
Mumps..................	51,52

N

	Table
National health expenditures,	
see Expenditures,	
national health.	
Neonatal mortality, see	
Infant mortality.	
Nurses, licensed practical ...	102,104
Full-time employees in	
community hospitals	102
Schools	104
Students	104

N—Con.	Table
Nurses, registered (see also	
Mental health	
resources).............	101,102, 104–106
Full-time employees in	
community hospitals	102
Geographic region.........	101
Schools	104
Students	104–106
Type of training.........	101,104, 105
Nursing home employees ...	97
Nursing home	
expenditures	116, 125–127, 134
Age and sex of	
residents	127
Amount in billions	125,134
Amount per capita	134
Average monthly	
charges	126,127
Facility characteristics ...	126,127
Geographic division and	
State	134
Source of funds	125,126
Nursing home utilization ...	91,92
Functional status of	
residents	92
Sex and race...........	91
Nursing homes	113

O

	Table
Occupational health	
(see also Deaths)........	75–77
Exposures, lead and	
noise	76
Health and safety	
services	77
Industry...............	75,76
Injuries with lost	
workdays.............	75
Size of facility	76,77
Optometrists..............	101, 104–106
Geographic region.......	101
Schools	104
Students	104–106
Osteopaths, see Physicians.	
Overweight persons........	73

P

	Table
Perinatal mortality, see	
Infant mortality.	
Personal health care	
expenditures, see	
Expenditures, national	
health.	

P—Con.	Table
Pertussis (whooping cough)	51,52
Pharmacists	101,102, 104–106
Employed in hospitals	102
Geographic region	101
Schools	104
Students	104–106
Physician expenditures (see also Consumer Price Index; Medicaid; Medicare)	125
Physician utilization	78–81
Family income	78,79
Geographic region	78,79
Interval since last physician contact	79
Office visits to physicians	80,81
Physician contacts per person	78
Place of physician contact	78
Residence within/ outside MSA	78,79
Visit characteristics	81
Physicians (see also Mental health resources)	97–101, 104–106
Doctors of osteopathy	99,101, 104–106
Employees in offices of	97
Geographic division and State	98
Geographic region	101
International medical school graduates	100
Primary specialty	98,100
Projections	99
Schools	104
Students	104–106
Type of activity	100
Podiatrists	101,105, 106
Geographic region	101
Students	105,106
Poliomyelitis	51,52
Pollution, see Air pollution.	
Population, resident	1
Postneonatal mortality, see Infant mortality.	
Poverty level, persons and families below	2
Prenatal care, see Births.	
Public health expenditures, State health agency	131

R	Table
Registered nurses, see Nurses, registered.	
Restricted-activity days	62
Age	62
Rubella (German measles)	51,52

S	
Salmonellosis	52
Self-assessment of health, see Health, self-assessment of.	
Shigellosis	52
Smoking, see Cigarette smoking.	
State data	
AIDS cases	57
AIDS deaths	58
Birth weight, low and very low	11,12
Expenditures, hospital care	133
Expenditures, nursing home care	134
Expenditures, personal health care	132
Expenditures, state mental health agency	145
Hospital beds	110
Hospital employees	112
Hospital occupancy rates	111
Infant mortality	21–24
Nursing home beds	113
Physicians	98
Stroke, see Deaths, Cerebrovascular disease; Hospital utilization.	
Surgery, see Hospital utilization.	
Syphilis	52

T	
Tetanus	51
Tuberculosis	52

V	
Vaccinations, ages 1 to 4	51
Veterans medical care	143
Veterinarians	101,105, 106
Geographic region	101
Students	105,106

W	Table
Women's health	
Abortion	13–15
AIDS cases	53,55
AIDS deaths	54,56
Alcohol consumption	66,67,69
Birth rates	3
Births, number	3,7
Blood pressure, elevated	70
Cancer incidence rates	59
Cancer survival, five year relative	60
Cholesterol, elevated serum	72
Cigarette smoking	64–67
Cocaine use	66–68
Completed fertility rates	5
Contraception	16,17
Death rates, all causes	28,31,34, 48
Death rates, selected causes	28,31, 35–45
Deaths, number, selected causes	30
Dental students	106
Dental visits	82
Education of mother	9
Educational attainment, death rates	32
Expected births	6
Fertility rates	4
Health, self-assessment of	63
Health insurance	135,136
Hospital utilization	83,84, 86–89
HIV	85
Hypertension	71
Life expectancy	26,27
Limitation of activity	61
Marijuana use	66,67
Medical students	106
Medicare	139
Mental health care utilization	95
Nursing home utilization	91
Nursing students	106
Optometry students	106
Overweight	73
Pharmacy students	106
Physician utilization	78–81
Population, resident	1
Poverty, families with female householder	2

	Table
W—Con.	
Women's health—Con.	
Prenatal care	9
Region, death rates.	32
Teenage mothers.	3,6,10
Unmarried mothers	10
Urbanization, death rates.	32
Veterinary students.	106
Years of potential life lost.	29

Y

Years of potential life lost . .	29

Health, United States, 1992 and Healthy People 2000 Review available on diskette

—— Spreadsheet files ——

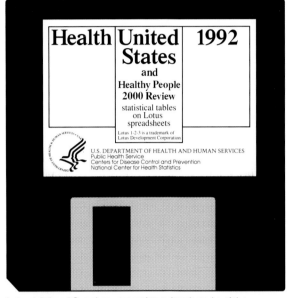

Lotus 1-2-3 and Symphony are registered trademarks of the Lotus Development Corporation.
Microsoft Excel is a registered trademark of the Microsoft Corporation

—— Text files ——

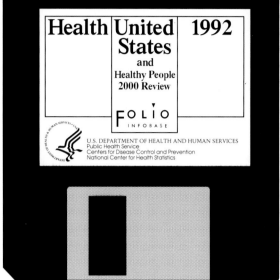

Folio is a registered trademark of the Folio Corporation

The 145 detailed tables and index from *Health, United States, 1992* and tabular data for 26 graphs from *Healthy People 2000 Review* are available on diskette from the Government Printing Office (GPO) and the National Technical Information Service (NTIS) for use with IBM-compatible personal computers. The tables are in Lotus 1-2-3 worksheet files. Lotus 1-2-3 version 2 or higher, or any program that can read WK1 files (e.g. Lotus Symphony and Microsoft Excel) is required to use these spreadsheets. The files have been compressed. To install these tables on your computer requires a minimum of 70 kilobytes of free memory, PC-DOS or MS-DOS version 2.0 or higher, and approximately 2 megabytes of hard disk space. Directions for decompression and copying the tables to your hard disk will be provided with the diskette(s).

Health, United States, 1992 and Healthy People 2000 Review, including text, charts, and tables is available as a Folio infobase from the Government Printing Office (GPO) and the National Technical Information Service (NTIS) for use with IBM-compatible personal computers. Keyword searches may be done using Folio Previews software, which is on the diskette(s). Other functions of the software are printing, marking and saving text as word processing files and saving tables as text files. Graphic files may be viewed in color, printed, and saved to view in graphics programs. Context-sensitive help and tutorials are also on the diskette(s). To install these files on your computer requires PC-DOS or MS-DOS 3.0 or higher and 5 megabytes of free memory. Directions for copying the files to your hard drive and a command card will be provided with the diskette(s).

3 1/2" disk: GPO Stock Number: 017-022-01214-6   Price: $15.00
NTIS Order Number: PB 93-505410   Price: $45.00
5 1/4" disk: GPO Stock Number: 017-022-01215-4   Price: $15.00
NTIS Order Number: PB 93-505428   Price: $45.00

3 1/2" disk: GPO Stock Number: 017-022-01217-1   Price: $14.00[*]
NTIS Order Number: PB 93-505436   Price: $65.00[*]
5 1/4" disk: GPO Stock Number: 017-022-01216-2   Price: $12.50[*]
NTIS Order Number: PB 93-505444   Price: $65.00[*]

[*] Set of 2 diskettes

U.S. DEPARTMENT OF HEALTH AND HUMAN SERVICES
Public Health Service
Centers for Disease Control and Prevention
National Center for Health Statistics

To order from GPO, call the order desk: (202) 783-3238
To order from NTIS, call the order desk: (703) 487-4650

For additional information, contact the Scientific and Technical Information Branch: (301) 436-8500